Pediatric Epilepsy

Pediatric Epilepsy

EDITORS

Michael Duchowny, MD
Director, Neurology Training and the Comprehensive Epilepsy Center
Miami Children's Hospital
Professor of Neurology and Pediatrics
University of Miami Miller School of Medicine
Clinical Professor, Department of Neurology
Florida International University College of Medicine
Miami, Florida

J. Helen Cross, MD
Professor of Pediatric Neurobiology
Prince of Wales's Chair of Childhood Epilepsy
University College of London
UCL Institute of Child Health
Great Ormond Street Hospital for Children
London, England
The Neville Epilepsy Centre
Young Epilepsy
Lingfield, Surrey, England

Alexis Arzimanoglou, MD
Head of the Epilepsy, Sleep, and Pediatric Neurophysiology Department
University Hospitals of Lyon (HCL)
Clinical Investigator
Translational and Integrative Group in Epilepsy Research (TIGER)
Lyon Neuroscience Research Center
INSERM, U1028; CNRS, UMR5292
Lyon, France

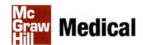

New York   Chicago   San Francisco   Lisbon   London   Madrid   Mexico City
Milan   New Delhi   San Juan   Seoul   Singapore   Sydney   Toronto

Pediatric Epilepsy

Copyright © 2013 by The McGraw-Hill Companies, Inc. All rights reserved. Printed in China. Except as permitted under the United States Copyright Act of 1976, no part of this publication may be reproduced or distributed in any form or by any means, or stored in a data base or retrieval system, without the prior written permission of the publisher.

1 2 3 4 5 6 7 8 9 0   CTP/CTP   17 16 15 14 13 12

ISBN 978-0-07-149621-6
MHID 0-07-149621-1

This book was set in Garamond by Aptara, Inc.
The editors were Anne M. Sydor and Peter J. Boyle.
The production supervisor was Catherine H. Saggese.
The art manager was Armen Ovsepyan.
Project management was provided by Shikha Sharma, Aptara, Inc.
China Translation & Printing Services, Ltd., was printer and binder.

Library of Congress Cataloging-in-Publication Data

Pediatric epilepsy / [edited by] Michael Duchowny, Helen Cross, Alexis
Arzimanoglou.—1st ed.
     p. ; cm.
Includes bibliographical references and index.
ISBN-13: 978-0-07-149621-6 (hardback : alk. paper)
ISBN-10: 0-07-149621-1 (hardback : alk. paper)
 I. Duchowny, Michael. II. Cross, Helen, 1961- III. Arzimanoglou, A.
 [DNLM: 1. Epilepsy. 2. Adolescent. 3. Child. 4. Infant. WL 385]
 LC classification not assigned
 618.92′853–dc23
                                                      2012014927

McGraw-Hill books are available at special quantity discounts to use as premiums and sales promotions, or for use in corporate training programs. To contact a representative please e-mail us at bulksales@mcgraw-hill.com.

This volume is dedicated to my wife Leslie for her enduring support and understanding which allowed me to bring this project to fruition. I am also indebted to my friends and mentors, Drs. Jean Aicardi and Cosimo Ajmone-Marsan who taught me throughout my professional life and inspired me to reach higher.
— Michael Duchowny —

CONTENTS

SECTION III   SEIZURES IN CHILDHOOD

SECTION IV   SEIZURES IN ADOLESCENCE

SECTION V   EPILEPSY SYNDROMES

SECTION VI   EPILEPSY AND NEUROLOGICAL DISORDERS

CONTRIBUTORS

Harry S. Abram, MD
Professor of Neurology
Mayo Clinic College of Medicine
Nemours Children's Clinic
Jacksonville, Florida
Chapter 20

Albert P. Aldenkamp
Epilepsy Center Kempenhaeghe
Heeze, The Netherlands
Department of Neurology
Research School Mental Health and
    Neurosciences
Maastricht University Medical Center
Maastricht, The Netherlands
Chapter 52

Israel Alfonso, MD
Director of Neonatal Neurology
Miami Children's Hospital
Miami, Florida
Chapter 8

Willem F. Arts, MD
Pediatric Neurologist
Department of Pediatric Neurology
Erasmus Medical Centre–Sophia Children's
    Hospital
Rotterdam, The Netherlands
Chapter 46

Alexis Arzimanoglou, MD
Head of the Epilepsy, Sleep, and Pediatric
    Neurophysiology Department
University Hospitals of Lyon (HCL)
Clinical Investigator
Translational and Integrative Group in
    Epilepsy Research (TIGER)
Lyon Neuroscience Research Center
INSERM, U1028; CNRS, UMR5292
Lyon, France
Chapters 1, 33

Christian G. Bien, MD
Chief Physician of Epilepsy Clinic
Bethel Epilepsy Center
Mara Hospital
Bielefeld, Germany
Chapter 37

Francesca Bisulli, MD
Department of Neurological Sciences
University of Bologna
Bologna, Italy
Chapter 44

W. T. Blume, MD, FRCP(C)
Professor of Neurology
London Health Sciences Centre
University of Western Ontario
London, Ontario, Canada
Chapter 3

Blaise F. D. Bourgeois, MD
Department of Neurology
Harvard Medical School
Boston, Massachusetts
Chapter 41

Lawrence W. Brown, MD
Associate Professor of Neurology and Pediatrics
Children's Hospital of Philadelphia
Philadelphia, Pennsylvania
Chapter 22

Roberto H. Caraballo, MD
Neurology Department
Hospital de Niños
Buenos Aires, Argentina
Chapter 26

Paul R. Carney, MD
Division of Neurology and Sleep Medicine
Department of Internal Medicine
University of Alabama, College of Community
    Health Sciences
Tuscaloosa, Alabama
Chapter 44

Mary B. Connolly, MB, BCh, FRCP(I), FRCP(Ed), FRCP(C)
Division of Pediatric Neurology
Department of Pediatrics,
University of British Columbia and
British Columbia's Children's Hospital
Vancouver, British Columbia, Canada
Chapter 13

J. Helen Cross, MD
Professor of Pediatric Neurobiology
Prince of Wales's Chair of Childhood Epilepsy
University College of London
UCL Institute of Child Health
Great Ormond Street Hospital for Children
London, United Kingdom
The Neville Epilepsy Centre
Young Epilepsy
Lingfield, Surrey, United Kingdom
Chapters 7, 10, 18, 19, 55

Patricia Dean, ARNP, MSN
Clinical Coordinator
Comprehensive Epilepsy Center
Miami Children's Hospital
Miami, Florida
Chapter 54

Christopher Derry, MD
Department of Clinical Neurosciences
Western General Hospital
Edinburgh, United Kingdom
Chapter 27

Dennis J. Dlugos, MD
Associate Professor of Neurology
Director of Pediatric Regional Epilepsy Program
Children's Hospital of Philadelphia
University of Pennsylvania School of Medicine
Philadelphia, Pennsylvania
Chapter 11

Charlotte Dravet, MD
Centre Saint-Paul-Hôpital Henri Gastaut
Marseille, France
Chapter 14

Michael Duchowny, MD
Director
Neurology Training and the Comprehensive
Epilepsy Center
Miami Children's Hospital
Professor of Neurology and Pediatrics
University of Miami Miller School of Medicine
Clinical Professor
Department of Neurology
Florida International University College of Medicine
Miami, Florida
Chapters 32, 36

Colin Dunkley, MD
Department of Pediatrics
King's Mill Hospital
Sutton-in-Ashfield, United Kingdom
Chapter 7

David W. Dunn, MD
Departments of Psychiatry and Neurology
Riley Hospital for Children
Indianapolis, Indiana
Chapter 41

Andrew Escayg, PhD
Associate Professor
Department of Genetics
Emory University School of Medicine
Atlanta, Georgia
Chapter 17

Natalio Fejerman, MD
Department of Neurology
Juan P. Garrahan Pediatric Hospital
Buenos Aires, Argentina
Chapter 25

David Friedman, MD
Epilepsy Specialist
Director of Epilepsy Surgery Program
Winthrop University Hospital
Mineola, New York
Chapter 45

Anne Gallagher, MD
Department of Psychology
University of Montreal
Montreal, Quebec, Canada
Chapter 40

William Davis Gaillard, MD
Professor of Neurology and Pediatrics
School of Medicine and Health Sciences
George Washington University
Professor of Neurology
Georgetown University
Washington, DC
Chapter 6

Eija Gaily, MD
Epilepsy Unit
Department of Pediatric Neurology
Helsinki University Central Hospital
Helsinki, Finland
Chapter 51

Aristea S. Galanopoulou, MD, PhD
Associate Professor
Saul R. Korey Department of Neurology
Dominick P. Purpura Department of Neuroscience
Albert Einstein College of Medicine
Bronx, New York
Chapter 2

James D. Geyer, MD
Departments of Pediatrics, Neurology, Neuroscience,
    and Biomedical Engineering
McKnight Brain Institute
University of Florida College of Medicine
Gainesville, Florida
Chapter 44

Frank G. Gilliam, MD, MPH
Caitlin Tynan Doyle Professor of Neurology
Director of the Comprehensive Epilepsy Center
The Neurological Institute
Columbia University
New York, New York
Chapter 45

Jamie T. Gilman, PharmD
Senior Neurology Scientific Affairs Liaison
Ortho-McNeil Janssen Scientific Affairs, LLC
Christiana, Tennessee
Chapter 50

B. G. Giráldez, MD
Epilepsy Unit
Neurology Service
Fundación Jiménez Díaz
Madrid, Spain
Chapter 23

Tracy A. Glauser, MD
Professor of Pediatrics and Neurology
Director of Comprehensive Epilepsy Center
Division of Neurology
Department of Pediatrics
Cincinnati Children's Hospital Medical Center
Cincinnati, Ohio
Chapter 29

Cristina Yip Go, MD
Department of Pediatrics (Neurology)
The Hospital for Sick Children
Toronto, Ontario
Chapter 28

Giuseppe Gobbi, MD
Child Neurology Unit
Neuroscience Department
Maggiore Hospital
Bologna, Italy
Chapter 25

Salvatore Grosso, MD
Pediatric Neurology Section
Department of Pediatrics
University of Siena
Siena, Italy
Chapter 25

Siobhan Hannan, RN, RSCN, MSc
Clinical Nurse Specialist
Epilepsy Surgery
Great Ormond Street Hospital
London, United Kingdom
Chapter 54

Yvonne Hart
Consultant Neurologist
Department of Neurology
Royal Victoria Infirmary
Newcastle upon Tyne, United Kingdom
Chapter 37

Sandra Helmers, MD
Associate Professor
Department of Neurology
Emory University School of Medicine
Atlanta, Georgia
Chapter 17

Bruce P. Hermann, PhD
Department of Neurology
University of Wisconsin School of Medicine and
    Public Health
Madison, Wisconsin
Chapter 42

Edouard Hirsch, MD
Department of Neurology HUS
CTRS INSERM
Strasbourg, France
Chapter 30

Gregory L. Holmes, MD
Dartmouth Medical School
Dartmouth-Hitchcock Medical Center
Lebanon, New Hampshire
Chapter 1

Dominique Ijff
Department of Behavioral Research and Clinical
    Neuropsychology
Epilepsy Center Kempenhaeghe
Heeze, The Netherlands
Chapter 52

Yushi Inoue, MD
National Epilepsy Center
Shizuoka Institute of Epilepsy and Neurological
  Disorders
Shizuoka, Japan
Chapter 31

Prasanna Jayakar, MD, PhD
Department of Neurology
Miami Children's Brain Institute
Miami Children's Hospital
Miami, Florida
Chapter 4

Jana E. Jones, PhD
Department of Neurology
University of Wisconsin School of Medicine and
  Public Health
Madison, Wisconsin
Chapter 42

Philippe Kahane, MD, PhD
Professor of Neurophysiology
Epilepsy Unit
Department of Neurology
University Hospital
Grenoble, France
Chapter 55

Sudha Kilaru Kessler, MD
Assistant Professor of Neurology
Children's Hospital of Philadelphia
Pereleman School of Medicine
University of Pennsylvania
Philadelphia, Pennsylvania
Chapter 11

Susan Koh, MD
Associate Professor
Department of Pediatrics and Neurology
University of Colorado School of Medicine
Denver, Colorado
Chapter 32

Eric H. Kossoff, MD
Associate Professor of Neurology and Pediatrics
Medical Director of Ketogenic Diet Center
Director of Pediatric Neurology Residency Program
Johns Hopkins Hospital
Baltimore, Maryland
Chapters 33, 53

Prakash Kotagal, MD
Head of Pediatric Epilepsy Section
Cleveland Clinic Epilepsy Center
Cleveland, Ohio
Chapter 57

Maryse Lassonde, MD
Department of Psychology
University of Montreal
Montreal, Quebec, Canada
Chapter 40

John A. Lawson, BMed, FRACP, PhD
Pediatric Neurologist
Sydney Children's Hospital
Randwick, Australia
Chapter 5

Dick Lindhout, MD
DBG-Department of Medical Genetics
University Medical Center, Utrecht
SEIN–Epilepsy Institute in the Netherlands
Hoofddorp, The Netherlands
Chapter 51

A. Marinas, MD
Epilepsy Unit
Neurology Service
Fundación Jiménez Díaz
Madrid, Spain
Chapter 23

Bruno Maton, MD
The Brain Institute
Miami Children's Hospital
Miami, Florida
Chapter 24

Ailsa McLellan, MBChB, MRCP, MRCPCH
Consultant Pediatric Neurologist
Department of Pediatric Neurosciences
Royal Hospital for Sick Children
Edinburgh, United Kingdom
Chapter 58

Joshua Mendelson, MD
Epilepsy Monitoring Program
Monmouth Medical Center
Long Branch, New Jersey
Chapter 17

Mohamad A. Mikati, MD
Department of Pediatrics
Duke University Medical Center
Durham, North Carolina
Chapter 49

Eli M. Mizrahi, MD
Professor of Neurology and Pediatrics
Comprehensive Epilepsy Center
Baylor College of Medicine
Houston, Texas
Chapter 9

Diego A. Morita, MD
Assistant Professor of Pediatrics and Neurology
Director of New Onset Seizure Program
Division of Neurology
Department of Pediatrics
Cincinnati Children's Hospital Medical Center
Cincinnati, Ohio
Chapter 29

Solomon L. Moshé, MD
Charles Frost Chair in Neurosurgery and Neurology
Director of Division of Pediatric Neurology and
    Clinical Neurophysiology
Saul R. Korey Department of Neurology
Director of Division of Neurology
Department of Pediatrics
Comprehensive Einstein/Montefiore Epilepsy Center
Albert Einstein College of Medicine
Bronx, New York
Chapter 2

Mona Nabulsi, MD, MSc
Department of Pediatrics
American University of Beirut Medical Center
Beirut, Lebanon
Chapter 49

Brian Neville, MD
Emeritus Professor of Pediatric Neurology
UCL Institute of Child Health
University College London
London, United Kingdom
Chapter 56

Yu-tze Ng, MD
Division of Pediatric Neurology
Barrow Neurological Institute
St. Joseph's Hospital and Medical Center
Phoenix, Arizona
Chapter 35

Douglas R. Nordli Jr., MD
Associate Professor of Neurology
Children's Memorial Hospital
Chicago, Illinois
Chapter 53

Shunsuke Ohtahara, MD, PhD
Department of Child Neurology
Okayama University Graduate School of Medicine,
    Dentistry, and Pharmaceutical Sciences
Kita-ku, Okayama Prefecture, Japan
Chapter 12

Shekhar G. Patil, MD
The National Centre for Young People with Epilepsy
Lingfield, United Kingdom
Senior Lecturer in Pediatric Neurosciences and
    Honorary Consultant Pediatric Neurologist
Neurosciences Unit
UCL Institute of Child Health
London, United Kingdom
Epilepsy Unit
Great Ormond Street Hospital for Children NHS Trust
London, United Kingdom
Chapter 39

John M. Pellock, MD
Professor and Chairman
Division of Child Neurology
Medical College of Virginia Hospital
Virginia Commonwealth University
Richmond, Virginia
Chapter 47

Ronit M. Pressler, MD
Department of Clinical Neurophysiology
UCL Institute of Neurology
London, United Kingdom
Chapter 9

Federica Provini, MD
Department of Neurological Sciences
University of Bologna
Bologna, Italy
Chapter 44

James J. Riviello Jr., MD
George Peterkin Endowed Chair in Pediatrics
Professor of Pediatrics and Neurology
Baylor College of Medicine
Director of Pediatric Neurocritical Care Service
Section of Neurology and Developmental Neuroscience
Chief of Neurophysiology
Texas Children's Hospital
Houston, Texas
Chapter 38

Philippe Ryvlin, MD, PhD
Hôpital Neurlogique
Lyons, France
Chapter 6

G. Lynette Sadleir, MD
Department of Pediatrics
Wellington School of Medicine and Health Sciences
University of Otago
Wellington, New Zealand
Chapter 21

Ingrid E. Scheffer, MD
Florey Neurosciences Institute
Departments of Medicine and Pediatrics
University of Melbourne
Austin Health and Royal Children's Hospital
Heidelberg, Victoria, Australia
Chapter 27

Rod C. Scott, MD
Senior Lecturer in Pediatric Neurosciences and
   Honorary Consultant Pediatric Neurologist
Neurosciences Unit
UCL Institute of Child Health
London, United Kingdom
Epilepsy Unit
Great Ormond Street Hospital for Children NHS Trust
London, United Kingdom
The National Centre for Young People with Epilepsy
Lingfield, United Kingdom
Radiology and Physics Unit
UCL Institute of Child Health
London, United Kingdom
Chapter 39

J. M. Serratosa, MD
Epilepsy Unit
Neurology Service
Fundación Jiménez Díaz
Madrid, Spain
Chapter 23

Raj D. Sheth, MD
Nemours Children's Clinic
Mayo Clinic College of Medicine
Jacksonville, Florida
Chapter 20

Mary Lou Smith, MD
Department of Psychology
University of Toronto Mississauga
Mississauga, Ontario, Canada
Chapter 40

O. Carter Snead III, MD
Faculty of Medicine
Department of Pediatrics (Neurology) and
Research Program in Neurosciences and Mental Health
The Hospital for Sick Children
University of Toronto
Toronto, Ontario
Chapter 28

John B. P. Stephenson, MA, BM, FRCP
Professor
Fraser of Allander Neurosciences Unit
Royal Hospital for Sick Children
Glasgow, United Kingdom
Chapter 16

Robert Surtees, MD
Neurosciences Unit
UCL Institute of Child Health
London, United Kingdom
Chapter 15

Paolo Tinuper, MD
Department of Neurological Sciences
University of Bologna
Bologna, Italy
Chapter 44

Roberto Tuchman, MD
Director of Developmental and Behavioral Neurology
Department of Neurology
Dan Marino Center
Miami Children's Hospital
Weston, Florida
Chapter 43

Kette D. Valente, MD, PhD
Associate Professor
Department of Clinical Neurophysiology
Institute of Psychiatry
Sao Paulo, Brazil
Chapter 34

Kim West, PharmD, MBA
Senior Neurology Scientific Affairs Liaison
Ortho-McNeil Janssen Scientific Affairs, LLC
Charlottesville, Virginia
Chapter 50

James W. Wheless, MD
Professor and Chief of Pediatric Neurology
LeBonheur Chair in Pediatric Neurology
University of Tennessee Health Science Center
Director of Neuroscience Institute and
   LeBonheur Comprehensive Epilepsy Program
LeBonheur Children's Hospital
Memphis, Tennessee
Chapter 48

Nicole I. Wolf, MD
Department of Child Neurology
VU University Medical Center
Amsterdam, The Netherlands
Chapter 15

Elaine Wyllie, MD
Professor of Pediatrics
Director of Center for Pediatric Neurology
Cleveland Clinic
Cleveland, Ohio
Chapter 55

Yasuko Yamatogi, MD
Department of Welfare System and Health Science
Faculty of Health and Welfare Science
Okayama Prefectural University
Soja-City, Okayama Prefecture, Japan
Chapter 12

PREFACE

The field of childhood epilepsy has witnessed a remarkable transformation over the past two decades. Once viewed as a handmaiden of adult epilepsy, the early-onset epilepsies have come into their own as a major area of medical importance. In many ways the diversity of pediatric epileptic seizures and epilepsy syndromes, the many etiologies of epilepsy presenting in the first two decades, and their far-reaching comorbidities surpass that of the adult-onset epilepsies. Advances in clinical semiology and diagnosis, epilepsy classification, methods of evaluation, and treatment have all played major roles. A perusal of any epileptology journal or attendance at an epilepsy symposium provides clear evidence of the growing number of research studies and intense clinical interest in pediatric epilepsy.

It is difficult to capture the entire spectrum of progress in childhood seizure disorders in a single volume. By itself, literature concerning brain development and epilepsy would constitute an enormous compendium of information. Similarly, advances in diagnostics, including imaging and electrophysiology, are sufficiently robust to require their own self-contained bodies of work. The pharmacology of antiepileptic drugs and surgical strategies for epilepsy management are also areas that have witnessed explosive growth.

Pediatric Epilepsy was developed in direct response to the clinical needs of the greater pediatric epileptology community. We have endeavored to distill core information about pediatric epilepsy and create a volume that is authoritative yet concise. By focusing on clinical treatment issues, we hope to provide useful guidelines for practical management that can be applied directly at the bedside and in the clinic. This information will hopefully not only be useful to epilepsy specialists but also to pediatricians, general neurologists, nurses, and allied professionals. It is our additional hope that the inclusion of management algorithms in many of the chapters will provide particularly valuable pointers for managing childhood epilepsy. While the algorithms should not be regarded as authoritative, they nevertheless are important starting points for the evaluation of epilepsy and treatment decision making.

Achieving these goals is not an easy task. Fortunately, the contributors are all distinguished experts in their respective fields. International in scope, they are drawn from 14 countries and 5 continents and bring a vast depth of experience to the project. Each chapter includes timely and informative information that is supported by figures, tables, and diagrams and followed by key references. These contributions form a solid foundation, and we are deeply appreciative of the authors' talents, efforts, and patience as the book was being assembled.

We sincerely believe that the collective efforts of everyone involved in bringing this volume to fruition—authors, editors, and publisher will together provide a fresh source of information and a reliable guide for clinicians involved in the care of children with epilepsy and related disorders. Knowledge changes every day, but a good "snapshot in time" can freeze that knowledge and allow an unhurried, in-depth look. If we can achieve this simple goal, we all will be richly rewarded.

SECTION I

Approach to the Child with Epilepsy

CHAPTER 1

Epileptic Seizures and Their Classification

Gregory L. Holmes and Alexis Arzimanoglou

▶ OVERVIEW

An epileptic seizure is a paroxysmal disorder characterized by an abnormal, excessive, hypersynchronous discharge of neurons which results in an alteration of function of the patient. This alteration of function can be quite dramatic such as during a generalized tonic–clonic (grand mal) seizure or much more subtle such as during an absence (petit mal) seizure. Epilepsy is a condition characterized by repeated, unprovoked seizures. If the seizures are consistently provoked, such as by fever or hypoglycemia, the term epilepsy should not be used. Epilepsy is not a single disorder, but rather a symptom of underlying brain dysfunction.

▶ EPILEPTIC SEIZURES

A classification of epileptic seizures and syndromes is an essential step in developing communication and provides a basis for an understanding of the underlying processes of epilepsy. A classification system provides guidance in determining the diagnostic evaluation, treatment, and prognosis (Table 1–1). However, no single classification code can cover the multiple aspects of epilepsy including behavioral and electroencephalographic (EEG) features, age of onset, and etiology (including genetic susceptibility and acquired insults). In addition, limited knowledge regarding the basic

mechanism does not permit classification on the physiopathology of the disorder.

The first modern classification system of seizures was proposed in 1969 by an ad hoc committee of the International League Against Epilepsy.[1] In 1981, the classification was revised.[2] It is based on two criteria: the clinical features and the EEG features of the seizures. Seizures are classified into two broad categories: (a) partial seizures (seizures beginning in a limited location in the brain) and (b) generalized seizures (seizures that are bilaterally symmetrical and without focal onset). Seizures are then further classified, depending on the exact clinical and EEG manifestations of the seizure. In 2010 the International League Against Epilepsy (ILAE) proposed a revision of the terminology and concepts for organization of seizures and epilepsies.[3] The ILAE felt they did not have enough data to support a new classification. Instead the ILAE provided new nomenclature for the seizures and epilepsies. In this chapter, the new terminology will be used with the older nomenclature in parentheses.

The various seizure types are described here and Fig. 1–1 provides a guide for correctly diagnosing seizure type.

FOCAL (PARTIAL) SEIZURES

Focal seizures are those that originate within networks limited to one hemisphere. Focal seizures may be

▶ **TABLE 1–1. CLASSIFICATION OF EPILEPTIC SEIZURES**

Focal (Partial) Seizures

Without impairment of consciousness or awareness (simple partial seizures)

With observable motor or autonomic components

  Motor
  Versive
  Postural

Phonatory (vocalization or arrest of speech)

Focal motor with march (Jacksonian)

Autonomic symptoms or signs (including epigastric sensation, pallor, sweating, flushing, piloerection, and pupillary dilation)

With selective sensory or psychic phenomena

Sensory

Somatosensory

Visual

Auditory

Olfactory

Gustatory

Vertiginous

Psychic symptoms (disturbance of higher cerebral function)

Dysphasic

Dysmnesic

Cognitive

Affective

Illusions

Structured hallucinations

With impairment of consciousness (complex partial seizures)

Focal followed by impairment of consciousness

With impairment of consciousness at onset

Focal seizure evolving to bilateral, convulsive seizures (involving tonic, clonic, or tonic and clonic complexes)

Generalized Seizures

  Tonic–clonic
  Absence
    Typical
    Atypical
    Absence with special features
    Myoclonic absence
    Absence with eyelid myoclonic
  Myoclonic
    Myoclonic atonic
    Myoclonic tonic
  Clonic
  Tonic
  Atonic

Unknown
  Epileptic spasms

Source: Data from (Commission on Classification and Terminology of the International League Against Epilepsy. Proposal for revised clinical and electroencephalographic classification of epileptic seizures. *Epilepsia* 1981;22:249–260) and (Berg AT, Berkovic SF, Brodie MJ, Buchhalter J, Cross JH, Van Emde BW, Engel J, French J, Glauser TA, Mathern GW, Moshe SL, Nordli D, Plouin P, Scheffer IE. Revised terminology and concepts for organization of seizures and epilepsies: report of the ILAE Commission on Classification and Terminology, 2005–2009. *Epilepsia* 2010;51:676–685).

classified further into those without impairment of consciousness or awareness (formerly termed simple partial seizures) and those with impairment of consciousness or awareness (formerly classified as complex partial seizures). Determining impaired consciousness may be quite difficult, particularly in patients in whom the seizures involve language cortex, patients with cognitive impairment, and in neonates or infants. In patients not demonstrating impairment of consciousness or awareness, further subdivision into seizures with: (i) observable motor or autonomic components and (ii) subjective sensory or psychic phenomenon. Focal seizures can evolve into a bilateral, convulsive seizure.

The signs or symptoms of focal seizures depend on the location of the focus. Seizures involving the motor cortex most commonly consist of rhythmic or semi-rhythmic clonic activity of the face, arm or leg. There is usually no difficulty in diagnosing this type of seizure. Seizures with somatosensory, autonomic, and psychic symptoms (hallucinations, illusions, déjà vu) may be more difficult to diagnose. Psychic symptoms usually occur as a component of a focal seizure with impaired consciousness or responsiveness. Focal seizures can occur at any age.

Focal seizures with impairment of consciousness or awareness (complex partial seizures), formerly termed temporal lobe or psychomotor seizures are one of the most common seizure types encountered in both children and adults. Focal seizures without impaired consciousness or awareness may evolve into seizures with impaired consciousness. The beginning of the focal seizure may serve as a warning to the patient (i.e., aura) that a more severe seizure is pending. It is important to recognize that the aura may enable the clinician to determine the cortical area from which the seizure is beginning.

The impairment of consciousness or awareness may be subtle. For example, the patient may either not respond to commands or respond in an abnormally slow manner. While focal seizures with altered consciousness or awareness may be characterized by simple staring and impaired responsiveness, behavior is usually more complex during the seizure. Automatisms, semipurposeful behaviors of which the patient is unaware and subsequently cannot recall, are common during the period of impaired consciousness. Types of automatism behaviors are quite variable and may consist of activities such as facial grimacing, gestures, chewing, lip smacking, snapping fingers and repeating phrases. The patient does not recall fully this activity following the seizure.

Although variable, focal seizures CPS usually last from 30 seconds to several minutes.[4] This should be contrasted to absence seizures, to be described below, which usually last less than 15 seconds. Most patients have some degree of postictal impairment, such as tiredness or confusion following a focal seizure in which consciousness or awareness is altered. Focal

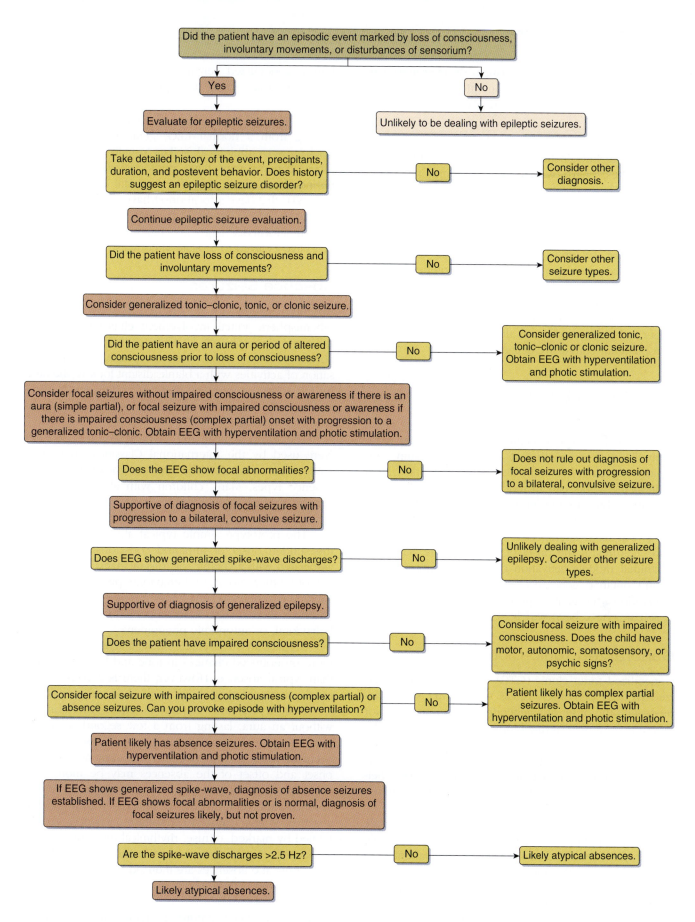

Figure 1–1. Take a detailed history of the description of the event, precipitants, duration, and postevent behavior. Does history suggest an epileptic seizure disorder?

seizures with altered consciousness or awareness can occur at any age, although as mentioned above, testing consciousness in infants and young children is difficult.

EEG.   The EEG in focal seizures is characterized by focal spikes, sharp waves, or less commonly, focal slowing. There is often a relationship between the location of the spikes and the seizure type, that is, occipital lobe spikes are associated with occipital lobe seizures while frontal lobe spikes are associated with frontal lobe seizures. However, patients with well-documented seizures may have normal interictal EEGs.

Different types of seizures may evolve in temporal succession in the same patient. For example, a focal seizure may begin with normal consciousness and awareness can be followed by an alteration in consciousness or a bilateral, convulsive seizure, or both.

GENERALIZED SEIZURES

Generalized seizures are those in which there is no discernible focal onset. Generalized seizures are conceptualized as originating at some point within, and rapidly engaging, bilaterally distributed networks.[3] Such bilateral networks can include cortical and subcortical structures, but do not necessarily include the entire cortex. Some patients with primary generalized epilepsy will have lateralized clinical,[5] EEG,[6] and blood flow[7] features at the onset of their seizures. Similarly, in animal models activation of cortex is not uniform during putative generalized seizures.[8,9] Despite these reservations, the general principles of this classification of seizures have been widely accepted.

Generalized Tonic–Clonic Seizures

Generalized tonic–clonic (GTC) seizures are characterized by loss of consciousness that occurs simultaneously with the onset of a generalized stiffening of flexor or extensor muscle (termed tonic phase). Following the tonic phase, generalized jerking of the muscles (clonic activity) occurs. The seizures are dramatic and there is rarely any difficulty in making the correct diagnosis. Seizures that begin with bilateral tonic posturing without a focal onset are classified as primary GTC.

Some patients may have a focal seizure (simple partial) preceding the loss of consciousness. While this is often described as an aura by the patient, it is important to note that the aura is a focal seizure. As the seizure spreads in the cortex the seizure develops into a GTC seizure. The seizure would then be classified as a focal seizure that evolves into a generalized tonic–clonic seizure. Other patients may have a focal seizure with impaired consciousness or awareness evolving into a generalized seizure. Generalized seizures are always associated with deep postictal sleep.

EEG.   Patients with GTC may have a variety of findings varying from a normal EEG, generalized spike-wave discharges or multifocal spikes usually in the frontal lobes. Patients may have photoconvulsive responses during photic stimulation. The interictal EEG in patients with GTC that have a focal onset have similar features to what is described above for patients with focal seizures. Persistent focal discharges are suggestive of focal seizures that have evolved to a bilateral convulsive seizure.

Absence Seizures

Absence seizures are generalized seizures, indicating bihemispheric initial involvement clinically and electroencephalographically.[10] Absence seizures have an abrupt onset and offset. There is typically a sudden cessation of activities with a blank, distant look to the face. As the seizure continues, there are often automatisms and mild clonic motor activity such as jerks of the arms and eye blinking.

The terms typical and atypical absence seizures were used by the International Classification of Epileptic Seizures to describe and categorize the various absence types. Many children with absence seizures can be further categorized as having a characteristic epileptic syndrome.

The prototype simple typical absence consists of the sudden onset of impaired consciousness, usually associated with a "blank" or "distant" facial appearance without other motor or behavioral phenomena. This subtype is actually relatively rare.[11] The complex typical absence, alternatively, is accompanied by other motor, behavioral, or autonomic phenomena.

Atypical absence seizures are characterized as having more pronounced changes in tone and longer duration than typical absence. However, there is a considerable overlap between typical and atypical absences.[12]

Both typical and atypical absences start abruptly without an aura, lasting from a few seconds to half a minute, and end abruptly. Since atypical absences often occur in patients with cognitive impairment, detecting onset and offset of the absences may be more difficult. Absences with special features include myoclonic absence and eyelid myoclonia. Epilepsy with myoclonic absences is characterized clinically by absences accompanied by marked, diffuse, rhythmical myoclonus, often associated with a progressive tonic contraction.[13,14] Eyelid myoclonia and absences are induced by eye closure and are associated with generalized polyspikes and waves.[15]

EEG.   The EEG signature of a typical absence seizure is the sudden onset of 3-Hz-generalized symmetrical spike- or multiple spike-wave complexes. The voltage of the discharge is often maximal in the frontal–central regions. The frequency tends to be faster, about 4 Hz, at the onset and slows to 2 Hz toward the end of discharges lasting longer than 10 seconds. The spike-and-wave discharge may be precipitated by hyperventilation or photic stimulation. The onset and offset of the spike-waves are usually abrupt although occasionally bifrontal spikes may precede the generalized discharge. EEG abnormalities other than generalized spike-wave are common. Holmes et al[12] reported that only 44% of 27 patients with typical absences had totally normal EEG backgrounds. Diffuse slowing was seen in 22%, paroxysmal spikes or sharp waves in 37%, and posterior rhythmic delta (less than 4 Hz) in 15%.

The spike-wave discharges are more numerous during all sleep states except REM. The spike-wave bursts have a modified appearance in sleep, and typically are briefer, irregular and slow to 1.5–2.5 Hz. Hyperventilation, photic stimulation, and hypoglycemia will activate typical absence seizures, but hyperventilation is the most effective procedure.

The ictal discharges during an atypical absence seizure are more variable. They typically occur at frequencies between 1.5–2.5 Hz and are irregular or asymmetrical in voltage. Only 11% of 27 patients with atypical absences had a normal interictal EEG in the study by Holmes et al.[12] Diffuse slowing and focal or multifocal spikes or sharp waves were seen in 85%. Sleep often activates spike-wave discharges.

Clinical effects are generally perceived accompanying discharges lasting longer than 3 seconds. Detailed neuropsychological investigations have demonstrated functional impairment from a spike-and-wave burst of any duration. Auditory reaction times were delayed 56% of the time when a stimulus was presented at the onset of the EEG paroxysm.[16,17] They were abnormal in 80% when the stimulus was delayed 0.5 seconds. Responsiveness may improve as the paroxysm continues.

Clonic Seizures

Clonic seizures are similar to GTC seizures, but only have rhythmic or semirhythmic contractions of a group of muscles. These jerks can involve any muscle group although the arms, neck, and facial muscles are most commonly involved. Clonic seizures are more common in children than adults.

EEG. The interictal EEG pattern seen in patients with clonic seizures is similar to those with GTCs. The ictal pattern usually consists of spike-wave discharges.

Myoclonic Seizures

Myoclonic seizures are characterized by sudden, brief (<350 milliseconds), shock-like contractions that may be generalized or confined to the face and trunk or to one or more extremities, or even to individual muscles or groups of muscles. Myoclonic seizures result in short bursts of synchronized electromyographic activity which often involves simultaneous activation of agonist and antagonist muscles. The muscle contractions are quicker than the contractions with clonic seizures. Any group of muscles can be involved in the jerk. Myoclonic seizures may be dramatic, causing the patient to fall to the ground or be quite subtle, resembling tremors. Because of the brevity of the seizures, it is not possible to determine if consciousness is impaired. Myoclonus may occur as a component of an absence seizure or at the beginning of a GTC seizure. Myoclonic seizures are usually associated with generalized spike-wave activity.

EEG. The interictal EEG pattern seen in patients with myoclonic seizures consists of generalized spike-wave, multifocal spikes or is normal.

Tonic Seizures

Tonic seizures are brief seizures (usually less than 60 seconds) consisting of the sudden onset of increased tone in extensor muscles. If standing, the patient typically falls to the ground. The seizures are invariably longer than myoclonic seizures. Electromyographic activity is dramatically increased in tonic seizures. There is impairment of consciousness during the seizure, although in short seizures this may be difficult to assess. Tonic seizures are frequently seen in patients with the Lennox–Gastaut syndrome, a disorder consisting of a mixed seizure disorder, mental retardation and the EEG findings of a slow spike-and-wave pattern.[18]

EEG. The EEG ictal manifestations of tonic seizures usually consist of bilateral synchronous spikes of 10–25 Hz of medium to high voltage with a frontal accentuation.[19] Marked suppression—termed desynchronization—may also occur. Occasional multiple spike-and-wave or diffuse slow activity may occur during a tonic seizure. The interictal EEG has features similar to those seen in the other generalized seizures.

Atonic Seizures

Atonic (astatic) seizures or drop attacks are characterized by a sudden loss of muscle tone. They begin without warning and cause the patient, if standing, to fall quickly to the floor. Since there may be total lack of tone, the child has no means to protect himself and injuries often occur. The attack may be fragmentary and lead to dropping of the head with slackening of the jaw or dropping of a limb. In atonic seizures there should be a loss of electromyographic activity. Consciousness is impaired during the fall, although the patient may regain alertness immediately upon hitting the floor. Atonic attacks are frequently associated with myoclonic jerks either before, during, or after the atonic seizure.[20,21] This combination has been described as myoclonic–astatic seizures (see below). Atonic seizures are rare. The majority of children with drop attacks will have myoclonic or tonic seizures.[22]

EEG. The interictal EEG has features similar to those seen in the other generalized seizures. Atonic seizures are usually associated with rhythmic spike-and-wave complexes varying from slow, 1–2 Hz, to more rapid, irregular spike- or multiple spike-and-wave activity. Many children with atonic seizures have background slowing as well.

REFERENCES

1. Gastaut H. Classification of the epilepsies. Proposal for an international classification. *Epilepsia* 1969;10(Suppl.): 14–21.
2. Commission on Classification and Terminology of the International League Against Epilepsy. Proposal for revised clinical and electroencephalographic classification of epileptic seizures. *Epilepsia* 1981;22:249–260.
3. Berg AT, Berkovic SF, Brodie MJ, Buchhalter J, Cross JH, Van Emde BW, Engel J, French J, Glauser TA, Mathern GW, Moshe SL, Nordli D, Plouin P, Scheffer IE. Revised terminology and concepts for organization of seizures and epilepsies: report of the ILAE Commission on Classification and Terminology, 2005–2009. *Epilepsia* 2010;51:676–685.
4. Holmes GL. Partial seizures in children. *Pediatrics* 1986; 77:725–731.
5. Casaubon L, Pohlmann-Eden B, Khosravani H, Carlen PL, Wennberg R. Video-EEG evidence of lateralized clinical features in primary generalized epilepsy with tonic–clonic seizures. *Epileptic Disord* 2003;5:149–156.
6. Holmes MD, Brown M, Tucker DM. Are "generalized" seizures truly generalized? Evidence of localized mesial frontal and frontopolar discharges in absence. *Epilepsia* 2004;45:1568–1579.
7. Blumenfeld H, Westerveld M, Ostroff RB, Vanderhill SD, Freeman J, Necochea A, Uranga P, Tanhehco T, Smith A, Seibyl JP, Stokking R, Studholme C, Spencer SS, Zubal IG. Selective frontal, parietal, and temporal networks in generalized seizures. *Neuroimage* 2003;19:1556–1566.
8. Nersesyan H, Herman P, Erdogan E, Hyder F, Blumenfeld H. Relative changes in cerebral blood flow and neuronal activity in local microdomains during generalized seizures. *J Cereb Blood Flow Metab* 2004;24:1057–1068.
9. Nersesyan H, Hyder F, Rothman DL, Blumenfeld H. Dynamic fMRI and EEG recordings during spike-wave seizures and generalized tonic–clonic seizures in WAG/Rij rats. *J Cereb Blood Flow Metab* 2004;24:589–599.
10. Pearl PL, Holmes GL. Absence seizures. In: Pellock JM, Dodson WE, Bourgeois BFD (eds), *Pediatric Epilepsy. Diagnosis and Treatment.* New York: Demos, 2001; pp. 219–231.
11. Penry JK, Porter RJ, Dreifuss FE. Simultaneous recording of absence sizures with videotape and electroencephalography. *Brain* 1975;98:427–440.
12. Holmes GL, McKeever M, Adamson M. Absence seizures in children: clinical and electroencephalographic features. *Ann Neurol* 1987;21: 268–273.
13. Bureau M, Tassinari CA. Epilepsy with myoclonic absences. *Brain Dev* 2005;27:178–184.
14. Bureau M, Tassinari CA. Myoclonic absences: the seizure and the syndrome. *Adv Neurol* 2005;95:175–183.
15. Caraballo RH, Fontana E, Darra F, Chacon S, Ross N, Fiorini E, Fejerman N, Dalla BB. A study of 63 cases with eyelid myoclonia with or without absences: type of seizure or an epileptic syndrome? *Seizure* 2009;18:440–445.
16. Porter RJ, Penry JK, Dreifuss FE. Responsiveness at the onset of spike-wave bursts. *Electroencephalogr Clin Neurophysiol* 1973;34:239–245.
17. Browne TR, et al. Responsiveness before, during, and after spike-wave paroxysms. *Neurology* 1974;24:659–665.
18. Arzimanoglou A, French J, Blume WT, Cross JH, Ernst JP, Feucht M, Genton P, Guerrini R, Kluger G, Pellock JM, Perucca E, Wheless JW. Lennox–Gastaut syndrome: a consensus approach on diagnosis, assessment, management, and trial methodology. *Lancet Neurol* 2009;8:82–93.
19. Yaqub HA. Electroclinical seizures in Lennox–Gastaut syndrome. *Epilepsia* 1993;34:120–127.
20. Doose H. Myoclonic-astatic epilepsy. In: Degen R, Dreifuss FE (eds), *Benign Localized and Generalized Epilepsies of Early Childhood.* Amsterdam: Elsevier Science Publishers, BV, 1992; pp. 163–168.
21. Oguni H, Fukuyama Y, Imaizumi Y, Uehara T. Video-EEG analysis of drop seizures in myoclonic astatic epilepsy of early childhood (Doose syndrome). *Epilepsia* 1992;33: 805–813.
22. Ikeno T, Shigematsu H, Miyakoshi M, Ohba A, Yagi K, Seino M. An analytic study of epileptic falls. *Epilepsia* 1985; 26:612–621.

CHAPTER 2

Networks and Systems in Epileptic Seizures

Aristea S. Galanopoulou and Solomon L. Moshé

▶ OVERVIEW

Epileptic seizures are stereotypical patterns of abnormal synchronized activity among different cellular populations. They are products of pathological activation of networks involved in controlling the temporal (initiation, maintenance, termination) or semiological evolution of these ictal events. Often seizure activity forms a reverberating circuit that can perpetuate and self-sustain, as is the case with temporal lobe seizures. Alternatively, a seizure can be paroxysmal but temporally confined, albeit with the potential to recur, such as in epileptic myoclonus or spasms. The basic elements of these networks may belong to a single or multiple systems, which are recognized based on well-identified physiological functions. As such, they are useful in localizing seizure activity and defining seizure propagation. Communications within a system or between different systems, during a seizure, can be via anatomical connections (i.e., afferent or efferent neuronal projections) or humoral (i.e., hormonal, metabolic or immune responses). A *sine qua non* of epilepsy is the propensity for unprovoked seizures to recur. In certain cases, this is already a predetermined feature of the original epileptic seizure network, as occurs in certain types of primary idiopathic epilepsies, that is, absence. The expression of the seizures, in such cases, appears to depend more on modifiers involved in the physiological maturation of the network, such as age or hormonal factors. In other types of epilepsy, the epileptic predisposition is not as strong initially, but dynamic changes of the network triggered by seizures or unrelated epigenetic factors promote epileptogenesis. The classical example is temporal lobe epilepsy (TLE), whereby initial precipitating events may increase the likelihood that TLE will manifest.

Epileptic networks include an *initiating circuit*, which, in certain cases, may be ignited by endogenous or exogenous triggers (such as stress, fever, photic stimulation, and sleep–wake cycle). Seizure activity may remain regionally contained or spread to *secondary domains*, via *propagation pathways*. Initiating networks

are different for generalized or localization-related epilepsies. Identification of the networks and systems involved in seizures and epilepsy is important for their correct localization, classification, and treatment, as well as the identification of methods to predict their recurrence and their outcome. In this review, we will summarize some of the known networks and systems implicated in common types of epileptic seizures and syndromes, discuss them in the context of specific types of epileptic seizures, and review factors that can modify them.

▶ BASIC NETWORKS IMPLICATED IN EPILEPTIC SEIZURES

CORTICAL–SUBCORTICAL NETWORKS

Temporal Lobe Network

Probably, the most popular focus of attention in epilepsy research has been the mesial temporal lobe structures, due to their high epileptogenicity and the high incidence of TLE. Medial temporal lobe structures are the dentate gyrus (DG), hippocampus, subiculum, pre- and parasubiculum, entorhinal, perirhinal, and parahippocampal cortices. These are normally involved in long-term memory formation, consolidating information obtained through connections with associational cortices. The basic circuit interconnects the subiculum, DG, and cornu ammonis regions of the hippocampus (CA3 and CA1) (a.k.a. *trisynaptic pathway*), with the entorhinal (EC) and amygdalar cortices (Fig. 2–1).[1] The major excitatory input to the DG originates at layer II of the EC and enters into the ipsilateral hippocampus through the *perforant pathway*. Granule neurons of the DG project onto area CA3 via the *mossy fiber pathway*. CA3 pyramidal neurons interact with CA1 pyramidal neurons through the *Schaffer collaterals*. Finally, CA1 neurons send axons to the subiculum, which in turn projects to cortical areas. The web of connections among different areas is actually more complex, as individual areas can project

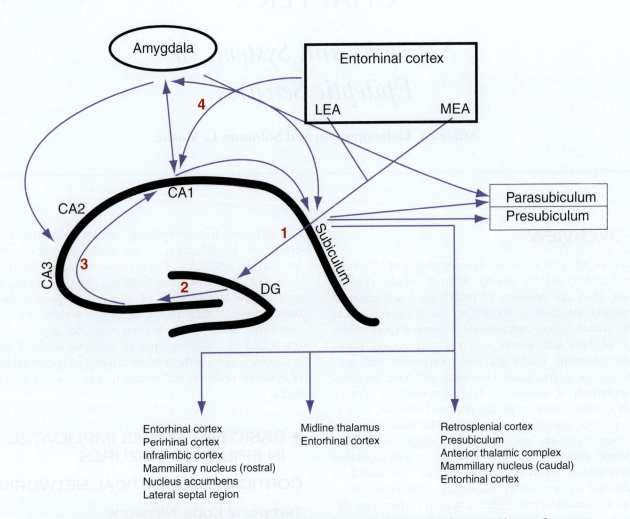

Figure 2–1. Schematic representation of hippocampal connections. 1, perforant pathway; 2, mossy fiber pathway; 3, Schaffer collaterals; 4, temporoammonic pathway; MEA, medial entorhinal cortex; LEA, lateral entorhinal cortex. (Based on information from Amaral D, Lavenex P. *Hippocampal Neuroanatomy*. New York: Oxford University Press, 2007.)

to contralateral hippocampus (i.e., CA3 neurons or hilar neurons) or have antidromic influences within the hippocampus (i.e., CA3 toward hilus or DG; CA1 toward CA3) or between the hippocampus and cortical areas (i.e., *temporoammonic pathway* connecting CA1–CA3 neurons to layer III of EC). Furthermore, local interneurons, classically operating via inhibitory signaling systems, such as gamma-aminobutyric acid (GABA), may modify the activity of this circuit. The medial temporal structures are also connected with the medial thalamus and inferior frontal lobes.[2] Midline thalamic nuclei act as synchronizers of the neuronal activity that reverberates through this network. Escape of seizure activity toward the cortex, directly or through the thalamus, or toward the brainstem allows seizure generalization and can impair consciousness.[3]

This network can be further modulated by subcortical influences. The *septohippocampal pathway* originates in the medial septal nucleus and diagonal band of Broca and enters the hippocampus through the fimbria/fornix, operating via cholinergic and GABAergic mechanisms. The cholinergic fibers interact with most hippocampal regions, whereas GABAergic ones modulate the basket cells of DG.[1] Cholinergic afferents from brainstem nuclei (pedunculopontine nucleus and pontomesencephalic reticular formation) participate in rapid eye movement (REM) sleep regulation. The septohippocampal is an important relay pathway, given its connections with the amygdala, hypothalamus, and brainstem, and plays critical role in the generation of the *theta rhythm*, which is important for learning and memory.[4] The *brainstem monoamine* pathways provide noradrenergic control from the locus coeruleus, targeting particularly CA3 and dentate hilar neurons, serotoninergic input from the raphe nuclei, and dopaminergic input from the ventral tegmental area. Noradrenergic input to the hippocampus enhances excitability and promotes long-term potentiation. Serotoninergic and dopaminergic pathways are primarily inhibitory and participate in sleep–wake transitions.[1]

OTHER NETWORKS INVOLVING CORTICAL REGIONS

In addition to the temporal lobe, functional neuroimaging, clinical, electrographic, and anatomic data have indicated the existence of additional distinct networks involving other cortical regions[2]: medial occipital–lateral temporal, superior parietal–medial frontal, bifrontal–pontine–subthalamic, and parietal–medial temporal.

Corticothalamic Network

The thalamus has central role in rhythm generation and sensory information trafficking in the brain.[5] First, it can act as a relay system forwarding information from multiple subcortical centers to the cerebral cortex. In seizures, this can lead to seizure spreading. Second, if the level of afferent information decreases, thalamus resumes its role as a generator of oscillatory rhythms observed in sleep, such as sleep spindles, by inducing neocortical cells to fire bursts.[6,7] These corticothalamic networks are important, as they can drive the expression of spike-wave (SW) discharges. Third, midline intralaminar thalamic nuclei project diffusely to the cortex, allowing diffuse activation of cortical areas. Utilization of this gateway may allow for seizure generalization. The principal sensory relay nuclei of the thalamus receive excitatory glutamatergic afferents from the cortex and send excitatory glutamatergic projections to the same cortical areas. Thalamic and cortical neurons both project to and excite the nucleus reticularis thalami (NRT) GABAergic interneurons, which in turn project onto and inhibit the thalamic relay neurons (GABAergic projections). Midline intralaminar thalamic nuclei project to the frontal, medial, and dorsolateral cortex in a more diffuse manner compared with relay neurons, as well as to the striatum; they receive afferents from cortex, globus pallidus, and NRT interneurons. In addition, thalamus receives afferents from brainstem structures (locus coeruleus, raphe nuclei, pedunculopontine, and lateral tegmental nuclei) and the basal forebrain and hypothalamus.[5]

During wakefulness, corticothalamic neurons fire continuously. When sensory input is diminished, thalamic neurons hyperpolarize, leading to deinactivation of low threshold calcium channels (T-channels), and this switches their mode of activity to a synchronized oscillatory pattern (spindles). These oscillations consist of sequential cycles of coactivation of cortical and thalamic relay neurons followed by NRT activation, which then inhibits thalamic neurons and leads to a new cycle of oscillation.[8] Bazhenov et al[9] have also proposed that sleep-induced NRT hyperpolarization may reverse $GABA_A$ergic inhibitory postsynaptic potentials (IPSPs)

and this in turn can trigger a low threshold spike and sleep oscillations.

SUBCORTICAL NETWORKS

The basal ganglia consist of the striatum (caudate and putamen), globus pallidus externa (GPe) and interna (GPi) (or entopeduncular nucleus), subthalamic nucleus (STN), and substantia nigra. They are extensively interconnected (Fig. 2–2) among themselves as well as with the rest of the cortical and subcortical neurons. As a result, they are involved in motor control, sleep, eye movement, cognitive functions, and affective disorders. Because of their central role in information trafficking and processing, as well as their synaptic organization in the form of loops, they play important role in seizure control. Among the first structures to be studied, in their role in seizure propagation, were the substantia nigra and lenticular nucleus (putamen, globus pallidus). A simplified form of the web of connections depicted in Fig. 2–2, as they pertain to seizure control, includes an input of cortical afferents (striatum), which either directly or indirectly (through the GPe and STN) reaches the output structures [GPi and substantia nigra pars reticulata (SNR)]. These in turn relay the information either to the striatum or the thalamus, superior colliculus, pedunculopontine nuclei, or other brainstem nuclei.

Apart from acting as secondary propagation pathways, experimental studies have suggested that certain of these nuclei have the ability to generate seizure-like behaviors. Electrical stimulation or excitation of the inferior colliculus or periaqueductal gray matter elicits running and bouncing clonic seizures; similar manipulations of the reticular system can generate extension or flexion spasms or tonic seizures.[10–14] Midbrain tegmental lesions increase the threshold for or prevent hindlimb tonic extension during maximal electroshock seizures (MES), but have no effect on electroshock, flurothyl, or pentylenetetrazole seizure thresholds.[15] In these studies (rats), damage to the superior cerebellar peduncle and/or reticular formation was responsible for inhibition of hindlimb extension.[13] Other supportive studies have shown that total cerebellectomy abolishes the hindlimb extension component of these seizures. Seizures have also been generated by penicillin injections in the midbrain tegmentum (myoclonic, tonic, and tonic–clonic).[16] However, the main focus of interest has been on exploiting the properties of this network to control seizure propagation, as will be discussed later on. Other popular brainstem structures involved in seizure networks are the raphe nuclei and the locus coeruleus. The raphe nuclei consist of serotoninergic neurons that are involved in the control of pain, sleep, and emotions. The noradrenergic projections of locus

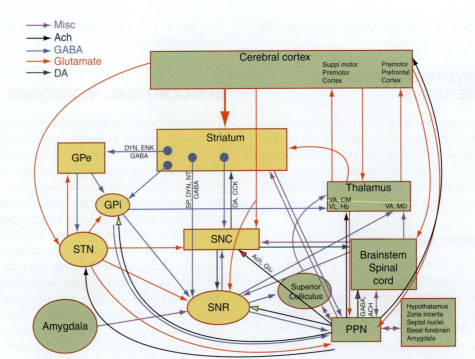

Figure 2–2. Network of basal ganglia connections. Supplementary Motor, supplementary motor cortex; STN, subthalamic nucleus; GPe, globus pallidus externa; GPi, globus pallidus interna; SNC, substantia nigra pars compacta; SNR, substantia nigra pars reticulata; PPN, pedunculopontine tegmental nucleus. *Thalamic nuclei*: VA, ventral anterior; CM, centromedian; VL, ventrolateral; Hb, habenular; MD, mediodorsal. *Neurotransmitters*: Ach, acetylcholine; Glu, glutamate; DA, dopamine; Misc, miscellanea.

coeruleus are involved in physiologic responses to stress and panic, REM sleep, autonomic functions, gaze control, and in most seizure models this pathway exerts anticonvulsant effects.[17]

NETWORKS IN THE CONTEXT OF SPECIFIC EPILEPTIC SEIZURES

Temporal Lobe Epilepsy

The best studied type of epilepsy is the mesial TLE (MTLE), which has been linked to characteristic histopathologic alterations in the mesial temporal lobe structures, often referred to as *mesial temporal or hippocampal sclerosis* (MTS). This is the preponderant histopathological abnormality in patients with intractable TLE, characterized by neuronal loss at specific hippocampal areas (hilar region, CA1, and CA3 pyramidal regions), gliosis, structural and functional reorganization of the hippocampus, including mossy fibers and granular DG cells, and the presence of dysplastic neurons. Although more widespread changes have been shown to occur outside the hippocampus, MTS has concentrated the greatest investigational interest, due to its linkage with intractable epilepsies, the excellent seizure

outcomes following temporal lobectomies, and experimental studies showing that prolonged seizures can induce mesial temporal lobe changes, including MTS, in animals that do progress to epilepsy. The initiating circuit in MTLE is thought to include the hippocampus, EC, and midline thalamic nuclei, and reverberates spreading to adjacent structures, such as the amygdala or the temporal neocortex (Fig. 2–3).[3] In neocortical TLE, the epileptogenic focus is thought to lie within temporal neocortex but may also spread to the mesial temporal lobe structures. It has been recently reported that the spread of amygdala-kindled seizures occurs first at the SNR, before it reaches the hippocampus or the STN, probably via direct propagation through the amygdalonigral pathway.[18] The extensive connectivity of the hippocampus and temporal lobe with other brain structures (Figs. 2–1 and 2–3) explains the diversity in semiology or associated symptoms observed in TLE patients. The sleep-induced aggravation of interictal and ictal events can be mediated by the brainstem connections with centers involved in sleep–wake cycle. Certain ictal signs have also been localized to different areas of the network, including fear or olfactory auras (amygdala, hippocampus, and parahippocampal areas), experiential auras or early unilateral somatic motor involvement

MTLE networks

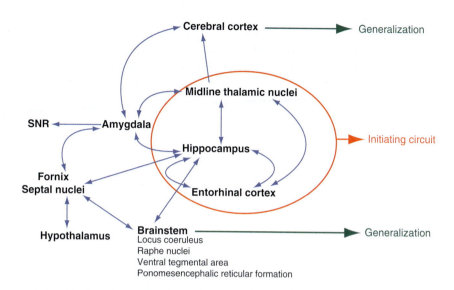

Figure 2–3. Networks involved in seizure generation in MTLE (initiating circuit), spread, and secondary generalization. MTLE, mesial temporal lobe epilepsy; SNR, substantia nigra pars reticulata. (Modified from Schwarcz R, Scharfman HE, Bertram EH. Temporal lobe epilepsy: renewed emphasis on extrahippocampal areas. In: Davis KL, Charney D, Coyle JT, Nemeroff C, (eds), *Neuropsychopharmacology: The Fifth Generation of Progress.* Lippincott Williams & Wilkins, 2002; pp. 1843–1855.)

without automatisms (temporal neocortex), and visceral sensations or automatisms (amygdala, hippocampus).[19] Impaired level of consciousness has been proposed to indicate spread to upper brainstem and medial thalamus and subsequent inhibition of bilateral frontoparietal association cortices.[20] Secondary generalization has been attributed to spread to corticothalamic networks.[3] TLE patients may also have reproductive endocrine abnormalities attributed to connections with the hypothalamus.[21]

Absences

The electrographic signature of typical absences is the generalized or frontally maximal SW complexes. The ictal behavior (*absence seizures*) consists of sudden behavioral arrest with loss of consciousness and rapid return to baseline toward the end of the ictus, without postictal confusion. Several lines of evidence from electrophysiological or functional neuroimaging studies support the involvement of the corticothalamic pathways in the generation of SW, as originally proposed by Jasper and Kershman,[22] although it has been debated whether the origin lies in the cortex or the thalamus.[5,7,23] Gloor[7] proposed that SW complexes are generated in the context of mild state of cortical hyperexcitability that increases the cortical responsiveness to excitatory thalamic volleys, which would otherwise produce spindle oscillations. In favor of the cortical origin of the SW are the occasional focality of these discharges with rapid bilateral synchrony; the ability of cortex to generate SW and absences in athalamic cats and monkeys; and the finding that thalamic excitation can produce oscillations but not SW.[24] In the penicillin model of SW seizures, SW activity was first noted in the cortex.[25] However, reports of SW generation following midline thalamic nucleus activation have been reported.[5] A SW complex consists of an early spike, corresponding to the cortical activation and a subsequent period of cortical inhibition (slow wave). Bursts of cortical activation (spike) excite the thalamic relay neurons, which depolarize, as well as the GABAergic interneurons in the NRT, which fire in bursts. The NRT neurons then directly inhibit the thalamic relay neurons leading to a fast $GABA_A$-driven IPSP and a slow $GABA_B$-driven IPSP. The hyperpolarization of thalamic neurons activates hyperpolarization-activated cation channels (Ih) and subsequently the low threshold calcium channels (T-channels) leading to a calcium spike that drives action potentials. This in turn activates both cortical neurons and NRT interneurons, leading to the next cycle.[5] In classical childhood absence, the SW frequency is around 3 Hz, but more rapid frequencies occur in juvenile absence (>3.5 Hz) and slower (<2.5 Hz) in atypical absences of the Lennox–Gastaut syndrome. It is not unusual that a fast rhythmic activity may precede the SW, reflecting the oscillatory spindle-like activity of the corticothalamic network, driving the SW.

As described earlier, this circuit is also the generator of spindles, that is, oscillatory 6–14 Hz activity that is set by $GABA_A$ and $GABA_B$ receptor-mediated IPSPs and low threshold calcium spikes. Inhibition of $GABA_A$ receptors in thalamocortical relay neurons can convert spindles to 3–4 Hz activity. Increase in the firing across the corticothalamic pathway activates NRT interneurons and thalamic relay activity by prolonging the duration of thalamoreticular bursts. This in turn favors $GABA_B$ over $GABA_A$ receptor-mediated IPSPs, prolongs the period of neuronal inhibition, and therefore decreases the SW frequency. It has been therefore proposed that the slow SW, typical of Lennox-Gastaut syndrome, reflects a greater degree of cortical excitability.[26] Similarly, the beneficial effects of $GABA_A$ receptor agonists, such as benzodiazepines, in absence have been attributed to the resultant decrease in cortical excitability.

The alteration of consciousness in absence is typically brief with rapid recovery. A possible explanation may be that absences selectively affect certain brain regions rather than the whole brain, as suggested by behavioral, imaging, and electroencephalographic (EEG) studies.[19] Projections to frontopolar or orbitofrontal regions have been proposed to contribute to impaired consciousness, based on observations that SW complexes are often maximal frontally and that focal seizures arising from the frontopolar cortex may present as "pseudo-absences."[8] In agreement, Marcus et al[27] have reported a rostrocaudal shift in the semiology of bilateral cortical epileptogenic foci: anterior foci triggered absences, whereas more posterior foci elicited motor phenomena, that is, myoclonic seizures or tonic–clonic seizures. During absences, diffuse decrease in blood flow, including the cortex,[28] has been reported, while the thalamus retains either a disproportionately higher[29] or relatively preserved blood flow.[28] Associative signs, such as myoclonias, may indicate activation of adjacent motor cortical areas. Perseverative automatisms are frequent, may break through prolonged SW bursts, and could reflect disinhibition or dysregulation of limbic areas during the ictal phenomena.[8] Tonic upgaze is common in absences but atypical in focal seizures and is thought to indicate activation of basal ganglia and brainstem, such as the striato–colliculo–thalamic network.[8,30]

Tonic Seizures

Tonic seizures consist of muscle contractions involving axial and/or limb muscles. They can be seen in symptomatic or cryptogenic epilepsies such as Lennox–Gastaut syndrome, in which nocturnal tonic seizures are its signature. The ictal EEG patterns may consist of either bilaterally synchronous slow SW complexes or fast rhythmic activity and polyspikes ("epileptic recruiting rhythm").[11] Slow SW complexes are usually maximal over the frontal regions, indicating that the frontal motor and premotor cortex participate in the initiating epileptic circuit. Activation of frontal cortical and subcortical structures (thalamus, brainstem) in generalized motor seizures was documented by Bancaud et al (1965) and Goldring (1972) with implanted electrodes.[11,31,32] Rodin et al[33] also provided electrographic recordings in which high frequency discharges were apparent at the pons, prior to the corticothalamic involvement, at the onset of generalized tonic seizures, in metrazol- or megimide-treated cats. Fast rhythmic activity has similarly been proposed to reflect increased cortical excitability, as it resembles "ripples," which have been linked to seizures.[23,26]

Alternatively, tonic seizures can be brief presenting as paroxysmal flexion or extension of limbs and trunk, as in infantile spasms. Infantile spasms are associated with the classical electrodecremental response on a hypsarrhythmic background. Infantile spasms manifest as clusters of sudden tonic flexion of extension of the axial and bilateral limb muscles, which correlate with characteristic electrodecremental responses on the EEG. The EEG background is typically hypsarrhythmic, indicating bilateral dysfunction with multifocal areas of epileptogenic potential. Both cortical and subcortical centers have been implicated in infantile spasms, as well as abnormal patterns of communications, attributed to white matter abnormalities.[34] In a significant number of patients with infantile spasms, a leading cortical spike, usually at the pre- or postcentral gyrus, preceded the ictus on electrocorticography.[35] Postoperative success was highest if the area of spike generation was excised. However, a leading spike cannot always be identified preictally. The resemblance of the ictal semiology to behaviors elicited by brainstem dysfunction has long suggested the involvement of subcortical structures, including brainstem. Case reports have described pathology in the brainstem of patients with history of infantile spasms, often isolated.[32] Experimentally, activation or electrical stimulation of the reticular system can generate extension or flexion spasms or tonic seizures.[10–13] In further support, positron emission tomography (PET) showed increased glucose metabolism at the lenticular nucleus (~72% of patients), and in 50%, an involvement of the pontomedullary reticular system was suggested.[36] Indeed, the high level of connectivity of the reticular activating system with the premotor, motor, and supplementary motor cortex (corticoreticular pathway), as well as with the thalamus, hypothalamus, and cortex via ascending fibers, and with the cerebellum and spinal cord could render it in a prime position to generate such ictal behaviors. Evidence for abnormal connectivity is the presence of periventricular leukomalacia and abnormal myelination on magnetic resonance imaging (MRI).[34]

Myoclonic Seizures

Myoclonic seizures are brief and sudden muscle contractions, which can appear in the context of idiopathic, generalized (i.e., juvenile myoclonic epilepsies), cryptogenic/symptomatic epilepsies (i.e., progressive myoclonic epilepsy, severe myoclonic epilepsy of infancy, and mitochondrial diseases). The ictal events can be either pure myoclonic jerks or may be followed by absences (myoclonic absence, perioral myoclonus with absence) or drop attacks (myoclonic astatic). Alternatively, sudden loss of tone may present as *negative myoclonus*, a symptom of epileptic, toxic, or metabolic encephalopathies. As myoclonus can often be a physiologic event, that is, benign nocturnal myoclonus, an EEG correlate is often sought to confirm its epileptic nature, and this consists of spikes or polyspikes or polyspike–slow waves complexes. The ictal events can occur spontaneously or may be triggered, as is the case in photosensitive epilepsies or reflex epilepsies. However, myoclonic seizures cannot only be generated by cortical areas but also by subcortical regions, implying that the EEG changes may be subtle.

The basic circuit that can generate myoclonus consists of the corticoreticular pathway and its efferent projections to the reticulospinal tract. This has been demonstrated by local stimulation of activation of cortical motor areas or the mesencephalic reticular formation, which suffice to induce myoclonic seizures.[16] Furthermore, using magnetoencephalography or EEG, ictal spikes or polyspikes have been localized at motor cortical areas. In negative myoclonus, the response to ethosuximide (T-type calcium channel blocker) has been interpreted as evidence of corticothalamic network involvement.[37] Using EEG, electromyography (EMG), and functional MRI co-registration in patients with reading reflex epilepsy and orofacial myoclonus, ictal patterns consisted of *blood oxygen level dependent* (BOLD) changes within cortical and subcortical regions, including striatum and thalami.[38]

Reflex Epilepsies

Reflex epilepsies are triggered by specific stimuli, such as photic, auditory, or tactile, or complex processes, such as thinking and reading. They are thought to be triggered by stimulus-induced increase in neuronal synchronization of an already hyperexcitable cortical area that is primarily involved in the processing of this stimulus or task. Seizures can be generalized tonic–clonic, absences, or myoclonic. The most common type is the photosensitive epilepsy. Propagation may involve a corticoreticular or corticocortical pathway.[39]

► NETWORKS INVOLVED IN SEIZURE CONTROL

Seizures may spread from the initiating circuits to other structures that determine whether they will spread further and generalize or stop. Spread to midline thalamic nuclei may synchronize neuronal activity, which then reverberates through the network. Escape of seizure activity toward the cortex, directly or through the thalamus, allows seizure generalization and can impair consciousness.[3] Seizure generalization can also be effected via spread to brainstem structures, as reported in patients with persistence of secondarily generalized tonic–clonic seizures, following anatomical hemispherectomies.[40]

A number of studies have detailed the role of basal ganglia and brainstem structures in seizure control. The basic elements of this network are depicted in Fig. 2–2. Among these structures, SNR deserves special mention, as it has been proposed to act as a gatekeeper for seizure propagation, in both focal onset and generalized models of seizures.[41] In adult rats, the SNR consists of two different regions, $SNR_{anterior}$ and $SNR_{posterior}$, which differ morphologically, functionally, as well as in regard to their connectivity with other regions.[41] SNR contains predominantly GABAergic neurons, but a small proportion of the $SNR_{posterior}$ neurons are dopaminergic. Silencing of the SNR activity by increasing $GABA_A$ergic, inhibiting glutamatergic input, or with deep brain stimulation has anticonvulsant effects when targeting the $SNR_{anterior}$.[42,43] The effects on SNR-mediated seizure control are therefore through disinhibition of output structures, such as superior colliculus, pedunculopontine tegmental nucleus, and possibly, in selected cases, the thalamus. In contrast, silencing of the $SNR_{posterior}$ has proconvulsant effects in males but no effect in females.[43] In addition, activation of the striatum also has anticonvulsant effects, which are thought to be mediated via inhibition of the SNR activity.[17] In patients with intractable epilepsy, attempts to alter this subcortical network using deep brain stimulation of the STN or anterior thalamus have resulted in positive effects on seizure control.[44–49]

► DEVELOPMENTAL FACTORS INVOLVED IN SEIZURE NETWORKS

Seizure incidence is highest during the very young and elder stages of life, with a mild preference for males. This is not just because males are more prone to accidents or other epigenetic factors predisposing to seizures. The immaturity of the developing brain, both in regard to signaling systems as well as to the morphological and structural organization of endogenous neuronal networks, appears to be key in rendering it more susceptible to seizures. This can influence not only the vulnerability to but also the phenotypic expression and consequences of seizures. For instance, among childhood epileptic encephalopathies with slow SW, tonic seizures were more prevalent in younger ages (16.6 months), atypical absences appeared around 32 months, myoclonic seizures at 39 months, and clonic or tonic–clonic seizures at 42 months.[50]

A lot of research has focused on the age- and gender-specific factors influencing the functional maturation of the subcortical centers controlling seizure control, such as the SNR. Early in life, increase in $GABA_A$ergic input into the infantile rat SNR [postnatal day (PN) 15] has proconvulsant effects in males but no effect in females.[43] The appearance of two functionally distinct SNR regions occurs earlier in females than in males, during the prepubertal period. The $SNR_{anterior}$, a predominantly GABAergic neuronal population, matures into a $GABA_A$-sensitive anticonvulsant center in both sexes; the $SNR_{posterior}$, which contains predominantly GABAergic and a minority of dopaminergic neurons, maintains its $GABA_A$-driven proconvulsant properties in males but has no effect in females.[43] The functional differentiation of the SNR in seizure control through development is also evident for the $GABA_B$ signaling pathway (functionally active only in infantile rats, where activation is anticonvulsive) and the N-methyl-D-aspartic acid (NMDA) signaling pathway (functionally active only in adult, but not in infantile male rats).[51] The changing function of the SNR through development and sexual maturation parallels changes in the expression and physiology of the molecular players involved in $GABA_A$ergic signaling.[52] The expression profiles of $GABA_A$ receptor $\alpha 1$ and $\gamma 2L$ subunit mRNA expression (subunits involved in benzodiazepine effects) increases with age, especially in $SNR_{anterior}$, and at least the $\alpha 1$ mRNA appears to be always higher in females. Content of glutamic acid decarboxylase-immunoreactivity (GAD-ir) is also higher in female SNR neurons, and particularly in the $SNR_{anterior}$ of juvenile and postpubertal rats. The kinetics of $GABA_A$ergic postsynaptic currents also accelerated with age due to a developmental switch from $\alpha 3$ to $\alpha 1$ subunit containing $GABA_A$ receptors in the $SNR_{anterior}$.[53] These indicate that $GABA_A$ergic signaling may become more efficient as a function of age, female gender, and localization at the $SNR_{anterior}$, that is, factors that also positively influence the appearance of $GABA_A$-sensitive anticonvulsant SNR effects.

An additional point of complexity is that neurotransmitter signaling, such as glutamatergic or GABAergic, changes during development.[54,55] Of particular interest is the switch of $GABA_A$ergic signaling from depolarizing to hyperpolarizing, as it is the primary inhibitory neurotransmitter in the adult brain. In most neuronal cells, during the early postnatal life, high intracellular chloride exists. Upon $GABA_A$ receptor activation, neurons depolarize, increase intracellular calcium, and activation of calcium-sensitive signaling cascades ensues. This is important for brain development, as it influences neuronal proliferation, migration, differentiation, synaptic integration, and communication.[55] During neuronal maturation, the balance between cation chloride cotransporters that export (i.e., the potassium chloride cotransporter KCC2) and those that import (i.e., the sodium potassium chloride cotransporter NKCC1) chloride shifts in favor of KCC2, decreasing intracellular chloride.[56] As a result, $GABA_A$ergic signaling becomes hyperpolarizing. The timing of switch is different among various brain regions, but usually is accomplished within the first 3 postnatal weeks. Based on ontogenetic patterns of developmental increase of KCC2 expression, it has been suggested that caudal regions, that is, spinal cord and brainstem, switch earlier than more rostral areas, such as the neocortex.[57] In actuality, each neuronal population has its own tempo of maturation, even compared with other neuronal groups in the same structure, adding further complexity to the evolution of communication protocols within the neuronal networks controlling seizures. Moreover, the maturation of KCC2/$GABA_A$ receptor system occurs earlier in females than in males, at least in the SNR.[58] Since $GABA_A$ergic signaling plays key role in the generation of normal rhythms and communication patterns, it is obvious that the operation protocols of seizure networks utilizing these rhythms will change through development and also between sexes. It is therefore interesting to postulate that the relative vulnerability of the very young brain to seizures, and particularly of males, may relate to the asynchronous maturation of networks controlling seizure onset and seizure spread, including the SNR. Furthermore, a number of endogenous or epigenetic factors, such as early life seizures, hormones, and $GABA_A$ergic drugs, may further alter the dynamics of $GABA_A$ receptor signaling.[59,60] It is possible therefore that one of the mechanisms through which early stressors may alter susceptibility to seizures may be by disrupting $GABA_A$-related neuronal differentiation and altering brain development.

▶ CONCLUSIONS

Epilepsy is a network disease. Epileptic networks may be activated by endogenous or exogenous precipitants. Different parts of the networks may be involved in the initiation of seizures, their spread or termination. The ictal semiology, EEG, and neuroimaging may provide insight on the brain regions involved in the epileptic focus and may help determine whether seizures have focal onset or are generalized from the start. Identification of subcortical structures involved in seizure control is important to design site-specific interventions, such as deep brain stimulation, to improve seizure control. Seizure networks undergo plastic changes through development, in a region-, gender-, and age-specific manner. The asynchronous maturation of their different components may contribute to the increased vulnerability of the developing brain to seizures. Epigenetic influences, such as stress, seizures, and drugs, may further alter the network dynamics by interfering both with signaling pathways, such as the GABA$_A$ergic, and with brain development. The design of effective treatments for seizures needs to be age-, gender-, and, possibly, region-specific. It is equally important to take into consideration the specific needs of the developing brain, so as to avoid long-lasting disruption of brain development.

▶ ACKNOWLEDGMENTS

The authors were supported by the following grants: NIH NINDS NS20253, NS45243, NS62947, NS43209, NS45911, the International Rett Syndrome Foundation, Autism Speaks, and the Heffer Family Medical Foundation. Dr. Solomon L. Moshé is the Charles Frost Chair in Neurosurgery and Neurology.

REFERENCES

1. Schwartzkroin PA, McIntyre DC. Limbic anatomy and physiology. In: Engel JJ, Pedley TA (eds), *Epilepsy: A Comprehensive Textbook*. Philadelphia: Lippincott-Raven Publishers, 1997; pp. 323–340.

2. Spencer SS. Neural networks in human epilepsy: evidence of and implications for treatment. *Epilepsia* 2002;43(3): 219–227.

3. Schwarcz R, Scharfman HE, Bertram EH. Temporal lobe epilepsy: renewed emphasis on extrahippocampal areas. In: Davis KL, Charney D, Coyle JT, Nemeroff C (eds), *Neuropsychopharmacology: The Fifth Generation Of Progress*. Philadelphia: Lippincott Williams & Wilkins, 2002; pp. 1843–1855.

4. Dutar P, Bassant MH, Senut MC, Lamour Y. The septohippocampal pathway: structure and function of a central cholinergic system. *Physiol Rev* 1995;75(2):393–427.

5. Coulter D. *Thalamocortical Anatomy and Physiology*. Philadelphia: Lippincott-Raven Publishers, 1997.

6. Buzsaki G, Traub RD. *Physiological Basis of EEG and Local Field Potentials*. Philadelphia: Lippincott-Raven Publishers, 2007.

7. Gloor P. Generalized epilepsy with bilateral synchronous spike and wave discharge. New findings concerning its physiological mechanisms. *Electroencephalogr Clin Neurophysiol Suppl* 1978;(34):245–249.

8. Hirsch E, Valenti M-P. Systems and networks in absence seizures and epilepsies in humans. In: Hirsch E, Andermann F, Chauvel P, Engel J, Lopes da Silva F, Luders H (eds), *Generalized Seizures: From Clinical Phenomenology to Underlying Systems and Networks*. Montrouge: John Libbey Eurotext, 2006; pp. 119–126.

9. Bazhenov M, Timofeev I, Steriade M, Sejnowski TJ. Self-sustained rhythmic activity in the thalamic reticular nucleus mediated by depolarizing GABA$_A$ receptor potentials. *Nat Neurosci* 1999;2(2):168–174.

10. Mori S, Iwakiri H, Homma Y, Yokoyama T, Matsuyama K. Neuroanatomical and neurophysiological bases of postural control. *Adv Neurol* 1995;67:289–303.

11. Blume WT. Systems and networks in tonic seizures and epilepsies in humans. In: Hirsch E, Andermann F, Chauvel P, Engel J, Lopes da Silva F, Luders H (eds), *Generalized Seizures: From Clinical Phenomenology to Underlying Systems and Networks*. Montrouge: John Libbey Eurotext, 2006; pp. 53–67.

12. Kreindler A, Zuckermann E, Steriade M, Chimion D. Electro-clinical features of convulsions induced by stimulation of brain stem. *J Neurophysiol* 1958;21(5):430–436.

13. Browning RA, Turner FJ, Simonton RL, Bundman MC. Effect of midbrain and pontine tegmental lesions on the maximal electroshock seizure pattern in rats. *Epilepsia* 1981;22(5):583–594.

14. Velisek L, Veliskova J, Giorgi FS, Moshe SL. Sex-specific control of flurothyl-induced tonic–clonic seizures by the substantia nigra pars reticulata during development. *Exp Neurol* 2006;201(1):203–211.

15. Browning RA, Simonton RL, Turner FJ. Antagonism of experimentally induced tonic seizures following a lesion in the midbrain tegmentum. *Epilepsia* 1981;22(5):595–601.

16. Jimenez F, Velasco F, Carrillo-Ruiz J, Villanueva FE, Velasco M, Ponce H. Seizures induced by penicillin microinjections in the mesencephalic tegmentum. *Epilepsy Res* 2000;38(1):33–44.

17. Proctor M, Gale K. *Basal Ganglia and Brainstem Anatomy and Physiology*. Philadelphia: Lippincott-Raven Publishers, 1997.

18. Shi LH, Luo F, Woodward DJ, McIntyre DC, Chang JY. Temporal sequence of ictal discharges propagation in the corticolimbic basal ganglia system during amygdala kindled seizures in freely moving rats. *Epilepsy Res* 2007; 73(1):85–97.

19. Gil-Nagel A, Risinger MW. Ictal semiology in hippocampal versus extrahippocampal temporal lobe epilepsy. *Brain* 1997;120(Pt 1):183–192.

20. Blumenfeld H. Consciousness and epilepsy: why are patients with absence seizures absent? *Prog Brain Res* 2005;150:271–286.

21. Herzog AG, et al. Interictal EEG discharges, reproductive hormones, and menstrual disorders in epilepsy. *Ann Neurol* 2003;54(5):625–637.

22. Jasper H, Kershman J. Electroencephalographic classification of the epilepsies. *Arch Neurol Psychiatry* 1941;45:903–943.

23. Timofeev I, Steriade M. Neocortical seizures: initiation, development and cessation. *Neuroscience* 2004;123(2):299–336.

24. Steriade M. Spike-wave seizures in corticothalamic systems. In: Hirsch E, Andermann F, Chauvel P, Engel J, Lopes da Silva F, Luders H (eds), *Generalized Seizures: From Clinical Phenomenology to Underlying Systems and Networks*. Montrouge: John Libbey Eurotext, 2006; pp. 127–144.

25. Rodin E, Kitano H, Nagao B, Rodin M. The results of penicillin G administration on chronic unrestrained cats: electrographic and behavioral observations. *Electroencephalogr Clin Neurophysiol* 1977;42:518–527.

26. Blume WT. Pathogenesis of Lennox–Gastaut syndrome: considerations and hypotheses. *Epileptic Disord* 2001;3(4): 183–196.

27. Marcus EM, Watson CW, Simon SA. An experimental model of some varieties of petit mal epilepsy. Electrical-behavioral correlations of acute bilateral epileptogenic foci in cerebral cortex. *Epilepsia* 1968;9(3):233–248.

28. Nehlig A, et al. Absence seizures induce a decrease in cerebral blood flow: human and animal data. *J Cereb Blood Flow Metab* 1996;16(1):147–155.

29. Prevett MC, Duncan JS, Jones T, Fish DR, Brooks DJ. Demonstration of thalamic activation during typical absence seizures using $H_2(15)O$ and PET. *Neurology* 1995;45(7):1396–1402.

30. Bhidayasiri R, Plant GT, Leigh RJ. A hypothetical scheme for the brainstem control of vertical gaze. *Neurology* 2000; 54(10):1985–1993.

31. Bancaud J, Talairach J, Bonis A, et al. La stereo-electroencephalographie dans l'epilepsie. *Arch Neurol* 1965;13(3):333.

32. Goldring S. The role of prefrontal cortex in grand mal convulsion. *Arch Neurol* 1972;26(2):109–119.

33. Rodin E, Onuma T, Wasson S, Porzak J, Rodin M. Neurophysiological mechanisms involved in grand mal seizures induced by metrazol and megimide. *Electro-encephalogr Clin Neurophysiol* 1971;30:62–72.

34. Lado FA, Moshe SL. Role of subcortical structures in the pathogenesis of infantile spasms: what are possible subcortical mediators? *Int Rev Neurobiol* 2002;49:115–140.

35. Asano E, et al. Origin and propagation of epileptic spasms delineated on electrocorticography. *Epilepsia* 2005;46(7): 1086–1097.

36. Chugani HT, Shewmon DA, Sankar R, Chen BC, Phelps ME. Infantile spasms: II. Lenticular nuclei and brain stem activation on positron emission tomography. *Ann Neurol* 1992;31(2):212–219.

37. Kubota M, Nakura M, Hirose H, Kimura I, Sakakihara Y. A magnetoencephalographic study of negative myoclonus in a patient with atypical benign partial epilepsy. *Seizure* 2005;14(1):28–32.

38. Koepp MJ, Hamandi K. Systems and networks in myoclonic seizures and epilepsies. In: Hirsch E, Andermann F, Chauvel P, Engel J, Lopes da Silva F, Luders H (eds), *Generalized Seizures: From Clinical Phenomenology to Underlying Systems and Networks*. Montrouge: John Libbey Eurotext, 2006; pp. 163–182.

39. Ferlazzo E, Zifkin BG, Andermann E, Andermann F. Cortical triggers in generalized reflex seizures and epilepsies. *Brain* 2005;128(Pt 4):700–710.

40. Lhatoo S, Luders H. The semiology and pathophysiology of the secondary generalized tonic clonic seizures. In: Hirsch E, Andermann F, Chauvel P, Engel J, Lopes da Silva F, Luders H (eds), *Generalized Seizures: From Clinical Phenomenology to Underlying Systems and Networks*. Montrouge: John Libbey Eurotext, 2006; pp. 229–246.

41. Veliskova J, Moshe SL. Update on the role of substantia nigra pars reticulata in the regulation of seizures. *Epilepsy Curr* 2006;6(3):83–87.

42. Velisek L, Veliskova J, Moshe SL. Electrical stimulation of substantia nigra pars reticulata is anticonvulsant in adult and young male rats. *Exp Neurol* 2002;173(1):145–152.

43. Veliskova J, Moshe SL. Sexual dimorphism and developmental regulation of substantia nigra function. *Ann Neurol* 2001; 50(5):596–601.

44. Lee KJ, Jang KS, Shon YM. Chronic deep brain stimulation of subthalamic and anterior thalamic nuclei for controlling refractory partial epilepsy. *Acta Neurochir Suppl* 2006; 99:87–91.

45. Lim SN, et al. Electrical stimulation of the anterior nucleus of the thalamus for intractable epilepsy: a long-term follow-up study. *Epilepsia* 2007;48(2):342–347.

46. Molnar GF, et al. Changes in motor cortex excitability with stimulation of anterior thalamus in epilepsy. *Neurology* 2006;66(4):566–571.

47. Shon YM, et al. Effect of chronic deep brain stimulation of the subthalamic nucleus for frontal lobe epilepsy: subtraction SPECT analysis. *Stereotact Funct Neurosurg* 2005;83(2–3):84–90.

48. Kerrigan JF, et al. Electrical stimulation of the anterior nucleus of the thalamus for the treatment of intractable epilepsy. *Epilepsia* 2004;45(4):346–354.

49. Chabardes S, Kahane P, Minotti L, Koudsie A, Hirsch E, Benabid AL. Deep brain stimulation in epilepsy with particular reference to the subthalamic nucleus. *Epileptic Disord* 2002;4(Suppl 3):S83–S93.

50. Chevrie JJ, Aicardi J. Childhood epileptic encephalopathy with slow spike-wave. A statistical study of 80 cases. *Epilepsia* 1972;13(2):259–271.

51. Wurpel JN, Sperber EF, Moshe SL. Age-dependent differences in the anticonvulsant effects of 2-amino-7-phosphono-heptanoic acid or ketamine infusions into the substantia nigra of rats. *Epilepsia* 1992;33(3):439–443.

52. Veliskova J, et al. Seizures in the developing brain. *Epilepsia* 2004;45(Suppl 8):6–12.

53. Chudomel O, Herman H, Nair K, Moshe SL, Galanopoulou AS. Age- and gender-related differences in $GABA_A$ receptor-mediated postsynaptic currents in GABAergic neurons of the substantia nigra reticulata in the rat. *Neuroscience* 2009;163(1):155–167.

54. Jensen FE. The role of glutamate receptor maturation in perinatal seizures and brain injury. *Int J Dev Neurosci* 2002;20(3–5):339–347.

55. Ben-Ari Y, Spitzer NC. Nature and nurture in brain development. *Trends Neurosci* 2004;27(7):361.

56. Rivera C, et al. The K^+/Cl^- co-transporter KCC2 renders GABA hyperpolarizing during neuronal maturation. *Nature* 1999;397(6716):251–255.

57. Wang C, et al. Developmental changes in KCC1, KCC2, and NKCC1 mRNA expressions in the rat brain. *Brain Res Dev Brain Res* 2002;139(1):59–66.

58. Galanopoulou AS, Kyrozis A, Claudio OI, Stanton PK, Moshe SL. Sex-specific KCC2 expression and GABA(A) receptor function in rat substantia nigra. *Exp Neurol* 2003;183(2):628–637.

59. Galanopoulou AS. Dissociated gender-specific effects of recurrent seizures on GABA signaling in CA1 pyramidal neurons: role of GABA(A) receptors. *J Neurosci* 2008; 28(7):1557–1567.

60. Galanopoulou AS. Sexually dimorphic expression of KCC2 and GABA function. *Epilepsy Res* 2008;80(2–3):99–113.

61. Amaral D, Lavenex P. *Hippocampal Neuroanatomy*. New York: Oxford University Press, 2007.

CHAPTER 3

EEGs: When, How, and Why

Warren T. Blume

▶ CLINICAL EVALUATION

Ictal symptoms and signs reflect area(s) of the brain involved in the seizure. Events early in the seizure have greater localizing value than later ones as these latter may result from propagation. As certain symptoms, such as a rising abdominal sensation in a focal seizure, may result from involvement of any one of two or more anatomically distinct regions usual accompanying phenomena may help to distinguish possible ictal areas of origin. Therefore, a cluster of patient- and observer-reported phenomena will more accurately chart seizure origin and propagation than will a single symptom or sign. Knowledge of cortical, thalamic, and brain stem physiology will equip the physician with insightful questions of the patient and associates and will allow perceptive evaluations of video-telemetry seizure depictions. Not only will such scrutiny localize most focal seizures but also it will often distinguish primary generalized from secondarily generalized seizures.[1]

Precipitating factors such as flashing lights or sleep deprivation need be sought. Enquiry about lifestyle may disclose potentially alternative diagnoses, such as excessive daytime sleep in a child thought to have absence or dyscognitive (temporal lobe) seizures. Epilepsy is likely more often overdiagnosed than underdiagnosed. Social and psychological consequences of incorrect diagnoses are difficult to reverse.[2]

As some phenomena will localize but not lateralize to a neural system, that is, visual or limbic, the neurological examination may help to determine the side of epileptogenesis. A decreased nasolabial fold or impaired fine finger movements are two of many physical signs of potential ictal lateralizing value. Moreover, normal aspects of the examination may eliminate certain regions, for example, full visual fields for calcarine occipital seizure onset. Therefore, thoughtful clinical evaluation will develop specific questions for electroencephalography (EEG), thus enhancing its value.

▶ EEG EVALUATION

Appropriate questions for EEG derive from the clinical evaluation and include: (1) does the child have epilepsy; (2) what type is present—focal, generalized, or secondarily generalized; (3) what is its severity and thus its prognosis; and (4) are there any avoidable precipitating factors?

In addition to an understandable concern about overlooking a significant EEG phenomenon, three factors can lead to overinterpretation of EEGs, particularly pediatric EEGs.

The first are sharply contoured artefacts such as muscle, sudden movement, electrode malfunction, and bottle-sucking. Before assigning any label to a waveform, think artefact first.

Secondly, nonartefactual apiculate (sharply contoured) waveforms usually appear in normal background activity of childhood, especially while awake or drowsy. These potentials are either apiculate in themselves or combine with other, smoother waveforms to create an apiculate morphology. As rich mixtures of waveforms appear in the posterior head, central and temporal regions; nonspike apiculate waveforms occur particularly often at these sites.

The following criteria help to identify real spikes in this apparent minefield: (1) the discharge should be paroxysmal, that is, clearly distinguished from background activity; (2) an abrupt change in polarity should occur in the waveform to produce a sharp contour; (3) the duration of the phenomenon should not exceed 200 ms; (4) the spike should have an electrical field that would conform to physiological principles; and (5) spikes usually exhibit two or more phases. Sleep recordings resolve some of these dilemmas as some sharply contoured potentials recede.

Thirdly, several spike-containing or otherwise apiculate normal phenomena appear frequently in the EEG of an awake child: six per second spike-waves, rhythmic midtemporal discharges ("psychomotor variant"), apiculate alpha or mu rhythm, "posterior slow of youth," and lambda waves. Those of non-REM sleep include: vertex sharp waves ("V-waves"), 14/6 per second positive spikes, and positive occipital sharp transients (POSTS).[2,3] For the more sustained of these normal features, two helpful principles can be applied: (1) *anything maintaining an invariably regular frequency is likely to be normal, and* (2) *apiculate waves that could result from the superimposition of background components should be considered normal.*[2]

Despite the aforementioned cautions, EEG spikes can confirm the presence of epilepsy, indicate whether it is focal or generalized, and help localize focal onsets. The following data will indicate the extent of EEG's value in these domains. Eeg-Olofsson[4] found spikes in 2% of 743 normal children. Cavazzuti et al[5] and Okubo et al[6] identified spikes in 3.5% and 4.5% of normal children, but most were spikes of the benign partial epilepsies of childhood (see further). In contrast, about 30% of children will demonstrate spikes after a first seizure,[7] and such discharges appear on 50%–75% of initial EEGs of children with epilepsy.[8,9] The latter study[9] found that spike sensitivity rose to 92% with three recordings. Several factors may increase the yield: younger age, sleep recording, generalized epilepsy, and recording the EEG after a seizure cluster.[8,10] However, focal spikes originating on inferior or mesial surfaces of the cerebral cortex may not appear on scalp recordings; thus no spikes does not equate with no epilepsy.

FOCAL SPIKES

Localization principles derived from adult studies apply equally to older children and adolescents.[11] However, focal epileptogenic lesions in children approximately 6-year old or less may be associated with multifocal or diffuse spikes, including hypsarrhythmia (HR).[12,13] The topographical lability of spikes in young children impairs their ability to localize epileptogenesis. However, this correlation improves if several recordings are performed; localization of most consistent spiking correlated with lobe of effective epilepsy surgery in 32 (67%) of 48 children.[14] Reliability in this regard further increases if accompanied by regional nonepileptiform phenomena.

TEMPORAL SPIKES

Anterior temporal spikes of children share features of those occurring in adults. These discharges may therefore involve M1, F7, T3, and A1 electrode positions.[15] Hyperventilation and non-REM sleep may be necessary to entice their appearance. Given the normally greater quantity of theta and delta activity in pediatric EEGs, identifying accompanying nonepileptiform abnormalities may more greatly challenge the EEGer but the effort should be undertaken. Compared to adults, EEGs of children with temporal lobe epilepsy (TLE) more commonly display multifocal spikes.[16] However, in our experience,[17] such multifocality almost always resides in the hemisphere ipsilateral to temporal seizure origin. Given a limbic seizure semiology and any MRI evidence of principally unilateral mesial temporal sclerosis (MTS), maximally ipsilateral spike activity may suffice to confidently identify the epileptogenic lobe in children.[17]

OCCIPITAL SPIKES

Eeg-Olofsson[4] found occipital spikes in only 2% of the 743 normal children in his study. Spikes appear more commonly in the occipital area than anywhere else among children less than 4 years of age and this is the age group in which they most commonly appear.[18] Of 31 children with occipital spikes in a Newfoundland population study, epilepsy was present in 29 (94%). Of these, 23 (74%) had benign, nonlesional epilepsy; lesion-based seizures occurred in 5 (16%). Others had less-defined conditions.[19]

Epileptogenic lesions may attenuate, distort, or slow the frequency of the abundant normal EEG features of the occipital lobe, such as alpha activity, "posterior slow of youth," and photic driving. Such features provide more confirmation of spike localization for epileptogenesis than is found for any other lobe. However, studies of occipital spike localization of occipital seizure origin have reached conflicting conclusions. Williamson et al[20] found interictal occipital epileptiform potentials of little localizing value; however, our studies[21,22] found the majority of spikes ipsilateral to epileptogenesis in 79%–94% of patients. Rarely, occipital spikes may appear contralaterally if their dipole is orientated in such a way that a contralateral electrode will best record it—a property seen principally in discharges from mesial structures.

Occipital spikes appear almost always with the eyes closed and immediately attenuate with eye opening while the opposite occurs with lambda, the other sharply contoured occipital paroxysm of wakefulness. While presenting as isolated or clusters of single spikes during wakefulness, polyspikes (multiple spikes) may occur from the same region in sleep.

A host of conditions may be associated with occipital spikes. They may appear in EEGs of young children blind from ocular abnormalities.[23] Several syndromes encompass migraine and occipital and other seizure disorders.[24] Occipital spikes, epilepsy, and calcifications in the occipital area can be associated with celiac disease.[25] A progressive myoclonus epilepsy, such as Lafora body disease, may produce occipital spikes and light-sensitive seizures.[26]

Associated EEG features largely influence the clinical significance of occipital spikes. An otherwise normal EEG suggests a benign partial epilepsy of childhood; the spike morphology resembles that of "Benign Rolandic Epilepsy" (see further). As indicated above, attenuated, or distorted alpha activity and focal excess delta may reflect a lesion-based epilepsy. Migraine-associated disorders may be associated with either a normal EEG or with focal abnormalities. Prominent epileptiform responses to photic stimulation raise the possibility of a progressive myoclonic epilepsy. The constellation of no alpha bilaterally and occipital spikes occurs in children with ocular abnormalities causing blindness from birth or infancy.

CENTRAL SPIKES

Several apiculate (sharply contoured) phenomena are recorded by central (C3,4) and adjacent electrodes during wakefulness and sleep. The apiculate nature of mu rhythm may challenge the EEG reader, particularly if a breach rhythm is present. V-waves, spindles, and beta, individually or superimposed, will create a normal apiculate appearance.

"Rolandic" spikes are stereotyped, distinct, abundant, high-voltage discharges whose location varies: central-parietal, occipital, frontal, and vertex in that approximate order. Thus, the label "Rolandic" refers as much to spike morphology as it does to location. A characteristic tangential dipole may be best displayed on an ear referential montage: electrode negativity of the major phase at C3–P3 with positivity at F3. This produces the prominent downward deflection of the F3–C3 derivation on bipolar recordings. Non-REM sleep augments their incidence. Such discharges occur most commonly at age 4–11 years and disappear between 15 and 18 years of age. The incidence of seizures in subjects with "Rolandic" spikes varies from 54% to 84%.[23,27,28] Thus, they may appear as incidental findings. However, their principal correlate is "Benign Rolandic Epilepsy" characterized by nocturnal generalized seizures and diurnal attacks usually implicating the lower Rolandic region.[29] "Rolandic" spikes are so prevalent in this disorder (a paradox, given the rarity of its seizures), that their lack on two awake and sleep recordings renders the diagnosis of "Benign Rolandic Epilepsy" untenable.

Lesion-based motor seizures are associated with a distinctly different EEG picture. Background awake and sleep rhythms, for example, mu and spindles, may be attenuated and often replaced by persistent delta or theta activity. Spikes lack the scalp-recorded dipole described above. However, some epileptogenic Rolandic lesions give little EEG evidence of their presence.

MULTIPLE INDEPENDENT SPIKE FOCI

This pattern, more common in children, can be defined as spike discharges that arise from three or more noncontiguous electrode positions with at least one focus in each hemisphere.[30] None of the 743 normal children in Eeg-Olofsson's study[4] had multiple independent spike foci (MISF). Seizures occur on over 90% of children with MISF of which 89% are generalized tonic–clonic.[30,31] Half the patients of these studies had more than one type of seizure.

PERIODIC PHENOMENA

Gross et al[32] measured interparoxysmal intervals of "periodic" lateralized epileptiform discharges (PLEDs)

and found their variability not to satisfy mathematical periodicity. "Repetitive" more accurately describes such complexes. Their presence indicates a physiologically acute process such as a recent seizure or viral encephalitis. Subacute lesions, such as regionally accentuated (Rasmussen's) encephalitis or subacute sclerosing encephalitis (SSPE), will also produce repetitive complexes if they are progressive.[33,34]

FOCAL SEIZURES

A focal seizure is represented by repetitive EEG activity from one region that is dissimilar to background rhythms and whose characteristics (sequential spikes, rhythmic waves, or both) evolve as progressive changes of morphology and/or frequency.[35] These criteria distinguish seizures from changes in state, that is, drowsiness or arousal, whose manifestations are more prominent and complex in children than in adults.[3,36]

► GENERALIZED EPILEPTIFORM PHENOMENA

When applied to epileptiform potentials, "generalized" applies to those occurring bisynchronously and involving a substantial portion of each hemisphere.[37] This corresponds to "generalized" seizures that can be described as those beginning without a specific warning, whose motor manifestations are bilateral, and which end without focal postictal manifestations.

Prognosis for intellectual development and for seizure control correlates well with background features and with characteristics of the epileptiform potentials (Table 3–1). A discontinuous background and one with excessive quantity of delta activity in wakefulness each augur poorly for seizure control and intellectual development. A slower spike-wave repetition rate and the presence of fast rhythmic waves each reflect enhanced corticothalamic excitation, medical intractability, and ultimately limited cognitive ability.[38] Except for the epilepsies of progressive conditions, these unfavorable EEG aspects usually occur among patients with an early age of seizure onset. Therefore, the generalized EEG phenomena will be presented in this chapter in order of usual age at first appearance.

BURST SUPPRESSION

A burst-suppression EEG pattern persists during both wakefulness and sleep. The high-voltage (150–350 μV) bursts consist of 1–3 Hz waves with intermixed multifocal spikes.[39] These are separated by 2–10 seconds of diffuse attenuation. The epileptic spasms are associated

▶ **TABLE 3–1.** GENERALIZED EPILEPSY SYNDROMES AND EEG

Syndrome	Onset	Principal Type(s)	EEG Background	EEG Epileptiform
Ohtahara	0–3 mo	Spasms	Discontinuous as burst-suppression	Bursts of: (1) multifocal spikes, (2) delta
Epileptic spasms	3 mo to 5 yr	Spasms	Excess delta	Multifocal spikes (with variants)
Severe myoclonic epilepsy of infancy (SMEI, Dravet)	2–12 mo	Bilateral myoclonus	Excess delta, theta	(1) bisynchronous polyspike-waves (PSWs) (2) photoparoxysmal response (PR)
Benign myoclonic epilepsy of childhood	4 mo to 3 yr	Myoclonus	Normal	SW, PSW, PR
Progressive myoclonus epilepsies (PME)	2 yr to adult	Myoclonus	Excess theta, delta or Normal	Spike-waves or PSW, PR to low flash rates
Lennox–Gastaut	2–5 yr	Tonic	Excess delta, theta	Slow spike-waves (SSWs), fast rhythmic waves = "epileptic recruiting rhythm" (FRW, ERR)
Secondary bisynchrony	Any age	Asymmetrical tonic; generalized tonic–clonic (GTC)	Focal delta, theta	Focal spikes leading to bisynchronous SW
Absence	3–12 yr	Absence; GTC	Normal or delta bursts	2.5–4 Hz SW; PR
Juvenile-myoclonic epilepsy and GTC on awakening	11–15 yr	Bisynchronous myoclonic; GTC	Normal	4.5 Hz SW; PR
Febrile seizures	3 mo to 5 yr	GTC	Normal or posterior delta postictally	None or rare SW with drowsiness

with diffuse desynchronization upon which low-voltage, high-frequency activity is occasionally superimposed. Although the spasms may be accompanied by bursts, only attenuation occurs during a series of spasms.

The OS proceeds to West syndrome, and thence to the Lennox–Gastaut syndrome. OS mortality is high. Survivors become mentally and physically handicapped.[40]

HYPSARRHYTHMIA (HR)

Described by Gibbs and Gibbs,[41] HR consists of a chaotic mixture of high-voltage 1–3 Hz waves with intermingled multifocal spikes, as though the bursts of OS became continuous. In fact, this virtually continuous pattern in wakefulness and light sleep may become discontinuous in deep non-REM sleep, thus resembling the OS burst-suppression.

Several HR variants have been encountered.[42] In "HR with episodic voltage attenuation" episodes of generalized or regional voltage attenuation occurs, thus resembling OS. "Asymmetrical HR" refers to a consistent amplitude asymmetry between the hemispheres, usually associated with asymmetrical structural abnormalities

of the brain. HR may be maximally expressed over the more abnormal or the more normal hemisphere. In the latter instance, activity over the more abnormal hemisphere will be attenuated.

"HR with a consistent focus of epileptiform activity" consists of an active focus of interictal spikes or of seizures along with the HR pattern. Persistence of this focus over several recordings would raise the possibility of surgical resection to improve the seizure disorder. A rare variant is "HR with sparse epileptiform activity," thus high-voltage 1–3 Hz waves with occasional multifocal spikes. Finally, "HR with increased interhemispheric synchronization" constitutes a transition to the Lennox–Gastaut syndrome.

HR is the most characteristic interictal pattern in patients with epileptic spasms, appearing in two-thirds of initial EEGs performed in such infants in one study,[43] but the proportion of infants with epileptic spasms whose EEGs contain HR varies from 7% to 75% in several studies.[44] Conversely, about two-thirds of patients with HR have epileptic spasms.[45] During spasms HR is replaced by diffuse attenuation, occasionally with superimposed low-voltage, high-frequency waves. If the etiology of HR and spasms is unclear, intravenous infusion of 50–100 mg of pyridoxine may be indicated; obliteration of HR would indicate a pyridoxine dependency or deficiency. HR is virtually confined to ages 3 months to 5 years, in parallel with the usual course of epileptic spasms. As HR resolves, the amplitude of its components declines and the spikes become less multifocal and more bilaterally synchronous as the transition to the slow spike-waves (SSWs) of the Lennox–Gastaut syndrome begins.[42]

POLYSPIKE-WAVES (PSWS) AND MYOCLONIC EPILEPSIES

Three 4 Hz bisynchronous polyspike-waves (PSWs) are the EEG correlates of the variety of myoclonic epilepsies. These complexes consist of two or more surface-negative spikes, an electropositive trough, then a 250–400 ms negative wave (additional aspects further). As with any "generalized" EEG phenomenon, hemispheric or even regional accentuation commonly occurs. See Section "Slow Spike-Waves (SSWs) and the Lennox–Gastaut Syndrome (LGS)" for additional data on spike-waves (further).

Reflecting a tendency for seizure precipitation by abrupt changes in ambient light intensity, EEG photosensitivity may be demonstrated although this may be inconsistent, even in the same patient on separate recordings. Pronounced photosensitivity at low flash rates raises the possibility of progressive myoclonus epilepsy (see further). Sleep enhances the incidence of PSW.

Except in the more severe forms, such as Dravet syndrome, background activity remains normal, including normal sleep potentials.[46,47] Initially in Dravet syndrome background activity is normal, then slows somewhat, likely reflecting arrest in CNS maturation, frequent seizures, and medication effect.

Abundance of the aforementioned EEG abnormalities approximates the position of a child on the broad continuum of the idiopathic myoclonic epilepsies, from severe to relatively benign.[46]

PROGRESSIVE MYOCLONUS EPILEPSIES

The several degenerative diseases in this category commonly share clinical characteristics of a worsening generalized seizure disorder, cognitive decline, ataxia, and—in some—deteriorating vision. Several EEG characteristics are also shared: (a) slowing and subsequent loss of normal background awake and sleep rhythms; (b) abundant generalized and multifocal spikes, spikewaves, and PSW; and (c) facile precipitation of epileptiform potentials by low-frequency photic stimulation.[48,49]

Therefore, follow-up EEGs should be performed in any patient with medically intractatable generalized seizures, seeking one or more of these features.

SLOW SPIKE-WAVES (SSWS) AND THE LENNOX–GASTAUT SYNDROME (LGS)

The LGS has been defined as a medically intractable seizure disorder, usually beginning in childhood, with multiple types of generalized seizures, principally tonic. Included in the definition are two EEG criteria: (1) interictal bilaterally synchronous slow (1–2.5 Hz repetition rate) spike-waves, and (2) runs of bilateral highfrequency activity, known as "paroxysmal fast rhythmic waves" or "epileptic recruiting rhythm."[50,51] This second criterion aids in making the clinically important distinction of LGS from secondary bilateral synchrony (SBS; see further). Each of these clinical and electrographic components reflects excessive corticothalamic excitation.[38]

Slow spike-waves (SSWs) occupy a greater proportion of the interictal awake EEG than the more common 3 Hz spike-waves. Although occasionally associated with absence-like attacks, they usually are unaccompanied by any discernible clinical change in these cognitively impaired children. The fast rhythmic waves have tonic seizures or absence as the clinical correlate.[15,38] SSWs appear most commonly and abundantly at age 1–5 years, but their presence extends into adulthood in some patients. SSW may occur in the first year of life, intermixed with hypsarrhythmia. In contrast to 3 Hz spike-waves (see further), background activity while awake is diffusely slow. In sleep, PSWs and fast rhythmic waves appear, possibly for the first time in the recording.[15,52]

Clinically apparent seizures occur in 98% of patients with SSWs.[53,54] Age of seizure onset varies from 12 to 48 months.[55] Tonic seizures begin earliest followed by atypical absence, myoclonic, atonic, and tonic–clonic attacks. Cognitive development is delayed, and may plateau or decline.[53,56]

SECONDARY BILATERAL SYNCHRONY (SBS)

Tukel and Jasper[57] defined this EEG complex as "bilaterally synchronous discharges which can be shown to arise from a single cortical focus." Blume and Pillay[58] adopted this approach by stipulating (a) a focal lead-in time of at least 2 seconds, and (b) the morphology of triggering spikes should resemble other focal spikes in the EEG and differ from that of the bisynchronous paroxysms in the second phase of the complex. The morphology distinction excludes bisynchrony emanating from hemispheric spike-waves as seen in hemispheric epilepsy.[59] Bisynchronous spike-waves of SBS may resemble those of SSW as the repetition rate is often less than 3 Hz, but the latter have no focal, morphologically distinct lead-in. As implied above, SBS is not associated with "fast rhythmic waves."

Patients with SBS have focal and asymmetrical secondarily generalized seizures that may begin at any age.[60] They occur less frequently than those of LGS. Atonic, symmetrical tonic, and atypical absence are very rare with SBS. On follow-up cognitive ability varies considerably among patients, and may be normal.

GENERALIZED SPIKE-WAVES (GWS)

Morphologically and clinically, these bilaterally synchronous complexes share many features with PSWs. Each SW or PSW complex consists of bisynchronous surface negative single or multiple spikes, then a deep positive "trough," then a negative 250–400 ms wave.[15] Sequential bilateral SWs or PSWs lasting 5 seconds or more are associated with a clinically evident absence seizure.[61] The first complex of a series may contain two or three spikes whereas subsequent ones could have single spikes. Repetition rate is fastest at onset of sequential SWs and subsequently slows; repetition rates as slow as 2 Hz may occur during absence status epilepticus giving the false impression of slow spike-waves (SSWs). Reflecting their physiology,[62] SWs and PSWs are principally expressed over association cortices, thus the superior frontal (F3,4) or parietal (P3,4) regions. As with all bisynchronous epileptiform phenomena, side-to-side shifts of maximum voltage may appear. Fragments of spike-waves, localized to one region, occur commonly, but their morphology will remain as spike-waves rather than as focal spikes.[15] Hyperventilation may elicit SWs or augment their incidence if already present. Eye closure may also precipitate SWs, especially in "light sensitive" patients. Photic stimulation may elicit a "photoparoxysmal response," that is, bisynchronous spikes, SWs, or PSWs, principally at 14–18 per second flash rate with eye closure or eyes closed.[15] SWs may appear more abundantly or only during non-REM sleep.

Four series of patients with SWs found generalized seizure disorders in 97%–98%[52,63–65] whereas Eeg-Olofsson[4] found no SW or PSW in the resting records of 743 normal children. About 60% of patients with SWs have absence attacks.[15] The proportion with generalized tonic–clonic seizures varies with age at recording, increasing as adolescence approaches. As the quantity of spike-waves on a routine outpatient EEG closely parallels absence frequency, EEGs monitor effectiveness of treatment.[66] However, incidence of generalized tonic–clonic seizures did not correlate with spike-wave quantity in that study.

Among patients with juvenile myoclonic epilepsy (JME), the EEG may contain 4- to 5-Hz SWs, or a single interictal EEG may be normal. A photoparoxysmal response may occur.[67] The entity "generalised tonic clonic seizures on awakening," very closely allied with JME, has identical EEG correlations.

LANDAU–KLEFFNER SYNDROME AND ELECTROGRAPHIC STATUS EPILEPTICUS OF SLEEP

Generalized or regional SWs, principally expressed over the parietal-temporal regions, occur in the Landau–Kleffner syndrome (LKS). Similar spike-waves, regional, general or both, may occupy substantial portions of sleep recordings in electrographic status epilepticus of sleep (ESES), a disorder whose manifestations overlap with LKS.[67]

► EEG IN CONDITIONS POTENTIALLY ASSOCIATED WITH EPILEPSY

FEBRILE SEIZURES

EEGs performed within the first week after a febrile seizure (FS) may contain excess delta activity diffusely, frequently maximally expressed over the posterior cortical regions, occasionally accentuated on one side.[68] Frantzen et al[68] found that delta quantity was greater if the FS exceeded 30 minutes, if the child was ill for more than 36 hours prior to the FS and if the gastrointestinal system was upset.

In most patients, the EEG beyond the acute phase is normal. However, sporadic spike-waves may occur in light sleep or with photic stimulation at 9–15 Hz flash rate.[68,69] However, such spike-wave activity does not portend epilepsy.[68,70,71]

Therefore, no EEG is needed in children with simple FS.[70,71] In practice, concern that FS represented an occult or overlooked ongoing neurological condition including epilepsy should arise if: (1) a prominent unilateral abnormality, such as excess delta activity, appeared in the acute phase or later, suggesting a focal lesion; (2) SWs or PSWs appeared abundantly suggesting a primary generalized epilepsy; or (3) low flash rate (1–3 Hz) photic stimulation evoked bisynchronous spikes or spike-waves, suggesting a progressive myoclonic epilepsy.[48]

FIRST AFEBRILE SEIZURE

Committees of The American Academy of Neurology and the Child Neurology Society[72] have indicated that EEG is useful in this circumstance as: (a) it helps to identify the epilepsy syndrome, (b) predicts risk of recurrence, (c) aids in determining the long term prognosis, (d) indicates the need for neuroimaging, and (e) aids in the differentiation of seizures from nonepileptic events. Shinnar et al[73] found an abnormal EEG to be among the few factors that, on multivariable analysis, predicted both early (<2 years) and late seizure recurrences.

CENTRAL NERVOUS SYSTEM INFECTIONS

Meningitis

Only mild excess, diffuse delta and theta are associated with meningitis if encephalitis is not also present. In fact, some of these diffuse abnormalities may simply reflect electrolytic derangements of an acutely ill child. In this clinical setting, any persistent focal delta activity raises the possibility of a complicating abscess or cortical vein thrombosis.[74]

Encephalitis

Predictably, considerable diffuse excess delta and theta accompany encephalitis. Magnitude of such abnormalities varies with severity of the infection, level of consciousness, degree of systemic abnormalities (electrolytes, hypoxia), and inversely with age. EEG may detect clinically subtle epileptic seizures consequent to the infection. Prolonged monitoring can assess therapeutic effectiveness if status epilepticus has occurred. EEG abnormalities described above are not specific as to etiology but "periodic" phenomena characterize the following two entities.

Herpes Simplex Encephalitis (HSE)

"Periodic" broad spikes repeating every 0.5 to 4 seconds (a form of PLEDs—see further) and delta activity appear in temporal-frontal regions or diffusely during the first 2 weeks of HSE[75] in most patients. ("Periodic" is kept in quotation marks as Gross et al[32] found interparoxysmal intervals of PLEDs to vary sufficiently that the metronomic rate of strict "periodicity" does not obtain in clinical practice). The diagnostic value for HSE of such acute temporal abnormalities is diminished by the very high specificity and sensitivity of polymerase chain reaction (PCR) for HSE in cerebrospinal fluid.[76] Each test—EEG, PCR—has limitations: (1) PCR results may not be immediately available and may be falsely negative in early CSF specimens, and (2) other acute conditions can produce PLEDs.

Subacute Sclerosing Panencephalitis (SSPE)

Effective measles immunization programs have decreased the incidence of this slowly progressive disorder. Although nonspecific EEG slowing accompanies an initial phase characterized by behavioral aberrations and deteriorating academic performances; a second phase is characterized by repetitive (every 4–15 seconds) EEG complexes of broad spikes and multiphasic delta waves appearing regionally or diffusely, associated with brief myotonic events of the trunk and proximal limbs. The repetitive nature of these complexes may require slow sweep speeds for their appreciation if the intervals are prolonged—as may occur initially. Progressive EEG attenuation accompanies the final clinical phase.[77]

Acquired Immunodeficiency Syndrome (AIDs)

Nonspecific slowing of EEG background activity occurs. Any focal abnormalities suggest a superimposed infection such as toxoplasmosis or a neoplasm such as a lymphoma.[77]

Brain Abscess

Although best detected and delineated by imaging, focal acute-appearing delta and background attenuation may represent a supratentorial abscess.[74]

TRAUMA

Trauma may cause many acute-appearing focal, multifocal, and diffuse EEG abnormalities whose severity parallels that of the injury, but whose prominence and persistence usually exceeds that occurring in adults.

Attenuation of "background" rhythms, marked arrhythmic delta activity, bursts of rhythmic delta, and "periodic" phenomena all may reflect a recent severe injury. Curiously, delta appears principally in the occipital region, even without other modality evidence of such accentuation. Over days or weeks, acute EEG signs gradually abate: alpha, theta, and mu may emerge, delta increases in frequency, rhythmicity and reactivity, and other acute phenomena, for example, rhythmic delta bursts and "periodic" patterns recede.[74,78,79]

Milder trauma may produce less prominent, higher frequency and more reactive delta, focal theta, and mild focal attenuation.[78] Spikes occur more commonly among children than adults[78] but apparently do not reliably herald posttrauma epilepsy.[79]

The unexpected appearance of the aforementioned features without an overt trauma history should raise suspicion of child abuse.[79]

Anoxia from attendant chest injury and electrolyte-acid/base derangements will prominently augment the severity of diffuse EEG abnormalities. Carotid artery trauma may cause dissection-related stroke; striking acute-appearing EEG abnormalities confined to one territory of vascular supply would suggest this. Fat embolism from fractured long bones may also evoke EEG abnormalities without direct head injury.

Importantly, the foregoing data indicate that even prominent EEG changes do not necessarily portend irreversible brain injury.

Turbulent conditions surrounding acute trauma and its care challenge even an experienced technologist; the following common artefacts should be considered when interpreting *any* waveform: muscle and movement in a delirious child, electrode artefact from sometimes unavoidable high-impedance scalp edema, pulse artefact, and electrical contamination from life support systems.

Even in an image-dominated era, sequential EEGs remain an essential component of the neurological evaluation of the traumatized child. Focal or generalized status-epilepticus complicates acute traumatic encephalopathy more commonly in children than adults.[80] Seizure activity can be subtle or clinically inapparent, particularly if neuromuscular blockade has been employed.[81] Secondly, with coma-producing brain stem injury, EEG best assesses cortical function.[82] Thirdly, any lack of congruence between location of EEG abnormalities and those disclosed by neuroimaging underscores the complexity of trauma rather than questioning EEG validity.[83] Additionally, EEG is useful in gauging depth of anesthesia produced by neuroprotective agents and antiepileptic drugs for status epilepticus administered in severe trauma.[84]

COMA

As the clinical neurological assessment of a comatose child is limited to the brain stem and the spinal cord, sequential EEGs provide essential therapeutic and prognostic information about cortical and thalamic function.[74,84]

Of EEG phenomena accompanying the severe degrees of coma, prominent diffuse delta and theta activity are the most common. Invariant persistence of such activity and lack of its modification by afferent stimuli indicate deep coma but not necessarily an irreversible state. Triphasic waves, rare in children, suggest a significant metabolic component. Periodic lateralizing epileptiform discharges indicate a superimposed acute regional process such as contusion, abscess or ischemia. Spindles, morphologically identical to those accompanying non-REM sleep, may appear in coma, thus "spindle" coma.[84] Often more abundant than those of sleep, they share the property of usual bilateral synchrony but may shift from one side to the other. Persistent spindle asymmetry usually reflects a greater dysfunction on the less abundant side.[85] As spindles result from integral function of both the thalamus and the nonspecific cortex, their presence reflects preservation of the widespread nonspecific activating system and thus augurs a favorable prognosis.[84,86]

A diffuse beta-/theta-dominated EEG likely indicates intoxication by benzodiazepines or barbiturates.

Inadequately treated nonconvulsive or minimally convulsive status epilepticus is best detected and monitored by continuous or frequent EEG. A variety of focal or bisynchronous ictal patterns may represent recurrent seizures.[84] Neglect of such seizure activity can prolong and deepen coma, thus worsening its prognosis.

Alpha/theta pattern coma consists of diffuse, persistent rhythmic, 4–12 Hz waves in various mixtures that typically do not react to external stimuli. Although the most common cause is anoxic-ischemic encephalopathy, other etiologies are possible, even intoxications.[87]

The burst-suppression pattern indicates deep coma. Bursts or brief runs of intermixed delta, theta, and spikes are separated by equal or longer periods of minimal or no EEG activity. "Suppression" thus refers to moderate loss or complete absence of spontaneous or evoked rhythms. This invariant and nonreactant pattern may appear diffusely, regionally or in one hemisphere. Again, etiologies vary from anoxia to intoxication.

Spontaneous variability and a rich mixture of waveforms suggest a relatively light coma. Moderate coma is characterized by less variability, but stimulation of the patient will attenuate or otherwise modify the unstimulated pattern. An invariant, nonreactive EEG represents deep coma.[82,84,88] In some instances, the left and right hemispheres may differ in patterns expressed, spontaneous variability, and modification by stimulation. Separate clinical interpretations and prognoses for each hemisphere may be required.

The prognosis of any of these patterns depends heavily on etiology, and the direction in which sequential EEGs are evolving. For a given EEG pattern, toxic and metabolic states usually have a better outcome than structural or anoxic encephalopathies. Within this framework, prognostically favorable aspects are: spontaneous variability, reaction to exogenous stimuli, and normal sleep potentials. An invariant, nonreactive EEG with low voltage, monorhythmic, or burst-suppression patterns augurs a grim outcome.

Studying EEGs of children 0–12 hours[89] and 12–24 hours[90] after cardiac arrest disclosed the following features and their prognoses: (1) when any normal activity is present, the outcome is favorable; (2) persistent high-voltage delta activity requires follow-up recordings in 2–3 days to determine whether prognostically favorable or unfavorable patterns will emerge; (3) very low voltage EEGs convey a poor outlook; and (4) patients whose EEGs show electrocerebral inactivity for 2–3 hours or burst-suppression succumb. These principles assume that reversible factors, such as metabolic abnormalities or sedative medication, are not present.

REFERENCES

1. Kotagal P, et al. Lateralizing value of asymmetric tonic limb posturing in secondarily generalized tonic–clonic seizures. *Epilepsia* 2000;41(4):457–462.

2. Engel J Jr. A practical guide for routine EEG studies in epilepsy. *J Clin Neurophysiol* 1984;1:109–142.

3. Blume WT, Kaibara M. Normal electroencephalogram. In: Blume WT, Kaibara M (eds), *Atlas of Pediatric Electroencephalography.* Philadelphia: Lippincott Raven, 1999; pp. 1–151.

4. Eeg-Olofsson O, Petersen I, Sellden U. The development of the electroencephalogram in normal children from the age of 1 through 15 years. *Neuropadiatrie* 1971;2(4):375–404.

5. Cavazzuti V, Winston K, Baker R, Welch K. Psychological changes following surgery for tumours of the temporal lobe. *J Neurosurg* 1980;53:618–626.

6. Okubo Y, et al. Epileptiform EEG discharges in healthy children: prevalence, emotional and behavioral correlates, and genetic influences. *Epilepsia* 1994;35:832–841.

7. Shinnar S, et al. EEG abnormalities in children with a first unprovoked seizure. *Epilepsia* 1994;35:471–476.

8. Carpay JA, et al. The diagnostic yield of a second EEG after partial sleep deprivation: a prospective study in children with newly diagnosed seizures. *Epilepsia* 1997;38:595–599.

9. Yoshinaga H, et al. Incidence of epileptic discharge in various epileptic syndromes. *Pediatr Neurol* 2001;25:38–42.

10. Fisch BJ. Interictal epileptiform activity: diagnostic and behavioral implications: 2002 ACNS Presidential Address. *J Clin Neurophysiol* 2003;20:155–162.

11. Blume WT. Interictal electroencephalography in neocortical epilepsy. In: Luders HO, Comair YG (eds), *Epilepsy Surgery.* Philadelphia: Lippincott Williams & Wilkins, 2001; 2nd edn: pp. 403–412.

12. Quesney LF, Risinger MW, Shewmon DA. Extracranial EEG evaluation. In: Engel J Jr (ed), *Surgical Treatment of the Epilepsies.* New York: Raven Press, 1993; pp. 173–195.

13. Blume WT, Girvin JP, Kaufmann JCE. Childhood brain tumors presenting as chronic uncontrolled seizure disorders. *Ann Neurol* 1982;12:538–541.

14. Blume WT, Kaibara M. Localization of epileptic foci in children. *Can J Neurol Sci* 1991;18:570–572.

15. Blume WT, Kaibara M. Abnormal electroencephalogram: epileptiform potentials. In: Blume WT, Kaibara M (eds), *Atlas of Pediatric Electroencephalography.* Philadelphia: Lippincott Raven, 1999; 2nd edn: pp. 153–297.

16. Franzon RC, et al. Interictal EEG in temporal lobe epilepsy in childhood. *J Clin Neurophysiol* 2007;24:11–15.

17. Blume WT, Girvin JP, McLachlan RS, Gilmore BE. Effective temporal lobectomy in childhood without invasive EEG. *Epilepsia* 1997;38:164–167.

18. Trojaborg W. Changes of spike foci in children. In: Kellaway P, Petersen I (eds), *Clinical Electroencephalography of Children.* New York: Grune & Stratton, 1968; pp. 213–225.

19. Maher J, Ronen GM, Ogunyemi AO, Goulden KJ. Occipital paroxysmal discharges suppressed by eye opening: variability of clinical and seizure manifestations in childhood. *Epilepsia* 1995;36:52–57.

20. Williamson PD, et al. Occipital lobe epilepsy: clinical characteristics, seizure spread patterns and results of surgery. *Ann Neurol* 1992;31:3–13.

21. Blume WT, Whiting SE, Girvin JP. Epilepsy surgery in the posterior cortex. *Ann Neurol* 1991;29:638–645.

22. Blume WT, Wiebe S, Tapsell LM. Occipital epilepsy: lateral versus mesial. *Brain* 2005;128:1209–1225.

23. Smith JMB, Kellaway P. The natural history and clinical correlates of occipital foci in children. In: Kellaway P, Petersen I (eds), *Neurological and Electroencephalographic Correlative Studies in Infancy.* New York: Grune & Stratton, 1964; pp. 230–249.

24. Andermann F. Clinical features of migraine-epilepsy syndromes. In: Andermann F, Lugaresi E (eds), *Migraine and Epilepsy.* Boston: Butterworth-Heinemann, 1987; pp. 3–30.

25. Gobbi G, et al. The malignant variant of partial epilepsy with occipital spikes in childhood. *Epilepsia* 1991;32(Suppl 1): 16–17.

26. Tassinari CA, et al. La maladie de Lafora. *Rev EEG Neurophysiol* 1978;8:107–122.

27. Beaussart M. Benign epilepsy of children with rolandic (centro-temporal) paroxysmal foci: a clinical entity. Study of 221 cases. *Epilepsia* 1972;13:795–811.

28. Blom S, Brorson LO. Central spikes or sharp waves (Rolandic spikes) in children's EEG and their clinical significance. *Acta Pediatr Scand* 1966;55:385–393.

29. Blom S, Heijbel J, Bergfors PG. Benign epilepsy of children with centro-temporal EEG foci. Prevalence and follow-up study of 40 patients. *Epilepsia* 1972;13:609–619.

30. Blume WT. Clinical and electroencephalographic correlates of the multiple independent spike foci pattern in children. *Ann Neurol* 1978;4:541–547.

31. Noriega-Sanchez A, Markand ON. Clinical and electroencephalographic correlates of independent multifocal spike discharges. *Neurology* 1976;26:667–672.

32. Gross DW, Wiebe S, Blume WT. The periodicity of lateralized epileptiform discharges. *Clin Neurophysiol* 1999;110: 1516–1520.

33. PeBenito R, Cracco JB. Periodic lateralized epileptiform discharges in infants and children. *Ann Neurol* 1979; 6:47–50.

34. Sternberg B, Lerique-Koechlin A, Mises J, Plouin P. Morphological study of so-called periodic abnomalies in children. *Rev Electroencephalogr Neurophysiol Clin* 1971;1:87–88.

35. Blume WT, Young GB, Lemieux JF. EEG morphology of partial epileptic seizures. *Electroencephalogr Clin Neurophysiol* 1984;57:295–302.

36. Kellaway P, Fox BJ. Electroencephalographic diagnosis of cerebral pathology in infants during sleep. *J Pediatr* 1952;41:262–287.

37. Blume WT, et al. Glossary of descriptive terminology for ictal semiology: Report of the ILAE Task Force on classification and terminology. *Epilepsia* 2001;42:1212–1218.

38. Blume WT. Pathogenesis of Lennox-Gastaut syndrome: considerations and hypotheses. *Epileptic Disord* 2001;3: 181–196.

39. Ohtahara S, et al. Early infantile epileptic encephalopathy with suppression-bursts. In: Roger J, et al (eds), *Epileptic Syndromes in Infancy, Childhood and Adolescence.* London: John Libbey, 1992; 2nd edn: pp. 25–34.

40. Ohtahara S, Yamatogi Y. Epileptic encephalopathy in early infancy with suppression–burst. *J Clin Neurophysiol* 2003;20:398–407.

41. Gibbs FA, Gibbs EL. *Atlas of Electroencephalography; Vol. 2: Epilepsy*. Reading: Addison-Wesley, 1952; pp. 214–290.

42. Hrachovy RH, Frost JD Jr, Kellaway P. Hypsarrhythmia: variations on the theme. *Epilepsia* 1984;25:317–325.

43. Jeavons PM, Bower BD. Infantile spasms. In: Vinken PJ, Bruyn GW (eds), *Handbook of Clinical Neurology; Vol. 15: The Epilepsies*. New York: Elsevier, 1974; pp. 219–234.

44. Hrachovy RH, Frost JD Jr. Infantile epileptic encephalopathy with hypsarrhythmia (Infantile spasms/West syndrome). *J Clin Neurophysiol* 2003;20:408–425.

45. Baird HW, Borofsky LG. Infantile myoclonic seizures. *J Pediatr* 1957;50:332–339.

46. Guerrini R, Aicardi J. Epileptic encephalopathies with myoclonic seizures in infants and children (severe myoclonic epilepsy and myoclonic astatic epilepsy). *J Clin Neurophysiol* 2003;20:449–461.

47. Dravet C, et al. Severe myoclonic epilepsy in infants. In: Roger J, et al (eds), *Epileptic Syndromes in Infancy, Childhood and Adolescence*. London: John Libbey, 1992; 2nd edn: pp. 75–88.

48. Pampiglione G, Harden A. Neurophysiological identification of a late infantile form of "neuronal lipidosis." *J Neurol Neurosurg Psychiatry* 1973;36:68–74.

49. Berkovic SF, Andermann F, Carpenter S, Wolfe LS. Progressive myoclonus epilepsies: specific causes and diagnoses. *N Engl J Med* 1986;315:296–305.

50. Aicardi J. Lennox–Gastaut syndrome and myoclonic epilepsies of infancy and early childhood. In: Aicardi J (ed), *Epilepsy in Children*. New York: Raven Press, 1986; pp. 39–65.

51. Genton P, Guerrini R, Dravet C. The Lennox–Gastaut syndrome. In: Meinardi H (ed), *Handbook of Clinical Neurology; Vol. 73 (29): The Epilepsies, Part II*. Amsterdam: Elsevier, 2000; pp. 211–222.

52. Blume WT. *Atlas of Pediatric Electroencephalography*. New York: Raven Press, 1982.

53. Blume WT, David RB, Gomez MR. Generalized sharp and slow wave complexes. Associated clinical features and long-term follow-up. *Brain* 1973;96:289–306.

54. Markand ON. Slow spike-wave activity in EEG and associated clinical features: often called "Lennox" or "Lennox–Gastaut " syndrome. *Neurology* 1977;27:746–757.

55. Chevrie JJ, Aicardi J. Childhood epileptic encephalopathy with slow spike-wave. A statistical study of 80 cases. *Epilepsia* 1972;13:259–271.

56. Oguni H, Hayashi K, Osawa M. Long-term prognosis of Lennox–Gastaut syndrome. *Epilepsia* 1996;37(Suppl 3):44–47.

57. Tukel K, Jasper H. The electroencephalogram in parasagittal lesions. *Electroencephalogr Clin Neurophysiol* 1952;4:481–494.

58. Blume WT, Pillay N. Electrographic and clinical correlates of secondary bilateral synchrony. *Epilepsia* 1985;26:636–641.

59. Blume WT. Hemispheric epilepsy. *Brain* 1998;121:1937–1949.

60. Gastaut H, Zifkin BG. Secondary bilateral synchrony and Lennox–Gastaut syndrome. In: Niedermeyer E, Degen R (eds), *The Lennox–Gastaut Syndrome*. New York: Alan R Liss, 1988; pp. 221–242.

61. Niedermeyer E. Epileptic seizure disorders. In: Niedermeyer E, Lopes da Silva F (eds), *Electroencephalography*. Philadelphia: Lippincott Williams & Wilkins, 2005; pp. 505–620.

62. Blume WT. Clinical and basic neurophysiology of generalised epilepsies. *Can J Neurol Sci* 2002;29:6–18.

63. Dalby MA. Epilepsy and 3 per second spike and wave rhythms. A clinical, electroencephalographic and prognostic analysis of 346 patients. *Acta Neurol Scand (Suppl)* 1969; 45:1–180.

64. Lundervold A, Henriksen GF, Fegersten L. The spike and wave complex: a clinical correlation. *Electroencephalogr Clin Neurophysiol* 1959;11:13–22.

65. Silverman D. Clinical correlates of the spike-wave complex. *Electroencephalogr Clin Neurophysiol* 1954;6:663–669.

66. Miller H, Blume WT. Primary generalized seizure disorder: correlation of epileptiform discharges with seizure frequency. *Epilepsia* 1993;34:128–132.

67. Stafstrom CE. The epilepsies. In: David RB (ed), *Child and Adolescent Neurology*. Malden: Blackwell Publishing Ltd., 2005; 2nd edn: pp. 172–222.

68. Frantzen E, Lennox-Buchtal M, Nygaard A. Longitudinal and clinical study of children with febrile convulsions. *Electroencephalogr Clin Neurophysiol* 1968;24:197–212.

69. Alvarez N, Lombroso CT, Medina C, Cantlon B. Paroxysmal spike and wave activity in drowsiness in young children. Its relationship to febrile convulsions. *Electroencephalogr Clin Neurophysiol* 1983;56:406–413.

70. Hirtz DG, Nelson KB. Febrile seizures. In David RB (ed), *Child and Adolescent Neurology*. Malden: Blackwood Publishing, 2005; 2nd edn: pp. 549–557.

71. Hwang P, Otsubo H, Riviello J Jr, Holmes GL. Age-specific seizure disorders. In: Holmes GL, Moshe SL, Jones HR (eds), *Clinical Neurophysiology of Infancy, Childhood and Adolescence*. Philadelphia: Butterworth Heinemann, 2006; pp. 219–251.

72. Hirtz D, et al. Practice parameter: treatment of the child with a first unprovoked seizure: Report of the Quality Standards Subcommittee of the American Academy of Neurology and the Practice Committee of the Child Neurology Society. *Neurology* 2003;60:166–175.

73. Shinnar S, et al. The risk of seizure recurrence after a first unprovoked afebrile seizure in childhood: an extended follow-up. *Pediatrics* 1996;98:216–225.

74. Blume WT, Kaibara M. *Atlas of Pediatric Electro-encephalography*. Philadelphia: Lippincott Williams & Wilkins, 1999; 2nd edn: pp. 361–367.

75. Upton A, Gumpert J. Electroencephalography in diagnosis of herpes-simplex encephalitis. *Lancet* 1970;1:650–652.

76. Bell WE, Henderson FW. Infections of the central nervous system. In: David RB (ed), *Child and Adolescent Neurology*. Malden: Blackwell Publishing Ltd., 2005; 2nd edn: pp. 247–273.

77. Riviello J Jr, Kovnar EH. Infectious diseases. In: Holmes GL, Moshe SL, Jones HR (eds), *Clinical Neurophysiology of Infancy, Childhood and Adolescence*. Philadelphia: Butterworth Heinemann, 2006; pp. 353–366.

78. Fisch BJ. *EEG Primer*. Amsterdam: Elsevier, 1999; pp. 276–277.

79. Brunquell PJ. Head trauma. In: Holmes GL, Moshe SL, Jones HR (eds), *Clinical Neurophysiology of Infancy, Childhood and Adolescence*. Philadelphia: Butterworth Heinemann, 2006; pp. 367–387.

80. Jennett B. Trauma as a cause of epilepsy in childhood. *Dev Med Child Neurol* 1973;15:56–62.

81. Hutchinson HT, Lebby PC. Traumatic encephalopathies. In: David RB (ed), *Child and Adolescent Neurology*. Malden: Blackwell Publishing Ltd., 2005; 2nd edn: pp. 147–171.

82. Young GB. The EEG in coma. *J Clin Neurophysiol* 2000; 17:473–485.

83. Hauser WA. EEG and head trauma. *Am J EEG Technol* 1979;19:145–151.

84. Young GB. EEG in the intensive care unit. In: Blume WT, Kaibara M, Young GB (eds), *Atlas of Adult Electroencephalography*. Philadelphia: Lippincott Williams & Wilkins, 2002; 2nd edn: pp. 469–499.

85. Blume WT, Kaibara M, Young GB. *Atlas of Adult Electroencephalography*. Philadelphia: Lippincott Williams & Wilkins, 2002; 2nd edn: p. 377.

86. Morison RS, Dempsey EW. A study of thalamocortical relations. *Am J Physiol* 1942;135:281–292.

87. Young GB, et al. Alpha, theta and alpha-theta coma: a clinical outcome study utilizing serial recordings. *Electroencephalogr Clin Neurophysiol* 1994;91:93–99.

88. Fischgold H, Mathis P. Obnubilations, comas, stupeurs: etudes electroencephalographiques. *Electroencephalogr Clin Neurophysiol*. Paris: Masson, 1959; (suppl 11): p. 124.

89. Pampiglione G, Harden A. Resuscitation after cardiocirculatory arrest. *Lancet* 1968;1:1261–1265.

90. Seshia SS, Chow PN, Sankaran K. Coma following cardiorespiratory arrest in childhood. *Dev Med Child Neurol* 1979;21:143–153.

CHAPTER 4

Sources of Error in EEG Interpretation

Prasanna Jayakar

An essential step in EEG interpretation is the identification of features that are statistically deviant compared to normative data, a process that defines abnormalities and establishes their significance in appropriate clinical context. EEG patterns evolve with maturation; neonates reveal distinct features that regress within 4–6 weeks after birth to be replaced by patterns characteristic of infancy and early childhood. The patterns also vary with the child's state at time of recording, the level of alertness during wakefulness, and cycling through stages of sleep. Recognizing the considerable variability of normative EEG features is thus a prerequisite to interpretation.

Once an abnormality is identified, the next goal of interpretation is to define its location and extent. While localization of abnormality is useful in most clinical settings, it gains particular relevance for patients with intractable epilepsy undergoing evaluation for resective surgery. Guidelines for localization were initially described by Adrian and Matthews[1] and have been subsequently addressed in several comprehensive reviews.[2–5] Principles of electric field theory were addressed by Nunez,[6] the physiological substrates of EEG sources became better appreciated after the introduction of intracranial recordings.[7,8] The pitfalls and caveats underlying many of the physical and physiological assumptions used in localization of epileptic sources were reviewed by Jayakar et al.[9]

The growing success of resective surgery over the past few decades increased the need for localizing accuracy. This led to the development of automated computational systems for 3-D source localization of spikes recorded on EEG. More recently, magnetoencephalography (MEG) and a hybrid technique where EEG spikes trigger activation of functional MRI signal have also been utilized. While these new methods are gaining popularity in many epilepsy surgery centers, the set of underlying assumptions are not generally well understood. The main focus of this review article is to discuss the principles of localizing seizure foci; the intent is not to reiterate the standard teachings of localization but rather to emphasize the limitations and pitfalls underlying many of the assumptions used in visual or automated analyses and the potential for misinterpretation.

▶ THE EPILEPTIC GENERATOR

Localization is facilitated by modeling the spike generator, the choice of a model is dictated by the distribution of the excitatory (negative) and inhibitory (positive) postsynaptic potentials within the generator. Since the majority of cortical neurons are arranged in parallel and activate synchronously by virtue of their interconnections, the respective potentials summate to generally produce layer of negativity on the superficial aspect of the cortex, and positivity on its deeper aspect, that is, a dipole layer.

The orientation of a generator greatly affects its field distribution on the scalp.[4] If a generator is located over a superficial gyrus, the dipole is oriented vertically to the scalp, that is, it is a "vertical dipole" and is the commonest orientation observed on the scalp EEG. Electrodes overlying the vertically oriented generator record negative spikes with a bell-shaped negative potential distribution field. The generator is interpreted to be located under the peak, that is, the electrode revealing spikes of maximum negativity. A bell distribution with restricted field implies a superficial generator; broad fields imply that the generator extends over a wider cortical region or is located deep.

Less frequently, the generator may be located in the bank of a sulcus or in the interhemispheric fissure and is oriented tangential to the scalp, that is, it is a "horizontal dipole." Its potential distribution curve is "S" shaped with a peak (negative) and a trough (positive). Unlike the scenario of a vertical dipole, the generator is not located under the peak or trough but lies in between; the wider apart are the peak and trough, and the deeper is its likely location. In children with benign rolandic epilepsy, the larger negative peak is distributed over the central/parietal region and the smaller trough over the frontal region consistent with an epileptic source in the rolandic sulcus.

Scenarios of surgical relevance include patients with interhemispheric foci such as those involving supplementary areas of the cortex. As a result of horizontal dipolar distribution, maximum spike negativity may project contralateral to the side of the focus. When the source is deep, the peak or trough may project at remote electrodes sites. For example, spikes from an

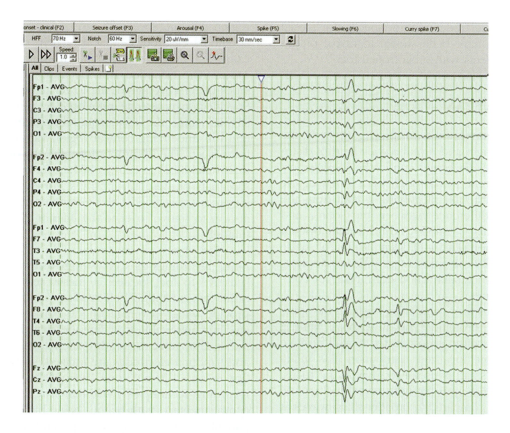

Figure 4–1. Scalp EEG recording using an average montage derivation showing spikes with negativity over the right temporal region (T4/F8) and a concomitant positivity over the vertex, a horizontal dipolar distribution seen in mesial temporal foci. The spikes also propagate and appear to be synchronous over the left temporal region.

anteromesial temporal focus may appear most prominent in frontopolar or supraorbital electrodes.[10] Likewise basal temporal foci may project a positive trough at the vertex (Fig. 4–1). Recognizing these pitfalls allays consternation and may avert the need for extensive implantation of intracranial electrodes.

In epileptic substrates of cortical malformations, the pyramidal neurons have a disorganized arrangement. Without the parallel alignment, the field potentials from neighboring neuronal groups may cancel each other instead of summating into an ordered dipole layer. Such spike foci behave as "closed" fields[11] to be undetectable on scalp recordings or present as several scattered "microfoci" within a region. Computation of these sources may require higher order or multiple dipole models.[6,12]

▶ VOLUME CONDUCTION

The magnitude of the field potential recorded on the scalp varies inversely to the square of the distance of the recording electrode from the generator. The drop-off is not uniform in all directions but depends on the inho-

mogeneity, that is, varying conductivities and shapes of the media (cerebrospinal fluid [CSF], skull, scalp) across which the current traverses. Whenever currents approach media with differing conductivity, they "bend" toward the path of least resistance. The CSF, skull, and the diploic space between the skull tables act to shunt current away from the scalp electrodes and further attenuate activity recorded on the scalp. Scalp amplitudes are generally 8- to 20-fold lower, the attenuation being greater for generators that involve only a small cortical surface.[6,13] As an estimate, spike discharges may not be seen on the scalp unless one square inch or more of cortex is synchronously involved.[13] The fast activity at ictal onset is even less likely to synchronize over adequately large cortical areas and thus often goes undetected on scalp recordings. This is potentially misleading since sites to which the seizure propagates may reveal higher amplitude slower seizure sequence; the focal "attenuation" of background at seizure onset may be the only clue to the focus.

Currents from the generator also preferentially flow toward skull defects and foramina because of their lower resistance. Mesial temporal foci may appear prominent over frontopolar regions or the ear reference may be significantly contaminated by distant generators.

Even sphenoidal electrodes are not specific for mesial temporal foci and have been shown to reveal prominent spikes in patients with orbitofrontal foci.[10]

▶ PROPAGATION

Interictal spikes are known to propagate from the primary sites of origin and reveal a wide field of distribution. Propagated discharges cannot be localized by defining an apparent peak/trough of a single-dipole source but must through identifying a lead from the focus. The time difference between the source and propagated sites may be subtle and not readily evident to visual examination (Fig. 4–1). Identification of subtle leads is facilitated by using faster speed screen displays, via use of a reference subtraction derivation[14] or computational techniques.[15]

Additional cues may come from studying the spike morphology. The prominent negative peak with a widespread field is often preceded by a small positive trough with a more localized distribution; this initial component albeit small is useful to identify the focus. Similarly, the focus is more likely to reveal multiphasic spike morphology compared to broader sharp waves at propagated sites.[7]

For computational 3-D source analyses of propagated discharges, more complex models such as moving dipoles, spatiotemporal dipole, or distributed current density models are better suited than a single-dipole model.

Propagated spike or seizure discharges have been shown to "skip" regions and appear as well-circumscribed "pseudofoci" at considerable distances from the primary focus.[16–18] Such propagations can occur along all known major fiber pathways and may even occur across regions without known anatomic connectivity. In situations where a primary focus located in basal or mesial regions propagates to the lateral convexity, the secondarily activated "pseudofocus" may easily be mistaken for the primary generator. Differentiating the primary focus from pseudofoci is not always possible.

The presence of background abnormalities, especially the lack of fast activity in the same region strongly suggests that the observed focus is the primary one. Likewise, the focal attenuation at or near ictal onset generally does not "skip" regions and unlike spike or beta discharges is a useful indicator of the primary focus.

▶ RECORDING TECHNIQUE

ELECTRODES

The standard 10–20 electrode placement may not always accurately define the spike potential distribution[19] making localization of a focus to a specific region difficult. Specificity can be increased by placing additional electrodes[20] that may help differentiate, for example, inferior frontal spikes from anterior temporal spikes. The extended 10% electrode placement[21] provides better coverage of the lower temporal convexity. Specificity may also be influenced by variations in skull shape[22] since the relationship between an electrode and the underlying cortical region varies from subject to subject. The disproportionately late maturation of the frontal lobes in young children further increases the variability of these relationships. For example, the F7/8 electrodes that overlie the temporal lobes in children appear to "move" over to the inferior frontal convexity in adults.

The choice of electrodes is important for intracranial recordings as well. Depth recordings are more sensitive to foci located in mesial temporal regions[23] or in sulci. Subdural electrodes, on the other hand, provide wider coverage of the cortical surface[18] and are thus better able to define the spatial boundaries of the epileptogenic region. In patients where both, depth and subdural electrodes are utilized, seizures are often first recorded in only one and not the other. The two recording techniques must therefore be regarded as complementary, with neither being ideally suited to all patients. The choice of the type and number of electrodes should be individualized from data obtained in the preoperative evaluation.[24]

MONTAGE DERIVATIONS

Recorded data is generally viewed on bipolar and referential montage derivations; each has its limitations. Bipolar derivations do not record absolute potentials, but display voltage differences between adjacent electrode positions; spike peaks (or troughs) are identified as "phase reversals" occurring simultaneously along anteroposterior and transverse chains of electrodes overlying the focus. However, potentials involving adjacent locations are subject to in-phase cancellation. Spikes with a diffuse field may thus be completely missed or only subtly evident on bipolar derivations.[15]

The opposite, namely out-of-phase addition is rare but may be a source of confusion. For example, if a spike is positive at F4 and negative at C4 (horizontal dipolar distribution), the F4–C4 channel records a spike of falsely high amplitude. Bipolar derivations may also distort shape. For example, if there is a time-phase difference between adjacent locations, the spike may falsely appear to be multiphasic. Bipolar derivations are thus ill-suited for voltage measurement or morphological analyses.

Referential derivations are better suited to analyze voltage and morphology. When plotting voltage fields, the spike amplitudes may be measured peak-to-peak or baseline-to-peak. Baseline-to-peak measurements reflect summated depolarizations. Peak-to-peak measurements are of unclear pathophysiological relevance and are best avoided. When the reference electrode is located within the field of a spike (contaminated reference), voltages at all electrodes referenced to it are altered. Electrodes less involved than the reference show apparent positivity that may be misinterpreted as a horizontal dipolar field distribution leading to a serious error of localization.[4,5]

The "pseudo horizontal dipole" caused by a contaminated reference can be differentiated from a true horizontal dipole by analyzing the field plot. Reference contamination changes absolute voltage values at all electrode locations equally and shifts the entire plot without changing its shape; that is, the plot shape is independent of reference choice. The pseudo positivity of a contaminated reference progressively increases away from the peak but never reverses to produce a trough. In contrast, a plot of a spike with a true horizontal dipole distribution reveals both a peak and a trough.

It is important to note that reference contamination can change apparent voltages of seizure discharges as well. Unlike spikes, seizure discharges propagate and do not generally involve all electrodes in their "field" synchronously. The choice of a reference thus may affect interpretation. For example, in patients with temporal lobe seizures, the use of ipsilateral ear reference may lead to in-phase cancellation over the temporal sites with higher amplitude seizure sequences being apparent over regions remote from the ear.

FILTERS

Use of appropriate filters often helps EEG interpretation. For example, low-frequency filters applied to seizure patterns dominated by high amplitude diffuse slowing may help emphasize spike/fast frequency components that are more focal. Conversely, application of high-frequency filters may help reduce muscle artifact that obscures slower seizure patterns. However, filtering can distort waveforms making muscle artifact simulate spikes or runs of fast activity and predispose to errors of localization.

▶ INTERPRETATION OF PATTERNS

Pattern recognition is only the first step of interpretation; analyzing patterns in their appropriate context is a key to minimizing errors. For example, localizing reliability of spike discharges is state dependent. Non-REM (NREM) slow-wave sleep often activates spike discharges facilitating their identification, but may also alter their morphology and distribution. Thus, focal epileptogenic processes may present diffuse discharges

or generalized epilepsies may reveal fragmented focal discharges. In general, spikes observed during REM sleep and wakefulness have greater localizing value than those during NREM sleep.[25–27]

Whether ictal localization is state dependent is unknown, but the ability to localize may be compromised by electrographic changes related to arousal, which mimic seizure discharges. Furthermore, seizures can occasionally present with generalized attenuation of the background activity: in these situations, it may be difficult to determine whether attenuation represents rapid ictal spread or is a nonspecific EEG response possibly related to arousal or alerting.

Spikes observed during anticonvulsant withdrawal may be falsely localizing since their field distribution can change and new independent foci appear.[28] A baseline EEG sample during wakefulness should therefore be obtained prior to anticonvulsant withdrawal. As with interictal discharges, a new seizure focus can appear during anticonvulsant withdrawal[29] and has a potential for misleading localization. Fortunately, however, such false activation is rare.[30]

Interictal spikes observed on the intraoperative electrocorticography (EcoG) may differ in location from those recorded on subdural electrodes extraoperatively (personal observations). It would thus be important to ascertain the effect of various types and depths of anesthesia on the localizing reliability of spikes on ECoG since they are often used to guide the plane of resection. Anesthesia may also influence "rim spikes" recorded along the edge following resection.

Many benign patterns simulate epileptiform discharges; most of these are commonly seen on routine EEG recordings and are easily recognized. However, some patterns such as frontal arousal rhythm (FAR) or sub-clinical rhythmic EEG discharge of adults (SREDA) are rare and may be mistaken for electrographic seizures. Also, there is little data on benign patterns observed on intracranial recordings. For example, mu rhythms in central regions can mimic epileptiform activity seen in cortical dysplasia (Fig. 4–2). Interpretation of intracranial data should therefore be tempered by an awareness of possibly benign patterns.[18]

The ability to generate robust seizure patterns is often dependent of tissue vitality. Severely damaged areas of cortex may be incapable of sustaining a characteristic ictal discharge and high-amplitude rhythmic seizure build-up may occur distant to the region of actual seizure onset.[17,31] The possibility of false ictal localization should be considered if the apparent ictal focus is divergent from areas revealing significant background abnormalities such as severe attenuation or burst suppression. These regions often reveal subtle transformation of ongoing "background" prior to the rhythmic build-up elsewhere, thus establishing the true location of ictal onset.[32]

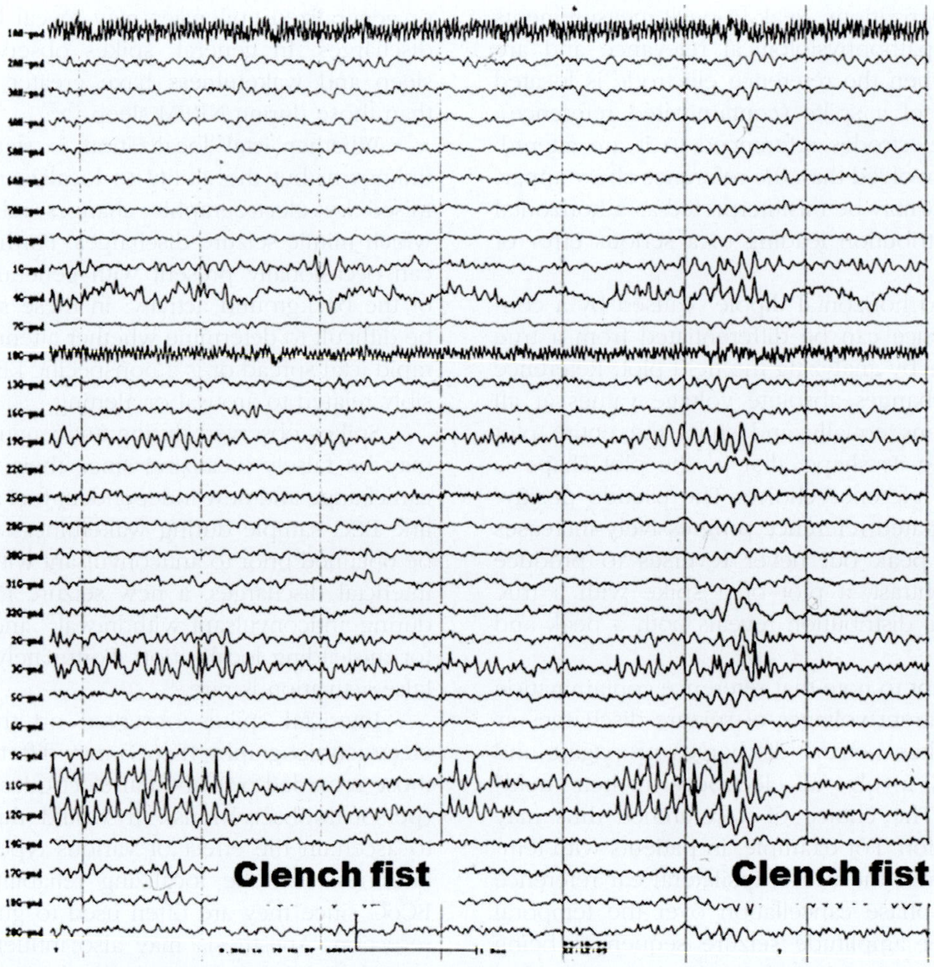

Figure 4–2. Subdural EEG recording showing prominent rhythmic activity at contacts 11 and 12 that attenuates with clenching of the fist that helps differentiate the physiological mu rhythm from epileptiform discharges that may have similar morphology.

The possibility for false localization also increases when there are several potentially epileptogenic regions. Seizures starting in one region can intraictally trigger other abnormal regions into prolonged discharges that outlast the primary focus.[33] Focal postictal background slowing, a sign that is generally useful for localization,[34] may be misleading under these circumstances since it may be more prominent over the secondary sites and outlast the slowing at the primary focus.

Seizures provoked by either electrical or pharmacologic stimulation are occasionally used to identify the focus. However, since the pathways of current spread and the population of neurons activated are not necessarily the same as during spontaneous seizures, provoked seizures should only be used to corroborate localization.[35] The localizing reliability of induced seizures is presumably greater if their clinical manifestations resemble the patient's spontaneous seizures. Similar considerations caution against the use of

afterdischarge thresholds during electrical stimulation to identify the focus.[36]

▶ SPECIAL METHODS

Automated systems for 3-D source localization of spike discharges allow the user to select a type of model for the EEG source and the head. The choice is generally based upon *a priori* knowledge of the source and its location. The single dipole within a spherical head model is computationally the simplest and reasonably robust for discrete stereotyped spikes located over the convexity. More complex source models such as moving dipole or distributed current density are better suited for pleomorphic discharges with variable fields. The realistic head model is appropriate for basal or deep foci.

When interpreting the results of 3-D source localization, it is useful to remember that the computed orientation is generally more reliable than the location; the extent of the generator is the least defined. The confidence in the results is higher if the computation of several spikes converges to the same location and if the temporal evolution of the spikes conforms to known propagation patterns.

Many studies have compared EEG and MEG for source localization accuracy. MEG is not affected by inhomogeneities and measures the "absolute" potential without requiring a reference electrode; however, MEG is mainly sensitive to horizontal dipolar sources such as those in a sulcus and may miss foci located over the crown of the gyrus. Comparative studies suggest that MEG complements the information obtained from EEG with some spikes seen on both, some only on MEG and some only on EEG.[37,38] The limited time for MEG generally does not allow capture of ictal events and the costs are much more prohibitive compared to EEG.

In a newer technique, EEG spikes recorded within the MRI unit are used to trigger the functional MRI; the blood-oxygen-level-dependent (BOLD) phenomenon identifies the location of the vascular response at the spike source.[39] This technique is promising but assumes a specific type of vascular coupling with the electrophysiological discharge, an assumption that may not hold true in epileptogenic tissue especially in the postictal period where vascular auto regulation may be compromised and affect the BOLD signal. Also, the method is technically challenging and yet not validated for widespread clinical use.

REFERENCES

1. Adrian ED, Matthews BHC. The Berger rhythm: potential changes from the occipital lobes in man. *Brain* 1934;57:355–385.
2. Magnus O. On the technique of localization by electro-encephalography. *Electroencephalogr Clin Neurophysiol* 1961;(Suppl. 19):1–35.
3. Osselton JW. Bipolar, unipolar and average reference recording methods. I. Mainly theoretical considerations. *Am J EEG Technol* 1966;5:53–64.
4. Gloor P. Neuronal generators and the problem of localization in electroencephalography: application of volume conductor theory of electroencephalography. *J Clin Neurophysiol* 1985;2:327–354.
5. Lesser RP, Luders H, Dinner DS, Morris H. An introduction to the basic concepts of polarity and localization. *J Clin Neurophysiol* 1985;2:45–62.
6. Nunez PL. *Electric Fields of the Brain. The Neurophysics of EEG*. New York: Oxford University Press, 1981.
7. Ajmone-Marsan C. Electrocorticography. In: Remond A (ed), *Handbook of Electroencephalography and Clinical Neurophysiology*. Amsterdam: Elsevier Scientific, 1973; 10C: pp. 1–49.
8. Engel J Jr (ed). *Surgical Treatment of the Epilepsies*. New York: Raven Press, 1987.
9. Jayakar P, Resnick TJ, Duchowny MS, Alvarez LA. Pitfalls and caveats of localizing seizure foci. *J Clin Neurophysiol* 1991;8:414–431.
10. Lesser RP, Luders H, Morris HH, Dinner DS, Wyllie E. Commentary: extracranial EEG evaluation. In: Engel J Jr (ed), *Surgical Treatment of the Epilepsies*. New York: Raven Press, 1987; pp. 173–179.
11. Klee M, Rall W. Computed potentials of cortically arranged populations of neurons. *J Neurophysiol* 1977; 40: 647–666.
12. Barth DS, Baumgartner C, Sutherling WW. Neuromagnetic field modeling of multiple brain regions producing interictal spikes in human epilepsy. *Electroenceph Clin Neurophysiol* 1989;73:389–402.
13. Cooper R, Winter AL, Crow HJ, Walter WG. Comparison of subcortical, cortical and scalp activity using chronically indwelling electrods in man. *Electroencephalogr Clin Neurophysiol* 1965;18:217–228.
14. Jayakar P, Duchowny MS, Resnick TJ, Alvarez LA. Localization of epileptogenic foci using a simple reference-subtraction montage to detect small interchannel time differences. *J Clin Neurophysiol* 1991;8:212–215.
15. Sharbrough FW. Commentary: extracranial EEG evaluation. In: Engel J Jr (ed), *Surgical Treatment of the Epilepsies*. New York: Raven Press, 1987; pp. 167–171.
16. Lieb JP, Walsh GO, Babb TL, Walter RD, Crandall PH. A comparison of EEG seizure patterns recorded with surface and depth electrodes in patients with temporal lobe epilepsy. *Epilepsia* 1976;17:137–160.
17. Quesney LF, Gloor P. Localization of epileptic foci. In: Gotman J, Ives JR, Gloor P (eds), *Long-Term Monitoring in Epilepsy*. Amsterdam: Elsevier Science Publishers, 1985; pp. 165–200.
18. Luders H, Lesser RP, Dinner DS, Morris HH, Hahn JF, Friedman L, Skipper G, Wyllie E, Friedman D. Commentary: chronic intracranial recording and stimulation with subdural electrodes. In: Engel J Jr (ed), *Surgical Treatment of the Epilepsies*. New York: Raven Press, 1987; pp. 297–321.
19. Morris HH III, Luders H, Lesser RP, Dinner DS, Klem GH. The value of closely spaced scalp electrodes in the localization of epileptiform foci: a study of 26 patients with complex partial seizures. *Electroencephalogr Clin Neurophysiol* 1986;63:107–111.
20. Quesney LF, Katsarkas A, Gloor P, Andermann F. Contribution of nasoethmoidal electrode recording in the electrographic exploration of frontal and temporal lobe epilepsy. In: Porter RJ, Mattson RH, Ward AA, Dam M (eds), *Advances in Epileptology: XIIth Epilepsy International Symposium*. New York: Raven Press, 1981; pp. 293–304.
21. American electroencephalographic society guidelines for standard electrode position nomenclature. *J Clin Neurophysiol* 1991;8:200–202.
22. Binnie CD, Dekker E, Smit A, Van der Linden G. Practical considerations in the positioning of EEG electrodes. *Electroencephalogr Clin Neurophysiol* 1982; 53:453–458.
23. Spencer S, Spencer D, Williamson P, Mattson R. The localizing value of depth electroencephalography in 32 patients with refractory epilepsy. *Ann Neurol* 1982;12:248–253.
24. Ojemann GA, Engel J Jr. Acute and chronic intracranial recording and stimulation. In: Engel J Jr (ed), *Surgical Treatment of the Epilepsies*. New York: Raven Press, 1987; pp. 263–288.

25. Lieb JP, Joseph JP, Engel J Jr, Walker J, Crandall PH. Sleep state and seizure foci related to depth spike activity in patients with temporal lobe epilepsy. *Electroencephalogr Clin Neurophysiol* 1980;49:538–557.

26. Montplaisir J, Laverdiere M, Saint-Hilaire JM. Sleep and focal epilepsy: contribution of depth recording. In: Sterman M, Passouant P (eds), *Sleep and Epilepsy.* New York: Academic Press, 1982; pp. 301–314.

27. Sammaritano M, Gigli GL, Gotman J. Interictal spiking during wakefulness and sleep and the localization of foci in temporal lobe epilepsy. *Neurology* 1991;41:290–297.

28. Ludwig BI, Ajmone-Marsan C. EEG changes after withdrawal of medication in epileptic patients. *Electroencephalogr Clin Neurophysiol* 1975;39:173–181.

29. Engel J Jr, Crandall PH. Falsely localizing ictal onset with depth EEG telemetry during anticonvulsant withdrawal. *Epilepsia* 1983;24:344–355.

30. Marciani MG, Gotman J. Effects of drug withdrawal on location of seizure onset. *Epilepsia* 1986;27:423–431.

31. Sammaritano M, de Lobtiniere A, Andermann F, Olivier A, Gloor P, Quesney LF. False lateralization by surface EEG of seizure onset in patients with temporal lobe epilepsy and focal cerebral lesions. *Epilepsia* 1984;25:664.

32. Jayakar P. Chronic intracranial EEG monitoring in children: when, where and what? *J Clin Neurophysiol* 1999;16(5): 408–418.

33. Jayakar P, Resnick TJ, Duchowny MS, Alvarez LA. Intra-ictal activation in the neocortex: a marker of the epileptogenic region. *Epilepsia* 1994;35(3):489–494.

34. Kaibara M, Blume WT. The postictal electroencephalogram. *Electroencephalogr Clin Neurophysiol* 1988;70:99–104.

35. Wieser HG, Bancaud J, Talairach J, Bonis A, Szikla G. Comparative value of spontaneous and chemically and electrically induced seizures in establishing the lateralization of temporal lobe seizures. *Epilepsia* 1979;20:47–60.

36. Cherlow DG, Dymond AM, Crandall PH, Walter RD, Serafetinides EA. Evoked response and after-discharge thresholds to electrical stimulation in temporal lobe epileptics. *Arch Neurol* 1977;34:527–531.

37. Kirsch HE, Mantle M, Nagarajan SS. Concordance between routine interictal magnetoencephalography and simultaneous scalp electroencephalography in a sample of patients with epilepsy. *J Clin Neurophysiol* 2007;24: 215–231.

38. Sharon D, Hämäläinen MS, Tootell RB, Halgren E, Belliveau JW. The advantage of combining MEG and EEG: comparison to fMRI in focally stimulated visual cortex. *Neuroimage* 2007;36:1225–1235.

39. Al-Asmi A, Bénar CG, Gross DW, Khani YA, Andermann F, Pike B, Dubeau F, Gotman J. fMRI activation in continuous and spike-triggered EEG-fMRI studies of epileptic spikes. *Epilepsia* 2003;10:1328–1339.

CHAPTER 5

Aims and Rationale of Anatomic Brain Imaging

John A. Lawson

▶ OVERVIEW

For any doctor looking after children with epilepsy, an essential skill is interpretation of the MRI. But, even in centers of imaging excellence, accurate clinical and EEG data are required to enable interpretation of an MRI abnormality or, alternatively, to allow a focused search for the common subtle abnormalities that may underlie symptomatic epilepsy. Brain imaging has become an essential part of the evaluation of most children with epilepsy. Yet, MRI has not taken over from the clinical basics. The pillars of a thorough evaluation of a child with seizures still remain; a good clinical assessment (detailed history and physical examination) supplemented by an interictal EEG.

As a consultant dealing with epilepsy, it is clearly a mistake to rely solely on imaging in the absence of good electroclinical data, ideally forming a diagnosis of the child's epilepsy syndrome. If the initial diagnostic question "Does this child have epilepsy?" is answered in the affirmative this should be followed by "what is the epilepsy syndrome?" The answer to the second question is the rational basis to determine which patients require brain imaging (Fig. 5–1).

This chapter will focus initially on the rationale, indications, and published clinical guidelines for imaging children with epilepsy. A brief discussion on the broad principles of optimal imaging methods for the epilepsy population will be followed by the application of imaging to more common specific clinical situations.

▶ RATIONALE FOR IMAGING IN CHILDREN WITH EPILEPSY

The rationale for neuroimaging in epilepsy is summarized in a position statement by the Commission on Neuroimaging of the International League Against Epilepsy (ILAE) (1997).[1,2] They provided two indications:

Diagnosis of Underlying Aetiology

"To identify underlying abnormalities such as vascular lesions, acute trauma and tumours that require specific treatment."

Syndrome Delineation and Prognosis

"To aid the formulation of syndromic and etiological diagnoses and to give patients, their relatives and physicians an accurate prognosis."

Other reasons for neuroimaging include:

Nonepilepsy Diagnoses

Metabolic diseases diagnosable on MRI can present with focal seizures such as adrenoleukodystrophy or mitochondrial encephalopathy. Other acute, nonepilepsy disorders such as hydrocephalus, trauma, infection, stroke, and acute-disseminated encephalomyelitis can clearly lead to change in management.

Potential Genetic Implications

Apart from the above hereditable metabolic and neurodegenerative conditions that have obvious genetic implications, an important group are the malformations of cortical development. An increasing number of the more common abnormalities such as polymicrogyria now have an underlying genetic diagnosis. Well-characterized recessive and X-linked disorders explain the majority of patients with lissencephaly.

Fear (Patient and Clinician)

One of the most common reasons driving families and clinicians to perform neuroimaging in childhood epilepsy is fear: "could there be a brain tumor?" If one looks at published imaging series low-grade or "benign" brain tumors are not an uncommon discovery. In an otherwise asymptomatic child presenting with epilepsy, the incidence of malignant brain tumors is very low. Looking from another angle, a description of the presenting symptoms of 200 consecutive children diagnosed with brain tumor was collected at one institution.[3] Seizures were the presenting symptom in 9% and were often the only symptom with no focal signs. It was not stated whether these children had low-or high-grade tumors.

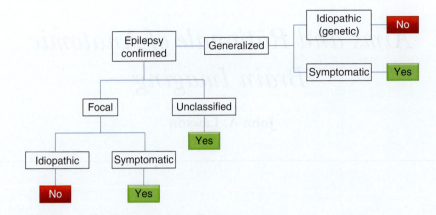

Figure 5–1. Decision-tree for neuroimaging based on epilepsy syndrome.

Ideally, it is recommended that one should obtain structural neuroimaging with MRI in all patients with epilepsy, except in patients with a definite electro-clinical diagnosis of idiopathic generalized or partial epilepsy. Those children with idiopathic epilepsy syndromes usually have a characteristic EEG and have a very low yield from imaging. Idiopathic partial epilepsies such as benign rolandic or idiopathic generalized, and childhood absence epilepsy are good examples where imaging is not indicated.

The authors of the ILAE statement[1,2] go on to say that MRI is particularly indicated in patients with one or more of the following:

1. Onset of seizures at any age with evidence of a partial onset on history, examination, or EEG unless clear evidence of a typical benign epilepsy.
2. Onset of unclassified or apparently generalized seizures in children under two years of age or in adulthood.
3. Difficulty in obtaining control of seizures with anti-convulsants worsening seizures, changes is seizure manifestations, or developmental regression also merit neuroimaging if not previously performed.
4. Loss of control of seizures with anticonvulsants or a change in the seizure pattern that may imply a progressive underlying lesion.
5. Children with characteristics of a symptomatic generalized epilepsy syndrome, including infantile spasms or early Lennox–Gastaut syndrome (e.g., tonic, atonic, mixed seizures), as focal MRI findings may be found in a substantial proportion of these children.
6. Finally, new-onset seizures/epilepsy presenting with evidence for a medical emergency such as increased intracranial pressure or status epilepticus always merit emergency imaging.

The latter recommendation highlights the need for reimaging in those patients who follow a negative course to exclude diseases such as Rasmussen encephalitis or inherited neurodegenerative condition.

► CLINICAL GUIDELINES

The American Academy of Neurology (AAN) published a practice parameter in 2000 for evaluating a first non-febrile seizure in children.[4] Class 1 and Class 2 evidence from studies of CT or MRI reports (all from the 1990s) in over 1290 children identified a low rate (1.9%) of relevant abnormalities that led to a change in clinical intervention. Consistently MRI had a far greater yield than CT on direct comparison. A well-known example of one of these studies is a prospective cohort[5] of 613 children with newly diagnosed epilepsy. Eighty-six percent had neuroimaging (predominantly MRI); 16% were abnormal but did not influence immediate management decisions.

The conclusions of the AAN practice parameter recommendations for imaging the first nonfebrile seizure were:

- If a neuroimaging study is indicated, MRI is the preferred modality.
- Urgent neuroimaging should be performed in a child of any age who exhibits a postictal focal deficit not quickly resolving, or who has not returned to baseline within several hours after the seizure.
- Nonurgent imaging with MRI should be seriously considered in any child with a significant cognitive or motor impairment of unknown etiology, unexplained abnormalities on neurologic examination, a seizure of focal onset, an EEG that does not represent an idiopathic partial or generalized epilepsy, or in children under 1 year of age.

The National Institute for Clinical Excellence (NICE) of Great Britain guidelines for epilepsy management[6] reaffirmed the AAN recommendations. In addition, they recommend that neuroimaging when indicated should be done within 4 weeks of being requested.

▶ NEGATIVE ASPECTS OF NEUROIMAGING

Given this rationale why not perform imaging on all children with epilepsy? There are negative aspects to neuroimaging including the risk of sedation or general anesthetic that is required for young or uncooperative children. Another common problem is the enormous anxiety that the family must go through waiting (sometimes) months for the exclusion of a potential life-threatening condition. Cost and access is the most important issue for most of the world's population.

Apart from these practical concerns, the identification of incidental findings on MRI is of limited or no relevance to the diagnosis of epilepsy and can have considerable negative consequences worsening seizures, changes is seizure manifestations, or developmental regression also merit neuroimaging if not previously performed.

The rates of MRI abnormality in normal children[7] and adults[8] are now recognized. A prospective study[8] of 2536 healthy young male military applicants, with a mean age of 20 years revealed potentially, clinically relevant abnormalities in 6.5% on limited sequences using 1.0T MRI. The most common findings were arachnoid cysts in 1.7%, Chiari malformations in 1.7%, vascular abnormalities in 0.5%, and tumors in 0.2%. Overall, 0.5% required "urgent" referral. In a pediatric study,[7] a 6% rate of brain abnormalities was found in 225 healthy children. These included posterior fossa abnormalities, focal white matter lesions of uncertain significance, and arachnoid cysts. Not reported in the pediatric series, benign pineal cysts are also very common and can raise unnecessary concern in families. At the minimum these findings often lead to a repeat or serial MRI's over months to years to ensure the benign nature of the incidental "abnormality" with clear potential for harmful psychological effects on families. Thus clinicians, when considering ordering MRI, as with other investigations, should anticipate and discuss the potential impact of the incidental finding as these are not rare.

The potential negative aspects of CT irradiation are beyond the scope of this chapter, but there have been several excellent reviews.[9] It is estimated that use of CT may be associated with 1.5% to 2% of all cancers in the United States and many authors are advocating that informed consent be obtained before imaging with CT.

▶ OPTIMAL IMAGING METHODS

Many studies have demonstrated the superior value of MRI over computed tomography. There are some exceptions to this, as in acute trauma and where calcification is prominent. Many studies[10] and reviews have suggested the optimum MRI acquisition sequences to try and increase yield. Collection of MRI sequences along or perpendicular to the longitudinal axis of the hippocampus enhances coronal and axial views of mesial temporal pathology. Sequences acquired perpendicular to the anterior–posterior commissural line are often used for extratemporal pathology. Emphasis is also placed on fine slice, contiguous MRI to include the whole brain utilizing both T1 and T2 weighted scans.

"Standard" MRI scans in most centers currently are of 1.5T strength and use quadrature head coils. Higher resolution is obtainable using *phased array coils* increasing the signal to noise ratio up to 4 times. In a small study,[11] five of nine children with previous normal standard MRI were found to have lesions using a four coil phased surface array. In an earlier prospective study[12] of 25 adults with refractory focal epilepsy, the use of phased array imaging at 1.5T improved lesion detection in comparison with standard imaging at 1.5T. New diagnostic information was obtained in half the cases, resulting in altered clinical management in two-thirds of these patients and new surgical referral in nearly one in five.

▶ 3T MRI VERSUS 1.5T MRI

Are there any advantages of higher strength magnets? Interestingly, there are very few head-to-head studies comparing the diagnostic yield of different strength MRI. One group[13] studied 40 patients with well-localized intractable focal epilepsy and normal 1.5T MRI. The authors used an 8-channel phased array head coil with 3T MRI. Fifteen of 25 with a normal 1.5T MRI had an abnormality detected on 3T. Most of these were diagnosed on imaging as focal cortical dysplasia. Only a small percentage of the patients had undergone surgery at the time of publication making it difficult to confirm that the additional information from imaging at 3T improved clinical outcomes.

Another study[14] looked at 120 adults with focal epilepsy who were not previously imaged and referred for 3T MRI without a phased array coil. A low rate of abnormalities was found (26%) with only 18% being of relevance to the epilepsy, the commonest being hippocampal sclerosis. Tumors, judged as low grade, on imaging were found in 4 (3%). The authors argued that there was a dearth of information on the rationale and health economics of recommending MRI "routinely" in this population.

Higher strength MRI clearly has a role in functional MRI and other experimental techniques such as diffusion tensor imaging and MR spectroscopy. However, it is not clear whether the yield of 3T structural MRI is significantly higher and justifies its additional cost. One large study[15] found higher rates of side effects with 3T magnets such as back pain and dizziness.

▶ PROGNOSIS

Several studies confirm a role for MRI in predicting the long-term outcome of epilepsy. Several adult studies reveal a relationship between pathology on MRI and the risk for intractable epilepsy. One of the largest series[16] examined the MRI of 1148 adults with partial epilepsy. Potentially epileptogenic lesions were identified in 71%—most commonly, hippocampal sclerosis (HS) in 25%, with gliosis being second most common. The highest rates of long-term seizure freedom were noted in 40% to 50% of patients with a normal MRI, poststroke, or low-grade gliomas. This compared to only 11% long-term seizure-freedom for patients with HS and 24% for patients with cortical dysplasia. In multivariate analysis, the presence of HS was the single biggest predictor of a low-seizure free outcome. In a separate study[17] of anticonvulsant withdrawal in 84 adults and adolescents with well-controlled epilepsy, the presence of hippocampal sclerosis was associated with a substantially higher risk of relapse (74% vs. 47%).

Another study[18] of 550 adult patients with epilepsy, including 43% with recurrent seizures, demonstrated similar findings. HS and malformations of cortical development were associated with the poorest prognosis, with 58% and 46% rates of drug resistance, respectively, followed by tumor (37%), stroke (33%), and arteriovenous malformations (22%).

A large pediatric cohort study[19] reported that a "remote symptomatic etiology" (often determined by neuroimaging) was a major factor as a predictor of recurrent seizures. A longitudinal study[20] followed 64 children with new-onset temporal lobe epilepsy (TLE) for a median of 14 years. Twenty-eight had a lesion with equal numbers of HS, tumor and focal cortical dysplasia. None were seizure-free long-term. The authors concluded that an MRI lesion was the only significant predictor of seizure outcome in childhood onset TLE.

▶ SPECIAL SITUATIONS

NEW TECHNIQUES FOR MRI NEGATIVE FOCAL EPILEPSY

The MRI negative patient with intractable partial epilepsy remains a major management problem in both children and adults. Several new MRI techniques have been developed in an attempt to evaluate the 20%–50% of patients with intractable epilepsy who do have an identifiable lesion. One study[21] of 93 adult surgical candidates with negative routine MRI studies had voxel-based comparisons of several novel contrasts that had been hypothesized in several smaller series to increase yield in MRI "negative" studies. These contrasts included T1-based voxel-based morphometry, double inversion recovery, magnetization transfer imaging, and fast FLAIR T2-mapping. The acquisition time for these additional tests was 60 minutes. The authors found a very poor yield from all of these contrasts with a low sensitivity and poor specificity correlating with the scalp EEG identified putative epileptogenic zone. This study emphasized that new techniques often trumpeted in small selective series need to be evaluated with larger patient numbers to truly establish their worth.

First Seizure

The prevalence of abnormalities from MRI must be lower in first seizure patients compared to a chronic epilepsy population. Reasons are that a large proportion will have an idiopathic generalized or partial epilepsy, or even a misdiagnosed nonepileptic event such as syncope. One of the leading papers[22] on patients presenting with first seizures found 38 lesions in 293 patients imaged (20% were aged <16 years). This rate of approximately 13% yield in this population is present across a number of predominantly adult studies.[23] The type of lesions found also differs from the intractable population in that there is a low rate of HS and higher rates of tumors.

A prospective study[24] of cognitive function in children aged 6–14 who had a first seizure enrolled 249 participants who also had MRI. The prevalence of epilepsy-related abnormalities was 14% of the sample. Half showed leukomalacia/gliosis, the rest were hippocampal sclerosis, encephalomalacia, and cortical dysplasias. Interestingly 16% had abnormalities considered nonsignificant such as posterior fossa abnormalities and nonspecific foci of T2 signal.

FEBRILE CONVULSIONS

An early prospective series[25] performed MRI in 27 infants who presented with complex febrile convulsions (CFC), and found acute T2 abnormalities in 4 of the 15 infants with focal seizures, and in none of the 12 infants with brief generalized seizures. Two of the four with acute changes had follow-up scans showing progressive hippocampal atrophy. This was the first prospective study to suggest that prolonged, focal febrile seizures can produce acute hippocampal injury evolving to hippocampal sclerosis.

Two recent large studies have addressed the role of urgent neuroimaging in complex febrile convulsions. The first[26] performed imaging in 45 of 159 children presenting with CFC (36 had CT, 9 MRI). Neuroimaging was performed in patients who had postictal neurologic deficit or focal seizures after their clinical status became stable. In these selected patients, 7 of 45 (16%) had an abnormality on imaging but none required a change in their management. A larger sample[27] from an emergency department presentation of complex febrile seizures in 79 children with no previous concerning history found that none required either urgent medical or surgical intervention. The majority of these children had an MRI evaluation. The authors suggested there was no evidence to support urgent imaging in these children.

Prolonged alteration in mental status, meningism, persisting postical focal deficits, and toxic appearance, among others, should raise clinical suspicion of a treatable condition where neuroimaging may play a diagnostic role.

THE EMERGENCY DEPARTMENT

Neuroimaging for seizures in the emergency department (ED) is almost certainly overutilized. This is definitely the case for individuals with known epilepsy who have been previously imaged. Many children with a first afebrile seizure presenting to an emergency department are scanned with no clear rationale. The majority who present with a single unprovoked seizure do not develop epilepsy. In a retrospective study[28] of 500 children with new-onset afebrile seizures (median age 4 years) presenting to an emergency department 95% had neuroimaging (91% of these CT only). Clinically insignificant neuroimaging results were reported in 9%, whereas clinically significant abnormalities were reported in only 8%. Acute intracranial hemorrhage was the most common finding, followed by acute or old cerebrovascular accident. A brain tumor or acute infarction was identified in only 1%. There were two factors that placed the child at highest risk of having a significant abnormality; those with a predisposing condition (e.g., sickle cell, malignancy) or focal seizures in those less than 33 months of age.

These rates of abnormality are lower than in adults and thus suggest different guidelines for urgent neuroimaging of children. In fact, of the 374 cases where CT was initially read as normal, 163 (43%) went on to have MRI performed. In six of these cases (3.7%), the MRI showed a clinically significant abnormality. It can thus be concluded that well-appearing children with new-onset afebrile seizures for whom these high-risk criteria do not apply can be safely discharged from the ED without neuroimaging, if follow-up is assured.

A report[29] of the "Therapeutics and Technology Assessment Subcommittee of the American Academy of Neurology" in 2007 provided an evidenced-based review of neuroimaging in the emergency patient with a seizure. Their conclusion was: "Immediate non-contrast CT is possibly useful for emergency patients presenting with a seizure to guide appropriate acute management especially where there is an abnormal neurologic examination, predisposing history, or focal seizure onset." Fifteen articles (4 pediatric) met criteria for review and were of level Class 2 to Class 3 of evidence. There is evidence that for adults with first seizure, cranial CT will change acute management in

9%–17% of patients. CT in the Emergency Department for children presenting with first seizure (excluding simple but including complex febrile seizures) will change acute management in approximately 3%–8%. These studies combined had over 600 children. The lesions that led to a change in management included cerebral hemorrhages, tumors, cysticercosis, and obstructive hydrocephalus. Abnormal neurologic examination, predisposing history, or focal seizure onset are probably predictive of an abnormal CT study in this context. There is no evidence that a CT is helpful for patients with chronic epilepsy.

An exception to the above guidelines may be the very young. One limited study[30] of 22 children less than age 6 months presenting with seizures showed clinically relevant abnormalities on CT scans 55% of the time. The diagnoses were Aicardi syndrome, lissencephaly, tuberous sclerosis, an infarct, and a depressed skull fracture. A separate study[31] of children with immediate posttraumatic seizures had a very low rate of CT abnormalities that led to a change in management. In the 62 patients studied, 16% had abnormal CT scans and 3 patients, about 5% had abnormalities that led to a surgical intervention.

BRAIN TUMORS

MRI is clearly the investigation of choice for children with brain tumors and epilepsy, assisting in diagnosis, surgical planning, and monitoring change.[32] It has not replaced histopathology on biopsy in terms of diagnosis or histological grading. Newer techniques such as MR Spectroscopy aide in distinguishing high-grade from low-grade tumors, but are insufficiently specific to be relied upon in clinical practice. Diffusion weighted imaging reveals restricted diffusion in dense cellular high-grade tumors and increased diffusion in low-grade gliomas but these findings await further confirmation.

Intraoperative MRI shows promise with real-time imaging enabling assessment of extent of resection offering a theoretical advantage. This benefit is yet to be shown in controlled trials and there is potential for increased morbidity through prolonged operating times.

INTRACTABLE EPILEPSY

A prospective study[10] of 385 adults and children (mean age 31 years) with drug-resistant epilepsy were imaged with 1.5T MRI. Potentially epileptogenic lesions were detected in 318 (83%) with hippocampal sclerosis being the most common finding in 52% of the cases. Glioneuronal tumors were next most common at 20% of cases and 10% had focal cortical dysplasia. Diagnostic errors by reporting neuroradiologists were most common in this group—several nonenhancing lesions labeled as dysplasia were subsequently proven to be low-grade gliomas on histology.

An earlier study by the same investigators[33] was titled "Standard MRI is inadequate for patients with refractory focal epilepsy." Consecutive adult epilepsy patients were evaluated with standard MRI/nonexpert radiologists (39% detected) and standard MRI/experts (50%). A third comparison was "epilepsy dedicated" MRI sequences read by experts with a lesion detection rate of 91%. In particular HS was missed in 86% of cases; dedicated MRI read by experts also doubled the rate of tumor detection.

EPILEPSY SURGERY AND FRAMELESS STEROTACTIC MRI

High-resolution T1 weighted images provide excellent anatomic resolution with isotropic voxels allowing reorientation in all planes. Many epileptogenic lesions including focal cortical dysplasia and its boundaries are either displayed poorly or overlooked. T2 weighted images (including FLAIR) have the inverse problem with less distinct structural morphology but excellent lesion definition. One group[34] addressed this by examining coregistration of FLAIR or T2 images coregistered with T1 in 50 patients utilizing frameless stereotactic MRI. This qualitative-uncontrolled study suggested improved complete lesional resection in this group.

► IDIOPATHIC GENERALISED EPILEPSY (IGE)

Although imaging is generally not recommended in IGE, there is only limited supporting data. In 134 mainly adults (age 9–50 years) with IGE evaluated with a 2.0T MR, 33 (24%) exhibited abnormalities including arachnoid cysts, nonspecific white matter abnormalities, diffuse cortical or hippocampal atrophy, and basal ganglia abnormalities.[35] The lesion could be considered potentially epileptogenic in only in four cases and influenced clinical management in none.

Imaging studies[36] in specific IGE syndromes such as juvenile myoclonic epilepsy demonstrate increased grey matter in the bilateral medial frontal grey matter by group "averaged" MRI utilizing statistical parametric mapping.

VALUE OF GADOLINIUM

Gadolinium enhancement is generally not recommended as a routine part of the initial MRI evaluation.[2] One study[37] has addressed particularly the value of IV gadolinium contrast in MRI in under 2-year olds. In 92% of 473 cases retrospectively reviewed, gadolinium did not add any further diagnostic information. Gadolinium was deemed essential in 1.8% of patients who had suspected acute meningitis or encephalitis. The authors concluded that IV contrast in MRI be reserved for suspected or documented infection or cases of known neoplasm.

► CONCLUSIONS

Although the majority of children in well-resourced countries include MRI as part of the investigation and management of their epilepsy evidence to support this practice is not strong. There is clearly little argument with the high yield of MRI abnormalities obtained in children with intractable epilepsy, but routine neuroimaging in children with a first seizure is more questionable. Clinicians must consider many factors, most importantly, the epilepsy syndrome and also to understand the potential negative effects of indiscriminate neuroimaging.

REFERENCES

1. Gaillard WD, Chiron C, Cross JH, Harvey AS, Kuzniecky R, Hertz-Pannier L, Vezina LG, for the ILAE, Committee for Neuroimaging, Subcommittee for Pediatric. Guidelines for imaging infants and children with recent-onset epilepsy. *Epilepsia* 2009;50(9):2147–2153.
2. Recommendations for neuroimaging of patients with epilepsy. Commission on neuroimaging of the international league against epilepsy. *Epilepsia* 1997;38(11):1255–1256.
3. Wilne SH, Ferris RC, Nathwani A, Kennedy CR. The presenting features of brain tumours: a review of 200 cases. *Arch Dis Child* 2006;91(6):502–506.
4. Hirtz D, Ashwal S, Berg A, Bettis D, Camfield C, Camfield P, Crumrine P, Elterman R, Schneider S, Shinnar S. Practice parameter: evaluating a first nonfebrile seizure in children: Report of the Quality Standards Subcommittee of the American Academy of Neurology, the Child Neurology Society, and the American Epilepsy Society. *Neurology* 2000;55:616–623.
5. Berg AT, et al. Neuroimaging in children with newly diagnosed epilepsy: a community-based study. *Pediatrics* 2003;111(1):194–196.
6. *The epilepsies. The diagnosis and management of the epilepsies in adults and children in primary and secondary care NICE guidelines*. National Institute for Health and Clinical Excellence. 2004, www.nice.org.uk.
7. Kim BS, Illes J, Kaplan RT, Reiss A, Atlas SW. Incidental findings on pediatric MR images of the brain. *Am J Neuroradiol* 2002;23:1674–1677.
8. Weber F, Knopf H. Incidental findings in magnetic resonance imaging of the brains of healthy young men. *J Neurol Sci* 2006;240:81–84.
9. Brenner DJ, Hall EJ. Computed tomography—an increasing source of radiation exposure. *N Engl J Med* 2007;357(22):2277–2284.
10. Urbach H, Hattingen J, von Oertzen J, Luyken C, Clusmann H, Kral T, Kurthen M, Schramm J, Blumcke I, Schild HH. MR imaging in the presurgical workup of patients with drug-resistant epilepsy. *Am J Neuroradiol* 2004;25:919–926.
11. Goyal M, Bangert BA, Lewin JS, Cohen ML, Robinson S. High resolution MRI enhances identification of lesions amenable to surgical therapy in children with intractable epilepsy. 8, *Epilepsia* 2004;45:954–959.

12. Grant PE, et al. High-resolution surface coil MR of cortical lesions in medically refractory epilepsy: a prospective study. *Am J Neuroradiol* 1997;18:291–301.

13. Knake S, Triantafyllou C, Wald LL, Wiggins G, Kirk GP, Larsson PG, Stufflebeam SM, Foley MT, Shiraishi H, Dale AM, Halgren E, Grant PE. 3T-phased array MRI improves the presurgical evaluation in focal epilepsies: a prospective study. *Neurology* 2005;65(7):1026–1031.

14. Griffiths PD, Coley SC, Connolly DJ, Hodgson T, Romanowski CA, Widjaja E, Darwent G, Wilkinson ID. MR imaging of patients with localization-related seizures: initial experience at 3.0T and relevance to the NICE guidelines. *Clin Radiol* 2005;60(10):1090–1099.

15. Weintraub MI, Khoury A, Cole SP. Biologic effects of 3 Tesla (T) MR imaging comparing traditional 1.5T and 0.6T in 1023 consecutive outpatients. *J Neuroimaging* 2007;17(3):241–245.

16. Semah F, Picot MC, Adam C, Broglin D, Arzimanoglou A, Bazin B, Cavalcanti D, Baulac M. Is the underlying cause of epilepsy a major prognostic factor for recurrence? *Neurology* 1998;51:1256–1262.

17. Cardoso TA, Coan AC, Kobayashi E, Guerreiro CA, Li LM, Cendes F. Hippocampal abnormalities and seizure recurrence after antiepileptic drug withdrawal. *Neurology* 2006;67:134–136.

18. Stephen LJ, Kwan P, Brodie MJ. Does the cause of localisation-related epilepsy influence the response to antiepileptic drug treatment? *Epilepsia* 2001;42:357–362.

19. Berg AT, Levy SR, Novotny EJ, Shinnar S. Predictors of intractable epilepsy in childhood: a case-control study. *Epilepsia* 1996;37(1):24–30.

20. Spooner CG, Berkovic SF, Mitchell LA, Wrennall JA, Harvey AS. New-onset temporal lobe epilepsy in children: lesion on MRI predicts poor seizure outcome. *Neurology* 2006;67(12):2147–2153.

21. Salmenpera TM, Symms MR, Rugg-Gunn FJ, Boulby PA, Free SL, Barker GJ, Yousry TA, Duncan JS. Evaluation of quantitative magnetic resonance imaging contrasts in MRI-negative refractory focal epilepsy. *Epilepsia* 2007;48:229–237.

22. King MA, Newton MR, Jackson GD, Fitt GJ, Mitchell LA, Silvapulle MJ, Berkovic SF. Epileptology of the first-seizure presentation: a clinical, electroencephalographic, and magnetic resonance imaging study of 300 consecutive patients. *Lancet* 1998;352:1007–1011.

23. Wiebe S, Tellez-Zenteno JF, Shapiro M. An evidence-based approach to the first seizure. *Epilepsia* 2008;49:50–57.

24. Byars AW, deGrauw TJ, Johnson CS, Fastenau PS, Perkins SM, Egelhoff JC, Kalnin A, Dunn DW, Austin JK. The association of MRI findings and neuropsychological functioning after the first recognized seizure. *Epilepsia* 2007;48(6):1067–1074.

25. Van Landingham KE, Heinz ER, Cavazos JE, Lewis DV. Magnetic resonance imaging evidence of hippocampal injury after prolonged focal febrile convulsions. *Ann Neurol* 1998;43(4):413–426.

26. Yucel O, Aka S, Yazicioglu L, Ceran O. The role of early EEG and neuroimaging in determination of prognosis in children with complex febrile seizures. *Pediatr Int* 2004;46:463–446.

27. Teng D, Dayan P, Tyler S, Hauser WA, Chan S, Leary L, Hesdorffer D. Risk of intracranial pathologic conditions requiring emergency intervention after a first complex febrile seizure episode among children. *Pediatrics* 2006;117(2):304–308.

28. Sharma S, Riviello JJ, Harper MB, Baskin MN. The role of emergent neuroimaging in children with new-onset afebrile seizures. *Pediatrics* 2003;111(1):194–196.

29. Harden CL, Huff JS, Schwartz TH, Dubinsky RM, Zimmerman RD, Weinstein S, Foltin JC, Theodore WH. Reassessment: neuroimaging in the emergency patient presenting with seizure (an evidence-based review): Report of the Therapeutics and Technology Assessment Subcommittee of the American Academy of Neurology. *Neurology* 2007;69(18):1772–1780.

30. Bui TT, Delgado CA, Simon HK. Infant seizures not so infantile: first-time seizures in children under six months of age presenting to the ED. *Am J Emerg Med* 2002;20(6):518–520.

31. Holmes JF, Palchak MJ, Conklin MJ, Kuppermann N. Do children require hospitalization after immediate posttraumatic seizures? *Ann Emerg Med* 2004;43(6):706–710.

32. Rees J. Advances in magnetic resonance imaging of brain tumours. *Curr Opin Neurol* 2003;16:643–650.

33. Von Oertzen J, Urbach H, Jungbluth S, Kurthen M, Reuber M, Fernández G, Elger CE. Standard magnetic resonance imaging is inadequate for patients with refractory focal epilepsy. *J Neurol Neurosurg Psychiatry* 2002;73(6):643–647.

34. Mahvash M, König R, Urbach H, von Ortzen J, Meyer B, Schramm J, Schaller C. FLAIR-/T1-/T2-co-registration for image-guided diagnostic and resective epilepsy surgery. *Neurosurgery* 2006;58:69–75.

35. Betting LE, Mory SB, Lopes-Cendes I, Li LM, Guerreiro MM, Guerreiro CA, Cendes F. MRI reveals structural abnormalities in patients with idiopathic generalized epilepsy. *Neurology* 2006;67:848–852.

36. Duncan JS. Brain imaging in idiopathic generalized epilepsies. *Epilepsia* 2005;46(Suppl 9):108–111.

37. Petrou M, Foerster B, Maly PV, Eldevik OP, Leber S, Sundgren PC. Added utility of gadolinium in the magnetic resonance imaging (MRI) workup of seizures in children under two years. *J Child Neurol* 2007;22(2):200–203.

CHAPTER 6

When and Why Perform Functional Brain Imaging: Medical and Surgical Treatment of Pediatric Epilepsy

William D. Gaillard and Philippe Ryvlin

▶ INTRODUCTION

Structural and functional imaging is employed to help identify candidates for surgery, to plan surgical approaches, and to inform likelihood of favorable outcome. The primary role of imaging is to help identify and to confirm the location of the seizures focus. This is the place of structural MRI, FDG-PET (fluoro-deoxy glucose positron emission tomography), and SPECT (single-photon emission computerized tomography). Surgical outcome is high when focal abnormalities are found with these imaging techniques. Newer techniques used in planning epilepsy surgery, fMRI, and DTI (diffusion tensor imaging) are used to identify areas to spare or to avoid during resection.

Outcomes from surgery are related to the certainty of successfully identifying the seizure focus. When MRI identifies a clear focal lesion—mesial temporal sclerosis (MTS), focal cortical dysplasia (FCD), tumor, vascular malformation—then excellent outcomes for surgery (Engel I–II) are high, in the order of 75%–90%, presuming that the entire lesion is removed. When motor, sensory, or eloquent areas known to be in the epileptogenic zone are not resected, then outcomes are less successful. In contrast, when MRI is normal and other functional imaging findings are also normal, then the likelihood for excellent outcomes is, at best, 40%–50%, and closer to 30%. Video EEG (vEEG) and high-resolution MRI are a prerequisite before pursuing functional imaging that is performed to confirm or identify the seizure focus when structural imaging is normal or ambiguous. Functional imaging is also used to help target and reduce invasive monitoring (Fig. 6–1). Finally, if imaging findings are discordant with surface vEEG, then caution is warranted; if surgery is to be pursued, invasive monitoring is essential and outcome success is reduced.

In the setting of a focal lesion, the seizure origin often arises from the margin of an identified tumor, FCD, stroke, or vascular malformation. In this circumstance, surgical planning may include functional imaging to target invasive monitoring to identify the adjacent epileptogenic cortex. Different approaches advocated by different epilepsy centers include: (1) removing the lesion, (2) perform intraoperative corticiography, or (3) conduct subdural grid monitoring.

▶ POSITRON EMISSION TOMOGRAPHY (PET)

There is extensive experience with FDG-PET in children and adults with childhood-onset epilepsy. FDG-PET is performed in the interictal state with EEG monitoring to assure an interictal study. Younger children, those less than 5 years, or significantly cognitively impaired, may require sedation before image acquisition, but after the period of ligand uptake, because sedating medications may reduce cerebral glucose metabolism. Abnormal findings, defined as greater than two standard deviations using quantitative measures, are usually focal. They are typically decreases in regional glucose uptake, representing decreased regional cerebral metabolism for glucose. Focal PET abnormalities are invariably ipsilateral to the seizure focus. However, the area of decreased metabolism is typically more widespread than the epileptogenic zone. While properly lateralizing, FDG-PET may not always provide lobar localization—proper lobar localization occurs in approximately 80%–90% of those with abnormal PET. FDG-PET does not provide additional information when MRI is unambiguously abnormal. When MRI is normal, FDG-PET will be abnormal in 60%–70% of temporal lobe epilepsy patients, and 30%–50% of extratemporal lobe epilepsy patients. Focal abnormality on FDG-PET is associated with good surgical outcomes in more than 90% of patients with temporal lobe epilepsy. Voxel-based morphometry methods may improve this yield, but are not clearly related to improved surgical outcome. The reasons for regional hypometabolism

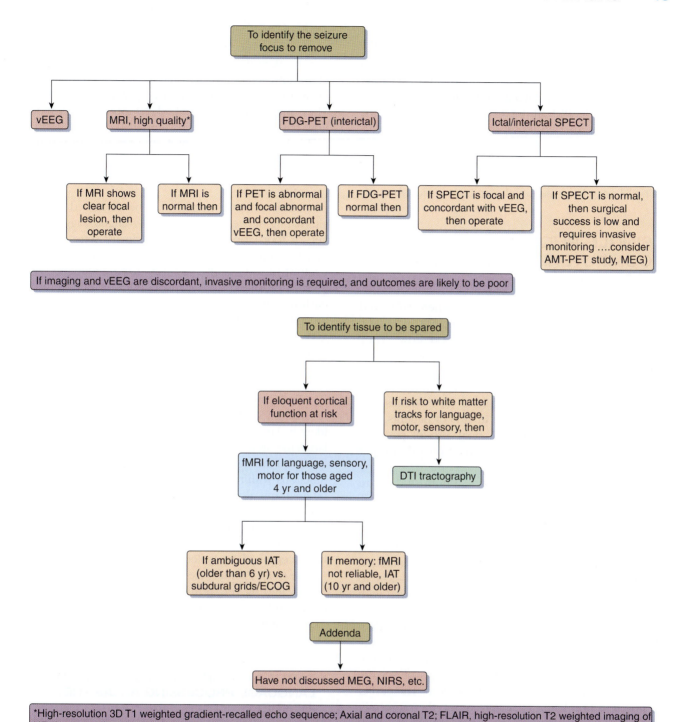

Figure 6–1. Imaging evaluation flow diagram.

are unknown, but may reflect neuronal loss in some patients and functional perturbations in others. As a consequence FDG-PET may help identify subtle dysplasia not apparent on MRI. In children less than 2 years old, before myelination is mature, FDG-PET may provide a valuable ability to identify abnormalities not seen on MRI. For children being evaluated for

hemispherectomy, FDG-PET abnormalities in the "good" hemisphere predict poor surgical outcome.

The role of other PET ligands in the evaluation of children with epilepsy is not yet fully established. Flumazinil is a benzodiazepine antagonist PET ligand that is used to identify GABAergic abnormalities. Flumazinil PET abnormalities may be more focal and restricted than

FDG-PET abnormalities but clear advantage in surgical planning has not been clearly demonstrated. Alpha-methyl tryptophan (AMT)-PET, a marker of serotonin synthesis or perhaps synthesis of neurokinin excitatory amino acids, may help identify the epileptic zone especially when FDG-PET shows a widespread abnormality; AMT-PET may also be useful in a minority of patients when FDG-PET and MRI are normal—mostly younger children, or children with failed resections. In the setting of multiple lesions, as occurs in tuberous sclerosis, then AMT-PET may help identify the epileptogenic tuber(s).

► SINGLE-PHOTON EMISSION COMPUTERIZED TOMOGRAPHY (SPECT)

Ictal/interictal SPECT may be useful when MRI, and FDG-PET are normal. The SPECT ligands, HMPAO, and ECD are markers of cerebral blood flow. They have advantages over PET given their longer half-life (6 hours vs. 20–90 minutes), but are not amenable to quantitation. Interictal SPECT is unreliable in identifying the seizure focus as interictal blood flow studies will provide false-lateralizing results in 10% of patients, and provide proper lateralization in only 50% of patients. However, ictal SPECT is more likely to provide proper lateralization and localization.

Ictal SPECT is most helpful when both studies are normalized and coregistered and the interictal SPECT is subtracted from the ictal study. When a clear focal lesion is present, then SPECT provides little additional information, unless lesion is large and one wishes further localization on the margin of the lesion. Subtraction SPECT is reported to improve yield from 35%–40% to 65%–75% when MRI is normal and is unassociated with improved surgical outcome.

If multiple structural lesions are present, then SPECT may help identify the focus. Ictal SPECT is only as reliable as the quality of the seizure captured. The ligand must be injected within 30 seconds of seizure cessation, and preferably during the seizure. The earlier the injection in relation to seizure onset, the more reliable and localizing the seizure focus. A potential confound is a given study may reflect propagation rather than seizure origin, a phenomena that likely accounts for the uncommon falsely lateralizing/localizing study. Also, if there are multiple seizure types, then any given study only reflects origin of that seizure type.

► FUNCTIONAL LOCALIZATION

After the seizure focus or epileptic zone has been identified, it may then be necessary to identify brain regions to be spared or avoided during surgery. While there is usually little disruption in the expression of primary and sensory functions, the cortex subserving language may be perturbed by epilepsy or its underlying causes. Motor and sensory cortex may be identified intraoperatively by evoked potentials or by cortical stimulation. They may also be identified by noninvasive blood-flow-based methods—^{15}O-water PET or fMRI. fMRI in pediatric populations is preferred because of radiation exposure, but some patients with implantable devices or extreme claustrophobia may not be studied with MRI for safety reasons.

Primary motor cortex may be identified by fMRI alternating between a motor task—tongue wiggling, finger, or foot tapping—and rest. Primary sensory cortex may be identified by brushing the face, hand, or foot in contrast to rest. Auditory cortex may be identified with a series of tones, and occipital cortex by checkerboard flash paradigms, again compared to rest. These studies are conducted when these areas are at risk during surgery. They usually are performed for planning resection of a lesion adjacent to, or within, motor sensory cortex, or for nonlesional frontal/parietal epilepsy when the margin of the resection may be unclear.

Epilepsy is associated with atypical language representation in 30% of patients. While it is uncommon to identify language processing outside of the traditional language areas in the left hemisphere and their homologues in the right hemisphere, the location of language functions within these broad areas cannot be predicted by anatomy alone. Often language is partially or completely shifted to the contralateral, typically nondominant (right) hemisphere for language.

Different aspects of language functioning can be ascertained by selection of the appropriate task (Table 6–1). Frontal "expressive" cortex (Broca's area) is activated by verbal fluency or decision tasks (generating a list of words to categories, letters, noun–verb, or deciding category or rhyme). Temporal "receptive"

► TABLE 6–1. FMRI PARADIGMS AND THE LANGUAGE PROCESSING AREAS THEY IDENTIFY

fMRI Paradigm	Targeted Area (Dominant)
Verbal fluency—words, letters	IFG (BA 44, 45)
Verbal fluency—noun–verb	IFG (BA 44, 45), STS (BA 22)
Semantic/phonological decision	IFG (BA 47, 44, 45), STS (BA 22, 37)
Story reading	IFG (BA 44, 45), STS (BA 21, 22, 39)
Story listening	STS (BA 22, 39)
Word definition, grammatical decision	IFG (BA 47, 44, 45), STS (BA 21, 22, 39)

cortex (Wernicke's area) is best identified by reading or auditory comprehension tasks using phrases, sentences, or stories. The more grammatically complicated or sophisticated the task the greater bilateral activation will be elicited. It is important to choose tasks that target the area at risk. A panel of tasks is advised to assure consistency of findings. These methods are reliable in 90% of patients and overt disagreement is rare. There is partial disparity between invasive tests such as intracarotid amobarbital test (IAT) and fMRI in up to 10% of patients; in these circumstances one method shows bilateral the other unilateral language dominance. fMRI-negative areas in general are safe to resect. fMRI cannot ascertain whether activated areas are critical to the function tested. There are some circumstances when fMRI may be unreliable as the blood oxygen level dependent (BOLD) response is disrupted, they include large tumors with edema and mass effect, vascular malformations with a vascular steal, critical carotid stenosis, and postictal states.

fMRI memory paradigms are as yet unreliable to lateralize memory functions in relation to postoperative outcomes. There is evidence, in adults, for material specificity (verbal tasks tend to activate left hippocampus) and visual tasks right HF, and some evidence for prediction of postoperative memory for experimental measures only but cannot be generalized to other memory measures. No memory studies have been reliably conducted in children.

Reliable and useful data can be obtained in 93% of patients with childhood epilepsy who are seven and older and who have normal intelligence. Eighty percent of typically developing 4 to 5 year olds can also be imaged. Obtaining image data in children with significant cognitive impairment (IQ 55–65) is possible in older children and teenagers. In contrast, obtaining useful information in children younger than nine with cognitive impairments, attention deficit hyperactivity disorder (off medications), or oppositional defiant disorder is challenging and may require several scanning sessions (50%–65% chance each session).

▶ DIFFUSION TENSOR IMAGING

DTI methods now allow identification of short- and long-fiber white matter tracts. This technology has been useful to identify, preoperatively, essential fiber tracts prior to lesion resection, usually tumor or dysplasia. Long tracts may be displaced by pathological lesions, and their identification informs surgical approach as well as areas to avoid. These issues are important for sensory-motor tracts, optic radiations, and long-fiber tracts connecting Wernicke's and Broca's areas.

REFERENCES

1. Chiron C, Vera P, Kaminska A, Hollo A, Cieuta C, Ville D, Dulac O. Single-photon emission computed tomography: ictal perfusion in childhood epilepsies. *Brain Dev* 1999;21: 444–446.
2. Gaillard WD. Functional MRI of language, memory and sensorimotor cortex. *Neuroimaging Clin N Am* 2004;14: 471–485.
3. Juhasz C, Chugani HT. Imaging the epileptic brain with positron emission tomography. *Neuroimaging Clin N Am* 2003;13:705–716.

CHAPTER 7

The Role of Guidelines in the Management of Childhood Epilepsy

Colin Dunkley and J Helen Cross

Epilepsy guidelines mean different things to different people, probably related to the wide variety of guidelines that are in existence. This chapter discusses the role that clinical guidelines can potentially play in contributing to the improved care of children and young adults with seizures and epilepsy. Examples from the United Kingdom are used to illustrate how guidelines can also have a wider role in supporting the development of services as part of a wider quality improvement agenda.

▶ DEFINITION

A clinical guideline can be thought of simply as set of recommendations designed to help a health professional deliver best practice. Field and Lohr provided a more formal definition stating that clinical practice guidelines are *"systematically developed statements to assist practitioner and patient decisions about appropriate health care for specific clinical circumstances."*[1] The Scottish Intercollegiate Guidelines Network (SIGN) adds the context *"they are intended as neither cookbook nor textbook but, where there is evidence of variation in practice which affects patient outcomes and a strong research base providing evidence of effective practice, guidelines can assist healthcare professionals in making decisions about appropriate and effective care for their patients.*[2] The challenge, therefore, for the epilepsies is translating the existing research base and range of professional opinions into effective guidelines. These guidelines must serve a population with a heterogeneous range of complex evolving diagnoses who interact with many different types of service in both hospital and community settings.

Epilepsy guidelines can vary in terms of their aims and scope, production method, subject matter, and subsequent implementation. Each will be considered in turn. In the first instance, subject matter may define the target of the guideline, in epilepsy this may be by seizure or syndrome, or by treatment. Illustrative UK examples are given in Table 7–1; a similar diversity is seen among the American Academy Practice Parameters.[3]

▶ DIFFERENT AIMS AND SCOPE

Often the aims and scope are of vital importance as they define the guideline's purpose and control the context in which the guideline should be used. Guidelines even for a given disease or problem can therefore vary considerably depending on this purpose and the intended user, healthcare setting and patient. This is important as ideally the role of a guideline should be intrinsically defined. These variations in aims and scope are illustrated in Table 7–2.

An example how these differences may manifest is illustrated using guidelines developed for the management of "status epilepticus." A guideline for "status epilepticus," using a standard definition of status as a convulsive seizure lasting longer than 30 minutes, is better framed operationally as a guideline for prolonged seizures such that steps can be recommended sooner than the 30-minute definition. If a guideline for management of prolonged convulsions is designed only for professionals in an Emergency Department, then it is likely to be inappropriate for paramedics on the way to hospital or professionals wishing to treat a child starting to seize on a pediatric ward. If the guideline is designed to manage the child's clinical course across multiple healthcare settings, for example, from the start of their seizure at school to intensive care, then the roles and actions for different professionals along the patient's course need to be explicit. It is easy to see given this how guidelines can have limited or detrimental effects if they are used in inappropriate patients or healthcare settings.

In an audit of the management of status epilepticus in North London, Chin et al highlighted significant deviation from well-established national guidelines.[9] The likelihood of an intensive care admission was associated with excessive numbers of doses of benzodiazepines and delayed administration of phenytoin. One response to these audit findings is to produce guidelines with a scope defining how prehospital and hospital teams can link their care, making the guideline more pragmatic, aiding timely, and accurate administration of phenytoin. The Children's Epilepsy Workstream in Trent (CEWT) and North Central London Epilepsy

▶ **TABLE 7–1.** UK EXAMPLES OF GUIDELINES DEFINED BY SEIZURE, TYPE OF EPILEPSY OR TREATMENT

- Childhood epilepsies[4,5]
- Febrile convulsion[6]
- First afebrile seizure[6]
- Prolonged convulsions[7]
- Specific epilepsy types, e.g., infantile spasms[8]
- For particular treatments (e.g., ketogenic diets, VNS adjustments, drug regimes)
- For investigations (e.g., melatonin for sleep EEGs)

Network for children have produced guidelines that account for these issues.[10,11]

▶ METHODOLOGY FOR GUIDELINE DEVELOPMENT

It is increasingly recognized that the production method of a guideline is an important determinant of its quality and acceptance by users. Guideline production should ideally involve all relevant stakeholders and use transparent and rigorous mechanisms for translating the evidence base and range of opinions into consensus recommendations. The user should be easily able to understand the "origins" of a guideline they may be using and the "weighting" of any recommendations made. The process of achieving consensus is of particular relevance in epilepsy as often the available evidence base is insufficient to provide comprehensive recommendations. The Delphi method, AGREE (Appraisal of Guidelines Research and Evaluation),[12] and consensus conferences[13] are examples of such approaches. Some of the difficulties of this process when applied to epilepsy are illustrated by a subsequent appraisal of the NICE guidelines for the management of the epilepsies.[14]

▶ DIFFERENT IMPLEMENTATION REQUIREMENTS

Some guidelines require little implementation; they already mirror current practice, are straightforward to

▶ **TABLE 7–2.** VARIATIONS IN AIMS AND SCOPE SEEN WITHIN GUIDELINES

- Diagnosis-based vs. problem-based
- Single service vs. multiple services
- Single professional vs. multiple professionals
- Single issue vs. multiple recommendations
- Immediately deliverable vs. aspirational
- Local vs. regional vs. national vs. international
- Reference guide-type recommendations vs. recommendations integrated into proformas, care pathways, electronic systems

follow, have no added cost, and are easily achievable. By contrast, other guidelines produce recommendations that contrast with current practice, are complex, may have cost issues, and may require extra interventions in order to be achieved. Guidelines for children with recurrent epileptic seizures often fall into the latter category.

▶ REASONS WHY GUIDELINES ARE USEFUL IN THE EPILEPSIES

Concerns regarding quality of care and misdiagnosis within seizures and epilepsy are part of the reason why there have been repeated calls for improvements made in media, political, and health settings.[15] Guidelines provide part of an essential response to this in terms of "articulating" what best practice looks like and prompting professionals to work together. Sometimes guidelines provide practical recommendations, for example, SIGN recommends a 12-lead ECG for all children with convulsive seizures. In other situations, for example prolonged convulsive seizures, clear guidelines can allow timely consistent team-based interventions where disagreement and deliberation may be detrimental.

▶ REASONS WHY GUIDELINES CAN BE DIFFICULT TO DEVELOP AS WELL AS ADOPT

The childhood epilepsies present significant diagnostic difficulties, heterogeneity, and variability in presentation. The terminology has guidelines of its own[16] and this language and thinking changes regularly making existing guidelines based on out-of-date classifications redundant or confusing. Many children with epilepsy have a number of conditions that can extend at different times beyond a single guideline. Also the population of children with epilepsy requires a large range of guidelines, and it can be difficult to choose which one is appropriate for a given child. This inter-relationship between guidelines is illustrated by the CEWT framework of guidelines that has attempted to provide initial guidance for any child, presenting with any seizure type, to any healthcare setting (Fig. 7–1).

There is an argument to be made against too much uniformity particularly where the evidence base is unclear. Variation and appropriate creativity can prompt valid research hypotheses and steps toward next year's evidence base.

In summary, the role of a guideline should therefore be defined within itself, within its own aims and scope. The ability of that guideline to achieve that role is strengthened by its "production pedigree" and this should be clear to the user. A guideline where required should prompt and define further implementation strategies to

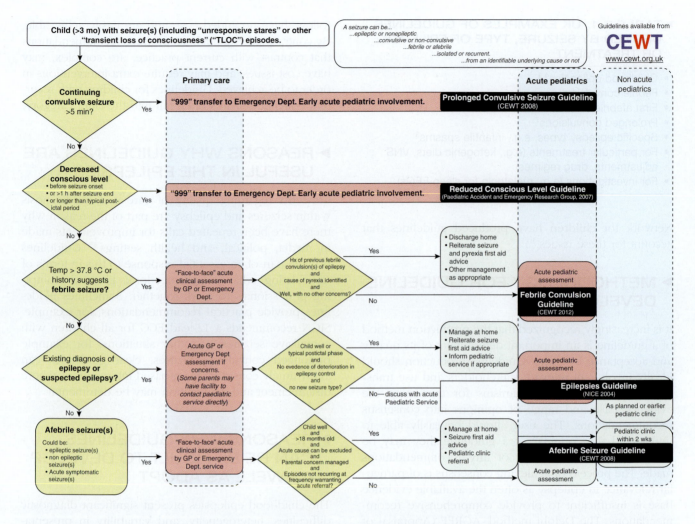

Figure 7–1. Seizure Guideline Framework, CEWT. (From Children's Epilepsy Workstream in Trent. Guideline for the management of prolonged convulsive epileptic seizures in children and young people. www.cewt.org.uk, 2008.)

achieve its intended role. There is a strong argument toward the need for an expanding portfolio of guidelines for children with epilepsy in line with an evolving and more specific evidence base, but we should not underestimate the challenges that this may present.

▶ THE ROLE OF UK NICE GUIDELINES FOR THE DIAGNOSIS AND MANAGEMENT OF THE EPILEPSIES IN PRIMARY AND SECONDARY CARE—AN EXAMPLE

The UK experience regarding the challenges of implementation of the NICE guideline is used as an example. As a response to continuing concerns regarding the care and provision for children and adults with epilepsies, NICE published recommendations for management of adults and children in October 2004, after 2 years of development.[4]

The Guideline Development Group used the AGREE.[12] The guideline aimed *"to provide best practice advice on the diagnosis, treatment and management of the epilepsies in children and adults."* Its scope included that it was *"intended for use by individual healthcare professionals, people with epilepsy and their carers and healthcare commissioning organisations and provider organisations."* They were designed for healthcare professionals in primary, secondary, tertiary centers, and emergency departments and covers diagnosis, treatment, and management of epilepsy in children and adolescents, but not neonates (Fig. 7–2).

Although the numerous recommendations were specific and practical, strategies for implementation were not included. The recommendations however implied changes not only in an individual's practice but also a change to the setting in which that practice was delivered. Many of the subsequent initiatives that have followed have been to clarify recommendations, support implementation, and develop parallel initiatives also centered on improving care and outcomes. The

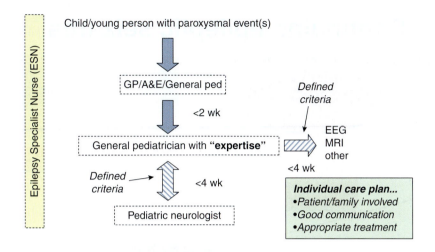

Figure 7–2. "NICE in a nutshell." A schemata summarizing NICE epilepsies guideline for children.

role of this guideline has been therefore not only to provide clinical recommendations but also to stimulate further service developments and catalyze change.

THE "PAEDIATRICIAN WITH EXPERTISE"

The NICE guidelines state that all children with a recent onset suspected seizure (or where there is diagnostic doubt) should see *"a specialist."* The definition of the specialist is stated as *"a paediatrician with training and expertise in the epilepsies."* This individual is defined as playing a key role in the diagnosis and management of epilepsy, but at the time of publication the exact definition of who this was and their required competencies were not stated. This has prompted a national education program developed by the British Paediatric Neurology Association (BPNA) (Paediatric Epilepsy Training, PET courses[17]) designed to help meet the training needs of such individuals and a proposed competencies package to support trainees working toward this consultant role.[18]

EPILEPSY SPECIALIST NURSES

"Epilepsy Specialist Nurses (ESNs) should be an integral part of the network of care of individuals with epilepsy. The key roles of the ESNs are to support both epilepsy specialists and generalists, to ensure access to community and multi-agency services and to provide information, training and support to the individual, families, carers and, in the case of children, others involved in the child's education, welfare and well-being."[4] Although the guidelines recommended every child with epilepsy should have access to a children's ESN, 3 years on

there were still only approximately 35 children's ESNs in the United Kingdom, a significant shortfall from the projected UK need of 300.[19] Despite this being a central recommendation, this has disappointingly proved insufficient incentive for providers or commissioners to fund such posts.

PEDIATRIC NEUROLOGISTS

There remain insufficient pediatric neurologists within the United Kingdom.[20] Recommendations on when referral to tertiary care should be considered are included and consequently should have resulted in a rationalization of tertiary involvement, but it remains unclear to what extent neurologists are seeing the appropriate children. This is an example of the difficulties that arise regarding assessing implementation where the outcome is difficult to measure and therefore potentially invisible. This also emphasizes the importance of systematic audit in order to evaluate the success of guideline implementation.

DEFINING COMPETENCIES

A "cookbook doesn't make a cook" and similarly a professional with a guideline in their hand does not make a competent professional; even the best guidelines are not sufficient to ensure competence in the user. Furthermore, there are risks if guideline recommendations are applied by professionals or services that do not have the relevant competence. The BPNA have worked with the royal college of paediatrics and child health (RCPCH) to develop a special study module and curriculum of competencies that define the knowledge and skills of "paediatricians with expertise" alongside those of a

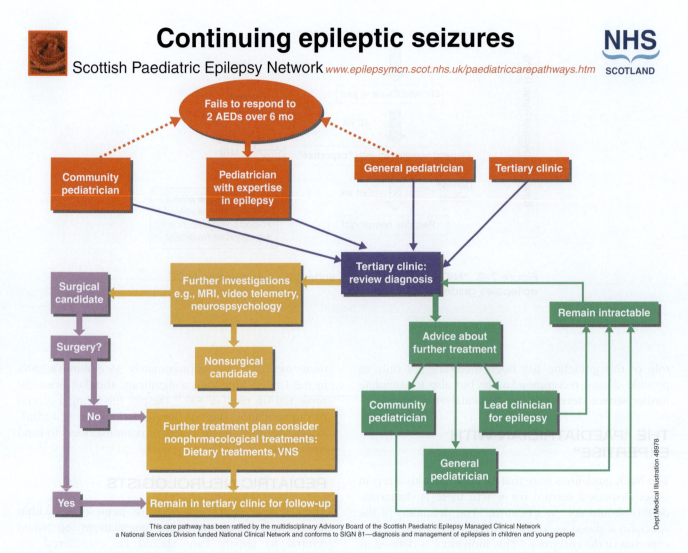

Continuing epileptic seizures

Scottish Paediatric Epilepsy Network www.epilepsymcn.scot.nhs.uk/paediatriccarepathways.htm

NHS SCOTLAND

This care pathway has been ratified by the multidisciplinary Advisory Board of the Scottish Paediatric Epilepsy Managed Clinical Network
a National Services Division funded National Clinical Network and conforms to SIGN 81—diagnosis and management of epilepsies in children and young people

Dept Medical Illustration 48978

Figure 7–3. Scottish Paediatric Epilepsy Network care pathway based on SIGN guidelines. From www.spen. scot.nhs.uk.

"paediatric neurologist."[18] It is acknowledged within such a curriculum that the service in which the professional works also requires "competencies" of its own.

MANAGED CLINICAL NETWORKS

Whereas the SIGN guidelines in Scotland have been followed up with a managed clinical network, this has not been the case for the rest of the United Kingdom.[21] Networks can potentially provide a number of activities to support implementation that cannot be achieved by an individual. They can create a perspective that considers the needs of the whole population and the "competencies" of all the steps in the whole care pathway. They can provide support for organization of educational and clinical meetings, communication between professionals, Websites with downloadable resources, coordinate audit and research, developing further guidelines,

specific-care pathways, and educational courses. It is difficult to imagine how epilepsy recommendations can be fully realized without such networks (Fig. 7–3).

TRAINING

Initial and continuing education for all those involved in the patient's journey is vital. A national educational program of Paediatric Epilepsy Training at three levels was established in 2004 in the United Kingdom.[17] PET1 is aimed at health professionals who anticipate clinical contact with children with suspected epileptic seizures. PET2 is for pediatricians and specialist nurses who provide clinical management, and are further developing expertise in epilepsy, and PET3 for those with tertiary level responsibilities. Standardized courses have been "rolled out" nationally allowing participants to obtain appropriate and continuing training that contributes to their competence. The NICE, SIGN, and **International League Against Epilepsy** guidelines have been an essential tool in providing a practical syllabus, translating how recommended practice might look in tutorial-based scenarios, and provide a consistent "educational" spine to underpin the learning aims throughout the courses.

AUDIT AND PERFORMANCE INDICATORS

NICE guidelines have identified standards against which audit can be conducted. In 2010 following a succession of pilots, a national audit was commissioned by the Department of Health.[22] Performance indicators mapped to specific recommendations within NICE and SIGN were defined. The audit systematically describes service provision, evidence of adherence to recommendations within rigorously defined patient groups and patient experience. It is designed as an audit of services rather than simply an individual's adoption of recommendations into their own practice.

► CONCLUSIONS

A guideline should hover restlessly among scientific evidence, expert opinion, local healthcare systems, and the patient population. A guideline need not be seen as a glossy document filed safely above an office desk. Even when appropriately produced and scoped, a guideline is rarely sufficient on its own; it needs to be digested, resourced, and implemented. Guidelines should not be seen as "rules," but "guidance" that should be adopted according to the local needs, utilized to the best of ability to improve practice. For a population's needs as broad and complex as children with epilepsies, good guidelines are only one important step toward what is needed. They need to be supported by a comprehensive package of supportive strategies. "What do I want my epilepsy guideline to do?" should be asked before a guideline is produced; "How do I ensure my epilepsy guideline delivers?" needs to be addressed when it has been produced.

REFERENCES

1. Field M, Lohr K. *Institute of Medicine Committee to Advise the Public Health Service on Clinical Practice Guidelines. Clinical Practice Guidelines: Directions for a New Program*. Washington, DC: National Academy Press, 1990.
2. Scottish Intercollegiate Guidelines Network. *SIGN 50: A Guideline Developer's Handbook*. Edinburgh, 2008.
3. American Academy of Pediatrics. *Pediatric Clinical Practice Guidelines & Policies*. Illinois, 2011; 11th edn.
4. National Institute for Clinical Excellence (NICE). *The Epilepsies: The Diagnosis and Management of the Epilepsies in Children and Young People in Primary and Secondary Care* Clinical Guideline20, 2004.
5. Scottish Intercollegiate Guidelines Network (SIGN). *Diagnosis and Management of Epilepsies in Children and Young People*. Edinburgh, 2005.
6. Armon K, Stephenson T, MacFaul R, Hemingway P, Werneke U, Smith S. Childhood seizure guideline an evidence and consensus based guideline for the management of a child after a seizure. *Emerg Med J* 2003;20:13–20.
7. Advanced Life Support Group. *Advanced Paediatric Life Support: The Practical Approach*. Massachusetts: Wiley-Blackwell, 2004; 4th edn.
8. Children's Epilepsy Workstream in Trent. Infantile spasms. www.cewt.org.uk, 2008.
9. Chin R, Verhulst L, Neville B, Peters M, Scott R. Inappropriate emergency management of status epilepticus in children contributes to need for intensive care. *J Neurol Neurosurg Psychiatry* 2004;75(11):1584–1588.
10. Children's Epilepsy Workstream in Trent. Guideline for the management of prolonged convulsive epileptic seizures in children and young people. www.cewt.org.uk, 2008.
11. Yoong M, Chin RFM, Scott RC. Management of convulsive status epilepticus in children. *Arch Dis Child Educ Pract Ed* 2009;94:1–9.
12. Appraisal of Guidelines Research and Evaluation. www.agreetrust.org.
13. Various consensus statements. www.rcpe.ac.uk.
14. Ferrie CD, Livingston JH. Epilepsy and evidence-based medicine: a vote of confidence in expert opinion from the national institute for clinical excellence? *Dev Med Child Neurol* 2005;47:204–206.
15. Clinical Standards Advisory Group (CSAG). *Services for Patients with Epilepsy*. London: Department of Health, 2000.
16. Engel J, ILAE Commission. A proposed diagnostic scheme for people with epileptic seizures and with epilepsy. *Epilepsia* 2001;42(6):796–803.
17. Paediatric Epilepsy Training. www.bpna.org.uk/pet.
18. A framework of competences for the Level 3 Training Special Study Module in Paediatric Epilepsy. www.rcpch.ac.uk, 2009.
19. Dunkley C, Cross JH. NICE guidelines and the epilepsies: how should practice change? *Arch Dis Chil* 2006;91:525–528.
20. A national approach to epilepsy management in children and adolescents. Submission by Royal College of Paediatrics and Child Health to Chief Medical Officer for England. www.bpna.org.uk, 2002.
21. Scottish Paediatric Epilepsy Network. www.spen.scot.nhs.uk.
22. Epilepsy12—United Kingdom collaborative clinical audit of health care for children and young people with suspected epileptic seizures. www.rcpch.ac.uk/epilepsy12.

SECTION II
Seizures in the Newborn and Infant

CHAPTER 8

Benign Neonatal Convulsions

Israel Alfonso

▶ OVERVIEW

Benign familial neonatal convulsions (BFNC) and benign nonfamilial neonatal convulsions (BNFNC) should be suspected in healthy-looking neonates with no interictal neurological deficit. These syndromes should be considered only after excluding benign nonepileptic paroxysmal motor events such as benign neonatal sleep myoclonus and behavioral movements, etiological-treatable seizures such as those due to sepsis and hypoglycemia, and more frequent causes of neonatal seizures associated with normal interictal neurological examinations such as subarachnoid bleed and hypocalcemia.

▶ BENIGN FAMILIAL NEONATAL CONVULSIONS

ETIOLOGY

The first description of BFNC was made by Rett and Teubel in 1964.[1] BFNC has an autosomal dominant mode of inheritance in most cases, but autosomal recessive and sporadic cases have been reported.[2] Patients with autosomal dominant BNFC have mutations in the two homologous genes: KCNQ2 (chromosome 20q) and KCNQ3 (chromosome 8q). These genes encode a subunit of the M-type voltage-gated potassium channel.[3] The autosomal recessive type of BFNC is associated with mutations of the sodium channel subunit gene SCN2A (chromosome 2q). In the later condition, some family members have neonatal-onset seizures whereas other members of the family have infancy-onset seizures.[4–6] Sporadic cases probably represent de novo mutations in the KCNQ2, KCNQ3, or SCN2A genes.

CLINICAL PRESENTATION

In patients with BFNC, seizures usually start between 2 and 15 days of birth, but most patients start having seizures at 2 or 3 days of age. Seizures tend to occur during sleep and are usually clonic. They may be focal or generalized. Generalized seizures tend to be asymmetrical due to immaturity of the corpus callosum. Seizures may be associated with apnea, vocalization, or chewing movements. The number of seizures during the first 2–3 months of age varies from a few to several dozen per day. The frequency of the episodes decreases during the following months and they are no longer present by 6 months of age.[2,7,8]

EEG FINDINGS

The interictal EEG is normal or may show minimal focal or multifocal abnormalities. A characteristic pattern named Theta Pointu Alternant has been reported, but it is not as frequently encounter as in benign idiopathic neonatal convulsions.[7] The ictal EEG consists of bilateral, symmetrical flattening for a few seconds followed by bilateral spikes and sharp waves discharges lasting for 1–2 minutes. This ictal pattern has led the authors to conclude that the convulsions of benign neonatal familial convulsions are a form of generalized seizure disorder.[8] Yet other authors consider the BNFC, a form of partial seizure disorder, based on their clinical manifestations.[9]

DIAGNOSIS

The clinical diagnosis of BNFC requires: (1) a family history of neonatal seizures in neurologically normal direct relatives, (2) a benign neonatal course, and (3) spontaneous cessation of seizures by 6 months of age.[2] Hence, the clinical diagnosis of BNFC cannot be made during the neonatal period. The diagnosis of BNFC can only be established in the neonatal period by detecting the gene mutations in KCNQ2, KCNQ3, or SCN2A. These mutations can be detected by using sequencing or multiplex ligation-dependent probe amplification.[4]

PROGNOSIS

The prognosis of BFNC is good. BFNC are not associated with mental retardation. The rate of febrile seizures in patients with BNFC is similar to the general population. Central temporal (rolandic) EEG foci without clinical manifestation have been reported in the follow-up of a few patients. Epilepsy occurs in 11%–14% of cases of BNFC.[2,10–12]

TREATMENT

Treatment of BNFC should be instituted when seizures are recurrent. The drug of choice is phenobarbital. The loading dose is from 20 to 40 mg/kg IV. Maintenance is 3–4 mg/kg per day PO or IV. The usual therapeutic range is 20–40 µg/mL. If seizures recur after achieving therapeutic levels, fosphenytoin should be added and later switched to phenytoin. The loading dose of fosphenytoin is from 10 to 20 mg/kg IV. Maintenance dose ranges from 2 to 4 mg/kg per day IV. The maintenance dose of phenytoin ranges from 2 to 4 mg/kg per day PO, but its absorption is erratic.[13,14] Vigabatrin decreased the frequency of seizures in patients who do not respond to phenobarbital or phenytoin.[15]

▶ BENIGN NONFAMILIAL NEONATAL CONVULSIONS

ETIOLOGY

BNFNC were first described by Dehan et al in 1977.[16] Other terms used to describe this condition are fifth day fits and benign idiopathic neonatal convulsions.[2,17]

The cause of BNFNC is unknown. The possibility of a viral etiology was initially considered.[16] Low zinc concentration in the CSF has been described.[17] More recently, a novel heterozygous mutation of KCNQ2 was

identified in a patient with benign nonfamilial neonatal seizures. The mutation was de novo verified by parentage analysis.[18] The classification of a patient with a mutation in the KCNQ2 as having benign nonfamilial neonatal seizures blurs the distinction between this entity and benign familial neonatal seizures.

CLINICAL PRESENTATIONS

In patients with BNFNC, seizures usually start between 4 and 6 days of age, but most patients start having seizures at 5 days of age. The seizures may be focal or generalized. The seizures are manifested by clonic movements or apnea. The presence of tonic seizures excludes the diagnosis of BNFNC. Status epilepticus may occur. The seizures tend to stop shortly after the neonatal period.[7,18,19]

EEG FINDINGS

The interictal EEG in these patients is normal. A characteristic pattern named Theta Pointu Alternant is frequently present. The presence of pathological paroxysmal patterns or any background abnormality including low voltage activity excludes the diagnosis.[7]

DIAGNOSIS

The diagnosis of BNFNC is established when the following criteria are met: (1) full-term birth, (2) normal pregnancy and delivery, (3) onset of seizures between 4 and 6 days of age, (4) normal neurological status before and between seizures, (5) clonic or apneic seizures or both, (6) no tonic seizures, (7) normal laboratory investigations, and (8) a normal interictal EEG. The presence of Theta Pointu Alternant supports the diagnosis.[7,18,19]

TREATMENT

Phenobarbital is probably the most used drug to manage BNFNC. In 1999, a French collaborative study recommended nonaggressive treatment aimed at controlling clinical seizures.[20]

▶ CONCLUSIONS

BFNC and BNFNC should be suspected in healthy-looking neonates with no interictal neurological deficit. Benign conditions such as benign neonatal sleep myoclonus, and common and treatable causes of epilepsy must be eliminated prior to considering either of these two age-dependent electroclinical syndromes. The diagnosis of BFNC can be made in the neonatal period by genetic studies. BNFNC is a diagnosis of exclusion. The first line of treatment of these disorders is phenobarbital.

REFERENCES

1. Rett A, Teubel R. Neugeborenen Krampfe im Rahmen einer epileptisch belasten familie. *Wiener Klinische Wochenschrift* 1964;76:609–613.

2. Plouin P. Benign idiopathic neonatal convulsions (familial and non-familial). In: Wolf P (ed), *Epileptic Seizures and Syndromes.* London: John Libbey, 1992; pp. 193–202.

3. Yalçin O, Cağlayan SH, Saltik S, Cokar O, Ağan K, Dervent A, Steinlein OK. A novel missense mutation (N258S) in the KCNQ2 gene in a Turkish family afflicted with benign familial neonatal convulsions (BFNC). *Turk J Pediatr* 2007; 49:385–389.

4. Heron SE, Cox K, Grinton BE, Zuberi SM, Kivity S, Afawi Z, Straussberg R, Berkovic SF, Scheffer IE, Mulley JC. Deletions or duplications in KCNQ2 can cause benign familial neonatal seizures. *J Med Genet* 2007;44:791–796.

5. Goutieres F. Convulsions neonatales familials benignes. In: *Congres de la societe de Neurologie infantile.* Marseille: Diffusion Generale de Librairie, 1977; pp. 281–286.

6. Herlenius E, Heron SE, Grinton BE, Keay D, Scheffer IE, Mulley JC, Berkovic SF. SCN2A mutations and benign familial neonatal-infantile seizures: the phenotypic spectrum. *Epilepsia* 2007;48:1138–1142.

7. Navelet Y, D'Allest AM, Dehan M, Gabilan JC. What's new about the fifth day seizures syndrome? *Rev Electroencephalogr Neurophysiol Clin* 1981;11:390–396.

8. Hirsch E, Velez A, Sellal F, Maton B, Grinspan A, Malafosse A, Marescaux C. Electroclinical signs of benign neonatal familial convulsions. *Ann Neurol* 1993;34:835–841.

9. Mizrahi EM, Kellaway P. *Diagnosis and Management of Neonatal Seizures.* Philadelphia: Lippincott-Raven, 1998.

10. Takebe Y, Chiba C, Kimura S. Benign familial neonatal convulsions. *Brain Dev* 1983;5:319–322.

11. Arzimanoglou A, Guerrini R, Aicardi J. *Aicardi's Epilepsy in Children.* Philadelphia: Lippincott Williams & Wilkins, 2004; pp. 188–209.

12. González Ipiña M, Roche Herrero MC, López Martín V, Hawkins Carranzo F, Sánchez Purificación MT, Pascual-Castroviejo I. Benign neonatal convulsions: review of 23 cases. *Neurologia* 1996;11:51–55.

13. Volpe JJ. *Neurology of the Newborn.* Philadelphia: WB Saunders Co, 1995; 3rd edn: pp. 172–207.

14. Painter MJ, Scher MS, Stein AD, Armatti S, Wang Z, Gardiner JC, Paneth N, Minnigh B, Alvin J. Phenobarbital compared with phenytoin for the treatment of neonatal seizures. *N Engl J Med* 1999;341:485–489.

15. Lee IC, Chen JY, Chen YJ, Yu JS, Su PH. Benign familial neonatal convulsions: novel mutation in a newborn. *Pediatr Neurol* 2009;40(5):387–391.

16. Dehan M, Quillerou D, Navelet Y, D'Allest AM, Vial M, Retbi JM, Lelong-Tissier MC, Gabilan JC. Convulsions in the fifth day of life: a new syndrome? *Arch Fr Pediatr* 1977;34:730–742.

17. Goldberg HJ, Sheehy EM. Fifth day fits: an acute zinc deficiency syndrome? *Arch Dis Child* 1982;57(8):633–635.

18. Ishii A, Fukuma G, Uehara A, Miyajima T, Makita Y, Hamachi A, Yasukochi M, Inoue T, Yasumoto S, Okada M, Kaneko S, Mitsudome A, Hirose S. A de novo KCNQ2 mutation detected in non-familial benign neonatal convulsions. *Brain Dev* 2009;31(1):27–33.

19. Pryor DS, Don N, Macourt DC. Fifth day fits: a syndrome of neonatal convulsions. *Arch Dis Child* 1981;56(10): 753–758.

20. Gautier A, Pouplard F, Bednarek N, Motte J, Berquin P, Billard C, Boidein F, Boulloche J, Dulac O, Echenne B, Humbertclaude V. Benign infantile convulsions. French collaborative study. *Arch Pediatr* 1999;6(1):32–39.

CHAPTER 9

Provoked and Nonprovoked Neonatal Seizures

Ronit M. Pressler and Eli M. Mizrahi

▶ OVERVIEW

Seizures are most common in the neonatal period (defined as the first 28 days of life or up to 44 weeks conceptional age) compared to any other period in life with an incidence of 1.5–3.5 per 1000 live births.[1–3] The incidence may vary according to birth weight, gestational age, and both antenatal and intranatal factors;[3–5] most notably, there is an increase risk for seizures in premature compared to full-term infants.

The time of seizure onset is usually within the first few days of life, with 80% of all neonatal seizures presenting within the first week of life.[1,4] Seizures in the neonatal period are also the most common neurological emergency and are associated with high potential mortality and morbidity.[6–10]

In contrast to seizures in infancy and childhood, most neonatal seizures are acute and symptomatic with suspected specific causes; relatively few seizures are idiopathic or symptomatic of a clearly defined epilepsy syndrome. Although neonatal seizures have many causes, a limited number account for most seizures (Table 9–1[11–15]). In term newborns, hypoxic–ischemic encephalopathy (HIE) is the most common underlying factor, typically beginning in the first 2 days of life. In preterm infants, intracranial hemorrhage (ICH) is the most common associated risk factor, although a direct relationship to seizure generation is unclear. Meningitis, focal cerebral infarction, transient metabolic disorders, and congenital abnormalities of the brain may cause seizures at any conceptional age.

The developing brain is particularly susceptible to developing seizures in response to injury; several mechanisms are likely to be involved. Overall the hyperexcitable state of the immature brain is based upon enhanced excitatory neurotransmission, paucity of inhibitory mechanisms, developmental expression of neuronal ion channels, age-dependent modulation of neuropeptides, and age-dependent early microglial activation.[16,17] An important contributing factor is that gamma-aminobutyric acid (GABA), considered the major inhibitory neurotransmitter in older children and adults, is initially excitatory in neonates and only later in development becoming inhibitory.[16,18] These mechanisms may also explain the different clinical semiology of neonatal seizures and the poor response to conventional antiepileptic drugs (AEDs) compared to older infants and children.

The immature brain was traditionally regarded to be less susceptible to seizure-induced injury. This has recently been challenged with the demonstration of long-term changes in behavior and cognition following seizures in animals with early-onset seizures.[19,20] This may in part may reflect cell death in specific neuronal populations, alteration of neuronal networks, and epigenetic changes that may contribute to neurodevelopmental disability and enhanced epileptogenesis following neonatal seizures in animals.[21–24] More recent clinical data present more conflicting data (see Prognosis below).[25,26]

▶ DIAGNOSTIC CRITERIA AND CLASSIFICATION

The clinical diagnosis of neonatal seizures may be difficult because clinical manifestations are highly variable with some features unique to that period of life.[27,28] Even among trained observers, clinical neonatal seizures may be difficult to recognize and differentiate from either normal behaviors or abnormal movements of nonepileptic origin.[29] Additional problems arise when the relationship between clinical and electroencephalographic (EEG) seizure are considered. There may be temporal overlap of the two (so-called "electroclinical seizures"). However, in some clinical settings up to 85% of electrographic seizures are clinically silent (i.e., EEG discharges with no clinical accompaniment, referred to as "electrical only seizures"), leading to significant underestimation of seizure burden.[30] In addition, some clinical seizures may occur in the absence of EEG seizure activity ("clinical only seizures"), but their clinical relevance is controversial.[31] For these reasons, in the broadest terms a seizure in this age group can be defined either in clinical terms as an abnormal paroxysmal event (with or without EEG seizure activity) or electrographically as a sustained epileptiform change in the EEG, which may or may not be accompanied by paroxysmal alteration in neurological function. However, unless all neonates at risk for seizures are

▶ **TABLE 9–1. COMMON CAUSES OF NEONATAL SEIZURES**

Cause	Frequency (%)
Hypoxic–ischemic encephalopathy	35–50
Intracranial hemorrhage	15–20
Cerebral infarction	5–20
Cerebral malformations	5–15
CNS infection	5–17
Acute	
Congenital	
Metabolic	5–30
Hypoglycemia	0.1–5
Hypocalcemia, hypomagnesemia	5–20
Hypo-/hypernatremia	
Inborn errors of metabolism	3–5
Maternal drug withdrawal	4
Neonatal epileptic syndromes	1–2
Early epileptic encephalopathy with suppression-burst (Ohtahara syndrome)	
Early myoclonic encephalopathy	
Benign familial neonatal convulsions	
Benign idiopathic neonatal convulsions (fifth day fits)	

Source: Adapted from Bergman I, Painter MJ, Crumrine PK. Neonatal seizures. *Semin Perinatol* 1982;6(1):54–67; Levene MI, Trounce JQ. Cause of neonatal convulsions. Towards more precise diagnosis. *Arch Dis Child* 1986;61(1):78–79; Estan J, Hope P. Unilateral neonatal cerebral infarction in full-term infants. *Arch Dis Child Fetal Neonatal Ed* 1997;76(2):F88–F93; and Mizrahi EM, Kellaway P. *Diagnosis and Management of Neonatal Seizures.* Philadelphia: Lippincott-Raven, 1998; 1st edn. Tekgul et al 2006.

subject to continuous neurophysiologic monitoring—an impractical strategy—clinicians must rely on bedside observation for initial recognition in susceptible infants, followed by diagnostic and then surveillance neurophysiologic studies.

Several features of seizure semiology in the neonatal period differ from those in infancy and childhood.

Neonatal seizures do not easily fit into traditional classification schemes.[27,28,32–34] While this continues to be a widely accepted tenant, the most recently proposed ILAE (The International League Against Epilepsy) classification suggested that neonatal seizures should not be considered a distinct seizure type, but could be classified within its more general, universal scheme—which would classify all neonatal seizures as either "focal seizures" or "other."[35]

There has been an evolution over several decades of the characterization and classification of neonatal seizures beginning with the pioneering work of French investigators utilizing clinical observation and EEG through the most recent work utilizing EEG-video monitoring. There was initial recognition that neonatal seizures had clinically distinct features,[32] then the development of standardized classification systems;[28,33,36] followed by more detailed characterization through initial EEG-video monitoring;[27,31] application of computer-assisted neurophysiological monitoring;[37–39] and most recently the use of EEG-video monitoring to refine techniques of clinical recognition and diagnosis.[29]

Neonatal seizures are classified by several different methods. They may be classified according to clinical features only: based upon either the most predominant clinical feature of the seizure or a more detailed description of the sequence of clinical events. A clinical classification includes: focal clonic, focal tonic, myoclonic, spasms, tonic, and motor automatisms (Table 9–2).[27] This scheme utilized the term "motor automatism" to refer to behaviors such as oral–buccal–lingual movements, ocular signs, and movements of progression including stepping, bicycling, and rotary limb movements. These events have also been referred to by as "subtle seizures" by Volpe.[28,33] In addition to these motor manifestations, some neonatal seizures may also have clinical features related to activation of the autonomic nervous system such as changes in heart rate, systemic blood pressure, and respirations,[28]

▶ **TABLE 9–2. CLASSIFICATION OF NEONATAL SEIZURES**

Seizure Type	Characterization	Pathophysiology
Focal clonic	Rhythmic muscle contractions; uni- or multifocal; cannot be restrained	Epileptic
Focal tonic	Sustained posturing of limb or trunk, sustained eye deviation; cannot be restrained	Epileptic
Myoclonic	Random single contractions; focal or generalized	May or may not be epileptic
Spasms	Flexor, extensor or mixed; may occur in clusters	Epileptic
Generalized tonic	Sustained symmetric posturing; flexor, extensor or mixed; may be stimulus sensitive; may be suppressed by restrain.	Nonepileptic, no EEG correlate
Motor automatism	Ocular (excluding tonic), oral–buccal–lingual, movements of progression	Nonepileptic, no EEG correlate
Electrographic seizures	By definition no clinical correlate	Epileptic

Source: Adapted from Mizrahi EM, Kellaway P. *Diagnosis and Management of Neonatal Seizures.* Philadelphia: Lippincott-Raven, 1998; 1st edn.

although these changes rarely occur in the absence of accompanying motor features.[27]

As discussed earlier, seizures may also be classified according to their electroclinical findings: the relationship between clinical and electrographic findings. When there is a temporal overlap of clinical and EEG seizures, the events are referred to as "electroclinical" seizures. Those events with only clinical manifestations are "clinical only" seizures, and those manifested only by EEG seizure activity are "electrical only" or subclinical.

Less frequently, seizures have also been classified according to their pathophysiology: epileptic or nonepileptic origin.[27] Seizures that are most clearly of epileptic origin are: focal clonic, focal tonic, some myoclonic, and spasms. Those that are more likely to be of nonepileptic origin are: generalized tonic, some myoclonic, and motor automatisms.

Traditionally, the ILAE has also included some neonatal epileptic syndromes in its classification.[34,40] Most recently, the ILAE proposed a revised syndromic classification that now includes: benign neonatal familial seizures, early myoclonic encephalopathy (EME), and Ohtahara syndrome (early infantile epileptic encephalopathy [EIEE]).[35] These syndromes will be discussed later.

Electrographically, all neonatal seizures have focal origin (except for epileptic spasms that are typically characterized by a generalized electrodetrimental event and some generalized myoclonic events, which may be generated at a subcortical level). The focal discharges may remain confined to one region or may spread to involve wider areas or the hemispheres opposite to the site of origin. One of the most common sites of seizure onset is the temporal lobe (Fig. 9–1), although they may arise from the frontal, occipital, central, or midline regions. Electrographic events may be brief, with 50% lasting less than a minute[41] and may tend to be shorter in preterm babies.[42] However, electrographic seizures may also be sustained over several minutes, with some even longer consistent with status epilepticus.

Clinical semiology is, for the most part, determined by site of origin and spread of electrographic seizures. When electrographic seizures remain confined to the neocortex, the clinical manifestations of seizures are predominantly motor; and most of neonatal seizure semiology is based upon these findings. However, in the neonate, the development within the limbic system with its connections to midbrain and brain stem is more advanced than the cerebral cortical organization, leading to a higher frequency of mouthing, ocular changes, apnea, and other clinical features related to the autonomic nervous system in neonates than in older children.

Electrographic seizures in the absence of clinical events may occur in a number of settings. The most obvious occurrence is in infants who have been pharmacologically paralyzed for respiratory care. These electrographic events may also occur in infants with

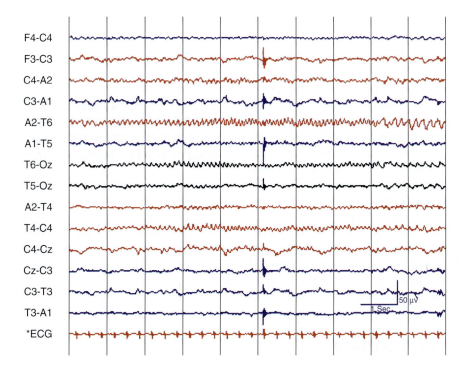

Figure 9–1. Term baby with late-onset streptococcal meningitis, now 7 days of age. Onset of seizures over right temporal region. The initial morphology is one of an "alpha seizure discharge," which evolves to rhythmic sharp waves.

severe encephalopathies and are characterized as "seizure discharges of the depressed brain"[43] and "alpha seizure discharges"[44,45] (Fig. 9–1).

In addition, the initial response to the therapy of electroclinical seizures with AEDs is characterized by control of the clinical events with the persistence of electrographic seizures—the clinical events is uncoupled from the electrographic events (see Section Treatment); also called electroclinical dissociation.[27,46] More recently, it has been suggested that hypothermia therapy for HIE may also uncouple electroclinical seizures, with a high incident of subclinical seizures in these cooled infants.[47,48]

▶ EPILEPSY SYNDROMES WITH ONSET IN THE NEONATAL PERIOD

Although by far the most neonatal seizures are acute and symptomatic, there are several well-defined syndromes which have their onset in the in the neonatal period including neonatal encephalopathies and errors of metabolism.[40]

BENIGN NEONATAL SEIZURES

Benign neonatal seizures (BNS) are also referred to as benign idiopathic neonatal convulsions and, historically, "fifth day fits." As the designation suggests, seizure onset occurs around the fifth day of life (day 1 to day 7, with 90% between day 4 and day 6) in otherwise healthy neonates. At present the etiology is unknown. Clinically, seizures are characterized as focal clonic variably accompanied by apneic.[49] The interictal EEG shows *theta pointu alternant* in approximately 60% of cases—although this finding is not unique to this disorder or diagnostic. In the remaining neonates, the background activity may be either discontinuous, with focal or multifocal abnormalities, or normal. Ictal recordings show unilateral or bilateral rhythmic spikes or slow waves. Treatment with AEDs may not be necessary, because of the self-limiting clinical course of the seizures. However, the diagnosis is one of exclusion. Seizures usually resolve within days. The outcome is good, but an increased risk of minor neurological impairment has been reported.[1] The incidence of BNS has diminished over the past several years to the point that ILAE in its recent proposed classification revision of epileptic syndromes did include BNS as a recognized syndrome.[35]

BENIGN FAMILIAL NEONATAL SEIZURES

Benign familial neonatal seizures (also referred to as benign familial neonatal convulsions [BFNC])[49] constitute a rare disorder with autosomal dominant inheritance with a mutation in the voltage-gated potassium channels genes (in most cases at 20q13.3, in a few families at 8q24).[50] Seizures occur mostly on the second or third day of life in otherwise healthy neonates and tend to persist longer than in benign idiopathic neonatal convulsions. They are mainly focal clonic, sometimes with apneic spells; tonic seizures have rarely been described. The background activity is normal with no specific pattern, although *theta pointu alternant* has also been associated with this disorder. Therapy is controversial and seizures usually resolve within weeks. The outcome is favorable, but secondary epilepsy may occur.

EARLY MYOCLONIC ENCEPHALOPATHY

EME is a syndrome often associated with inborn errors of metabolism, but cerebral malformations have also been reported.[51] Onset is nearly always in the first month of life. The clinical ictal manifestations include: (1) partial or fragmentary myoclonus, (2) massive myoclonias, (3) partial motor seizures, and (4) tonic spasms. Background EEG activity is characterized by a suppression–burst pattern—bursting consisting of complex bursts of spikes and sharp waves lasting for 1–5 seconds and periods of suppression lasting from 3 to 10 seconds in both waking and sleep. The EEG may later evolve toward atypical hypsarrythmia. Seizures are typically resistant to AED treatment, although hormonal therapy such as ACTH has been reported to may have some temporary effect. All infants are severely neurologically abnormal and half of them die before the age of 1 year.

EARLY INFANTILE EPILEPTIC ENCEPHALOPATHY WITH BURST–SUPPRESSION PATTERN (OHTAHARA SYNDROME)

Age of onset of EIEE is in the first 3 months of life with frequent tonic spasms (100–300 per day), often occurring in clusters. Partial seizures may also occur.[51] The EEG is characterized by a burst-suppression pattern, both in sleep and waking. It may be asymmetric, in part reflecting underlying etiologic factors. This syndrome is usually associated with cerebral malformations. Seizures are resistant to AED treatment, although it has been reported that ACTH may have some temporary effect. The prognosis is serious, but may be somewhat better than for EME. Evolution into infantile spasms is common. Both EME and EIEE have clinically and electrographically distinct features. However, there are also similarities, which have prompted some to suggest that they are not two syndromes, but rather part of a spectrum of a single disorder.[51]

▶ DIFFERENTIAL DIAGNOSIS

The differential diagnosis of clinical neonatal seizures includes: normal movements of the awake neonate (mouthing, jitteriness, random limb jerks, fisting, and stretching), REM sleep behavior, benign neonatal sleep myoclonus, excessive jitteriness, motor hyperexcitability associated with mild HIE, and abnormal nonepileptic events such as tonic posturing and motor automatisms (so-called brain stem release phenomenon). Typically, nonepileptic motor events stop with gentle restrain and are more likely to be stimulus sensitive, these criteria may not always be reliable and recently stimulus-sensitive seizures in infants with stroke have been described.[52] When changes in the measured parameters of autonomic nervous system function occur in the neonate, seizures may be suspected. However, changes in heart rate, system blood pressure, and respirations as seizure manifestations are rare, and other physiologic causes should be considered.

▶ MANAGEMENT (FIG. 9–2)

The overall strategy in management of neonatal seizures typically includes: addressing the infant's acute immediate medical needs (airway and circulatory access); initiation of assessment for treatable causes of seizures; initiation of etiologic-specific therapy; and initiation of AEDs if needed. Following medical stabilization, the identification of treatable causes of neonatal seizure is the next critical step in the management of seizures in

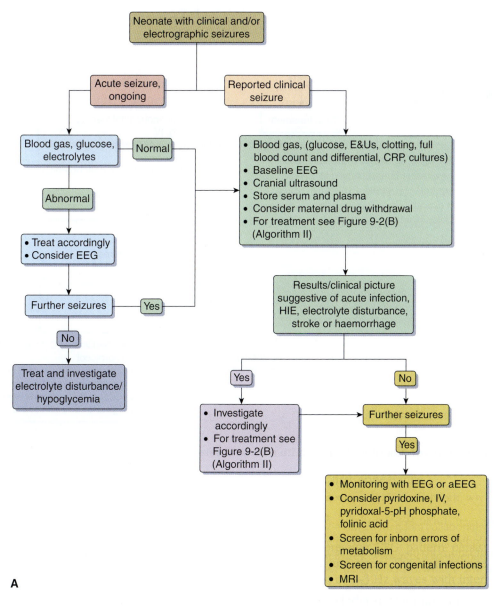

A

Figure 9–2. Algorithm I. (**A**) Acute neonatal seizures: investigations. *(continued)*

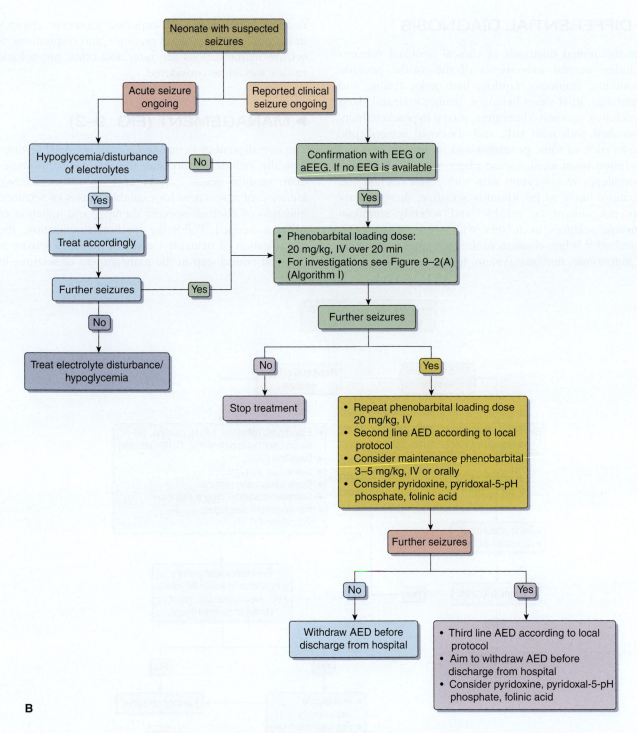

B

Figure 9–2. *(Continued)* Algorithm II. (**B**) Acute neonatal seizures: treatment.

this age group (see Table 9–3[53] and Fig. 9–2). Assessment is directed toward both major cause and toward the less frequent but more clearly treatable causes. Thus, assessment for the following etiological factors is initiated early after seizure recognition: HIE, central nervous system (CNS) infection, transient metabolic disturbances, and intracranial structural abnormalities.

With acute seizure onset routine studies to determine the infants metabolic status is performed. This includes assessment of arterial blood gas, serum glucose, and electrolytes including calcium and magnesium. This is followed by other basic laboratory screens. Septic screening will help to diagnose infections such as meningitis, septicemia, or encephalitis.

► **TABLE 9–3.** TREATMENT OF NEONATAL SEIZURES

Drug	Loading Dose	Route	Maintenance/Day	Route	Levels
Phenobarbital	20 mg/kg, may be repeated	IV	3–5 mg/kg	PO	90–180 µmol/L 20–40 mg/L
Phenytoin	15–20 mg/kg	IV/20 min	3–4 mg/kg	IV/PO	40–80 µmol/L 10–20 mg/L
Midazolam	60 µg/kg	IV	100–400 µg/kg/h	IV	
Lignocaine[a]	2 mg/kg	IV over 10 min	6 mg/kg/h for 6 h 4 mg/kg/h for 12 h 2 mg/kg/h for 12 h	IV	3–6 mg/L
Lorazepam	0.05–0.1 mg/kg	IV	Repeat BD or TDS		
Diazepam	0.2–1 mg/kg	IV			
Clonazepam	0.1 mg/kg	IV/30 min	Repeat OD	IV	30–100 mg/L
Pyridoxine (B6)	50–100 mg	IV	15–500 mg/kg/d (BD)		
Pyridoxal phosphate	100 mg	PO	10–50 mg/kg/d	PO	
Folinic acid (Ca folinate)	2.5 mg/kg	IV	2.5–5 mg BD	PO	
Biotin			5–20 mg/d	PO	
L-Serine (Serine deficiency)	400–600 mg/kg/d				
Creatine monohydrate (Creatine deficiency)	0.5–2 g/kg/d				

Note: Drug doses vary between countries and between hospitals. Local protocols and guidelines have to be considered. OD, once per day; BD, twice per day; TDS, three times per day; IV, intravenously; PO, per os (orally).
[a]For dosing recommendation, see Malingre MM, van Rooij LG, Rademaker CM, Toet MC, Ververs TF, van Kesteren C, de Vries LS. Development of an optimal lidocaine infusion strategy for neonatal seizures. *Eur J Pediatr* 2006;165(9):598–604.

Cranial ultrasound remains the first-line neuroimaging investigation in neonatal seizure because of its ready accessibility at the bedside. A head ultrasound scan (HUS) is typically performed at the first opportunity and repeated frequently thereafter, since some abnormalities only appear after several days, and in other cases the appearances evolve over time.[54] HUS may be normal or show one of the following abnormalities: ICH, focal cerebral infarction, cerebral edema, cerebral malformation, abnormalities of the deep gray matter or watershed areas, enlarged ventricles, or changes within the ventricles suggesting infection. Computerized axial tomography (CT) or magnetic resonance imaging (MRI) may be needed to compliment HUS studies, although somewhat less practical in the acute setting. The diagnosis of HIE is based upon historical and clinical data. Because of emerging evidence of the efficacy of acute hypothermia therapy in reducing morbidity and mortality of HIE, rapid diagnosis has become increasing more important.[55]

Following assessment for the more common and treatable causes of neonatal seizures, the potential of additional etiologies are explored. Family history, clinical presentation, EEG features (true suppression-burst pattern), and lack of response to AED treatment suggest the possibility of inborn error of metabolism and should be investigated accordingly. There are also a group of metabolic disturbances, which may present as otherwise medically intractable seizures (Table 9–4). Neonates with persistent seizures or suggestive EEG background abnormalities should all undergo a therapeutic trial with pyridoxine, pyridoxal-5-phosphate, and folinic acid.[56,57] Unexplained and persistent hypoglycemia should be thoroughly investigated (lactate, ammonia, amino acids, urine organic acids, urine ketones, insulin, cortisol, free fatty acids, and B-hydroxybutyrate). In addition, depending on the history other etiologic considerations should include congenital infections (TORCH), drug withdrawal (maternal toxicology screen), and genetic disorders.

Neurophysiological testing is important both in diagnosis and management. This may include: electroencephalography (EEG), continuous EEG monitoring (cEEG), EEG-video monitoring, and amplitude integrated EEG (aEEG) that is also referred to as cerebral function monitoring (CFM). Each technique has advantages and limitations in diagnosis and management,

► **TABLE 9–4.** TREATABLE METABOLIC SYNDROMES PRESENTING WITH NEONATAL SEIZURES

Pyridoxine dependency
Pyridoxal phosphate dependency
Folinic acid responsive seizures
Serine deficiency
Glucose transporter 1 deficiency
Biotinidase deficiency
Creatine deficiency
Untreated phenylketonuria

Source: Adapted from Pearl PL. New treatment paradigms in neonatal metabolic epilepsies. *J Inherit Metab Dis* 2009;32:204–213.

and application is dependent upon availability of both instrumentation and interpretive expertise. As seizures are difficult to diagnose clinically and a significant proportion of the total seizure burden in a given infant may be subclinical, neurophysiological testing is essential for the management of neonatal seizures. Neurophysiologic monitoring, with EEG or an EEG-reduced seizure burden.[58] However, consensus about what constitutes appropriate monitoring technique and duration is lacking, although raw EEG is considered the so-called "gold standard" with noted limitations of aEEG.[59] In addition, there is some controversy over what constitutes a true electrographic neonatal seizure. Some workers have chosen an arbitrary duration of 10 seconds, while others have chosen 5 seconds. The minimum duration, according to the latest IFCN (The International Federation of Clinical Neurophysiology recommendations,[60] is 5 seconds if the background activity is normal and 10 seconds if it is abnormal; although 10 seconds is most universally accepted as the minimum.[42] There is usually evolution of frequency, amplitude, and morphology over time, typically with an increase in amplitude and a decrease of frequency. At the other extreme, neonatal status epilepticus is defined as a total seizure time occupying 50% of a 30 minutes recording[5] although, here too, there is not consensus about the definition of status epilepticus. Abnormal background activity is associated with an increased risk of subsequent seizures and poor neurodevelopmental outcome.[61–63]

The amplitude-integrated EEG (aEEG) has the advantage that it is widely available, and interpretation using pattern recognition can easily be learned.[64] However, short seizures (<30 seconds) are often not detected, low amplitude or focal seizures are easily missed, and movement artefacts are difficult to exclude and may look like seizures. Thus, in neonates aEEG is prone to false-negative and false-positive errors.[37] Nonexperts are prone to false-negative errors and the interobserver agreement is low.[39,65]

▶ TREATMENT (FIG. 9–2)

Treatment of neonatal seizures involves initial consideration of etiologic-specific therapies and then consideration

of AEDs. Etiologic-specific therapy is guided by laboratory findings of transient metabolic disorders (e.g., hypoglycemia, hypocalcemia, hypomagnesemia; see Table 9–5) and clinical concern of CNS bacterial or viral infection.

Metabolic disorders are associated with otherwise medically intractable seizures, some of which are deficiencies of pyridoxine, folic acid, or biotinidase (Table 9–4). These should be treated accordingly (Table 9–3).

The decision to initiate AEDs is based upon the certainty of the diagnosis of clinical seizures and then on seizure duration, frequency, and severity. Clinicians must decide whether to treat with AEDs based either upon clinical observation alone, or may require confirmation of electrographic seizure activity in association with clinical events. For the most part, focal clonic seizures are the most reliably diagnosed clinical seizure type.[29] Thus, in the absence of EEG availability AED therapy may be initiated if these clinical events are present. For other types of clinical events, AED treatment may be started if and when EEG confirms that suspicious movements are indeed seizures or reveals subclinical seizures.

The AEDs available for treatment of neonatal seizures have not significantly changed over the last 50 years, although there have been recent reports of the use of newer medications (see later). Recently published surveys from Israel, Australia, United States, and Europe indicated a rather unanimous use of phenobarbitone as a first-line drug worldwide despite the fact that it has limited efficacy.[66–69] The choice of second- and third-line drugs vary, but in general include a benzodiazepine (midazolam or lorazepam), phenytoin (or fosphenytoin), and lidocaine.

A recent Cochrane report has reviewed the treatment of neonatal seizures.[70] Only two randomized controlled studies were identified using adequate methodology,[71,72] both indicating that current first-line treatment with phenobarbitone was only effective in about 40%–50% of babies. Furthermore, phenobarbitone increases the electroclinical uncoupling (or dissociation) of the clinical event from the electrographic event. Thus, while the number of electroclinical seizures decreases, the number of electrographic seizures may increase, making EEG monitoring necessary to optimize treatment.[73,74] It has been suggested that this

▶ **TABLE 9–5.** TREATMENT OF TRANSIENT METABOLIC DISTURBANCES ASSOCIATED WITH ACUTE NEONATAL SEIZURES

Metabolic Disturbances	Level	Route	Drug	Loading Dose
Hypoglycemia	BM <2.5 mmol/L	IV	10% dextrose	2 mL/kg bolus
Hypocalcemia	Ionized Ca <1.1 mmol/L	IV	10% calcium gluconate	2 mL/kg over 10 min
Hypomagnesemia	Mg <1.0 mmol/L	IV, IM	50% $MgSO_4$	0.2 mL/kg over 10 min

Note: Doses vary between countries and between hospitals. Local protocols and guidelines have to be considered. IV, intravenously; IM, intramuscular.

is due to a time difference of the GABA switch, which is earlier in thalamic compared to neocortical neurons.[75] In addition, with the increasing use of hypothermia to manage infants with HIE becomes another factor to consider when phenobarbitone is used to treat neonatal seizures. When phenobarbitone is administered to newborns under whole-body hypothermia, it results in higher plasma concentration and longer half-lives than expected compared to normothermic newborns.[76] There may also be an increased incidence of electroclinical dissociation seizures during therapeutic hypothermia and an increased risk of seizures during rewarming.[47,48,77]

Phenytoin (or fosphenytoin) and benzodiazepines (midazelam, lorazepam, or clonazepam) are used as second-line AED. Phenytoin can cause significant myocardial depression and should be avoided in babies requiring inotropic support. Clonazepam may achieve better EEG control. Midazolam has a shorter half-life than clonazepam and does not accumulate, and it avoids the side effect of increased oropharyngeal secretions. Others have reported success with lignocaine: between 70% and 92% of newborns responded to lignocaine as second-line AED. However, all these studies were uncontrolled, apart from one with small numbers. Lignocaine has a narrow therapeutic range and can induce seizures in high doses. Off-label use of antiepileptic drugs is not uncommon among American pediatric neurologists, despite a lack of information about safety or efficacy in newborns.[78] However, there are more recent studies providing information concerning safety and efficacy of topiramate[79,80] and leviteractam[81–84] in neonates.

There is little experience with carbamazepine, vigabatrin, and lamotrigine in the neonatal period.[69,79]

Although there appears to be several different potential AED strategies for neonatal seizure treatment, it is still possible to develop and implement a focused, well-designed plan of therapy. A first-line AED should be selected—typically phenobarbitone in an appropriate loading dose, followed by adequate maintenance dosing. Therapeutic serum levels should be achieved. If seizures persist, additional phenobarbitone dosing is given to achieve high therapeutic levels. If seizures still persist, a second-line drug is used—typically a benzodiazepine. This may be given as single boluses, repeated maintenance doses, or as a continuous infusion.[85] If seizures continue an additional drug is given—typically lignocaine[53] or phenytoin (up to high therapeutic levels). It should be noted that in some cases, even with aggressive AED therapy, neonatal seizures will not be effectively controlled. It is important to determine the relative risk/benefit ratio of further AED therapy compared to iagtrogenic generation of hypotension, respiratory depression, or cardiac arrhythmias. When pyridoxine

dependency is suspected, 100 mg of pyridoxine is given intravenously under EEG control. If the etiology is pyridoxine-related, the seizures will abruptly stop (within minutes) and the EEG will normalize during the next few hours. Acute suppression of EEG activity occurs occasionally and may be associated with acute cardiovascular collapse.[86] A subgroup of affected babies responds only to very high doses given for 2 weeks. A closely related disorder with a similar clinical picture has now been identified as pyridoxal-5-phosphate-dependent seizure.

In the United Kingdom and at some centers in the United States, babies are usually weaned of AED before they are discharged from hospital. Phenobarbitone treatment is maintained only if the infant is continuing to experience seizures. In the United States, only few neonatologists would stop antiepileptic drugs prior to discharge and treatment is continued for several months. Overall is unclear whether continuing AED treatment beyond the phase of acute seizures reduces the risk of secondary epilepsy later in childhood.

▶ PROGNOSIS

The outcome of infants who have experienced neonatal seizure is usually described in terms of survival and in the presence and degree of subsequent developmental delay, neurological motor impairment, and postneonatal epilepsy. Reported outcomes vary with study populations and methodology.[87–91] Approximately 25% of those with neonatal seizures die, and of the survivors, about 40% exhibit abnormal neurological examination, and about 50% experience some degree of developmental delay. In addition, approximately 25% have postneonatal epilepsy. These conditions may coexist.[10] Prognosis is mainly determined by the etiology, although other factors include antenatal and maternal factors and gestational age and birth weight with an overall better outcome for term than for preterm babies.[9,88] In HIE, the prognosis depends very much on the grade (overall 30%–50% normal), while CNS malformations are generally associated with poor outcome. Both animal and clinical studies suggest that neonatal seizures have an adverse effect on neurodevelopmental outcome, and predispose to cognitive, behavioral, or epileptic complications in later life.[15,92] However, recent clinical studies provide conflicting data. Glass and colleagues[26] report that clinical neonatal seizures in the setting of birth asphyxia are associated with worse neurodevelopmental outcome, independent of hypoxic–ischemic injury. However, Kwon and colleagues[25] did not find such an association in a population of infants with HIE treated with hypothermia. There is evidence that electrographic seizures have similar impact on long-term outcome as electroclinical seizures.[93]

There is also increasing concern about the potentially adverse effects of antiepileptic drugs on the developing nervous system. In animal models, phenobarbitone has been shown to cause additional brain injury by increasing neuronal death (apoptosis),[94,95] although some AEDs do not have this affect.[94] Better treatments for neonatal seizures have been identified as a high priority for research by several international expert groups with emphasis on new innovative strategies targeted specifically to the needs of babies with the ultimate aim to improve long-term outcome.[78,96]

Currently, the most effective way to limit adverse outcomes in terms of developmental delay, neurological disability, and epilepsy following neonatal seizures, it to identify the underlying etiology and identify and implement etiology-specific therapies.

REFERENCES

1. Ronen GM, Penney S, Andrews W. The epidemiology of clinical neonatal seizures in Newfoundland: a population-based study. *J Pediatr* 1999;134:71–75.
2. Saliba RM, Annegers JF, Waller DK, Tyson JE, Mizrahi EM. Incidence of neonatal seizures in Harris County, Texas, 1992–1994. *Am J Epidemiol* 1999;150(7):763–769.
3. Glass HC, et al. Antenatal and intrapartum risk factors for seizures in term newborns: a population-based study, California 1998–2002. *J Pediatr* 2009a;154:24–28.
4. Lanska MJ, et al. A population-based study of neonatal seizures in Fayette County, Kentucky. *Neurology* 1995;45:724–732.
5. Scher MS, Hamid MY, Steppe DA, Beggarly ME, Painter MJ. Ictal and interictal electrographic seizure durations in preterm and term neonates. *Epilepsia* 1993;34(2):284–288.
6. Holden KR, Mellits ED, Freeman JM. Neonatal seizures. I. Correlation of prenatal and perinatal events with outcomes. *Pediatrics* 1982;70(2):165–176.
7. Miller SP, et al. Seizure-associated brain injury in term newborns with perinatal asphyxia. *Neurology* 2002;58:542–548.
8. Pisani F, et al. A scoring system for early prognostic assessment after neonatal seizures. *Pediatrics* 2009;124:e580–e587.
9. Davis AS, et al. Seizures in extremely low birth weight infants are associated with adverse outcome. *J Pediatr* 2010;157:720–725.
10. Garkinfle J, Shevell MI. Cerebral palsy, developmental delay, and epilepsy after neonatal seizures. *Pediatr Neurol* 2011;44:88–96.
11. Bergman I, Painter MJ, Crumrine PK. Neonatal seizures. *Semin Perinatol* 1982;6(1):54–67.
12. Levene MI, Trounce JQ. Cause of neonatal convulsions. Towards more precise diagnosis. *Arch Dis Child* 1986;61(1):78–79.
13. Estan J, Hope P. Unilateral neonatal cerebral infarction in full-term infants. *Arch Dis Child Fetal Neonatal Ed* 1997;76(2):F88–F93.
14. Mizrahi EM, Kellaway P. *Diagnosis and Management of Neonatal Seizures.* Philadelphia: Lippincott-Raven, 1998; 1st edn.
15. Tekgul H, et al. The current etiologic profile and neurodevelopmental outcome of seizures in term newborn infants. *Pediatrics* 2006;117(4):1270–1280.
16. Ben Ari Y, Holmes GL. Effects of seizures on developmental processes in the immature brain. *Lancet Neurol* 2006;5:1055–1063.
17. Jensen FE. Neonatal seizures: an update on mechanisms and management. *Clin Perinatol* 2009;36(4):881–900.
18. Rakhade SN, Jensen FE. Epileptogenesis in the immature brain: emerging mechanisms. *Nat Rev Neurol* 2009;5(7):380–391.
19. Holmes GL. Effects of seizures on brain development: lessons from the laboratory, Pediatr. *Neurol* 2005;33:1–11.
20. Sayin U, Sutula TP, Stafstrom CE. Seizures in the developing brain cause adverse long-term effects on spatial learning and anxiety. *Epilepsia* 2004;45(12):1539–1548.
21. Wasterlain CG, Niquet J, Thompson KW, Baldwin R, Liu H, Sankar R, Mazarati AM, Naylor D, Katsumori H, Suchomelova L, Shirasaka Y. Seizure-induced neuronal death in the immature brain. *Prog Brain Res* 2002;135:335–353.
22. Holmes GL. The long-term effects of neonatal seizures. *Clin Perinatol* 2009;36(4):901–914.
23. Karnam HB, Zhou JL, Huang LT, Zhao Q, Shatskikh T, Holmes GL. Early life seizures cause long-standing impairment of the hippocampal map. Exp Neurol 2009;217:378–387.
24. Auvin S, Shin D, Mazarati A, Sankar R. Inflammation induced by LPS enhances epileptogenesis in immature rat and may be partially reversed by IL1RA. *Epilepsia* 2010;51(Suppl 3):34–38.
25. Kwon JM, et al. Clinical seizures in neonatal hypoxic-ischemic encephalopathy have no independent outcome: secondary analysis of data from the Neonatal Research Network Hypothermia Trial. *J Child Neurol* 2011;26:322–328.
26. Glass HC, et al. Clinical neonatal seizures are independently associated with outcome in infants at risk for hypoxic-ischemic brain injury. *J Pediatr* 2009b;155b:318–323.
27. Mizrahi EM, Kellaway P. Characterization and classification of neonatal seizures. *Neurology* 1987;37:1837–1844.
28. Volpe JJ. *Neurology of the Newborn.* Philadelphia: Saunders, 1987; 2nd edn.
29. Malone A, et al. Interobserver agreement in neonatal seizure identification. *Epilepsia* 2009;50(9):2097–2101.
30. Murray DM, Boylan GB, Ali I, Ryan CA, Murphy BP, Connolly S. Defining the gap between electrographic seizure burden, clinical expression and staff recognition of neonatal seizures. *Arch Dis Child Fetal Neonatal Ed* 2008;93:F187–F191.
31. Boylan GB, Pressler RM, Rennie JM, Morton M, Leow PL, Hughes R, Binnie CD. Outcome of electroclinical, electrographic, and clinical seizures in the newborn infant. *Dev Med Child Neurol* 1999;41(12):819–825.
32. Dreyfus-Brisac C, Monod N. Electroclinical studies of status epilepticus and convulsions in the newborn. In: Kellaway P, Petersen I (eds), *Neurological and Electroencephalographic Correlative Studies in Infancy.* New York: Grune and Stratton, 1964; pp. 250–272.

33. Volpe JJ. *Neurology of the Newborn*. Philadelphia: Elsevier, 2008; 5th edn.

34. ILAE: Proposal for revised classification of epilepsies and epileptic syndromes. Commission on Classification and Terminology of the International League Against Epilepsy. *Epilepsia* 1989;30(4):389–399.

35. Berg At, et al. Revised terminology and concepts for organization of seizures and epilepsies: Report of the ILAE Commission on Classification and Terminology, 2005–2009. *Epilepsia* 2010;51(4):676–685.

36. Rose AL, Lombroso CT. A study of clinical, pathological, and electroencephalographic features in 137 full-term babies with a long-term follow-up [or is it neonatal seizure states]. *Pediatrics* 1970;45:404–425.

37. De Vries LS, Hellström-Westas L. Role of cerebral function monitoring in the newborn. *Arch Dis Child Fetal Neonatal Ed* 2005;90(3):F201–F207.

38. De Vries LS, Toet MC. Amplitude integrated electroencephalography in the full-term newborn. *Clin Perinatol* 2006; 33(3):619–632.

39. Shellhaas RA, Soaita AI, Clancy RR. Sensitivity of amplitude-integrated electroencephalography for neonatal seizure detection. *Pediatrics* 2007;120(4):770–777.

40. Tharp BR. Neonatal seizures and syndromes. *Epilepsia* 2002;43(Suppl 3):2–10.

41. Patrizi S, Holmes GL, Orzalesi M, Allemand F. Neonatal seizures: characteristics of EEG ictal activity in preterm and full-term infants. *Brain Dev* 2003;25(6):427–437.

42. Clancy RR, Legido A. The exact ictal and interictal duration of electroencephalographic neonatal seizures. *Epilepsia* 1987;28(5):537–541.

43. Kellaway P, Hrachovy RA. Status epilepticus in newborns: a perspective on neonatal seizures. *Adv Neurol* 1983; 34:93–99.

44. Knauss TA, Carlson CB. Neonatal paroxysmal monorhythmic alpha activity. *Arch Neurol* 1978;35(2): 104–107.

45. Watanabe K, Hara K, Miyazaki S, Hakamada S. Rhythmic alpha discharges in the EEGs of the newborn. *Clin Electroencephalogr* 1982;13(4):245–250.

46. Weiner SP, et al. Neonatal Seizures: electroclinical dissociation. *Pediatric Neurol* 1991;7:363–368.

47. Yap V, Engel M, Takenouchi T, Perlman JM. Seizures are common in term infants undergoing head cooling. *Pediatr Neurol* 2009;41(5):327–331.

48. Nash KB, et al. Video-EEG monitoring in newborns with hypoxic-ischemic encephalopathy treated with hypothermia. *Neurology* 2011;76:556–562.

49. Plouin P, Anderson VE. Benign familial and non-familial neonatal seizures. In: Roger J, et al (eds), *Epileptic Syndromes in Infancy, Childhood and Adolescence*. London: John Libbey, 2005; 4th edn: pp. 3–15.

50. Berkovic SF, Scheffer IE. Epilepsies with single gene inheritance. *Brain Dev* 1997;19(1):13–18.

51. Aicardi J, Ohtahara S. Severe neonatal epilepsies with burst suppression pattern. In: Roger J, Bureau M, Dravet C, Dreifuss A, Perrot A, Wolf P (eds), *Epileptic Syndromes in Infancy, Childhood and Adolescence*. London: John Libbey, 2005; 4rth edn: pp. 39–50.

52. Takenouchi T, Yap VL, Engel M, Perlman JM. Stimulus-induced seizure in sick neonates—novel observations with potential clinical implications. *Epilepsia* 2010;51(2):308–311.

53. Malingre MM, van Rooij LG, Rademaker CM, Toet MC, Ververs TF, van Kesteren C, de Vries LS. Development of an optimal lidocaine infusion strategy for neonatal seizures. *Eur J Pediatr* 2006;165(9):598–604.

54. Rennie JM, Hagman CF, Roberson NJ (eds). *Neonatal Cerebral Investigations*. Cambridge: Cambridge University Press, 2008.

55. Azzopardi DV, Strohm B, Edwards AD, Dyet L, Halliday HL, Juszczak E, Kapellou O, Levene M, Marlow N, Porter E, Thoresen M, Whitelaw A, Brocklehurst P; TOBY Study Group. Moderate hypothermia to treat perinatal asphyxial encephalopathy. *N Engl J Med* 2009;361(14):1349–1358.

56. Pearl PL. New treatment paradigms in neonatal metabolic epilepsies. *J Inherit Metab Dis* 2009;32:204–213.

57. Wolf NI, Bast T, Surtees R. Epilepsy in inborn errors of metabolism. *Epileptic Disord* 2005;7:67–81.

58. Van Rooij LGM, Toet MC, van Huffelen AC, Groenendaal F, Laan W, Zecic A, de Hann T, van Straaten ILM, Vrancken S, van Wezel G, van der Sluijs J, ter Horst H, Gavilanes D, Laroche S, Naulaers G, de Vries LS. Effects of treatment of subclinical neonatal seizures detected with a EEG: randomized, controlled trial. *Pediatrics* 2010;125;e358–e366.

59. Clancy RR, Dicker L, Cho S, Cook N, Nicolson SC, Wernovsky G, Spray TL, Gaynor JW. Agreement between long-term neonatal background classification by conventional and amplitude-integrated EEG. *J Clin Neurophysiol* 2011;28(1): 1–9.

60. de Weerd AW, Despland PA, Plouin P. Neonatal EEG. The international federation of clinical neurophysiology. *Electroencephalogr Clin Neurophysiol Suppl* 1999;52:149–157.

61. Laroia N, Guillet R, Burchfiel J, McBride MC. EEG background activity as predictor of electrographic seizures in high-risk neonates. *Epilepsia* 1998;39(5):545–551.

62. Pezzani C, Radvanyi-Bouvet MF, Relier JP, Monod N. Neonatal electroencephalography during the first twenty-four hours of life in full-term newborn infants. *Neuropediatrics* 1986;17(1):11–18.

63. Khan RL, Nunes ML, Garcias da Silva LF, da Costa JC. Predictive value of sequential electroencephalogram (EEG) in neonates with seizures and its relation to neurological outcome. *J Child Neurol* 2008;23(2):144–150.

64. Hellstrom-Westas L. Comparison between tape recorded and amplitude integrated EEG monitoring in sick newborn infants. *Acta Paediatr* 1992;81:812–819.

65. Rennie JM, et al. Non-expert use of the cerebral function monitor for neonatal seizure detection. *Arch Dis Child* 2004;89:F37–F40

66. Bassan H, Bental Y, Shany E, Berger I, Froom P, Levi L, Shiff Y. Neonatal seizures: dilemmas in workup and management. *Pediatr Neurol* 2008;38(6):415–421.

67. Carmo KB, Barr P. Drug treatment of neonatal seizures by neonatologists and paediatric neurologists. *J Paediatr Child Health* 2005;41(7):313–316.

68. Guillet R, Kwon JM. Prophylactic phenobarbital administration after resolution of neonatal seizures: survey of current practice. *Pediatrics* 2008;122(4):731–735.

69. Vento M, de Vries LS, Alberola A, Blennow M, Steggerda S, Greisen G, Boronat N. Approach to seizures in the neonatal period: a European perspective. *Acta Paediatr* 2010;99(4):497–501.

70. Booth D, Evans DJ. Anticonvulsants for neonates with seizures. *Cochrane Database Syst Rev* 2004;18(4):CD004218.

71. Painter MJ, et al. Phenobarbital compared with phenytoin for the treatment of neonatal seizures. *N Eng J Med* 1999; 341:485–489.

72. Boylan GB, Rennie JM, Chorley G, Pressler RM, Fox GF, Farrer K, Morton M, Binnie CD. Second-line anticonvulsant treatment of neonatal seizures: a video-EEG monitoring study. *Neurology* 2004;62(3):486–488.

73. Boylan G B, Rennie JM, Pressler RM, Wilson G, Morton M, Binnie CD. Phenobarbitone, neonatal seizures and Video-EEG. *Arch Dis Child Fetal Neonatal Ed* 2002;86(3):F165–F170.

74. Scher M, et al. Uncoupling of EEG-clinical neonatal seizures after antiepileptic drug use. *Pediatr Neurol* 2003; 28:277–280.

75. Glykys J, Dzhala VI, Kuchibhotla KV, Feng G, Kuner T, Augustine G, Bacskai BJ, Staley KJ. Differences in cortical versus subcortical GABAergic signaling: a candidate mechanism of electroclinical uncoupling of neonatal seizures. *Neuron* 2009;63(5):657–672.

76. Filippi L, la Marca G, Cavallaro G, Fiorini P, Favelli F, Malvagia S, Donzelli G, Guerrini R. Phenobarbital for neonatal seizures in hypoxic-ischemic encephalopathy: a pharmacokinetic study during whole body hypthermia. *Epilepsia* 2011;52:795–801.

77. Wusthoff CJ, Dlugos DJ, Gutierrez-Colina A, Wang A, Cook N, Donnelly M, Clancy R, Abend NS. Electrographic seizures during therapeutic hypothermia for neonatal hypoxia-ischemia encephalopathy. *J Child Neurol* 2011;26 (6):724–728.

78. Silverstein FS, Jensen FE, Inder T, Hellstrom-Westas L, Hirtz D, Ferriero DM. Improving the treatment of neonatal seizures: National Institute of Neurological Disorders and Stroke workshop report. *J Pediatr* 2008b;153(1):12–15.

79. Silverstein FS, Ferriero DM. Off-label use of antiepileptic drugs for the treatment of neonatal seizures. *Pediatr Neurol* 2008a;39(2):77–79.

80. Soul J. Novel medications for neonatal seizures: bumetanide and topiramate. *J Pedia Neurol* 2009;7:85–93

81. Sharpe C, Haas RH. Levetiracetam in the treatment of neonatal seizures. *J Pedia Neurol* 2009;7:79–83, 79.

82. Abend NS, Gutierrez-Colina AM, Monk HM, Dlugos DJ, Clancy RR. Levetiracetam for treatment of neonatal seizures. *J Child Neurol* 2011;26(4):465–470.

83. Khan O, Chang E, Ciprian C, Wright C, Crisp E, Kirmani B. Use of intravenous levetiracetam for management of acute seizures in neonates. *Pediatr Neurol* 2011;44:265–269.

84. Khan O, Chang E, Cipriani C, Wright C, Crisp E, Kirmani B. Use of intravenous levetiracetam for management of acute seizures in neonates. *Pediatr Neurol* 2001;44:265–269.

85. Riviello JJ Jr. Drug therapy for neonatal seizures: part 2. *Neo Reviews* 2004;5:262–268.

86. Baxter P. Epidemiology of pyridoxine dependent and pyridoxine responsive seizures in the UK. *Arch Dis Child* 1999;81:431–433.

87. Ellenberg JH, Nelson KB. Cluster of perinatal events identifying infants at high risk for death or disability. *J Pediatrc* 1988;113:546–552.

88. Ronen GM, Buckley D, Penney S, Streiner DL. Long-term prognosis in children with neonatal seizures: a population-based study. *Neurology* 2007;69:1816–1822.

89. Ortibus EL, Sum JM, Hahn JS. Predictive value of EEG for outcome and epilepsy following neonatal seizures. *Electroencephalogr Clin Neurophysiolog* 1996;98:175–185.

90. Mizrahi EM, et al. Neurologic impairment, developmental delay and post-natal seizures two years after video-EEG documented seizures in near-term and full-term neonates: Report of the Clinical Research Centers for Neonatal Seizures. *Epilepsia* 2001;102:47.

91. Pisani F, Barilli AL, Sisti L, Bevilacqua G, Seri S. Preterm infants with video-EEG confirmed seizures: outcome at 30 months of age. *Brain Dev* 2008;30:20–30.

92. Cornejo BJ, et al. A single episode of neonatal seizures permanently alters glutamatergic synapses. *Ann Neurol* 2007;61(5):411–426.

93. McBride MC, Laroia N, Guillet R. Electrographic seizures in neonates correlate with poor neurodevelopmental outcome. *Neurology* 2000;55:506–513.

94. Bittigau P, et al. Antiepileptic drugs and apoptotic neurodegeneration in the developing brain. *Proc Natl Acad Sci USA* 2002;99(23):15089–15094.

95. Kim JS, Kondratyev A, Tomita Y, Gale K. Neurodevelopmental impact of antiepileptic drugs and seizures in the immature brain. *Epilepsia* 2007;48(Suppl 5):19–26.

96. Chiron C, Dulac O, Pons G. Antiepileptic drug development in children: considerations for a revisited strategy. *Drugs* 2008;68(1):17–25.

CHAPTER 10

Focal Seizures in Infancy

J. Helen Cross

Focal seizures are the most common seizure type presenting in childhood. They may present as the occurrence of a single seizure type, or as part of a wider spectrum of seizure types integral to an epilepsy syndrome. By definition and implication, such seizures arise from one area of the brain. The most recent proposal by the ILAE (The International League Against Epilepsy) defined a focal seizure *"as one that originates within networks limited to one hemisphere. They may be discretely localised or more widely distributed and may also arise in subcortical structures. For each seizure type, ictal onset is consistent from one seizure to another, with preferential propagation patterns that can involve the contralateral hemisphere. In some cases however there is more than one network, and more than one seizure type, but each individual seizure type has a consistent site of onset."*[1]

Focal seizures can then be described on the basis of semiology (the clinical presentation of the event), which depends on the area of brain origin and propagation pattern, both of which define the localization of seizure onset. By recognizing the clinical seizure pattern, with or without EEG confirmation, seizure onset may be attributed to one particular lobe (e.g., temporal lobe) or localized brain region (e.g., supplementary motor area). Further, they may be described according to whether consciousness (awareness) is retained (see Table 10–1). The terms "complex" and "simple" may be confusing; therefore, it has been recommended that these terms should no longer be used. The term "dyscognitive" has been proposed for impaired awareness (if this can be determined).[1]

EVALUATION: GENERAL PRINCIPLES (SEE FIG. 10–1)

The evaluation should begin with a detailed description of the attack by an eyewitness. Any indication of a warning, focal motor components, or stereotyped changes in behavior suggest focal onset. An EEG is likely to show interictal epileptic abnormalities (sharp waves, spikes, spike, and slow wave) in the awake state in approximately 50% (see Fig. 10–2); this may rise to 85% if a sleep recording is obtained. The EEG is often localizing in children presenting with focal epilepsy, particularly in the older child. Where seizure manifestations and the EEG suggest a particular epilepsy syndrome, particularly in a developmentally normal child, further investigation

may not be required. However, most children presenting with focal epilepsy require detailed MR imaging to exclude a structural brain abnormality.[3]

Further evaluation may be necessary to determine if the seizure and EEG pattern are consistent with a specific epilepsy syndrome. This information will result in optimal medication, more accurate prognosis for seizure control and neurodevelopmental outcome. If imaging is negative, with seizure control by medication no further investigation may be required. If a unilateral lesion on imaging is identified, referral for evaluation for epilepsy surgery should be considered early in the natural history (see Chapter). Ictal video-EEG telemetry will be required to determine the area of seizure onset; further investigation that may help in determining whether surgery may be an option includes fluorodeoxyglucose (FDG) positron emission tomography (that may reveal an area of hypometabolism consistent with a structural area responsible for seizures), magnetoencephalography (which may point to a focal area with dipole localization), or other functional studies (e.g., ictal and interictal single-photon emission computed tomography, functional MRI). Such investigations are only useful in presurgical evaluation, in the hands of those experienced in surgical assessment.

In rare circumstances, the pattern of seizures and EEG may suggest genetic causes; this may be seen where focal seizures may be the presenting feature in the first year of life as prolonged lateralized convulsions (SCN1A mutation) or frontal lobe seizures in early life in the context of normal imaging with episodes of nonconvulsive status epilepticus (ring chromosome 20). However, research now reveals an increasing number of the epilepsies likely to have a genetic etiology.

▶ FOCAL SEIZURES IN INFANCY

FOCAL SEIZURES IN THE NEONATE

Most epileptic seizures in the neonatal period are focal[4] and may present as focal clonic or focal tonic movement.[5] Further, paroxysmal changes in autonomic function have also been reported including changes in heart rate, respiration, and blood pressure associated with flushing, salivation, and pupillary dilatation.[6,7] These features are rare as isolated manifestations of epileptic events and are more consistently observed in association

▶ **TABLE 10–1. DESCRIPTORS OF FOCAL SEIZURES ACCORDING TO DEGREE OF IMPAIRMENT DURING SEIZURE**[a]

- Without impairment of consciousness or awareness.
  - With observable motor or autonomic components.
    - This roughly corresponds to the concept of "simple" partial seizure.
    - "Focal motor" and "autonomic" are terms that may adequately convey this concept depending on the seizure manifestations).
  - Involving subjective sensory or psychic phenomena only.
    - This corresponds to the concept of an aura, a term endorsed in the 2001 Glossary.
  - With impairment of consciousness or awareness.
    - This roughly corresponds to the concept of complex partial seizure. "Dyscognitive" is a term that has been proposed for this concept.[2]
  - Evolving to a bilateral, convulsive[b] seizure (involving tonic, clonic, or tonic and clonic components).
    - This expression replaces the term "secondarily generalized seizure."

[a]For more descriptors that have been clearly defined and recommended for use. See Blume WT, Luders HO, Mizrahi E, Tassinari C, van Emde BW, Engel J Jr. Glossary of descriptive terminology for ictal semiology: Report of the ILAE Task Force on Classification and Terminology. *Epilepsia* 2001;42:1212–1218.
[b]The term "convulsive" was considered a lay term in the Glossary; however, we note that it is used throughout medicine in various forms and translates well across many languages. Its use is, therefore, endorsed.
Source: From Berg AT, Berkovic SF, Brodie MJ, Buchhalter JR, Cross JH, Van Emde Boas W, Engel J, French J, Glauser TA, Mathern GW, Moshe SL, Nordli D, Plouin P, Scheffer IE. Revised terminology and concepts for organisation of seizures and epilepsies: Report of the ILAE Commission on Classification and Terminology, 2005–2009. *Epilepsia* 2010;51:676–685.

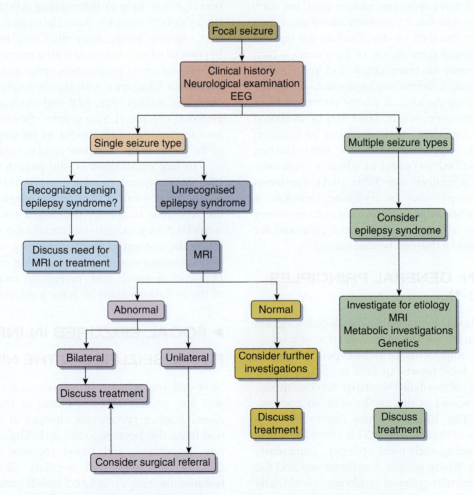

Figure 10–1. Suggested algorithm to be followed in the management of focal seizures in all age groups.

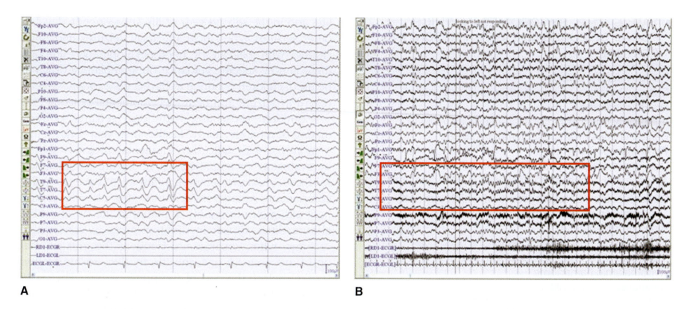

A   B

Figure 10–2. Interictal (**A**) and ictal (**B**) EEG of boy with temporal lobe seizures. Interictal EEG shows spike- and slow-wave activity over left temporal electrodes (T7, T9). Ictal EEG shows rhythmic activity with onset over the same electrodes, suggesting left temporal origin.

with other clinical evidence of epileptic seizures. EEG recordings of neonatal seizures have wide-ranging features; the frequency, voltage, and morphology of the discharges may change within an individual seizure; EEG transients commonly arise focally and may either remain confined to that region or spread (see Chapter 9).

FOCAL SEIZURES IN INFANCY

In the very small child, where networks have not fully matured, components of focal seizures may be subtle and simple in their manifestation. Generalized seizures are rarely documented in video-EEG studies in infants under age 2 years.[8,9] Secondarily generalized clinical manifestations may arise from focal lesions, and seizures may evolve into infantile spasms even with evidence of focality in the original presentation (see Fig. 10–3),[10,11] whereas others may retain focal symptomatology.

CLINICAL EVALUATION

There is a limited repertoire of semiological presentation in the very young.[12] In one study of children presenting under the age of 3 years only four seizure types accounted for 81% of total symptomatologies (epileptic spasms, tonic seizures, clonic seizure, and hypomotor seizures).[12] The frequency of aura, limb automatisms, dystonic posturing, secondary generalization, and unresponsiveness increases with age.[13] In seizures of temporal lobe onset, there is an apparent evolution with age where all children younger than 42 months have a high ratio of motor features whereas children older than 4 years demonstrate a higher rate of adult semiology with behavioral arrest and automatisms.[11] Auras are not documented in

the younger group; a further study has suggested an aura is unlikely to manifest less than 2.5 years in seizures of focal onset.[14] The degree of awareness is almost impossible to determine in most younger children; for this reason, it has been suggested that the terminology simple and complex (relating to degree of awareness retained) be omitted from the current ILAE classification.[1,15]

Lateralizing signs in infants and young children are also lacking.[14] It is therefore extremely difficult to comment on locality of onset dependent on semiology without video-EEG telemetry in this age group. An important exception is gelastic seizures that may present early in the first year of life and should alert the clinician to the possibility of a hypothalamic hamartoma (see Chapter 35).

Difficulties remain thereafter in determining the likely epilepsy syndrome. Focal seizures may manifest as one of several seizure types (as in genetic epilepsy syndromes such as Dravet; see Chapter 14), or may manifest as a single seizure type. Confusion may remain if focal seizures and spasms arise from the same area in lesional epilepsy (see Fig. 10–3). However, if focal seizures are seen independently, it should be presumed to be a symptom of lesional epilepsy until proven otherwise (see Chapter 55).

SYNDROME DIAGNOSIS (SEE TABLE 10–2)

Early-onset stereotyped focal or lateralized seizures should suggest a structural brain lesion and should lead to an early referral to an epilepsy surgery center. Recurrent lateralized and prolonged seizures with variability in the side involved may suggest Dravet syndrome (see Chapter 14). Affected children present with prolonged febrile or afebrile-lateralized seizures in the first year of

▶ **TABLE 10–2. SYNDROMES IN WHICH FOCAL SEIZURES MAY BE A PRESENTING FEATURE**

Benign infantile epilepsy
Epilepsy of infancy with migrating focal seizures
Dravet syndrome
Autosomal dominant frontal lobe epilepsy (ADFLE)
Benign epilepsy with centrotemporal spikes
Panayiotopolous syndrome
Late-onset occipital epilepsy of Gastaut type
Autosominal dominant epilepsy with auditory features

Recognizable etiologies (some of which currently referred to as "distinctive constellations"):
Ring chromosome 20
Lesional focal epilepsy (malformations of cortical development, developmental tumors)
Hypothalamic hamartoma
Rasmussen encephalitis

Source: From Berg AT, Berkovic SF, Brodie MJ, Buchhalter JR, Cross JH, Van Emde Boas W, Engel J, French J, Glauser TA, Mathern GW, Moshe SL, Nordli D, Plouin P, Scheffer IE. Revised terminology and concepts for organisation of seizures and epilepsies: Report of the ILAE Commission on Classification and Terminology, 2005–2009. *Epilepsia* 2010;51:676–685.

life, and in the second year of life subsequently develop other seizures types including focal seizures and myoclonus, with plateau of neurodevelopment. Although there is now specific guidance on antiepileptic drugs to be used, children continue to have a poor prognosis with regard to seizure and neurodevelopmental outcome.

Children presenting with focal seizures of fluctuating semiology, early in the first year (mean age 3 months), with little developmental progress should be evaluated for migrating partial seizures of infancy.[16] In these children seizures often also have a motor component. Autonomic features may also be prominent although not readily apparent at the onset.[17] EEG abnormalities appear in different areas in consecutive seizures; when seizures are frequent the area of ictal onset moves from one area to another, seizures often starting before the end of the previous one. The prognosis is extremely poor both for neurodevelopment and seizure control with a high rate of fatality.

EVALUATION AND INVESTIGATIONS

All children presenting with events likely to be seizures warrant an EEG. Further, all children under 2 years of age presenting with at least two epileptic seizures should

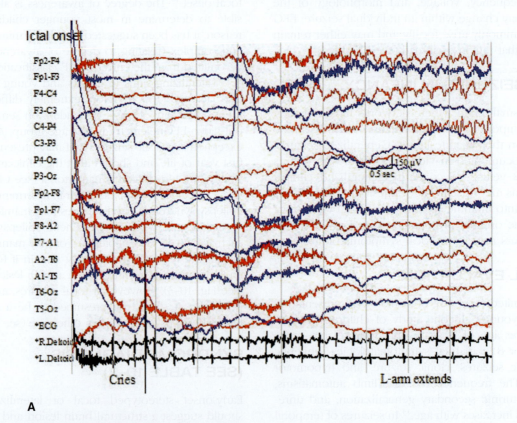

A

Figure 10–3. Infant presented with focal seizures at 5 days involving shaking of all limbs, whole body becoming stiff, eyes rolled upward, smacking of lips lasting about 1 minute, with associated grunting. EEG demonstrated origin from the right frontal region (**A**); *(continued)*

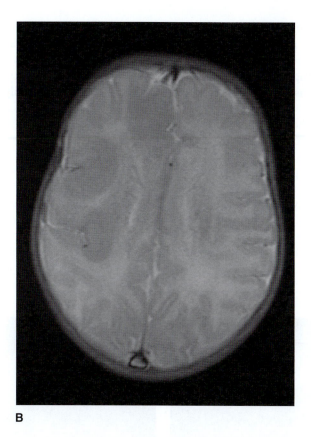

B

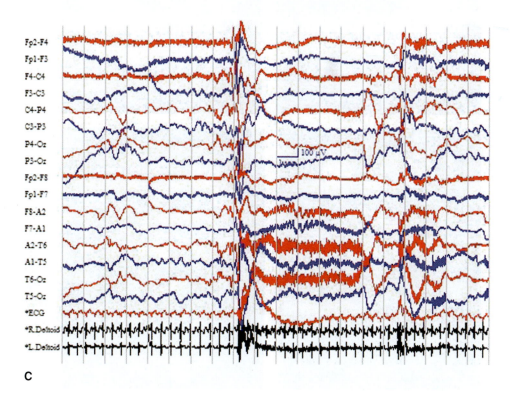

C

Figure 10–3. *(Continued)* MRI demonstrated extensive frontal polymicrogyria (**B**). At 3 m, seizures evolved into asymmetric infantile spasms with EEG demonstrating rhythmic activity immediately prior to generalized sharp and slow wave (**C**).

undergo MRI[3] (www.nice.org.uk/cg20). Studies have suggested a high yield of abnormality in this age group, albeit difficult at times to interpret the relevance of the abnormality (see Fig. 10–4).[18] The diagnosis of a focal brain abnormality has major implications for early consideration for epilepsy surgery.

The dilemma often remains however as to how far to pursue neurometabolic investigation. A trial of pyridoxine should be considered in all cases to exclude pyridoxine dependency.[19] Many early-onset epilepsies have a genetic etiology, which should be considered early to save excessive investigations that are likely to be negative. For example, a child presenting with two prolonged lateralized febrile seizures should be evaluated for the SCN1A mutation (see Chapter 14). A further form of early-onset multifocal epilepsy has also been reported in association with SCN1A mutations.[20] However, there is no question that neurometabolic evaluation in infants presenting with seizures, including for mitochondrial disease, is more likely to be positive in yield in this age group and therefore should be carefully considered, especially if other neurological symptoms and signs emerge.

TREATMENT

There is little evidence supporting first-line medications in infants with focal seizures. First-line therapy for infantile spasms, regardless of etiology includes steroids or vigabatrin,[21] the latter preferred for patients in whom tuberous sclerosis complex is the underlying cause (see Chapter 32).[22] Physicians are reluctant to administer sodium valproate due to concerns about liver dysfunction.[23] This risk

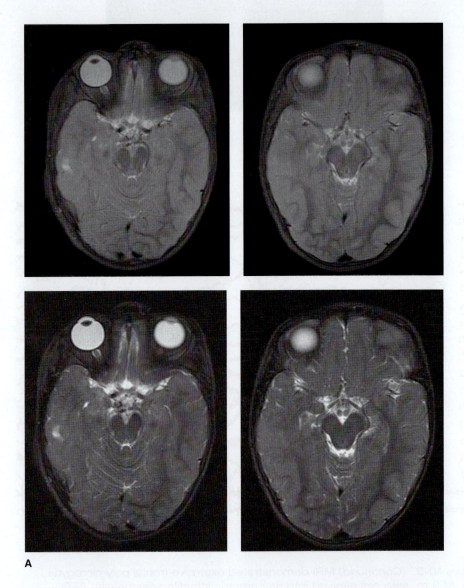

A

Figure 10–4. Child presented at 15 m with brief head nods, evolving into frequent episodes of behavioral arrest with and without clusters of head-nodding episodes. MRI showed right temporal cortical dysplasia (**A**). *(continued)*

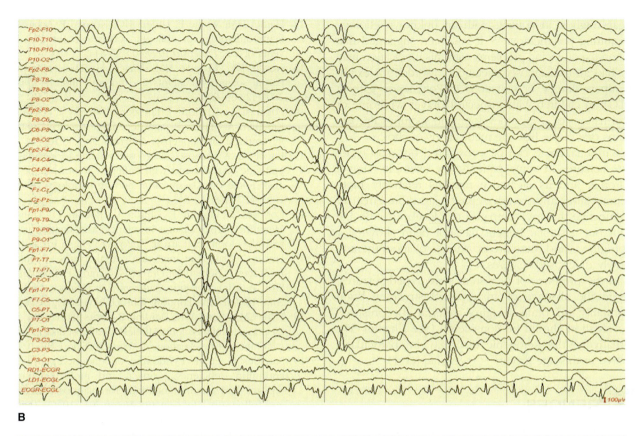

B

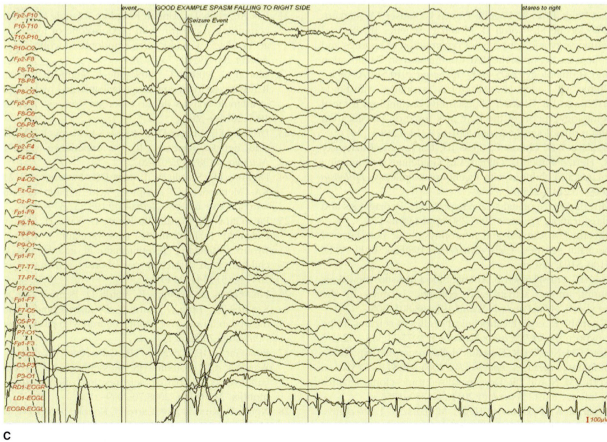

C

Figure 10–4. *(Continued)* Clinical semiology suggested focality of onset, and lateralization to the right. Interictal and ictal recordings were nonlocalizing (**B, C**); subsequent temporal resection led to seizure freedom.

appears highest in patients with an unknown etiology or requiring polytherapy.[23,24] It has been suggested that children experiencing problems with this medication may have had an undiagnosed metabolic disorder, for example, Alpers disease or mutations in Polymerase gamma (POLG). In children with suspected Dravet syndrome or malformations of cortical development, sodium valproate remains one of the first-line medications of choice.

Carbamazepine can be considered but may exacerbate seizures in some patients, for example, Dravet syndrome, and its clearance remains relatively high. Levetiracetam[25] and oxcarbazepine[26] are more effective as adjunctive therapy compared to placebo in this age group, but a similar benefit has not been shown for lamotrigine,[27] and there are no studies of monotherapy in newly diagnosed seizures.

In the presence of persistent stereotyped seizures, even in the absence of an apparent structural brain abnormality on brain imaging, referral for presurgical evaluation should be considered (see Chapter 55). Alternatively, the ketogenic diet may be particularly effective in this age group[28,29] (see Chapter 53).

REFERENCES

1. Berg AT, Berkovic SF, Brodie MJ, Buchhalter JR, Cross JH, Van Emde Boas W, Engel J, French J, Glauser TA, Mathern GW, Moshe SL, Nordli D, Plouin P, Scheffer IE. Revised terminology and concepts for organisation of seizures and epilepsies: Report of the ILAE Commission on Classification and Terminology, 2005–2009. *Epilepsia* 2010;51:676–685.

2. Blume WT, Luders HO, Mizrahi E, Tassinari C, van Emde BW, Engel J Jr. Glossary of descriptive terminology for ictal semiology: report of the ILAE task force on classification and terminology. *Epilepsia* 2001;42:1212–1218.

3. Gaillard WD, Chiron C, Cross JH, Harvey AS, Kuzniecky R, Hertz-Pannier L, Gilbert VL. Guidelines for imaging infants and children with recent-onset epilepsy. *Epilepsia* 2009;50:2147–2153.

4. Mizrahi EM. Neonatal seizures: problems in diagnosis and classification. *Epilepsia* 1987;28(Suppl 1):S46–S55.

5. Mizrahi EM. Clinical and neurophysiologic correlates of neonatal seizures. *Cleve Clin J Med* 1989;56(Suppl Pt 1): S100–S104; discuss.

6. Lou HC, Friis-Hansen B. Arterial blood pressure elevations during motor activity and epileptic seizures in the newborn. *Acta Paediatr Scand* 1979;68:803–806.

7. Watanabe K, et al. Electroclinical studies of seizures in the newborn. *Folia Psychiatr Neurol Jpn* 1977;31:383–392.

8. Korff CM, Nordli DR. The clinical-electrographic expression of infantile seizures. *Epilepsy Res* 2006;70S:S116–S131.

9. Korff CM. Nordli DR. Do generalised tonic–clonic seizures in infancy exist. *Neurology* 2011;65:1750–1753.

10. Fogarasi A, Tuxhorn I, Hegyi M, Janszky J. Predictive clinical factors for the differential diagnosis of childhood extratemporal seizures. *Epilepsia* 2005;46:1280–1285.

11. Fogarasi A, Jokeit H, Faveret E, Janszky J, Tuxhorn I. The effect of age on seizure semiology in childhood temporal lobe epilepsy. *Epilepsia* 2002;43:638–643.

12. Hamer HM, Wyllie E, Luders HO, Kotagal P, Acharya JN. Symptomatology of epileptic seizures in the first three years of life. *Epilepsia* 1999;40:837–844.

13. Nordli DR, Kuroda MM, Hirsch LJ. The ontogeny of partial seizures in infants and young children. *Epilepsia* 2001;42:986–990.

14. Fogarasi A, Tuxhorn I, Janszky J, Janszky I, Rasonyi G, Kelemen A, Halasz P. Age dependent seizure semiology in temporal lobe epilepsy. *Epilepsia* 2007;48:1697–1702.

15. Engel J Jr. A proposed diagnostic scheme for people with epileptic seizures and with epilepsy: Report of the ILAE Task Force on Classification and Terminology. *Epilepsia* 2001;42:796–803.

16. Coppola G, Plouin P, Chiron C, Robain O, Dulac O. Migrating partial seizures in infancy: a malignant disorder with developmental arrest. *Epilepsia* 1995;36:1017–1024.

17. Dulac O. Malignant migrating partial seizures in infancy. In: Roger J, Bureau M, Dravet C, Genton P, Tassinari CA, Wolf P (eds), *Epileptic Syndromes in Infancy, Childhood And Adolescence*. London: John Libbey, 2005: p. 73.

18. Eltze CM, Chong WK, Harding B, Cross JH. Focal cortical dysplasia in infants: some MRI lesions almost disappear with maturation of myelination. *Epilepsia* 2005;46:1988–1992.

19. Stockler S, et al. Pyridoxine dependent epilepsy and antiquitin deficiency. Clinical and molecular characteristics and recommendations for diagnosis, treatment and follow-up. *Mol Genetics Metab* 2011;104(1–2):48–60.

20. Harkin LA, et al. The spectrum of SCN1A-related infantile epileptic encephalopathies. *Brain* 2007;130:843–852.

21. Lux AL, et al. The United Kingdom Infantile Spasms Study comparing vigabatrin with prednisolone or tetracosactide at 14 days: a multicentre, randomised controlled trial. *Lancet* 2004;364:1773–1778.

22. Chiron C, Dumas C, Jambaque I, Mumford J, Dulac O. Randomized trial comparing vigabatrin and hydrocortisone in infantile spasms due to tuberous sclerosis. *Epilepsy Res* 1997;26:389–395.

23. Dreifuss FE, Langer DH, Moline KA, Maxwell JE. Valproic acid hepatic fatalities. II. US experience since 1984. *Neurology* 1989;39:201–207.

24. Dreifuss FE, Santilli N, Langer DH, Sweeney KP, Moline KA, Menander KB. Valproic acid hepatic fatalities: a retrospective review. *Neurology* 1987;37:379–385.

25. Pina-Garza JE, Nordli DR, Rating D, Yang H, Schiemann-Delgardo J, Duncan B. Levetiracetam N01009 Study Group. Adjunctive levetiracetam in infants and young children with refractory partial-onset seizures. *Epilepsia* 2009;50(5):1141–1149.

26. Pina-Garza JE, Espiniza R, Nordli D, Bennett DA, Spirito S, Stites TE, Tang D, Sturm Y. Oxcarbazepine adjunctive therapy in infants and young children with partial seizures. *Neurology* 2005;65:1370–1375.

27. Pina-Garza JE, Levisohn P, Gucuyener K, Mikati MA, Warnock CR, Conklin HS, Messenheimer J. Adjunctive lamotrigine for partial seizures in patients aged 1–24 months. *Neurology* 2008;70:2099–2108.

28. Nordli D, Kuroda MM, Carroll J, Koenigsberger DY, Hirsch LJ, Bruner HJ, Seidel WT, De Vivo DC. Experience with the ketogenic diet in infants. *Pediatrics* 2002;108:129–133.

29. Kossoff EH, Hedderick EF, Turner Z, Freeman JM. A case-control evaluation of the ketogenic diet versus ACTH for new-onset infantile spasms. *Epilepsia* 2008;49:1504–1509.

CHAPTER 11

Generalized Seizures in Early Childhood (2–4 Years of Age)

Sudha K. Kessler and Dennis J. Dlugos

▶ OVERVIEW

As discussed in Chapter 1, classification of epileptic seizure types has practical importance but also significant limitations. Historically used terms may not accurately reflect the complex pathophysiology or phenomenology of seizures. Generalized seizures involve synchronous epileptic discharges throughout the cerebral cortex, and are further distinguished by the terms *primary* or *secondarily*. Seizures that appear to have synchronous bihemispheric involvement at initiation (based on clinical and electrographic evidence) are primary generalized seizures and those that begin in a focal area of cortex and subsequently spread to involve both hemispheres are secondarily generalized. This distinction is not always straightforward, and a high index of suspicion should be maintained for focal onset seizures that appear generalized, because evaluation and treatment differs between generalized and focal epilepsies.

By age 2–4 years, children can manifest all of the generalized seizure types that are seen in older age groups—generalized tonic–clonic seizures (GTCs), absence seizures, myoclonic seizures, tonic seizures, and atonic/astatic seizures. Infantile spasms do not typically present at this age, and the occasional cases of late-onset infantile spasms are reviewed in Chapter 28.

Generalized seizures presenting in early childhood often fail to meet criteria for an epilepsy syndrome, or the syndrome may not be obvious at presentation.

The process of evaluation for a child in this age group, as with any child with epilepsy, begins with an accurate diagnosis of seizure, seizure classification, and, when possible, determination of etiology. A series of questions (see Box 11–1) should lead to the most appropriate diagnosis, which then guides further diagnostic evaluation and treatment decisions. This chapter is organized by clinical seizure type, and will focus on young children presenting with two or more unprovoked generalized seizures who do not fit into a definitive epilepsy syndrome.

▶ GENERALIZED TONIC–CLONIC SEIZURES (GTCs)

CLASSIFICATION AND DIAGNOSIS (FIG. 11-1)

History

Most GTCs in this age group are, in fact, something else. The first step in approaching the young child presenting with an event reported to be a GTC is to *obtain a detailed description of the episode*. Witnesses may describe a wide variety of clinical events (epileptic and nonepileptic) as "grand mal seizures" or "convulsions." In early childhood, events mimicking GTCs include breath-holding spells, syncope with subsequent convulsive movements, and gastroesophageal reflux. A careful description is essential for distinguishing epileptic from nonepileptic events. For example, breath-holding spells may be provoked by crying or a sudden fright, and are characterized by a respiratory pause in expiration resulting in loss of consciousness or limpness, sometimes followed by opisthotonic posturing or clonic limb movements.[1]

A common cause of a GTC in a 2–4-year old is a focal onset seizure with rapid secondary generalization, so the diagnostic evaluation should carefully evaluate this possibility. Distinguishing primary from secondarily generalized seizures based on the history of the event is often challenging. Clues to focal onset may be missed because young children are often unable to articulate an aura, and parents may be so overwhelmed by seeing the convulsion that they are unable to describe details of seizure onset or postictal findings such as weakness. Requesting a demonstration of what the parent or other witness saw may reveal clues not apparent in a verbal description of the events.

The next step in seizure classification is taking a careful *developmental and medical history*, focusing on risk factors for epilepsy such as premature birth, neonatal hypoxic–ischemic encephalopathy, neonatal seizures, significant head trauma, CNS infection, stroke, or developmental delays. While these factors do not exclude the possibility of a primary GTC, their presence should raise suspicion for symptomatic focal or multifocal epilepsy characterized by rapidly secondarily generalized seizures. Similarly, the *neurologic exam* should be directed toward identifying focal neurologic deficits suggesting focal epilepsy. Though handedness is established by age 36 months in most children, significant

functional asymmetries and developmental reflex asymmetries (e.g., the parachute reflex) should raise red flags about the possibility of an underlying focal lesion.

When clues to seizure classification are not forthcoming from a description of the event, medical history, and neurologic exam, further diagnostic studies are needed.

Electroencephalography (EEG)

EEG is a helpful tool for refining basic seizure classification. Every child with an unprovoked GTC should have a routine EEG searching for background abnormalities, focal epileptiform features, or generalized epileptiform abnormalities. The recording should include photic stimulation, and, in cooperative older children, hyperventilation. In our experience, it is possible to coax a child as young as 3 years into blowing on a pinwheel for a short period of time, and children 4 years and older are able

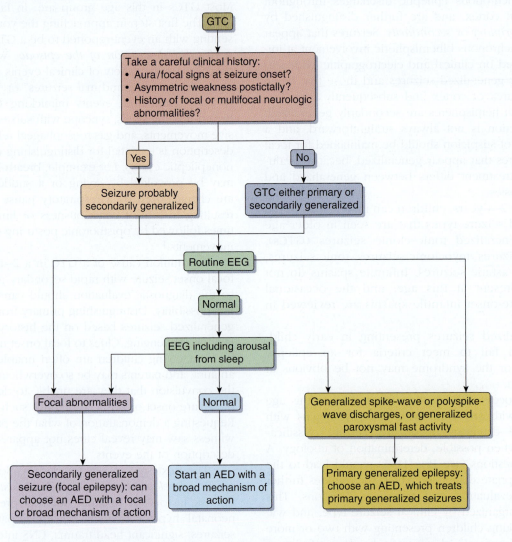

Figure 11–1. Algorithm for classifying a generalized tonic–clonic seizure (GTC) as primary generalized, or secondarily generalized.

to cooperate more reliably with hyperventilation. A focal EEG abnormality strongly implies that a presumed GTC was a focal seizure with secondary generalization. A normal EEG, particularly if sleep and arousal from sleep were recorded, may also suggest a focal onset seizure. The presence of generalized epileptiform abnormalities such as spike-wave discharges, polyspike-wave discharges, or generalized paroxysmal fast activity, suggests a true primary generalized seizure.

If basic seizure classification remains unclear and response to initial antiepileptic drug (AED) treatment is suboptimal, then ictal recordings in an epilepsy monitoring unit may be needed. If seizures are too infrequent for ictal recording on an inpatient unit to be practical, a longer recording in the monitoring unit may still yield interictal clues not seen on routine EEG. While ictal recording with an ambulatory EEG may be attempted, it is often challenging to obtain high-quality recordings using ambulatory EEG in this age group.

Differential Diagnosis

Most idiopathic generalized epilepsy (IGE) syndromes that are characterized by GTCs do not present between 2 and 4 years of age. Identifying a recognized syndrome often depends on characterizing the *other* seizure types in a child with GTCs. The most likely syndrome diagnosis for a child presenting with a GTC at this age may be myoclonic–astatic epilepsy (MAE; Doose syndrome), which often begins with a febrile or afebrile GTC followed by typical myoclonic or myoclonic–astatic seizures days to months later.[2] Thus, the syndrome may not be initially obvious.

The syndrome of primary GTCs upon awakening (PGTCA) typically presents after age 6 years.[3] Juvenile absence epilepsy (JAE) and juvenile myoclonic epilepsy (JME), syndromes in which children may have GTCs, also present later in life. Typical childhood absence epilepsy (CAE) rarely presents under age 3 or 4, and does not involve early GTCs.[4] IGE with absences of early childhood, an epilepsy syndrome distinct from CAE, may involve early GTCs in two-thirds of patients. Some children with a form of "borderline severe myoclonic epilepsy of infancy (SMEB)" may have only GTCs—this rare epilepsy type, labeled "severe idiopathic generalized epilepsy of infancy with GTCs" presents before age 2 years.[5] GTCs are not the predominant seizure type in Lennox–Gastaut syndrome (LGS).

After thorough evaluation, many children with GTCs between 2 and 4 years of age will not meet criteria for any recognized epilepsy syndrome and will not have a clear symptomatic etiology. These children can be described as having "generalized epilepsy characterized by GTCs, etiology unknown." This diagnosis is imprecise, but recognizes the many uncertainties surrounding the clear diagnosis of GTCs in this age group.

The search for an etiology of GTCs also begins with a thorough history, and general physical and neurologic examination. The same points of the history and exam that aid in seizure classification also provide information for assisting the search for an underlying cause.

Imaging Studies

Brain imaging is recommended for children presenting with a GTCs if a focal abnormality is found on neurologic exam or EEG. In the developmentally normal child with a normal neurologic exam, and EEG characteristic of an IGE, imaging may not be required.[6] Children presenting to an emergency room with a first GTC are often imaged with computed tomography (CT) scan to rule out hemorrhage, mass lesions, or hydrocephalus, although such studies are low yield except in certain high-risk groups, such as children with general medical problems or closed head injury.[7] In the nonemergent setting, when imaging is indicated, an MRI is the modality of choice. With a high-quality MRI, some children with GTCs and generalized epileptiform EEG patterns may actually have evidence of unilateral or bilateral structural lesions, often malformations of cortical development (MCDs). It is unclear why some children with focal or multifocal structural lesions have apparently generalized epilepsy on clinical and EEG evaluation. Possibilities include an age-related susceptibility to rapid secondary synchrony of focal epileptic activity, or the limitation of current diagnostic techniques to distinguish among focal, multifocal, and generalized epilepsy.

Other Tests

Beyond EEG and MRI, other diagnostic studies are generally not required in a normal toddler or preschool age child with new-onset, self-limited unprovoked GTCs. In children with abnormal examinations or developmental delays, the clinical presentation will dictate which laboratory tests are needed to evaluate for genetic or metabolic disorders. The role of epilepsy-specific genetic testing in a normal child presenting with GTCs is presently unknown. The spectrum of clinical manifestations of SCN1A mutations in childhood epilepsy is increasingly wide, extending beyond the already broad boundaries of generalized epilepsy with febrile seizures plus (GEFS+), and Dravet syndrome.[8] The potential clinical utility of SCN1A testing for probands, parents, and siblings must be carefully considered if such testing is to be performed on young children with isolated GTCs.[9]

▶ TREATMENT

If a diagnosis of "generalized epilepsy—characterized by GTCs" is established, then treatment with antiepileptic

▶ **TABLE 11–1. DRUG DOSES FOR MEDICATIONS COMMONLY USED TO TREAT GENERALIZED SEIZURES**[a]

Drug	Dose Range for Maintenance Therapy
Valproate	15–30 mg/kg/d
Lamotrigine	Without VPA: 5–15 mg/kg/d
	With VPA: 5 mg/kg/d
Levetiracetam	30–100 mg/kg/d
Topiramate	5–10 mg/kg/d (in the 2–4-yr age group, doses as high as 20 mg/kg/d)
Ethosuximide	20–40 mg/kg/d
Felbamate	15–45 mg/kg/d
Zonisamide	4–12 mg/kg/d
Clobazam	0.5–1 mg/kg/d
Rufinamide	15–45 mg/kg/d

[a]Recommended starting doses and titration schedules can be found in Chapter XX.

drugs (AEDs) taken daily is usually indicated (Table 11–1). There is little data specific to GTCs in young children. In general, valproic acid (VPA), lamotrigine (LTG), topiramate (TPM), and levetiracetam (LEV) are preferred, due to their broad spectrum of efficacy against multiple seizure types. Zonisamide (ZNS), clobazam (CLB), rufinamide (RFM), and phenobarbital are additional options. Carbamazepine (CBZ), oxcarbazepine (OXC), and gabapentin (GBP) are less useful, because they may precipitate other generalized seizure types, such as absence or myoclonic seizures.[10]

The goal of AED treatment in children with GTCs is to prevent seizure recurrence while minimizing adverse effects. Since there is no data comparing the efficacy of AEDs for the treatment of GTCs in early childhood, decisions regarding specific AEDs are based on available evidence for efficacy, safety, tolerability, titration schedule, ease of administration, and cost. Because knowledge about the effectiveness of individual AEDs on specific seizure types and patient populations changes rapidly, we advise that the information here be used only as a guide to current practice.

LEV is a commonly used AED in children with new-onset seizures of many types, including GTCs in primary generalized epilepsies and focal epilepsies. It is often preferred over other AEDs for its broad range of efficacy, its favorable tolerability profile, its ability to be titrated quickly, and its lack of drug–drug interactions. LEV has US FDA indications for use in primary GTCs in children as young as 4 years of age,[11] and its efficacy in children under the age of 2 with refractory partial or generalized seizures has also been demonstrated.[12] The use of LEV as initial monotherapy in children has been described, but largely in retrospective studies that include generalized and focal seizure types, with very few patients in the 2–4-year-age range.[13,14] Nevertheless, based on extrapolation to this population from

available data, and because of its excellent tolerability profile, LEV is often preferred as the first-line drug for new-onset GTCs in children. Its efficacy against a broad range of seizure types is particularly appealing because, as discussed earlier, the primary versus secondary nature of GTCs in this age group is often unclear. The side effect most often reported is behavioral disturbances or irritability, which can occur in as many as 30% of children under age 4, but leads to discontinuation of the medication in only 16%.[15]

LTG also has efficacy for a broad range of seizure types including GTCs, and has been shown to be efficacious in treating primary generalized seizures in children as young as age 2 years.[16] LTG is generally well tolerated, but titration to a therapeutic dose must be slow to minimize the risk of a serious rash. Serious rashes due to LTG are rare, particularly with the recommended titration schedules, but children have a three-fold greater risk than adults.[17] The requirement for slow titration may limit the use of LTG in children with frequent GTCs, unless another medication such as a long-acting benzodiazepine is used as a bridge during the initiation period.

TPM is also efficacious in treating newly diagnosed epilepsy, including epilepsies characterized by GTCs in children as young as 2 years.[18] Most side effects are dose dependent, and include weight loss, difficulties with attention or concentration, sleepiness, and paresthesia. Rare idiosyncratic side effects include glaucoma and urolithiasis. An issue of practical importance in using TPM in this age group is the rapid rate of clearance,[19] which can necessitate using dosing ranges far higher than in older age groups (as high as 20 mg/kg per day in some toddlers in our experience), and three times daily dosing schedules.

VPA until recently was often used as the first-line treatment for GTCs, particularly when a primary generalized epilepsy was suspected or could not be ruled out. Though decades of experience with this agent have established it as a safe medication in most populations, certain idiosyncratic and dose-related side effects merit comment. The most serious is irreversible hepatotoxicity, an idiosyncratic reaction with an incidence of less than 1:16,000 in children aged 3–10 years on monotherapy, and less than 1:8000 in children over age 2 years on multiple medications.[20] Infants under the age of 2 years on multiple AEDs are at greatest risk, with a 1:600 incidence of hepatotoxicity. Underlying metabolic disease is believed to contribute to the risk of hepatotoxicity, and at least one specific mitochondrial disorder is known to be highly associated with valproate-related liver toxicity.[21] Routine laboratory surveillance can help identify dose-related toxicities such as thrombocytopenia, but is unlikely to identify idiosyncratic reactions like liver failure if the patient is not symptomatic. Close clinical follow-up and parental education about red-flag symptoms are more important than frequent laboratory testing for identifying idiosyncratic hepatic dysfunction in high-risk patients. No studies have clearly defined a role for the preventative use of levocarnitine in children treated with valproate, but some recommend routine oral supplementation, particularly those with the highest risk category.[22]

▶ OUTCOME AND PROGNOSIS

Once a diagnosis of GTCs has been made, further distinguishing whether the child has IGE or symptomatic generalized epilepsy (SGE) is not crucial for choosing the initial AED, but is important for understanding the child's prognosis. In general, children with GTCs due to IGE have a more favorable AED response and neurodevelopmental outcome than children with SGE.[23] However, many children presenting with GTCs between age 2 and 4 years will have epilepsy of unclear etiology and their long-term prospects for epilepsy remission and normal cognitive function are uncertain.

▶ ABSENCE SEIZURES

CLASSIFICATION AND DIAGNOSIS

History

Typical absence seizures are characterized clinically by brief (10–30 seconds) lapses in consciousness with behavioral arrest and staring, variably associated with facial myoclonus, eye blinking, or subtle facial and limb automatisms. Onset and offset are abrupt, with immediate return to baseline behavioral state and activity. Seizures are classically triggered by hyperventilation. In the untreated state, seizures occur many times per day, and sometimes many times per hour.

Absence seizures may be mistaken by parents and teachers for inattentiveness or daydreaming. Conversely, inattentive children and normal daydreamers are often referred to neurologists for evaluation of absence seizures. Tics that involve blinking or subtle facial movements may also be mistaken for absence seizures, particularly when they occur in a child with concurrent attention deficit disorder. Absence seizures must also be distinguished from complex partial seizures which are also characterized by impairment of consciousness and behavioral arrest, but are generally longer, less frequent, and may be associated with a preceding aura, complex automatic behaviors, and postictal confusion or focal neurologic deficits (such as aphasia).

Atypical absence seizures are longer, have less distinct onsets and offsets, and may be associated with more complex ictal behaviors. They occur in the context of symptomatic generalized epilepsies.

EEG

Diagnosing typical absence seizures is not difficult. In the majority of untreated children with absence seizures, a routine EEG with hyperventilation is adequate for capturing the typical electrographic finding of 3 Hz generalized spike-wave discharges. EEG background is normal, though occipital intermittent rhythmic delta activity (OIRDA) can be seen. In a neurologically normal child, other diagnostic studies are rarely warranted.

Atypical absence seizures are accompanied by a slow spike-wave electrographic pattern, and may also be associated with background abnormalities frequently seen in symptomatic epilepsies, such as generalized slowing.

Differential Diagnosis

Typical absence seizures are the hallmark of CAE, but CAE rarely begins before the age of 4 years. Most children presenting with absence seizures in very early childhood do not appear to have typical CAE, and some studies suggests that early age of onset is associated with more difficult to control seizures and greater neurodevelopmental impairment.[24] Epilepsy mainly characterized by absence seizures (but often including GTCs and myoclonic seizures) presenting under the age of 4 years has been labeled as "absence epilepsy of early childhood," "IGE with absences of early childhood," and "intermediate petit mal."[25]

A specific etiology is rarely identified and brain imaging is unlikely to be helpful. As with GTCs in this age group, history, and physical exam will dictate the need for genetic or metabolic evaluation.

A specific etiology warranting comment is GLUT-1 glucose transporter deficiency, a recently characterized disorder caused by mutations in the SLC2A1 gene that can present in early childhood with absence or other generalized seizure types, and is associated with 2.5–4 Hz generalized spike-wave discharges superimposed on a normal EEG background.[26,27] Because treatment with the ketogenic diet (KD) is highly efficacious for this disorder and standard AEDs are usually ineffective, and because diagnosis can be made in most cases with gene testing (with no need for lumbar puncture to show low cerebrospinal fluid glucose, as was previously required), we recommend evaluation for this disorder when a child in the 2–4-year age range presents with epilepsy primarily characterized by absence seizures.

▶ TREATMENT

The goal of treatment with absence seizures is to eliminate clinically apparent seizures and minimize electrographic spike-wave discharge frequency without significant AED side effects. Bursts of generalized spike-wave complexes, particularly if longer than 3 seconds, may cause transient cognitive impairment, even when a discrete seizure is not externally apparent.[28] Follow-up EEGs are recommended once the child's parents report that they have ceased to see seizures. Though routine EEGs with hyperventilation are probably adequate, prolonged EEG recordings (such as ambulatory EEG) may yield a more accurate picture of the frequency of unrecognized absence seizures and interictal epileptiform discharges.

Information on the most effective AEDs for treating absence seizures in very young children, under the age of 4, is lacking. Evidence from a large randomized controlled clinical trial on the treatment of CAE in children ages 4–10 indicates that ethosuximide (ETX) should be the first-line AED, because it is effective in two-thirds of children and may have less of an impact on cognition (attention) than VPA, which also has efficacy against seizures in two-thirds of children with CAE.[29] However, in a child with absence epilepsy who has had one or more GTCs, ETX alone is not recommended. LTG appeared to be less effective in this double-blinded randomized clinical trial, but in a child with GTCs in addition to absence seizures who does not tolerate VPA, LTG would be a reasonable next option.

Many children with CAE achieve adequate seizure control on monotherapy, but children with early-onset absence seizures (who usually do not have CAE) are often treatment-resistant. If control is not achieved with trials of monotherapy with ETX, VPA, or LTG, a combination of these agents is appropriate. TPM and ZNS for absence seizures have been less well studied, but may have a role as second-line agents. In a randomized, placebo-controlled trial of LEV for newly diagnosed CAE and JAE, LEV appeared modestly effective at a relatively low-target dose, and thus should not be considered first-line therapy but may have a role as second line or adjunctive therapy.[30] Other options for treatment resistant epilepsy with absence seizures in this age group include Clobazam (CBZ), Acetazolamide (ACZ), Felbamate (FBM), and the KD. As discussed earlier, a child with absence seizures due to GLUT-1 glucose transporter deficiency should be referred for KD treatment, a first-line treatment for this disorder.

► OUTCOME AND PROGNOSIS

The natural history of absence seizures with onset under age 4 years is not well studied, but outcome is considered to be less favorable than typical CAE. However, a child who has been seizure-free on AED therapy for 2 years, particularly if the EEG has normalized, merits a medication discontinuation trial. There is no evidence that seizures that recur off of medication will be more difficult to treat when medication is restarted.

The discovery of an underlying disorder may offer more specific prognostic information. Many children with absence seizures in this age group will have other generalized seizure types, such as myoclonic seizures or GTCs.

► MYOCLONIC SEIZURES

CLASSIFICATION AND DIAGNOSIS

History

Myoclonic seizures, momentary jerks of the head, trunk, or limbs without apparent loss of consciousness, may be difficult for parents to recognize initially. As normal movements may also be confused with myoclonic seizures, the behavioral state during these movements is important for accurate diagnosis. During wakefulness, myoclonic seizures must be distinguished from an exaggerated startle response, pronounced clonus, and complex motor tics. During sleep, myoclonic seizures must be distinguished from nearly ubiquitous benign sleep myoclonus. As with any seizure type, a detailed description of the event, including circumstances and possible triggers, is critical. Many children with myoclonic seizures have other seizures types as well, which may be less frequent but more disabling. In fact, myoclonic seizures may not be diagnosed until the child presents with falls related to tonic or atonic seizures or GTCs. Myoclonic seizures occur singly or in clusters, and spontaneously or reflexively in response to sound or tactile stimuli.

EEG

The characteristic EEG pattern in patients with myoclonic seizures is a generalized spike-wave or polyspike-wave complex with a wide range of possible frequencies, from less than 2 Hz to greater than 5 Hz.

Differential Diagnosis

The key diagnostic issue when evaluating a young child with new-onset myoclonic seizures is whether the seizures are symptomatic of an underlying metabolic or progressive neurodegenerative disorder, or whether they are part of a nonprogressive epilepsy syndrome. Making this distinction is challenging initially because the cognitive deterioration typical of the progressive myoclonic epilepsies may also occur in MAE (Doose syndrome) and LGS, epilepsy syndromes with multiple seizure types including myoclonus.

Many of the progressive myoclonic epilepsies present in older childhood or adolescence, but some present in early childhood—specifically, some types of neuronal ceroid lipofuscinosis (NCL) and myoclonic epilepsy with ragged red fibers (MERRF) or other mitochondrial disorders. Genetic testing to confirm these diagnoses is often available (www.genetests.org). Other genetically determined disorders presenting myoclonus in this age group include Dravet syndrome and GEFS+, discussed previously in this chapter, which are associated with mutations in the SCN1A gene, and sometimes other sodium channel mutations.

Diagnostic Testing

The question of how far to pursue diagnostic testing for the progressive myoclonic epilepsies when a child initially presents with epileptic myoclonus has no straightforward answer. The presence of cerebellar signs, movement disorders, visual impairment, myopathy, cardiac abnormalities, or deafness should certainly prompt further investigation. If these signs or symptoms are absent initially, the clinician should look for them at each subsequent evaluation. EEG findings are not likely to be diagnostic early on, but neurophysiologic abnormalities such as background slowing, occipital spike discharges (in NCL), and giant somatosensory evoked potentials may become apparent later in the course of several of the myoclonic epilepsies. For all children 2–4 years of age with new-onset epilepsy with myoclonus, MRI is recommended to assess for MCDs or evidence of prior insults. Further genetic or metabolic testing depends on other clinical features, associated cognitive or developmental abnormalities, and family history. Since the development of new-onset myoclonic seizures is an unusual presentation of epilepsy in a 2–4-year old, a comprehensive evaluation can be justified, because some of these disorders have implications for genetic counseling.

▶ TREATMENT

Treatment considerations for a young child with myoclonic epilepsy are similar to those for GTCs, with little high-quality data for treatment decisions. VPA is a commonly employed first-line agent, but TPM, ZNS, LEV, and LTG are also options. LTG appears effective for myoclonic seizures in some patients, but may exacerbate myoclonic seizures in others.[31,32] If AEDs used alone or in combination are ineffective, clonazepam or other benzodiazepines should be considered, although the side effect of sedation may limit their usefulness. The KD is another treatment option for children with myoclonic seizures refractory to medication (see Chapter 53).

▶ OUTCOME AND PROGNOSIS

The outcome of myoclonic seizures presenting in a 2–4-year old is often poor, and clearly linked to the underlying etiology or epilepsy syndrome. Children who are developmentally normal at presentation (and remain so) and have a normal EEG background and MRI often do well, but long-term data on cases without a specific etiology is lacking. Even cases with the specific syndrome diagnosis of MAE have an unpredictable outcome, with epilepsy remitting in some cases but developing along the lines of LGS in other cases.[33]

▶ TONIC AND ATONIC SEIZURES

CLASSIFICATION AND DIAGNOSIS

History

Tonic seizures are characterized by sustained muscle contraction leading to stiffening of the trunk and sometimes the limbs, typically lasting 10–60 seconds. Extension of the trunk or flexion of the legs, if the child is standing, may cause the child to fall, risking injury. Contraction of the respiratory muscles may lead to brief vocalization or apnea. Tonic seizures occur with increased frequency during non-REM sleep and may occur in clusters.

Atonic seizures, also called astatic seizures if loss of station (falling) occurs, are characterized by a sudden loss of postural muscle tone. Onset is without warning and seizures are usually brief. If loss of tone is restricted to the neck or upper trunk, a head drop will occur. If loss of tone is more widespread, the child may collapse to the ground. Falls from atonic seizures carry a risk of injury, particularly when multiple falls occur daily. The term "drop attack" is generally applied to any seizure that causes a fall. A "drop attack" may refer to a tonic seizure, an atonic seizure, or even a myoclonic seizure.

As with other seizure types, a detailed description, or even a demonstration of the events by the parents, is helpful in determining the nature of these seizures. Muscle contraction is sustained for a longer period of time in tonic seizures than in infantile spasms (called epileptic spasms when they occur outside of infancy), but both seizure types form a semiological continuum. When a fall is involved, tonic seizures can be distinguished by a rigid fall, where atonic seizures may be characterized by loss of limb or truncal tone resulting in slumping over. Nonepileptic events, including gastroesophageal reflux and opisthotonic posturing also mimic tonic seizures. A child with tonic seizures is highly likely to have other seizure types including atypical absence, GTCs, atonic, myoclonic, nonconvulsive status epilepticus, or even focal seizures. A tonic seizure may also occur in combination with another seizure type, particularly a myoclonic seizure (where a myoclonic jerk may precede stiffening of the trunk and limbs), and atypical absence seizure (where ictal discharges and behavioral arrest may continue after the tonic posturing has stopped).

EEG

The electroencephalographic pattern during a tonic seizure is typically a paroxysm of diffuse high-amplitude fast activity (10–25 Hz) that is sometimes preceded or followed by a series of generalized spike-wave or polyspike-wave complexes. Alternatively, tonic seizures may be accompanied only by diffuse flattening of the electrographic tracing without obvious fast activity.[34] Atonic seizures are usually accompanied electrographically by generalized spike-wave or polyspike-wave discharges.

Differential Diagnosis

Tonic seizures almost always occur in the context of symptomatic generalized epilepsy, and are a major seizure type in LGS, which is discussed in greater detail in Chapter XX. Less commonly, tonic seizures may occur in SMEI and MAE, but are not the prominent seizure type in either disorder. Atonic seizures, like tonic seizures, are most commonly seen in the symptomatic generalized epilepsies, but are also a major component of MAE.

The diagnostic evaluation in a young child presenting with tonic or atonic seizures depends on the individual clinical situation. MRI is always warranted to evaluate for underlying developmental or acquired abnormalities. The need for further genetic or metabolic evaluation depends on associated signs and symptoms, as discussed previously in this chapter.

▶ TREATMENT

Tonic and atonic seizures, particularly in the context of LGS, are frequently medically refractory, and children with these seizure types are often treated with a combination of medications. However, a multiple AED regimen should be employed with caution because of the increased potential for side effects, particularly sedation, without improved seizure control.

Traditionally, VPA is considered first-line therapy for these seizure types.[35] A recently introduced drug, Rufinamide, has been approved for use specifically for the seizures associated with LGS, including tonic and atonic seizures, in children as young as 4 years.[36] There is no body of evidence for its use in younger children, but studies are expected in the next few years. Rufinamide appears to be generally well tolerated, with side effects chiefly involving the CNS (sedation, dizziness) or GI systems (nausea, emesis). One issue that warrants special comment is the interaction between VPA and Rufinamide. VPA can substantially lower Rufinamide clearance.[37] When these two medications are used in combination, particularly in children, the target Rufinamide dose should be 50%–60% of what is used in the absence of VPA.

Other AED options include LTG, TPM, and felbamate (FBM), which have all been shown to have some efficacy for tonic and atonic seizures, though mostly in small open-label studies or in adjunctive therapy trials in refractory patients, which included children but not young children specifically.[38–40] In a placebo-controlled study of 28 children with LGS, FBM led to a 34% reduction in atonic seizures compared to a 9% reduction in the placebo group.[38] Tonic seizures were not studied separately. Though rare but potentially serious hepatic and hematologic side effects have limited its use, FBM is a reasonable option for tonic and atonic seizures in children when first-line agents have not been effective.

Treatment alternative for refractory tonic and atonic seizures also include the KD, vagus nerve stimulation, and corpus callosotomy. Though the KD can be effective over a broad range of ages, patients in the 2–4-year age group may be particularly good candidates for the KD because their dietary intake is largely controlled by their parents and they are less apt to seek out restricted foods. A number of studies demonstrating KD efficacy have shown a reduction in seizure frequency in children with tonic and atonic seizures, though no trials have looked at these seizures types separately.[41–43] Corpus callosotomy, most often limited to sectioning of the anterior two-thirds of the corpus callosum, appears to be an effective treatment for drop attacks, although efficacy for other seizure types is limited. Up to 85% of patients achieve 90% or better reduction in seizures producing falls.[44] An important consideration in caring for children with drop attacks is minimizing injury incurred by falls. Helmets with face protection are almost universally indicated, and care should be taken to avoid situations in which a fall may cause catastrophic injury.

▶ OUTCOME AND PROGNOSIS

Prognosis for seizure control and cognitive development in a child with tonic or atonic seizures will depend on the underlying etiologies, other comorbidities, and associated seizure types. As discussed earlier, children with symptomatic generalized epilepsy, which includes most patients with tonic seizures, have a poorer outcome than children with idiopathic epilepsy, which includes some children with atonic seizures (such as those with MAE). A high frequency of tonic seizures has been proposed as a predictor of poorer prognosis in LGS.[45] If a clear epilepsy syndrome or etiology is not obvious, then prognostic data are very limited but important features likely include baseline cognitive and developmental status, EEG background, brain imaging, and response to initial AED trials.

REFERENCES

1. DiMario FJ Jr. Prospective study of children with cyanotic and pallid breath-holding spells. *Pediatrics* 2001;107(2):265–269.

2. Kilaru S, Bergqvist AG. Current treatment of myoclonic astatic epilepsy: clinical experience at the Children's Hospital of Philadelphia. *Epilepsia* 2007;48(9):1703–1707.

3. Genton PGSM, Thomas P. Epilepsy with Grand Mal on awakening. In: Roger JBM, Dravet C, Genton P, Tassinari CA, Wolf P (eds), *Epileptic Syndromes in Infancy, Childhood and Adolescence*. London: John Libbey, 2005; 4th edn: pp. 389–394.

4. Loiseau P, Pestre M, Dartigues JF, Commenges D, Barberger-Gateau C, Cohadon S. Long-term prognosis in two forms of childhood epilepsy: typical absence seizures and epilepsy with rolandic (centrotemporal) EEG foci. *Ann Neurol* 1983;13(6):642–648.

5. Doose H, Lunau H, Castiglione E, Waltz S. Severe idiopathic generalized epilepsy of infancy with generalized tonic-clonic seizures. *Neuropediatrics* 1998;29(5):229–238.

6. Camfield C, Camfield P. Management guidelines for children with idiopathic generalized epilepsy. *Epilepsia* 2005;46(Suppl 9):112–116.

7. Sharma S, Riviello JJ, Harper MB, Baskin MN. The role of emergent neuroimaging in children with new-onset afebrile seizures. *Pediatrics* 2003;111(1):1–5.

8. Gambardella A, Marini C. Clinical spectrum of SCN1A mutations. *Epilepsia* 2009;50(Suppl 5):20–23.

9. Ferraro TN, Dlugos DJ, Buono RJ. Role of genetics in the diagnosis and treatment of epilepsy. *Expert Rev Neurother* 2006;6(12):1789–1800.

10. Thomas P, Valton L, Genton P. Absence and myoclonic status epilepticus precipitated by antiepileptic drugs in idiopathic generalized epilepsy. *Brain* 2006;129(Pt 5):1281–1292.

11. Berkovic SF, Knowlton RC, Leroy RF, Schiemann J, Falter U. Placebo-controlled study of levetiracetam in idiopathic generalized epilepsy. *Neurology* 2007;69(18):1751–1760.

12. Krief P, Li K, Maytal J. Efficacy of levetiracetam in children with epilepsy younger than 2 years of age. *J Child Neurol* 2008;23(5):582–584.

13. Perry S, Holt P, Benatar M. Levetiracetam versus carbamazepine monotherapy for partial epilepsy in children less than 16 years of age. *J Child Neurol* 2008;23(5):515–519.

14. Khurana DS, Kothare SV, Valencia I, Melvin JJ, Legido A. Levetiracetam monotherapy in children with epilepsy. *Pediatr Neurol* 2007;36(4):227–230.

15. Perry MS, Benatar M. Efficacy and tolerability of levetiracetam in children younger than 4 years: a retrospective review. *Epilepsia* 2007;48(6):1123–1127.

16. Trevathan E, Kerls SP, Hammer AE, Vuong A, Messenheimer JA. Lamotrigine adjunctive therapy among children and adolescents with primary generalized tonic–clonic seizures. *Pediatrics* 2006;118(2):e371–e378.

17. Guberman AH, et al. Lamotrigine-associated rash: risk/benefit considerations in adults and children. *Epilepsia* 1999;40(7):985–991.

18. Glauser TA, Dlugos DJ, Dodson WE, Grinspan A, Wang S, Wu SC. Topiramate monotherapy in newly diagnosed epilepsy in children and adolescents. *J Child Neurol* 2007;22(6):693–699.

19. Dahlin MG, Ohman IK. Age and antiepileptic drugs influence topiramate plasma levels in children. *Pediatr Neurol* 2004;31(4):248–253.

20. Bryant AE, Dreifuss FE. Valproic acid hepatic fatalities. III. U.S. experience since 1986. *Neurology* 1996;46(2):465–469.

21. McFarland R, et al. Reversible valproate hepatotoxicity due to mutations in mitochondrial DNA polymerase gamma (POLG1). *Arch Dis Child* 2008;93(2):151–153.

22. de Vivo DC, et al. L-carnitine supplementation in childhood epilepsy: current perspectives. *Epilepsia* 1998;39(11):1216–1225.

23. Sullivan JE 3rd, Dlugos DJ. Antiepileptic drug monotherapy: pediatric concerns. *Semin Pediatr Neurol* 2005;12(2):88–96.

24. Chaix Y, Daquin G, Monteiro F, Villeneuve N, Laguitton V, Genton P. Absence epilepsy with onset before age three years: a heterogeneous and often severe condition. *Epilepsia* 2003;44(7):944–949.

25. Hirsch EPC. Childhood absence epilepsy and related syndromes. In: Roger JBM, Dravet C, Genton P, Tassinari CA, Wolf P (eds), *Epileptic Syndromes in Infancy, Childhood and Adolescence*. London: John Libbey, 2005; 4th edn: pp. 315–335.

26. Leary LD, Wang D, Nordli DR Jr, Engelstad K, De Vivo DC. Seizure characterization and electroencephalographic features in GLUT-1 deficiency syndrome. *Epilepsia* 2003;44(5):701–707.

27. Mullen SA, Suls A, De Jonghe P, Berkovic SF, Scheffer IE. Absence epilepsies with widely variable onset are a key feature of familial GLUT1 deficiency. *Neurology* 2010;75(5):432–440.

28. Aldenkamp AP, Arends J. Effects of epileptiform EEG discharges on cognitive function: is the concept of "transient cognitive impairment" still valid? *Epilepsy Behav* 2004;5(Suppl 1):S25–S34.

29. Glauser TA, et al. Ethosuximide, valproic acid, and lamotrigine in childhood absence epilepsy. *N Engl J Med* 2010;362(9):790–799.

30. Fattore C, et al. A multicenter, randomized, placebo-controlled trial of levetiracetam in children and adolescents with newly diagnosed absence epilepsy. *Epilepsia* 2011;52(4):802–809.

31. Guerrini R, Dravet C, Genton P, Belmonte A, Kaminska A, Dulac O. Lamotrigine and seizure aggravation in severe myoclonic epilepsy. *Epilepsia* 1998;39(5):508–512.

32. Crespel A, et al. Lamotrigine associated with exacerbation or de novo myoclonus in idiopathic generalized epilepsies. *Neurology* 2005;65(5):762–764.

33. Neubauer BA, Hahn A, Doose H, Tuxhorn I. Myoclonic-astatic epilepsy of early childhood—definition, course, nosography, and genetics. *Adv Neurol* 2005;95:147–155.

34. Chatrian GE, Lettich E, Wilkus RJ, Vallarta J. Polygraphic and clinical observations on tonic-autonomic seizures. *Electroencephalogr Clin Neurophysiol Suppl* 1982;(35):101–124.

35. Wheless JW, Clarke DF, Carpenter D. Treatment of pediatric epilepsy: expert opinion, 2005. *J Child Neurol* 2005;20(Suppl 1):S1–S56; quiz S9–S60.

36. Glauser T, Kluger G, Sachdeo R, Krauss G, Perdomo C, Arroyo S. Rufinamide for generalized seizures associated with Lennox–Gastaut syndrome. *Neurology* 2008;70(21): 1950–1958.

37. Perucca E, Cloyd J, Critchley D, Fuseau E. Rufinamide: clinical pharmacokinetics and concentration-response relationships in patients with epilepsy. *Epilepsia* 2008;49 (7): 1123–1141.

38. The Felbamate Study Group in Lennox–Gastaut Syndrome. Efficacy of felbamate in childhood epileptic encephalopathy (Lennox–Gastaut syndrome). *N Engl J Med* 1993;328(1):29–33.

39. Motte J, Trevathan E, Arvidsson JF, Barrera MN, Mullens EL, Manasco P. Lamotrigine for generalized seizures associated with the Lennox–Gastaut syndrome. Lamictal Lennox–Gastaut Study Group. *N Engl J Med* 1997;337(25):1807–1812.

40. Sachdeo RC, Glauser TA, Ritter F, Reife R, Lim P, Pledger G. A double-blind, randomized trial of topiramate in

Lennox–Gastaut syndrome. Topiramate YL Study Group. *Neurology* 1999;52(9):1882–1887.

41. Neal EG, et al. The ketogenic diet for the treatment of childhood epilepsy: a randomised controlled trial. *Lancet Neurol* 2008;7(6):500–506.

42. Freeman JM, Vining EP, Pillas DJ, Pyzik PL, Casey JC, Kelly LM. The efficacy of the ketogenic diet—1998: a prospective evaluation of intervention in 150 children. *Pediatrics* 1998;102(6):1358–1363.

43. Bergqvist AG, Schall JI, Gallagher PR, Cnaan A, Stallings VA. Fasting versus gradual initiation of the ketogenic diet: a prospective, randomized clinical trial of efficacy. *Epilepsia* 2005;46(11):1810–1819.

44. Maehara T, Shimizu H. Surgical outcome of corpus callosotomy in patients with drop attacks. *Epilepsia* 2001; 42(1):67–71.

45. Roger J, Dravet C, Bureau M. The Lennox–Gastaut syndrome. *Cleve Clin J Med* 1989;56(Suppl Pt 2):S172–S180.

CHAPTER 12

Neonatal Epilepsies with Suppression–Burst Pattern

Shunsuke Ohtahara and Yasuko Yamatogi

▶ OVERVIEW

In 2001, ILAE Commission on Classification and Terminology proposed a diagnostic scheme of epilepsy that included a new concept of epileptic encephalopathy in which epileptic abnormalities contribute to a progressive disturbance in cerebral function.[1] Also called catastrophic epilepsy, the earliest form of epileptic encephalopathies are Ohtahara syndrome (OS) and early myoclonic encephalopathy (EME).[2–4] This chapter outlines OS and EME, referring to their treatment and prognoses.

PRINCIPLES OF DIAGNOSIS

EEG

The suppression–burst pattern (SB) is a unique EEG pattern in which bursts of high voltage paroxysmal activity and near-flat suppression appear alternately, and likely represents disconnection of the cortex from subcortical structures.[2,3] Clinically, SB is also observed in (1) neonatal hypoxic–ischemic encephalopathy, in which it is usually called burst–suppression pattern, (2) deep anesthesia/sedation, and (3) neonatal epileptic encephalopathy such as OS and EME. SB in these latter disorders differs from the former two conditions; SB in the epileptic encephalopathy includes active epileptic discharges in bursts and has a shorter suppression phase than the former two transient nonepileptic conditions. To separate from other conditions with transient SB, Aicardi and Ohtahara[3] considered that SB in the severe neonatal epilepsies must be stable or "invariant" for more than two weeks. As OS and EME share similar features besides SB such as very early onset, frequent and intractable seizures and severe prognoses, they are sometimes inclusively described such as early infantile epileptic syndromes with suppression–burst[5] or severe neonatal epilepsies with suppression–burst pattern.[3]

DIFFERENTIAL DIAGNOSIS

Differential Diagnosis of Ohtahara and West Syndromes

The age at onset of the two syndromes is different: OS appears from the neonatal period to early infancy and West syndrome (WS) in middle infancy (Table 12–1).

The main seizure type is tonic spasms in both syndromes, but tonic spasms in OS appear not only while awake but also during sleep, and not always in clusters. Focal seizures also occur in some cases of both syndromes, but are much less frequent in WS.

OS usually has more severe cortical pathology, often displaying asymmetric lesions in neuroimaging, and some asymmetry or focal features in EEG, that is, SB, subsequent hypsarrythmia or focal spikes.

The EEG helps discriminate SB in OS from hypsarrhythmia in WS. SB in OS differs from the periodic type of hypsarrhythmia, in which periodicity becomes remarkable only during sleep.

Seizures are more intractable in OS, and adrenocorticotrophic hormone (ACTH) is usually much less effective. Furthermore, OS has a poorer developmental prognosis than WS.

Differential Diagnosis Between EME and OS

As EME and OS share some clinicoelectrical characteristics, such as very early onset and SB on EEG, differentiation may be challenging in atypical cases (Table 12–1). The cardinal seizure type in OS is tonic spasms whereas myoclonias are rare. However, myoclonias, especially erratic myoclonias, and frequent partial seizures are the main seizure types in EME.[3,4,6–8]

SB differs considerably in both syndromes in the age of its appearance and its relation to the circadian cycle. SB in OS appears at the onset of the disorder, with the onset of tonic spasms, and is consistently observed during both the awake and sleep states. In contrast, SB in EME becomes distinct at age 1–5 months in some cases and is enhanced by sleep and often not apparent in waking records.[2,4,6,8,9]

The age-related EEG evolution also differs considerably between OS and EME.[4,8] In OS the transition from SB to hypsarrhythmia occurs within 6 months of life in many cases and may progress to diffuse slow spike-waves or multiple independent spike foci (MISF) in some cases.[2,4,10–13] In EME, however, SB persists for a longer time, at least in sleep although atypical hypsarrhythmia may appear transiently in some cases.[4,8]

OS is the earliest age-dependent epileptic encephalopathy and may sequentially evolve to WS and

► **TABLE 12–1. ELECTROCLINICAL FEATURES OF NEONATAL ENCEPHALOPATHIES**

Characteristics		Ohtahara Syndrome	Early Myoclonic Encephalopathy	West Syndrome
Age of onset		Early infancy (mainly neonatal)	Early infancy (mainly neonatal)	Middle infancy
Etiology		Polyetiology; mainly organic, malformative brain lesion (organic/static encephalopathy)	Some metabolic disorders (metabolic encephalopathy)	Polyetiology
Initial seizure type		Tonic spasms, partial seizures	Myoclonia, partial seizures	Tonic spasms
Clinical seizure	Nonepileptic myoclonia	+ (erratic)	+++ (erratic, fragmentary)	–
	Tonic spasms	Main seizure type (single/in series)	Transiently in middle or late infancy (single/in series)	Main seizure type (usually in series)
	PS	+	+++ (main seizure type)	±
	Sleep-wake cycle	Diffuse	Diffuse	Awake
EEG	Interictal	SB	SB (burst-suppression type in neonate)	Hypsarrhythmia
	Burst–burst interval	Relatively regular	Irregular (shorter burst and longer suppression in neonatal period)	
Sleep-wake cycle		Consistently, regardless of sleep-wake cycle	Enhanced by sleep (after neonate)	Periodic in sleep
	Course of SB	Transition to hypsarrhythmia or spike foci after middle infancy	Persist even after 1 yr of age (in sleep)	Transition to diffuse slow spike-waves, spike foci from late infancy
	Ictal EEG	Desynchronization (tonic spasm)	Focal rhythm (PS), myoclonia sometimes concordant with burst	Desynchronization (tonic spasm)
Treatment		Intractable; ACTH, ZNS	Extremely intractable, PAL-P	ACTH, PAL-P, VPA, BZP, ZNS
Evolution		To WS, LGS, SE-MISF, SPE	Long-term persistence with regression, WS, SE-MISF, SPE	To LGS, SE-MISF, SPE
Prognosis		Very poor	Extremely poor	Variable

BZP, benzodiazepines; LGS, Lennox–Gastaut syndrome; PAL-P, pyridoxal phosphate; PS, partial seizure; SB, suppression–burst; SE-MISF, severe epilepsy with multiple independent spike foci; SPE, symptomatic partial epilepsy; VPA, valproate; WS, West syndrome; ZNS, zonisamide.

Lennox–Gastaut syndrome (LGS) in accordance with EEG transition, while EME shows no age-specific evolution.

Etiologically, OS usually occurs on the basis of gross organic brain lesions including brain malformations and cerebral dysgenesis, while EME may associate with some verified or undetermined inborn errors of metabolism.[2–4]

Differential Diagnosis of EME from Malignant Migrating Partial Seizures in Infancy (MMPSI)

MMPSI is a recently recognized epileptic syndrome that begins in the first 6 months of life in which frequent partial seizures involve multiple independent areas of both hemispheres with arrest of psychomotor development.[14] EME and MMPSI share some characteristics such as onset in early infancy, no evidence of organic brain lesion, various types of partial seizures with ictal EEG features migrating from one cortical area to the other. Decisive difference is absence of myoclonias or tonic spasms and SB in MMPI.

► OHTAHARA SYNDROME: EARLY INFANTILE EPILEPTIC ENCEPHALOGRAPHY WITH SUPPRESSION–BURST

EPIDEMIOLOGY

OS is a rare syndrome compared with WS and LGS. An epidemiologic study on childhood epilepsy carried out in Okayama Prefecture, Japan, detected one case of OS (0.04%), 4 cases of EME (0.17%), and 40 cases (1.68%) of WS among 2378 epileptic children younger than 10 years of age in 1980.[15] Compared to WS, the prevalence of OS is 1/40. A similar study in 1999 observed two cases of EME (0.09%), no cases of OS, and 59 cases of WS (2.7%) among 2222 epileptic children younger than 13 years of age.[16] Similarly, Kramer et al[17] described one case of OS (0.2%) and 40 cases of WS (9.1%) in a cohort of 440 consecutive children with epilepsy under 15 years of age in Tel Aviv. The incidence rates of OS and WS were estimated as 0.1 and 4.2/10,000 live births, respectively, in Miyagi Prefecture, Japan. Thus, the relative incidence of OS and EME to WS is nearly 1/40 or less and 1/10–30, respectively. There are no obvious sex differences.

ETIOLOGY

Among the heterogeneous causes of OS, static structural brain lesions including brain malformations and cerebral dysgenesis are often found; it may be reasonably called an organic encephalopathy.[2,12] Documented etiologies are porencephaly, Aicardi syndrome, olivary–dentate dysplasia,[18] olivary–dentate dysplasia with agenesis of the mamillary bodies,[19] hemimegalencephaly,[5,20–23] lissencephaly, linear sebaceous nevus syndrome.[2,3,10,12] Pathologic analysis has sometimes disclosed significant abnormalities not demonstrated on neuroimagings.[18,19,24] Metabolic disorders have not been reported except mitochondrial respiratory chain complex IV[25] and I[26,27] deficiency or Leigh encephalopathy, in which OS may be caused by secondary neuronal migration disorders or extensive brain damage rather than the metabolic disorder itself.[3]

No etiology has been identified in nearly one-third of cases.[12,28] However, these cryptogenic cases may have undetectable microdysgenesis or migration disorders that cause the progressive atrophy during the follow-up.

Recently, mutations have been identified in the aristaless-related homeobox gene (ARX) at Xp22.13, involving in the development of GABAergic interneurons,[29] STXBP1 (MUNC18–1) gene at 9q34.1, relating synapse vesicle release,[30] and SLC25A22 gene at 11p15.5 encoding a mitochondrial glutamate carrier,[31,32] mainly in cryptogenic OS. ARX gene mutations are also reported in familiar cases of OS[33,34] and each one boy with OS and WS are found in a family.[35] STXBP1 gene mutations were identified in as many as 14 of 43 cryptogenic OS cases by Saitsu et al,[36] one of 10 cases (10%) by Otsuka et al,[37] but none of 9 cases by Deprez et al.[38] One mutation of SLC25A22 gene had been reported in a family with 4 children with "EME",[39] but later it was regarded to be responsible for OS as well as another mutation of this gene.[31,32] A precise and accurate acquisition or diagnosis of clinicoelectrical features will be fundamentally important for the proper interpretation of the results of molecular genetic studies.

As the expression of these genes is essential for early brain development such as neuronal progenitor cells proliferation and migration, and neurotransmitter regulation, their dysfunction could cause migration disorders or microdysgenesis, and neuronal miscommunication or hyperexcitability.[32] Further investigation of these gene functions is expected to elucidate the manifestation mechanism of OS and WS.

CLINICAL PRESENTATION

OS is an intractable and severe epileptic syndrome that begins within the first few months of life that is characterized by frequent tonic spasms/epileptic spasms, either in clusters or sporadic, with SB in the EEG, in both the awake and sleep states

EIEE was initially described by Ohtahara et al in 1976 and was designated as the earliest form of the age-dependent epileptic encephalopathy that was proposed as the inclusive concept of OS, WS, and LGS.[2,4,10] Each of these syndromes is an independent clinicoelectrical entity with unique features; OS is characterized by clustering and/or single tonic spasms and SB in early infancy, while WS evidences tonic spasms in cluster and hypsarrhtymia in middle infancy, while LGS is distinguished by multiple types of generalized minor seizures and a diffuse slow spike-wave pattern in late infancy or childhood.

The three syndromes share several common features: (1) age dependency, (2) frequent minor generalized seizures, (3) severe and continuous epileptic EEG abnormalities, (4) etiological heterogeneity, often causing gross organic brain damage and developmental/mental deficit, and (5) seizure intractability and severe psychomotor prognoses.[2,4,10] Mutual transition is often observed among three syndromes; many patients with OS evolve into WS and more than half of WS to LGS.[11,12] The shared characteristics and transition with age support the concept of age-dependent epileptic encephalopathy for these syndromes. "Epileptic encephalopathy" was applied to the group of disorders according to (1) the presence of a serious underlying disorder, (2) extremely frequent clinical seizures, (3) continuous and widespread epileptic EEG abnormalities and (4) catastrophic features of cognitive stagnation or deterioration associated with seizure persistence.[2,4,10] These features are compatible with the concept of epileptic encephalopathy formulated by the ILAE.[1]

As heterogeneous etiologies are observed in all three syndromes, maturational status appears to be a primary determinant for the expression of individual characteristics. These syndromes, therefore, may be an age-specific epileptic reaction of the brain at certain developmental stages to various nonspecific exogenous brain insults.

Clinical Seizure Manifestations

Seizure onset occurs within 3 months of birth, usually within the first month[2–4,10,12] Prenatal seizure onset has been described.[28] The main seizure type is tonic, lasting up to 10 seconds, with or without clustering. Clusters of 10 to 40 spasms may occur at intervals of 5 to 15 seconds. Epileptic spasms occur in wakefulness and sleep. Daily seizure frequency is high, ranging from 10 to 300 single spasms or 10 to 20 clusters of spasms. In addition to tonic spasms, partial seizures such as focal motor seizures, hemiconvulsions, or tonic seizures are observed in about one-third to one-half of patients. Combination of focal seizures and epileptic spasms as single ictal event (combined seizures) may be characteristic, particularly in patients with focal cortical pathology.[40,41] In contrast to EME, myoclonic seizures or erratic myoclonias are rare in OS.

Developmental Aspects

Age-dependent evolution is another remarkable characteristic of OS; the transition from OS to WS in the middle infancy, particularly during 3 to 6 months of age, in many cases, and further from WS to LGS in early childhood, about 1 to 3 years of age, in some cases.[4,10–12] Others transform to severe epilepsy with multiple independent spike foci (MISF)[13] and symptomatic generalized and partial epilepsies.

The EEG evolves from SB to hypsarrhythmia at around 3 to 6 months of age, and to diffuse slow spike-waves at around 1 year of age.[4,10,12] The transition from SB to hypsarrhythmia begins with a gradual increase in the amplitude of the suppression phase. Both SB and hypsarrhythmia disappear in wakefulness before sleep, suggesting that evolution proceeds in a close relation with the wake–sleep cycle.[10]

DIAGNOSIS

EEG Findings

The most characteristic and diagnostically important EEG feature is SB that persists throughout the wake–sleep cycle, and through all sleep stages including REM sleep.[10] SB is characterized by high voltage bursts alternating with nearly flat patterns at an approximately regular rate. Bursts of 150 to 350 microvolt high-voltage slow waves intermixed with multifocal spikes and sharp waves last between 1 to 5 seconds. The duration of suppression is typically 2 to 5 seconds. The burst–burst interval, measured from onset-to-onset, ranges from 5 to 15 seconds. Presumably reflecting underlying pathology, asymmetry in SB is observed in approximately two-thirds of cases, but without marked asynchrony or asymmetry except in Aicardi syndrome or hemimegalencephaly. Tonic spasms usually appear with

bursts, accompanied by EEG desynchronization with or without initial rapid activity superimposed on slow waves.[11,12,42] A low-voltage fast activity is also often superimposed on the attenuated/desynchronized part. SB gradually disappears to the midst of the cluster of spasms at a regular rate and then gradually regains to the end of the cluster.

Focal seizures usually show repetitive or rhythmic discharges from fixed foci and sometimes combined with tonic spasms in series.

Other Findings

Affected patients show marked developmental and neurological abnormalities after birth, although very early seizure onset makes it difficult to evaluate developmental profiles before onset. CT and MRI reveal structural lesions, even at disease onset, in many cases. Asymmetric or cortical lesions are more prominent in OS than WS. Progressive brain atrophy may accompany seizure persistence, particularly during infancy. Routine laboratory examinations of blood, urine, cerebrospinal fluid, bone marrow and liver functions and metabolic studies including amino acids, lysosomal enzymes, pyruvate and lactate, and organic acids, or immunological and virological examinations are normal.

TREATMENT AND PROGNOSIS

ACTH, corticosteroids, vitamin B6, valproate, vigabatrin, zonisamide, and benzodiazepines are often tried in patients with OS with limited success.[12] Zonisamide,[12,43] vigabatrin,[44,45] high dose phenobarbital[28,46] may be useful in some cases. The ketogenic diet,[27,28] thyrotropin releasing hormone or its analogue, chloral hydrate, lidocaine or mexiletine, liposteroid are reportedly effective in isolated cases.[2,3] Therapeutic responsiveness tends to be better in cryptogenic cases.

As transition to WS with brain maturation may alter the response to therapeutic agents, it may be worthwhile to retry them.

Successful resection of focal cortical dysplasia[47,48] and hemispherectomy for hemimegalencephaly[20,21,49] is reported. Considering the catastrophic course of OS, it is important to consider surgical treatment as early as possible.

The prognosis of OS is poor due to seizure intractability, high mortality and severe psychomotor retardation. Although intractable, seizures moderate by school age in nearly half of patients. In our series, half of affected patients died, in infancy or early childhood.[12] All survivors were mentally and physically handicapped. Life expectancy or prognoses may be better in cryptogenic cases or in cases with focal cortical pathology involved in producing asymmetry or focal feature in SB and transition to focal spike pattern.[10,12] Exceptionally favorable cases are reported sporadically, including cases with pyridoxine dependency[21] or with immediate response to vigabatrin.[45]

▶ EARLY MYOCLONIC EPILEPSY

EPIDEMIOLOGY

EME is as rare as OS or slightly more frequent than OS; the relative incidence of EME to WS is approximately 1/10–30. There is no sex difference.

ETIOLOGY

The high incidence of familial cases, as found in 4 of 12 families in the series of Aicardi[7] and 2 of 8 families in the series of Dalla Bernardina et al,[6] and 1 case of Schulumberger et al[5] indicates a genetic component or inborn errors of metabolism as the most likely cause of EME. This hypothesis is supported by the unremarkable prenatal and perinatal histories, and progressive brain atrophy. Autosomal recessive inheritance is suggested by the morbidity in siblings, the normality of parents, and equal sex distribution.[3] Glycine encephalopathy or nonketotic hyperglycinemia,[50–52] propionic acidemia, methylmalonic acidemia and D-glyceric acidemia,[50] sulphite and xanthine oxidase deficit resulting from molybdenum cofactor deficiency,[7] Menkes disease, and Zellweger syndrome[53] have similar clinicoelectrical features with EME[3] Typically however, the etiology of EME cases remains unknown and postmortem examination reveal variable findings that are nonspecific and affect both cortical and subcortical structures including the brainstem.[3,6,7,54]

Epilepsy phenotype of pyridoxine dependency,[55,56] pyridoxine phosphate oxidase deficiency,[56–58] or impaired mitochondrial glutamate transport[31,39] may include EME or other types of neonatal or infantile epileptic encephalopathy. Phenotype- and genotype-/mutation-type correlation and other modifying factors remain to be clarified for the understanding of gray zone between OS and EME.

CLINICAL PRESENTATION

EME is a rare epilepsy syndrome of very early onset with frequent myoclonias and partial seizures, and SB in the EEG. Seizures, particularly partial seizures, are intractable, and the life expectancy and psychomotor prognosis are very poor. EME was first described by Aicardi and Goutières in 1978; to date, over 50 cases have been reported under a variety of names, such as early myoclonic epileptic encephalopathy,[6] myoclonic encephalopathy with neonatal onset, neonatal myoclonic encephalopathy, early myoclonic encephalopathy with epilepsy.[3]

Identification of OS and EME has long been controversial in the cases with SB and early onset seizures including myoclonia and tonic spasms; some cases reported as OS may be EME[28] and many cases published as neonatal metabolic disorders such as nonketotic hyperglycinemia probably had EME.[3]

Seizure onset occurs within the first three months of life, but usually in the neonatal period. Fragmentary or segmental erratic myoclonias and various partial seizures are the cardinal seizure symptom in most cases and may occur within the first several hours of life or perhaps even prenatally.[59] In some cases, myoclonia is unclear at seizure onset and only becomes apparent 1–2 months later. Massive myoclonias and tonic spasms are seen in the middle infancy.

Myoclonias are often nonepileptic and consist of isolated twitching of the distal extremities, eyelids, and mouth, and may be subtle and unreported without careful observation. The frequency, localization, and severity of these jerks are variable and may fluctuate from several times a day to several dozen times a minute, may occur during sleep, and often tend to shift asynchronously.[3,7,9]

Focal seizures are the main seizure type and include focal seizures with eye-deviation or autonomic symptoms such as apnea and facial flushing, clonic seizures involving various parts of the body or migrating from one part to another in the same seizure, and asymmetric tonic posturing with or without generalization. They occur in both awake and sleep. Dalla Bernardina et al[6] considered focal seizures simultaneously associated with erratic myoclonias to be particularly characteristic to EME. The frequency of focal seizures is remarkably high, ranging from 7–8 times to 30–100 times a day, and have a tendency to cluster in the early stages, but decreases with age.[3,6]

Tonic spasms are also often observed, but massive myoclonias and tonic spasms are not necessarily observed in all cases. When tonic spasms appeared, usually at around 3 to 4 months of age, but ranging 5 days to 9 months of age,[8] cases are considered to have evolved to WS. The coexistence of myoclonic jerks, focal seizures and tonic axial spasms are more characteristic of WS developed from EME.[6] As WS is transient, EME typically recurs in late infancy or early childhood and may persist for a considerable period in childhood thereafter.[8]

Developmental Aspects

EME manifests little electroclinical development throughout its course, except for the EEG which changes from SB to a disorganized pattern with frequent multifocal spikes within the first several months of life[2–4,7,9] and to atypical hypsarrhythmia with WS transiently from 3 months to 2.5 years of age at the latest.[6,8] Focal seizures and SB in sleep often remain throughout childhood.[2,4,8] Symptomatic partial epilepsy with MISF may develop in some affected patients.[4]

DIAGNOSIS

EEG Findings

SB is diagnostically indispensable; bursts last 1 to 5 seconds and isoelectric suppression lasts 3–10 seconds or longer.[5,9] SB is more pronounced as sleep deepens.[6,8] The burst–burst interval is often irregular, longer than OS, with lower burst amplitude.[9] In some cases, SB in neonatal period may resemble the burst-suppression pattern with less active bursts and very long suppression phase, which shortens with age.[9] SB may first appear a few months after onset.[6,8]

Ictal EEG of focal seizures has the similar characteristics with neonatal seizures; various patterns of focal onset fast activity, alphoid or theta rhythm, rhythmic spikes or sharp waves, and irregular spike-waves, usually migrating from two or more foci (multifocal onset) even in one seizure.[3,6–9]

Tonic spasms show desynchronization preceded by slow waves, similar to tonic spasms in WS. Myoclonic seizures or massive myoclonias occur during bursts, but not strictly synchronous with spikes or spike-waves.[7,9,42] Erratic myoclonias usually show no consistent EEG change, although some coincidentally occur with bursts.[6–9]

Other Findings

Neuroimaging is often normal at the onset, but progressive brain atrophy is verified in some cases.[6,7,9] Abnormalities are often detected from 3 to 10 months of age, that is, 3–8 months after the onset. Diffuse cortical atrophy is noted in all, often with delayed myelination, and with ventricular dilatation in some, but focal structural abnormalities are exceptional. Signs of peripheral neuropathy with slowing of motor and sensory conduction velocities are reported in a familial case.[3,7] Frequent abnormality in various evoked potential studies suggests the diffuse progressive brain pathology including brainstem.[2] Neurological status is very poor at birth or soon after seizure onset, even though appeared healthy at birth, and probably show deterioration, but difficult to confirm due to a very early onset.[3,6,7] In addition to initially observed hypotonia, various pyramidal or extrapyramidal symptoms may appear later, including dystonia or choreoathetosis.[3]

TREATMENT AND PROGNOSES

Even symptomatic, treatment is directed toward the specific metabolic error, if present.[52,60] The target of antiepileptic treatment is usually partial seizures which

are multifocal and migratory. Accordingly, a similar therapeutic strategy for OS may be applied. Vitamins such as pyridoxal phosphate should be tried first.[60] Pyridoxine dependency or pyridoxal 5′-phosphate dependency with the clinical features of EME and atypical SB has been reported.[51,55–58] AEDs that might interfere with metabolic disorders, such as valproate, should be started with care. Surgery is rarely indicated due to widespread brain involvement in most cases. Myoclonias gradually decrease with age but partial seizures often persist and remain intractable.[3,6]

EME has an extremely poor prognosis including a high mortality, with death within two years of life in about half of the patients. Survivors have persistent partial seizures and stagnation of development or progressive psychomotor deterioration to a vegetative state,[3,5,7,8] excepting pyridoxine or pyridoxal phosphate responsive cases.

REFERENCES

1. Engel J. A proposed diagnostic scheme for people with epileptic seizures and with epilepsy: report of the ILAE task force on classification and terminology. *Epilepsia* 2001;42: 796–803.
2. Ohtahara S, Yamatogi Y. Epileptic encephalopathies in early infancy with suppression–burst. *J Clin Neurophysiol* 2003;20:398–407.
3. Aicardi J, Ohtahara S. Severe neonatal epilepsies with suppression–burst pattern. In: Roger J, Bureau M, Dravet C, Genton P, Tassinari CA, Wolf P (eds), *Epileptic Syndromes in Infancy, Childhood and Adolescence.* Montrouge: John Libbey Eurotext, 2005; 4th edn: pp. 39–50.
4. Ohtahara S, Yamatogi Y. Ohtahara syndrome: with special reference to its developmental aspects for differentiating from early myoclonic encephalopathy. *Epilepsy Res* 2006;70 (Suppl 1):S58–S67.
5. Schlumberger E, Dulac O, Plouin P. Early infantile epileptic syndrome(s) with suppression–burst: nosological considerations. In: Roger J, Bureau M, Dravet C, Dreifuss FE, Perret A, Wolf P (eds), *Epileptic Syndromes in Infancy, Childhood and Adolescence.* London: John Libbey, 1992; 2nd edn: pp. 35–42.
6. Dalla Bernardina B, et al. Early myoclonic epileptic encephalopathy (EMEE). *Eur J Pediatr* 1983;140:248–252.
7. Aicardi J. Early myoclonic encephalopathy (neonatal myoclonic encephalopathy). In: Roger J, Bureau M, Dravet C, Dreifuss FE, Perret A, Wolf P (eds), *Epileptic Syndromes in Infancy, Childhood and Adolescence.* London: John Libbey, 1992; 2nd edn: pp. 13–23.
8. Murakami N, Ohtsuka Y, Ohtahara S. Early infantile epileptic syndromes with suppression–bursts: early myoclonic encephalopathy vs. Ohtahara syndrome. *Jpn J Psychiatry Neurol* 1993;47:197–200.
9. Otani K, Abe J, Futagi Y, Yabuuchi H, Aotani H, Takeuchi T. Clinical and electroencephalographical follow-up study of early myoclonic encepahlopathy. *Brain Dev* 1989;11: 332–337.
10. Ohtahara S, Ohtsuka Y, Yamatogi Y, Oka E, Inoue H. Early-infantile epileptic encephalopathy with suppression–bursts. In: Roger J, Bureau M, Dravet C, Dreifuss FE,

Perret A, Wolf P (eds), *Epileptic Syndromes in Infancy, Childhood and Adolescence.* London: John Libbey, 1992; 2nd edn: pp. 25–34.

11. Yamatogi Y, Ohtahara S. Age-dependent epileptic encephalopathy: a longitudinal study. *Folia Psychiatr Neurol Jpn* 1981;35:321–331.

12. Yamatogi Y, Ohtahara S. Early-infantile epileptic encephalopathy with suppression–bursts, Ohtahara syndrome: its overview referring to our 16 cases. *Brain Dev* 2002;24:13–23.

13. Yamatogi Y, Ohtahara S. Multiple independent spike foci and epilepsy, with special reference to a new epileptic syndrome of "severe epilepsy with multiple independent spike foci". *Epilepsy Res* 2006;70S:S96–S104.

14. Coppola G, Plouin P, Chiron C, Robain O, Dulac O. Migrating partial seizures in infancy: a malignant disorder with developmental arrest. *Epilepsia* 1995;36: 1017–1024.

15. Oka E, Ishida S, Ohtsuka Y, Ohtahara S. Neuro-epidemiological study of childhood epilepsy by application of international classification of epilepsies and epileptic syndromes (ILAE, 1989). *Epilepsia* 1995;36:658–661.

16. Oka E, Ohtsuka Y, Yoshinaga H, Murakami N, Kobayashi K, Ogino T. Prevalence of childhood epilepsy and distribution of epileptic syndromes: a population-based survey in Okayama, Japan. *Epilepsia* 2006;47:626–630.

17. Kramer U, Nevo Y, Neufeld MY, Fatal A, Leitner Y, Harel S. Epidemiology of epilepsy in childhood: a cohort of 440 consecutive patients. *Pediatr Neurol* 1998;18:46–50.

18. Harding BN, Boyd SG. Intractable seizures from infancy can be associated with dentato-olivary dysplasia. *J Neurol Sci* 1991;104:157–165.

19. Trinka E, et al. A case of Ohtahara syndrome with olivary-dentate dysplasia and agenesis of mamillary bodies. *Epilepsia* 2001;42:950–953.

20. Bermejo AM, et al. Early infantile epileptic encephalopathy: a case associated with hemimegalencephaly. *Brain Dev* 1992;14:425–428.

21. Fusco L, Pachatz C, Di Capua M, Vigevano F. Video/EEG aspects of early-infantile epileptic encephalopathy with suppression–bursts (Ohtahara syndrome). *Brain Dev* 2001;23:708–714.

22. Guzzetta F, et al. Epileptic negative myoclonus in a newborn with hemimegalencephaly. *Epilepsia* 2002;43: 1106–1109.

23. Sasaki M, et al. Clinical aspects of hemimegalencephaly by means of a nationwide survey. *J Child Neurol* 2005;20:337–341.

24. Miller SP, Dilenge M-E, Meagher-Villemure K, O'Gorman AM, Shevell MI. Infantile epileptic encephalopathy (Ohtahara syndrome) and migrational disorder. *Pediatr Neurol* 1998;19:50–54.

25. Williams AN, Poulton K, Ramani P, Whitehouse WPA. A case of Ohtahara syndrome with cytochrome oxidase deficiency. *Dev Med Child Neurol* 1998;40:568–570 (refer to 2000;42:785–787).

26. Lee YM, et al. Mitochandrial respiratory chain defects: underlying etiology in various epileptic conditions. *Epilepsia* 2008;49:685–690.

27. Seo JH, Lee YM, Lee JS, Kim SH, Kim HD. A case of Ohtahara syndrome with mitochondrial respiratory chain complex I deficiency. *Brain Dev* 2010;32:253–257.

28. Clarke M, Gill J, Noronha M, McKinlay I. Early infantile epileptic encephalopathy with suppression–burst: Ohtahara syndrome. *Dev Med Child Neurol* 1987;29:520–528.

29. Kato M, et al. A longer polyalanine expansion mutation in the ARX gene causes early infantile epileptic encephalopathy with suppression–burst pattern (Ohtahara syndrome). *Am J Hum Genet* 2007;81:361–366.

30. Saitsu H, et al. De novo mutations of the gene encoding STXBP1 (MUNC18–1) cause early infantile epileptic encephalopathy. *Nat Genet* 2008;40:782–788.

31. Molinari F, et al. Mutations in the mitochondrial glutamate carrier SLC25A22 in neonatal epileptic encephalopathy with suppression–bursts. *Clin Genet* 2009;76:188–194.

32. Molinari F. Mitochondria and neonatal epileptic encephalopathy with suppression–burst. *J Bioenerg Biomembr* 2010;42:467–471.

33. Kato M, Koyama N, Ohta M, Miura K, Hayasaka K. Frameshift mutations of the ARX gene in familiar Ohtahara syndrome. *Epilepsia* 2010;51:1679–1684.

34. Giordano L, et al. Familial Ohtahara syndrome due to a nobel ARX gene mutation. *Am J Med Genet* 2010; 152A:3133–3137.

35. Fullston T, et al. Ohtahara syndrome in a family with an ARX protein truncation mutation (c.81C>G/p.Y27X). *Eur J Hum Genet* 2010;18:157–162.

36. Saitsu H, et al. STXBP1 mutations in early infantile epileptic encephalopathy with suppression–burst pattern. *Epilapsia* 2010;51:2397–2405.

37. Otsuka M, et al. STXBP1 mutations cause not only Ohtahara syndrome but also West syndrome—result of Japanese cohort study. *Epilepsia* 2010;51:2449–2452.

38. Deprez L, et al. Clinical spectrum of early-onset epileptic encephalopathies associated with STXBP1 mutations. *Neurology* 2010;75:1159–1165.

39. Molinari F, et al. Impaired mitochondrial glutamate transport in autosomal recessive neonatal myoclonic epilepsy. *Am J Hum Genet* 2005;76:334–339.

40. Akiyama T, Kobayashi K, Ohtsuka Y. Electroclinical characterization and classification of symptomatic epilepsies with very early onset by multiple correspondence analysis. *Epilepsy Res* 2010;91:232–239.

41. Kobayashi K, et al. Clinical spectrum of epileptic spasms associated with cortical malformation. *Neuropediatrics* 2001;32:236–244.

42. Kobayashi K, et al. Relation of spasms and myoclonus to suppression–burst on EEG in epileptic encephalopathy in early infancy. *Neurogenetics* 2007;38:244–250.

43. Ohtahara S. Zonisamide in the management of epilepsy: Japanese experience. *Epilepsy Res* 2006;68(Suppl 2):S25–S33.

44. Baxter PS, Gardne-Medwin D, Barwick DD, Ince P, Livingston J, Murdoch-Eaton D. Vigabatrin monotherapy in resistant neonatal seizures. *Seizure* 1995;4:57–59.

45. Cazorla MR, Verdu A, Montes C, Ayuga F. Early infantile epileptic encephalopathy with unusual favourable outcome. *Brain Dev* 2010;32:673–676.

46. Ozawa H, Kawada Y, Noma S, Sugai K. Oral high-dose phenobarbital therapy for early infantile epileptic encephalopathy. *Pediatr Neurol* 2002;26:222–224.

47. Pedespan JM, Loiseau H, Vital A, Marchal C, Fontan D, Rougier A. Surgical treatment of an early epileptic

encephalopathy with suppression–bursts and focal cortical dysplasia. *Epilepsia* 1995;36:37–40.

48. Komaki H, Sugai S, Maehara T, Shimizu H. Surgical treatment of early-infantile epileptic encephalopathy with suppression–bursts associated with focal cortical dysplasia. *Brain Dev* 2001;23:727–731.

49. Hmaimess G, et al. Impact of early hemispherotomy in a case of Ohtahara syndrome with left parieto–occipital megalencephaly. *Seizure* 2005;14:439–442.

50. Lombroso CT. Early myoclonic encephalopathy, early infantile epileptic encephalopathy, and benign and severe infantile myoclonic epilepsies: a critical review and personal contributions. *J Clin Neurophysiol* 1990;7:380–408.

51. Chen P-T, Young C, Lee W-T, Wang P-J, Pen SS, Shen Y-Z. Early epileptic encephalopathy with suppression–burst electroencephalographic pattern; an analysis of eight Taiwanese patients. *Brain Dev* 2002;23:715–720.

52. Suzuki Y, Kure S, Oota M, Hino H, Fukuda M. Nonketotic hyperglycinemia: proposal of diagnostic and treatment strategy. *Pediatr Neurol* 2010;43:221–224.

53. Spreafico R, et al. Burst suppression and impairment of neocortical ontogenesis: electroclinical and neuropathologic findings in two infants with early myoclonic encephalopathy. *Epilepsia* 1993;34:800–808.

54. Itoh M, Hanaoka S, Sasaki M, Ohama E, Takashima S. Neuropathology of early-infantile epileptic encephalopathy with suppression–bursts; comparison with those of early myoclonic encephalopathy and West syndrome. *Brain Dev* 2001;23:721–726.

55. Mills PB, et al. Genotypic and phenotypic spectrum of pyridoxine-dependent epilepsy (ALDH7A1 deficiency). *Brain* 2010;133:2148–2159.

56. Schmitt B, et al. Seizures and paroxysmal events: symptoms pointing to the diagnosis of pyridoxine-dependent epilepsy and pyridoxine phosphate oxidase deficiency. *De Med Child Neurol* 2010;52:e133–e142.

57. Mills PB, et al. Neonatal epileptic encephalopathy caused by mutations in the PNPO gene encoding pyridox(am)ine 5′-phosphate oxidase. *Hum Mol Genet* 2005;14:1077–1086.

58. Veerapandiyan A, et al. Electroencephalographic and seizure manifestations of pyridoxal 5′-phosphate-dependent epilepsy. *Epilepsy Behav* 2011;20(3):494–501.

59. du Plessis AJ, Kaufmann WE, Kupsky WJ. Intrauterine-onset myoclonic encephalopathy associated with cerebral cortical dysplasia. *J Child Neurol* 1993;8:164–170.

60. Pearl PL. New treatment paradigms in neonatal metabolic epilepsies. *J Inherit Metab Dis* 2009;32:204–213.

CHAPTER 13

Benign Myoclonic Epilepsy in Infancy

Mary B. Connolly

▶ OVERVIEW

Benign myoclonic epilepsy in infancy (BMEI), first described by Dravet and Bureau in 1981, is a rare epilepsy syndrome.[1] It is classified among the idiopathic generalized epilepsies and typically begins by the age of 3 years.[2] BMEI is characterized by brief myoclonic seizures without other seizure types in developmentally normal children. The myoclonic seizures may occur spontaneously or be provoked by contact or noise. A history of simple febrile seizures may be present. In a series of 88 patients with BMEI, 26.1% had a history of simple febrile seizures.[3] There is a family history of epilepsy or febrile seizures in 50% or more of patients. Myoclonic seizures are easily controlled with medication and usually remit later in childhood. Generalized tonic–clonic seizures may occur in late childhood or adolescence. Neurodevelopmental outcome is variable; most children have normal development but may experience educational difficulties.

▶ CLINICAL AND EEG MANIFESTATIONS

The most common age of onset of BMEI is between 4 months and 3 years of age, but later onset up to 4 years 8 months has been reported.[4,5] The myoclonic seizures are brief, and typically involve the upper limbs and head, and less frequently the lower limbs. Seizures may be extremely subtle or may be characterized by head nodding or spasm-like events. The frequency of myoclonic seizures gradually increases over time. Studies using video-EEG recordings have demonstrated that the myoclonic jerks involve the axis of the body and the arms, provoking a head drop, and commonly result in an upward and outward movement of the upper limbs with flexion of the lower limbs. As a consequence, the patient may drop objects from the hand during the seizures or there may be a loss of posture. However, it is uncommon for the child to fall to the ground unless the lower limbs are involved. In some instances, there may be involvement of the eyeball resulting in eye rolling. Seizures typically last 1–3 seconds but are always

shorter than 10 seconds. They occur multiple times daily and their onset is unpredictable. In contrast to infantile spasms, they do not occur in clusters. They tend to occur most frequently during periods of drowsiness and may be triggered by intermittent photic stimulation or a sudden noise.

Reflex myoclonic seizures, triggered particularly by noise or touch, may represent a separate clinical entity, which has been called reflex myoclonic epilepsy.[6–8] There is, however, controversy as to whether reflex myoclonic epilepsy in infants should be characterized separately or as part of BMEI. Capovilla and colleagues described eight children with photosensitive benign myoclonic epilepsy of infancy and proposed that this was a subgroup of children with benign myoclonic epilepsy of infancy in whom, myoclonic seizures were always triggered by photic stimulation.[9] However, it is likely, that reflex myoclonic epilepsy is not a separate entity.

The interictal EEG background is typically normal in waking, drowsy, and sleeps states. Paroxysmal slowing, however, has been reported rarely over the central areas. Generalized spike-wave or polyspike-wave discharges may occur in drowsiness or sleep (Fig. 13–1) and these may be precipitated by intermittent photic stimulation in 20% of cases (Fig. 13–2). The ictal correlate of the myoclonic seizure is a generalized spike-wave discharge, or polyspike-wave discharges or occasionally a central spike-wave discharge (Fig. 13–3).

Limited epidemiological data are available. BMEI is rare and thought to represent less than 1% of all epilepsies and 2% or less of all genetic generalized epilepsies. There is a slight predominance in males. No familial cases have been described. However, a family history of epilepsy or febrile seizures is present in 50% of patients.[3] A family history of epilepsy was reported in 27% of patients in this series, most commonly idiopathic epilepsy. In one case, the proband's brother had the electroclinical features of myoclonic–astatic epilepsy.[10]

▶ DIFFERENTIAL DIAGNOSIS

The differential diagnosis is summarized in Table 13–1.

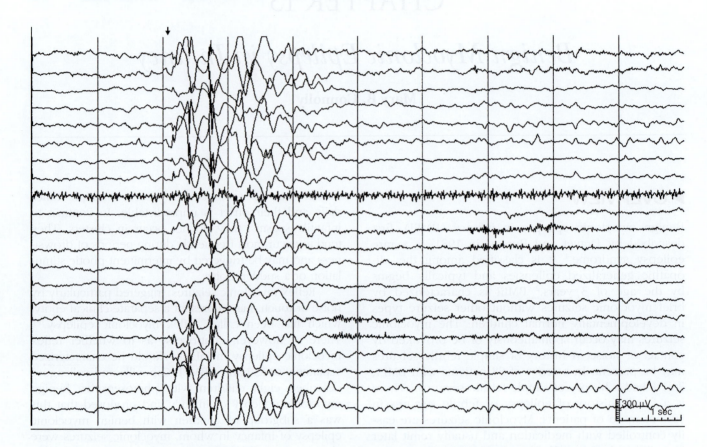

Figure 13–1. Spontaneous generalized spike and wave viewed on a longitudinal bipolar montage.

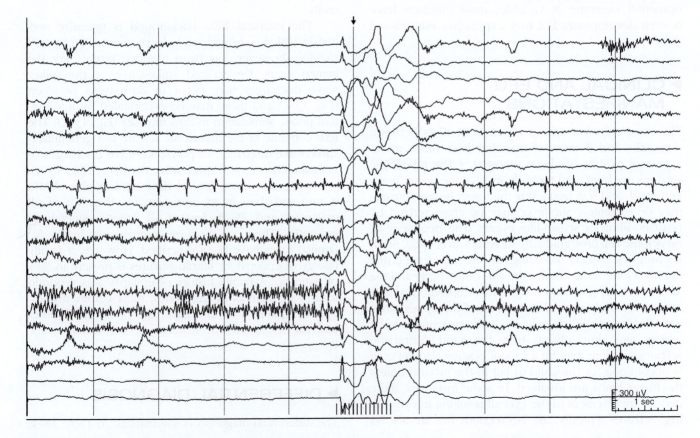

Figure 13–2. Generalized spike and wave with photic stimulation viewed on a longitudinal bipolar montage.

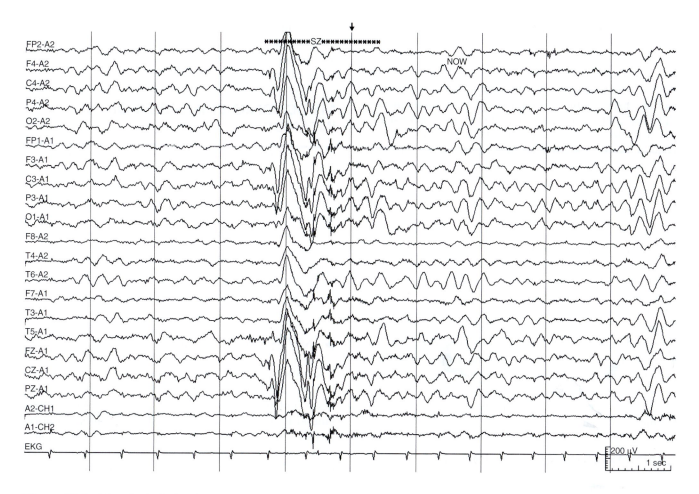

Figure 13–3. Myoclonic jerk of arms with generalized spike and wave viewed on a referential montage.

SHUDDERING SPELLS

Shuddering spells are benign events that occur in children during the first year of life. They occur in the waking state when the infant is excited and usually involve tremulous movements of the body. The infants are normal on neurological examination and their development is normal. The EEG shows no abnormality during the events. This condition may be associated with a family history of essential tremor.

▶ **TABLE 13–1.** DIFFERENTIAL DIAGNOSIS OF BENIGN MYOCLONIC EPILEPSY OF INFANCY

Nonepileptic myoclonus
Shuddering spells
Benign essential myoclonus
Myoclonus–dystonia
Infantile spasms
Epileptic myoclonus
Dravet syndrome
Lennox–Gastaut syndrome
Myoclonic–astatic epilepsy
Familial infantile myoclonic epilepsy
Symptomatic myoclonic epilepsies of infancy

BENIGN MYOCLONUS OF INFANCY

Benign myoclonus of infancy is a nonepileptic phenomenon that occurs in normal children and is characterized by spasms that resemble infantile spasms but are not associated with an EEG abnormality.[11]

MYOCLONUS–DYSTONIA

Myoclonus–dystonia is an autosomal dominant movement disorder characterized by myoclonus and/or dystonia that most often involves the neck, trunk, and upper limbs, and less commonly the legs. Symptom onset is usually in childhood or adolescence but has been reported to begin in the first 3 years of life. The disorder is caused by mutations in the SGCE gene or mutations in DRD1 and DYT1 genes. A proband with myoclonus–dystonia may have the disorder as a result of a de novo gene mutation and the proportion of de novo mutations is unknown. Almost all children who inherit the mutation from their fathers develop symptoms in contrast to only 15% of children who inherit the mutation from their mothers. Benzodiazepines, particularly clonazepam, divalproex sodium, and topiramate may improve the myoclonus.

INFANTILE SPASMS

The most important disorder to exclude in the differential diagnosis of BMEI is infantile spasms. Patients with infantile spasms demonstrate a tonic component to the seizure, which is appreciated with simultaneous EEG and EMG recordings. Infantile spasms also usually occur in clusters over time. The EEG during a cluster of spasms most commonly shows an electrodecremental pattern with or without suppression and fast activity. The interictal EEG classically shows hypsarrhythmia or demonstrates multifocal slowing and epileptiform discharges (see Chapter 28).

DRAVET SYNDROME

Dravet syndrome or severe myoclonic epilepsy of infancy is also an important differential diagnostic consideration.[12] This condition generally presents with prolonged focal seizures in the context of a febrile illness and myoclonic seizures usually begin during the second year of life. Psychomotor development, which is usually normal in the first year of life, gradually slows during the second year. SCN1A mutations have been identified in most, but not all, patients with Dravet syndrome (see Chapter 14).[13,14]

LENNOX–GASTAUT SYNDROME

Myoclonic seizures can be seen in the Lennox–Gastaut syndrome. However, classically Lennox–Gastaut syndrome is characterized by tonic seizures, atonic seizures, and atypical absence seizures. The interictal EEG may be normal at the onset, but gradually over time shows a slowing of the background and generalized slow spike-wave discharges, which are often maximal in the bifrontal regions. During sleep in patients with Lennox–Gastaut syndrome, there are frequently subtle tonic seizures with suppression of the EEG and superimposed fast activity or fast rhythmic spikes (see Chapter 29).

MYOCLONIC–ASTATIC EPILEPSY

Myoclonic–astatic epilepsy should also be considered in the differential diagnosis but this condition, is characterized by myoclonic seizures with atonic seizures and absence seizures. Typically affected children fall to the ground and the EEG demonstrates generalized spike-and-wave discharges.

FAMILIAL INFANTILE MYOCLONIC EPILEPSY

A familial type of infantile myoclonic epilepsy with an autosomal recessive inheritance has been described in one large kindred.[15] In the affected individuals, myoclonic seizures occur in clusters and generalized tonic–clonic seizures are common and persist into adulthood. The gene locus associated in this family has been mapped to chromosome 16p13.[16]

MYOCLONIC EPILEPSIES OF INFANCY

There are also several rare epilepsies with an onset in the first year of life where myoclonic seizures are the main seizure type. These heterogeneous conditions are often associated with abnormal development and often do not respond to medical therapy. The associated conditions include neurometabolic disorders, such as mitochondrial disorders, storage disorders, neuronal ceroid lipofucinosis, infantile hexoseaminidase deficiency, and biopterin deficiency. These conditions are often associated with developmental arrest or regression.

► INVESTIGATIONS

The most important investigation in patients suspected to have BMEI is a polygraphic video-EEG recording to document myoclonic seizures. They may occur spontaneously, or in drowsiness or sleep, or after auditory, tactile or intermittent photic stimulation. Neuroimaging should also be considered to rule out a neurometabolic disorder or structural brain lesion. However, neuroimaging is not usually necessary if the electroclinical features are classical, the child is developmentally normal and the seizures respond rapidly to medical therapy. However, the differential diagnosis of symptomatic mycolonic epilepsy in infancy is extensive and if there is any evidence of developmental delay, extensive neurometabolic and genetic investigations are indicated.

► MANAGEMENT

There have been no controlled studies of any of the antiepileptic drugs in BMEI. Divalproex sodium or valproic acid, however, have been the most commonly reported medications for BMEI and are recommended by Dravet and Bureau.[3] However, consideration of the risk of hepatoxicity that is highest in children under the age of 2 years may influence the choice of treatment.[17] In 62 cases of BMEI where sodium valproate was the first medication tried, 77% became seizure free on monotherapy. The remaining 12 children became seizure free with the addition of benzodiazepines, phenobarbital, lamotrigine, or ethosuximide. Daily doses of 30 mg/kg or higher sodium valproate were used in some instances.[5] However, it would seem prudent to titrate the dose of sodium valproate to seizure control and maintain the lowest dose that controls seizures

▶ **TABLE 13–2.** MEDICATIONS FOR TREATMENT OF BENIGN MYOCLONIC EPILEPSY OF INFANCY

Divalproex sodium or valproic acid
Clonazepam
Ethosuximide
Levetiracetam or topiramate

without side effects. In a series of six children with BMEI, three responded well to valproic acid, but the other cases did not respond to the addition of clobazam or lamotrigine.[18] One child was not treated with medication at the parent's request and development was normal 9 months following seizure onset. There is limited information about the use of newer antiepileptic medications such as topiramate or levetiracetam for BMEI. However, failure to respond to valproic acid or benzodiazepines should prompt a reevaluation of the diagnosis and consideration of a diagnosis symptomatic myoclonic epilepsy. A treatment logarithm is proposed in Table 13–2.

▶ NATURAL HISTORY AND COGNITIVE OUTCOME

Other seizure types are not observed in children with BMEI even if untreated. In particular, absence, tonic–clonic and tonic seizures have not been reported. The long-term follow-up of BMEI patients, suggest that the natural history is that the myoclonic seizures disappear.[3] In this published series, follow-up ranged from 9 months to 27 years in 79 patients. In most patients, the myoclonic seizures lasted less than 1 year. However, with longer follow-up of patients, the myoclonic seizures had disappeared, but rare generalized tonic–clonic seizures were reported in 11 of 79 patients during drug withdrawal; these tended to occur between the ages of 11 and 15 years and were easily controlled by divalproex sodium. Photosensitivity was observed in some of these patients. EEG evolution has been reported in a total of 55 cases.[3–5,19–24] Twenty-seven patients had normal EEGs, thirteen had spontaneous generalized spike-wave, six photosensitivity, three focal abnormalities, and five had focal and one generalized abnormalities during sleep.

Cognitive outcome has been described in 77 of 116 children reported in the literature. Thirty-five of sixty-seven (37%) were reported to have cognitive problems. Rossi et al and Mangano et al provided details of the neuropsychological outcome in their patients.[25,26] Five of eleven children reported by Rossi had educational difficulties, two had executive dysfunction with attention and concentration problems.[25] One had a specific learning

disability, one had mild intellectual impairment, and one had moderate intellectual impairment. In seven patients reported by Mangano et al, all of whom responded to medical therapy, six had neuropsychological problems at follow-up, with a mean age of 6 years 9 months (range of follow-up 4 years 9 months to 9 years 2 months).[26] It is noteworthy that all children had normal psychomotor development at presentation, and treatment was initiated 18 days to 5 months following onset of myoclonic seizures. Seizure control was achieved within 6 months of initiation of treatment in six patients, and in one patient seizure control was not achieved until 28 months following initiation of treatment. At follow-up, two children had intellectual impairment, three had borderline intellectual function, and one had low normal intellectual quotient. Six had attention difficulties or language impairment. Zuberi and O'Regan reported their experience of cognitive outcome in six patients all of whom had normal cognitive development at a minimum of 1 year follow-up.[18] In a long-term multicenter follow-up study of 34 children with BMEI in France, two children developed juvenile myoclonic epilepsy and one cryptogenic partial epilepsy.[27] Cognitive outcome was evaluated in 20 of 34 children and was normal in 17 children.

Thus, it would seem prudent to follow up children with BMEI for a minimum of 5 years or longer to assess cognitive outcome.

The reason for educational or cognitive difficulties in children with BMEI is unclear. However, it is likely that there is genetic heterogeneity and many children with genetic epilepsies may have cognitive and executive difficulties. Furthermore, delay in initiation of treatment or poor response to treatment may provide a partial explanation for the relatively poor cognitive outcome in some children.

BMEI belongs to the group of genetic generalized epilepsy syndromes and it is likely that the syndrome forms part of a disease spectrum and the late occurrence of other seizure types especially generalized tonic–clonic seizures should be expected. It has been emphasized that in the genetic generalized epilepsies, there is likely to be considerable overlap and the inheritance is likely to be polygenic.

REFERENCES

1. Dravet C, Bureau M. L'epilepsie myoclonique benigne du nourrisson. *Rev EEG Neurophysiol* 1981;11:438.
2. Commission on Classification and Terminology of the International League Against Epilepsy. Proposal for revised classification of epilepsies and epileptic syndromes. *Epilepsia* 1989;30:389.
3. Dravet C, Bureau M. Myoclonic epilepsies. *Adv Neurol* 2005; 95:127.

4. Giovanardi Rossi P, et al. Benign myoclonic epilepsy: long-term follow-up of 11 new cases. *Brain Dev* 1997;19:473.

5. Lin YP, et al. Benign myoclonic epilepsy in infants: video-EEG features and long-term follow-up. *Neuropediatrics* 1998;29:268.

6. Ricci S, et al. Reflex myoclonic epilepsy in infancy: a new age dependent idiopathic epileptic syndrome related to startle reaction. *Epilepsia* 1995;36:341.

7. Vigevano F, et al. In: Engel J, Pedley TA (eds), *Epilepsy: A Comprehensive Textbook*. Philadelphia: Lippincott-Raven, 1997; p. 2267.

8. Carballo R, et al. Epilepsias en el primer ano de vida. *Rev Neurol (Paris)* 1997;25(146):1521–1524.

9. Capovilla G, et al. Photosensitive benign myoclonic epilepsy in infancy. *Epilepsia* 2007;48(1):96.

10. Arzimanoglou A, Prudent M, Salefranque F. Epilepsie myoclono-astatique benigne du nourisson dans une meme famille: quelques reflexions sur la classification des epilepsies. *Epilepsies* 1996;8:307.

11. Lombroso CT, Fejerman B. Benign myoclonus of early infancy. *Ann Neurol* 1977;1:138.

12. Dravet C, et al. Severe myoclonic epilepsy in infancy (Dravet syndrome). In: Roger J, et al (eds), *Epileptic Syndromes in Infancy, Childhood Adolescence*. London: John Libbey, 2002; 3rd edn: p. 81.

13. Claes L, et al. De novo mutations in the sodium-channel gene SCN1A cause severe myoclonic epilepsy of infancy. *Am J Hum Genet* 2001;68:1327.

14. Scheffer IE, et al. Clinical and molecular genetics of myoclonic astatic epilepsy and severe myoclonic epilepsy in infancy (Dravet syndrome). *Brain Dev* 2001;23:732.

15. De Falco FA, et al. Familial infantile myoclonic epilepsy: clinical features in a large kindred with autosomal recessive inheritance. *Epilepsia* 2001;42(12):1541–1548.

16. Zara F, et al. Mapping of a locus for a familial autosomal recessive myoclonic epilepsy of infancy to chromosome 16p13. *Am J Hum Genet* 2000;66:1552–1557.

17. Dreifuss FE. Fatal liver failure in children on valproate. *Lancet* 1987;1(8523):47–48.

18. Zuberi SM, O'Regan ME. Developmental outcome in benign myoclonic epilepsy in infancy and reflex myoclonic epilepsy in infancy: a literature review and six new cases. *Epilepsy Res* 2006;70:S110–S115.

19. Salas-Puig J, et al. Benign myoclonic epilepsy of infancy. Case report. *Acta Paediatr Scand* 1990;79:1128–1130.

20. Todt H, Muller D. The therapy of benign myoclonic epilepsy in infants. In: Degen R, Dreifuss FE (eds), *Epilepsy Research, S6. The Benign Localized and Generalized Epilepsies in Early Childhood*. Amsterdam: Elsevier Science, 1992; p. 137.

21. Deonna T, Despland PA. Sensory-evoked (touch) idiopathic myoclonic epilepsy of infancy. In: Beaumanoir A, Naquet R, Gastaut H (eds), *Reflex Seizures and Reflex Epilepsies*. Geneva: Medecine et Hygiene, 1989; p. 99.

22. Revol M, et al. Touch evoked myoclonic seizures in infancy. In: Beaumanoir A, Naquet R, Gastaut H (eds), *Reflex Seizures and Reflex Epilepsies*. Geneva: Medecine et Hygiene, 1989; p. 103.

23. Cuvellier JC, et al. Epilepsie myoclonique benigne reflexe du nourrison. *Arch Pediatr* 1997;8:775.

24. Ribacoba-Montero R, Salas-Puig J. Benign myoclonic epilepsy in childhood. A case report. *Rev Neurol* 1997;25:1210–1212.

25. Rossi PG, et al. Benign myolconic epilepsy: long-term follow-up of 11 new cases. *Brain Dev* 1997;19:473–479.

26. Mangano S, Fontana A, Gusumano L. Benign myoclonic epilepsy in infancy: neuropsychological and behavioural outcome. *Brain Dev* 2005;27:218–223.

27. Auvin S, et al. Benign myoclonic epilepsy in infants: electroclinical features and long-term follow-up in 24 patients. *Epilepsia* 2006;47(2):387–393.

CHAPTER 14

Severe Myoclonic Epilepsy of Infancy (Dravet Syndrome)

Charlotte Dravet

► OVERVIEW

Recognized as a syndrome by the International League Against Epilepsy in the last classification,[1] severe myoclonic epilepsy of infancy (SMEI) has been placed among the "epileptic encephalopathies", defined as conditions in which the epileptiform abnormalities are believed to contribute to a progressive disturbance in cerebral function, whether seizures are generalized, localized, symptomatic, idiopathic or cryptogenic.[2] Since 2001[3] its etiology is regarded to be genetic as the majority of affected patients carry a mutation in the sodium-channel gene *SCN1A*. However, it remains unproven whether the cognitive decline observed in the first stages of the disease is a consequence of the epilepsy. In this new scheme, SMEI is renamed "Dravet syndrome" because of the lack of myoclonic seizures in many patients.

► EPIDEMIOLOGY

The frequency in the general population is not well known but has been estimated at 1/40,000 births.[4] Since 1990, knowledge of the disease has grown considerably and it is likely its frequency is higher, but there is no other epidemiological data.

► CLINICAL DESCRIPTION

The typical features of the core syndrome are present in the majority of the patients, although variations exist in semiology and outcome.

ONSET

Seizures typically begin in the first year of life in a normal infant without pathological antecedents. A family history of epilepsy and febrile seizures is frequent. Seizures begin between ages 4 and 9 months, accompanied by mild hyperthermia, and last longer than the simple febrile seizures (10 minutes or more). They are clonic, generalized, unilateral or predominating on one side of the body, and change from one seizure to the next. They may have localized onset. In some patients, isolated episodes of focal myoclonia are observed before the appearance of the first convulsive seizure. Purely focal complex seizures are exceptional at the onset.

The first convulsive seizure can be afebrile, after a vaccination, a bath, or during a cold. Usually, afebrile seizures are quickly associated with febrile seizures. This first seizure is considered as an occasional seizure that does not require a treatment. But, shortly thereafter, other seizures occur, with or without fever, and persist in spite of the institution of a chronic treatment.

STEADY STATE

Seizure frequency increases during the second year of life. Affected patients have many upper respiratory tract infections and are repeatedly hospitalized. Some seizures are resistant to acute treatment and evolve to status epilepticus (SE) requiring intensive care. Other seizure types appear and psychomotor development slows.

Ictal Semiology

Convulsive seizures are reported to be generalized by the parents but have variable features. They may be truly generalized, clonic or tonic clonic. Others are "falsely generalized" or "unstable" with some focal elements, clinical or EEG, and localize to different areas during the course of the same seizure (Fig. 14–1). The most typical variants are *unilateral and hemiclonic*. *Myoclonic seizures* appear between ages 1 and 5 years in approximately 85% of the cases. They are generalized, involving the body axis and the proximal parts of the limbs. They occur several times a day and may be focal or secondarily generalized. Seizures are accompanied by diffuse spike-waves (SWs) in the EEG and are often associated with interictal segmental myoclonia.

Atypical absences may present up to age 12 years. Their frequency is difficult to assess due to a frequent myoclonic component that makes them difficult to differentiate from myoclonic seizures. Atonic

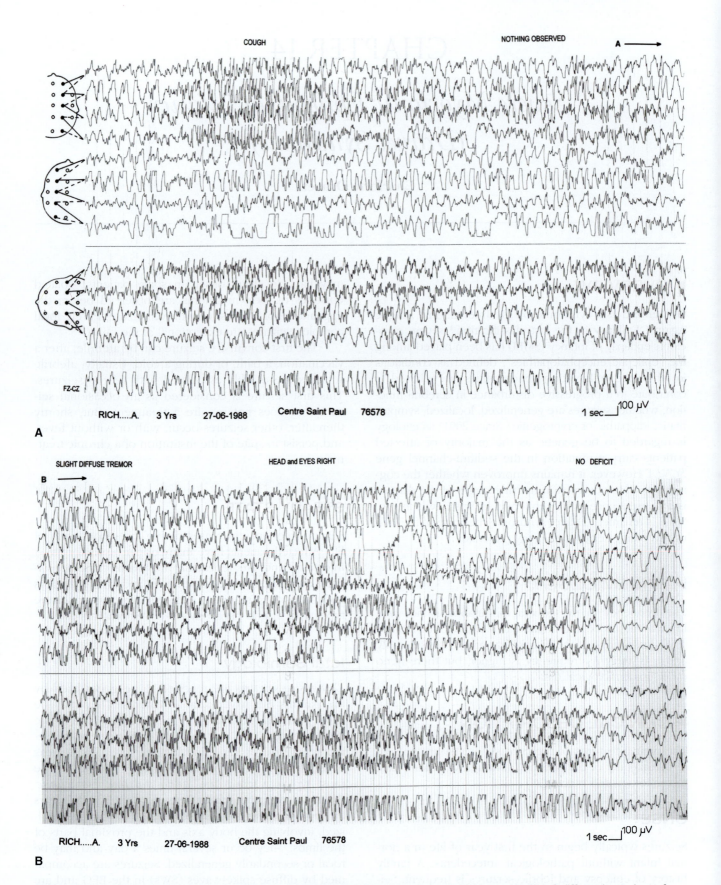

COUGH

NOTHING OBSERVED

A ⟶

FZ-CZ

RICH.....A.   3 Yrs   27-06-1988   Centre Saint Paul   76578   1 sec⌐ 100 µV

A

SLIGHT DIFFUSE TREMOR ⟶

HEAD and EYES RIGHT

NO DEFICIT

B

RICH.....A.   3 Yrs   27-06-1988   Centre Saint Paul   76578   1 sec⌐ 100 µV

B

Figure 14–1. An unstable seizure occurring during slow sleep in a 3-year-old boy. (**A**) Brief diffuse lowering of voltage, intermixed, in the right hemisphere, with high-voltage fast activity, then spikes and slow waves during 10s, followed by a more or less rhythmic activity around 10 Hz in the right centroparietal area. (**B**) 20 s after the onset of that activity, a similar one appears in the left fronto-centrotemporal region, progressively associated with slow waves, while slow waves and spike-waves persist on the right side. (From Roger J, et al. *Epileptic Syndromes in Infancy, Childhood, and Adolescence.* London: John Libbey Eurotext, 2005; 4th edn.)

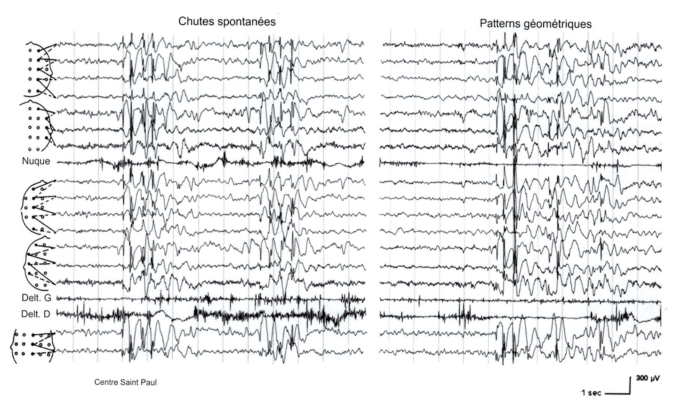

Figure 14–2. Atypical absences with the head nodding in a 2-year-9-month-old girl. High-voltage, diffuse, slow spike-waves during spontaneous absences (left). The same discharge with more slow waves elicited by geometrical patterns (right). The muscular recording does not show well-defined correspondence. Nuque, neck muscle; Delt. G, left deltoid muscle; Delt. D, right deltoid muscle. (From Crespel A, et al. *Atlas of Electroencephalography.* John Libbey Eurotext, 2006; Vol. 2.)

components with a head drop are not uncommon and are accompanied by more or less regular diffuse spike-wave discharges and slow waves (Fig. 14–2). Peculiar *obtundation status* is observed in 40% of cases and consists of impaired consciousness accompanied by segmental and fragmentary erratic myoclonia, involving the limbs and the face, sometimes associated with a slight increase in the muscular tone. According to their degree of consciousness, patients may react to stimuli and continue simple activities (e.g., eat, manipulate toys). They last from 30 minutes to several hours and can be intermixed with short episodes of complete loss of consciousness or convulsive seizures. Clinically they may be difficult to distinguish from focal complex SEs, which are rarer and usually shorter. The EEG is associated with mixed diffuse slow waves, notched slow waves, sharp waves and spike-wave discharges without rhythmicity or less commonly, repeated diffuse spike-wave discharges (Fig. 14–3).

Focal seizures with and without loss of awareness appear between ages 4 months to 4 years or later. SPS are either versive seizures, with or without clonic jerks limited to a limb or one hemiface, or a combination of the two. CPS are characterized by loss of consciousness, autonomic phenomena (pallor, cyanosis, rubefaction, res-

piratory changes, drooling, sweating), oral automatisms, hypotonia, rarely stiffness, sometimes eyelid or distal myoclonia. When the symptomatology is mild, they are difficult to distinguish from atypical absences without concomitant EEG and the parents report them as "absences".

Tonic seizures are exceptional and were recorded in nine patients.[5] They differ from the tonic seizures of Lennox–Gastaut syndrome as they are sporadic, do not repeat in series and have variable EEG features.

Parents rarely describe *polymorphic paroxysmal events* which do not fit with usual epileptic seizures and which remain unclassifiable.

Triggering Factors

Fever and Temperature Variations Sensitivity.   Patients are remarkably sensitive to infections and may experience numerous hyperthermic episodes accompanied by epileptic seizures. However, seizures can also be triggered by slight variations of body temperatures that do not rise above 38°C and are not caused by infection. Thus, it is more appropriate to substitute the term "temperature variation" for "fever". Patients are also sensible to the ambient temperature, having more seizures when it is hot. The triggering

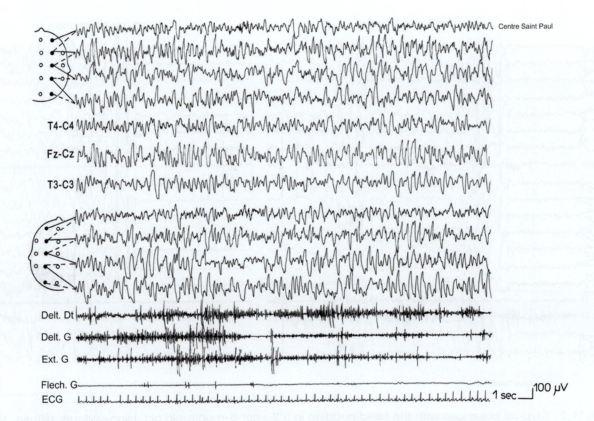

Figure 14–3. Obtundation status in a 3-year-old boy. Slow and irregular background with isolated notched slow waves predominantly on median and posterior areas. The muscular recording shows a slightly increased tone. Delt. Dt, right deltoid muscle; Delt. G, left deltoid muscle; Ext. G, left wrist extensor muscle; Flech. G, left wrist flexor muscle; ECG, electrocardiogram. (From Crespel A, et al. *Atlas of Electroencephalography.* John Libbey Eurotext, 2006; Vol. 2.)

effect of hot baths was first noted in Japan where hot baths are a custom.[6] Physical exercise is also a frequent triggering factor.

Photosensitivity can appear at different stages, from infancy to adolescence. It is not constant in the same patient and can disappear either transiently or definitively. Patients may present with myoclonia, absences and convulsive seizures when exposed to a bright environment, particularly after a dark one. A discrepancy between the EEG response to intermittent photic stimulation (IPS) and clinical photosensitivity has been observed. The quantity of light may have a more important role than wavelength.[7] Patients with constant light sensitivity represents the most treatment-resistant form of SMEI. Eye closure, patterns, and television are also recognized as triggering factors; autostimulation may aggravate the situation.

Interictal Semiology

The interictal EEG is usually normal at the onset. It may display a diffuse or unilateral slow background if recorded after a prolonged seizure. In some patients, generalized spike-wave discharges are elicited by intermittent photic

stimulation. Rhythmic 4–5-Hz theta activity may be present in the centroparietal areas and the vertex.[8] The EEG changes progressively with the appearance of generalized, focal and multifocal abnormalities; specific features are lacking.

The waking background is either near-normal with slowing present only after a seizure, or constantly slow and poorly organized. Rhythmical theta activity may be present, but paroxysmal abnormalities are highly variable and consist of notched slow waves, sharp waves, spikes, spike-wave discharges and multispike-wave discharges. Discharges may be generalized or localized, mainly in the frontocentral and vertex areas, but also in the temporal and occipital areas, and may spread throughout the hemisphere. Eye closure facilitates their occurrence. The sleep EEG is usually well organized, with physiological patterns and cyclic organization, except after nocturnal seizures. In photosensitive patients, the IPS provokes generalized discharges (Fig. 14–4).

Psychomotor Development

Psychomotor delay becomes evident after age 2 years. Children begin walking at the normal age of 12–18 months,

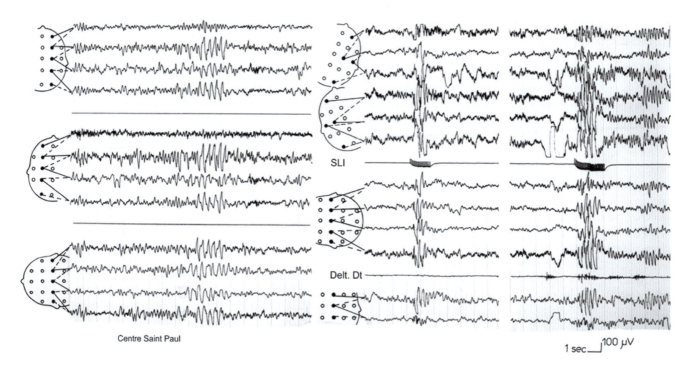

Figure 14–4. Photosensitivity in a 4-year-old girl. Background activity at rest with association of fast rhythms and one burst of generalized sharp waves (left). Brief trains of light stimulation provoke generalized SWs and poly-SWs of highest voltage on the left hemisphere, accompanied by slight myoclonic jerks (right). SLI, intermittent light stimulation; Delt. Dt, right deltoid muscle. (From Crespel A, et al. *Atlas of Electroencephalography.* John Libbey Eurotext, 2006; Vol. 2.)

but an unsteady gait persists for an unusually long time. About 60% of the children are ataxic and 20% show mild pyramidal signs. Language begins at the normal time (lallation and first words) but progresses slowly and often does not reach the stage of elementary sentence construction. Affected patients develop hyperactivity, oppositional behavior and major learning problems. Relationships with adults and other children are often bizarre and autistic features may appear. In a single neuropsychological study of 20 patients[9,10] the neuropsychological deficits were global with motor, linguistic and visual abilities being more strikingly affected. Deterioration was related to the severity of the epilepsy during the first two years of life. However, no genetic analysis was performed and establishing a link to the *SCN1A* mutation was not possible.

We recently studied 11 patients aged 15 months to 9 years who were regularly followed with neuropsychological evaluations.[11] Slowing of psychomotor development was observed between ages 2 to 4 years and was more evident in eye–hand coordination, visual attention, expressive language, memory and executive functions. Partial recovery of language functions and, to a lesser degree, visual attention occurred subsequently. Only one girl has reached a borderline IQ level at the age of eight and could write, read and count. All patients older than age 3 years evidenced motor impairment and

behavior disorders. Distractibility, hyperactivity, and oppositional behaviors were observed in all patients at first evaluation, which subsequently improved. Signs of withdrawal were present in only two patients, and one girl was psychotic.

Comorbidities

Comorbid conditions are frequent in SMEI and include orthopedic conditions (including pes planus/pes valgus, foot deformities, and neurogenic scoliosis), chronic upper respiratory infections, otitis media, low humoral immunity, and growth and nutrition issues.

▶ NEUROIMAGING

Until recently, magnetic resonance imaging (MRI) was reported as normal, even when serially repeated. In 2005, Siegler et al[12] found hippocampal sclerosis (HS) in 10 of 14 investigated patients. However, a more recent study[13] of 58 patients, 60% carrying SCN1A mutations, investigated by MRI after the age of 4, found only one case of HS. In one Argentinian study,[14] signs compatible with unilateral HS were found in 3/53 patients. In this series one patient presented with unilateral brain atrophy following unilateral febrile SE.

▶ ATYPICAL OR BORDERLINE PRESENTATIONS

Atypical or borderline presentations of Dravet syndrome were first reported by Japanese investigators.[15] The presentations were characterized by a lack of one or several signs, mainly myoclonic seizures. Subsequently it was noted that patients lacking myoclonic seizures who were otherwise similar shared the same prognosis: 21% for Dravet et al.[16] However, most of those lacking myoclonic seizures had interictal segmental myoclonus which compromised their motor abilities. In other patients myoclonic fits were transitory. A report of two siblings, one with and the other lacking myoclonic seizures has been reported[15,16] suggesting that both presentations are part of the same disorder.

With the advent of genetic investigations, it is now apparent that patients with borderline presentations also harbor the *SCN1A* mutation, although generally less severe and less frequent. Conversely, patients with only refractory grand mal seizures described in Japan[17,18] and Germany[19] should not be included in SMEI, even if the genetic studies reveal the *SCN1A* mutation in some, demonstrating that they are a part of the GEFS+ syndrome.

▶ GENETICS

In 2001, Claes and colleagues found new mutations in the sodium-channel gene *SCN1A* in all seven probands with SMEI.[3] Subsequent studies have confirmed the presence of this mutation in most, but not all patients. Approximately 70% of patients are mutationally positive.[20] Frameshift and nonsense mutations are most frequent. Correlations between phenotype and genotype suggest a higher frequency of truncating mutations in the typical patients, including patients with myoclonia.[21,22] Mutations have also been identified in borderline forms[23] but are less frequent (7/27) than in the typical forms (19/31) and less severe (no truncating mutations). Likewise, missense mutations were found in patients presenting exclusively with refractory grand mal seizures.[18]

More often, mutations are *de novo*, but may be detected in one of the parents.[21,24,25] Parental mosaicism was recently demonstrated.[26,27] With other more sensitive techniques (multiplex ligation-dependent probe amplification, multiplex amplicon quantification), approximately 15% of screened negative cases were found to carry a deletion or duplication of pathogenic significance on the *SCN1A* gene.[28] Recently, mutations in *PCDH19*, the gene encoding the protocadherin 19 on the X chromosome, were discovered in *SCN1A*-negative female patients presenting with a clinical picture resembling the borderline SMEI.[29] The authors estimated that 16% or 25%, if only females were included in the

calculation, of their *SCN1A*-negative SMEI patients had *PCDH19* mutations and that this gene might overall account for 5% of SMEI. Clinical similarities between *PCDH19* mutation positive patients and SMEI, including febrile and afebrile seizures, occurrence of hemiclonic seizures, regression following seizure onset, suggest that *PCDH19* should be tested in those patients in whom no *SCN1A* abnormalities can be found. Further studies should elucidate the possible role of other genes or of *SCN1A* promoters in the pathogenesis of this syndrome.

▶ DIFFERENTIAL DIAGNOSIS

Patients with Dravet syndrome must be distinguished from patients with routine *febrile seizures* (FS). FS are usually simple, i.e. brief, generalized, triggered by a temperature higher than 38° 5, and rarely occur before age 6 months. In an infant less than 1 year of age who lacks predisposing factors prolonged seizures (more than 15 minutes) that are lateralized, accompanied by a temperature lower than 38° should lead to a diagnostic consideration of SMEI. SMEI should also be considered when the seizures repeat frequently with or without hyperthermia, and sometimes evolve to SE, in spite of chronic treatment.

The EEG does not assist in diagnosis because it is often normal, unless it displays photosensitivity.

Because SMEI is characterized by polymorphic seizures, pharmacoresistency, psychomotor regression and behavioral disturbances, the diagnosis of *Lennox–Gastaut syndrome* is sometimes considered. However, early-onset LGS is rare and often follows infantile spasms. Seizures are axial and tonic, mainly nocturnal, not clonic or myoclonic; patients have drop attacks due to tonic and atonic seizures. The EEG is specific revealing interictal diffuse slow spike-wave discharges that increase in sleep and are associated with polyspikes and fast rhythms. LGS is related to a known etiology in about 60% of the cases.

Epilepsy with myoclonic astatic seizures (Doose syndrome) may present with recurrent febrile and nonfebrile convulsive seizures, but rarely does so before the age of 1 year. The initial presentation is quickly followed by atypical absences and drop attacks due to myoclonic–atonic seizures which are not observed in SMEI. Absences and myoclonic statuses may occur, but focal seizures are extremely rare. The EEG reveals numerous bursts of generalized SWs and poly SWs, without focal abnormalities. In some patients, the outcome can be favorable after an initial catastrophic period.

When neurological and behavioral signs appear in the second year of life, a diagnosis of *progressive myoclonus epilepsy* is often considered, predominantly *ceroïd lipofuscinosis (Jansky Bielschowski)*. Ceroïd lipofuscinosis may produce abnormal findings on ophthalmologic examination (fundus oculi, electroretinogram, visual evoked potentials), which are normal in SMEI; induced low frequency IPS-induced posterior large evoked potentials in the EEG are absent in SMEI. Skin or rectal mucous biopsy and genetic study confirm the diagnosis.

In very severe cases, *mitochondrial encephalomyopathy* should be excluded by biological examinations and muscle biopsy.

Lesional focal epilepsy may present similarly to FS, followed by focal seizures. These patients do not manifest atypical absences or myoclonic jerks. Their EEG is often normal at the onset. The diagnosis of SMEI is probable when clonic seizures change lateralization and the EEG becomes multifocal.

In some patients with family antecedents of FS and epilepsy with a variety of seizure patterns, FS may be part of *the GEFS+ syndrome.*[30] However, prolonged FS, febrile and afebrile SEs, and drug resistance are unusual in patients with GEFS+. Their psychomotor development is normal and cognitive deficits are rare. Confusion may arise from the genetic analysis since the *SCN1A* mutation is present in the two forms. But mutations in SMEI are more severe and usually occur *de novo*. If mutations are also present in one parent and other family members, the patient may be diagnosed as affected by SMEI in a GEFS+ family.

▶ TREATMENT

In spite of recent progress, the treatment of SMEI remains disappointing. This may be explained by the polymorphism of the seizures and the lack of drugs medical therapy for generalized convulsive, focal, absence and myoclonic seizures when they occur together. A recent meta-analysis of AED therapy in SMEI underscores the scarcity of controlled studies.[31]

WHICH AEDs ARE USEFUL?

Bromides (Br) have been used successfully in Germany and Japan,[32] with significant results against convulsive seizures and SE. In the Japanese study, five of 22 patients had ≥75% and two experienced ≥50% reduction of their GTCS at 12 months. Myoclonic seizures were not improved. Side effects occurred in 12 children (loss of appetite, drowsiness, ataxia and snoring). They gradually disappeared after slow increase in Br dosage or after reduction of the other AEDs. Three patients presented a skin rash, which required reduction of the Br dosage with loss of seizure control. An initial dosage of 30 mg/kg per day and a slow titration up to 100 mg/kg per day facilitates better tolerance. The maximum serum levels ranged from 64 to 159 mg/dl. Br may be administered to infants before age one year.

Valproate (VPA) and *benzodiazepines (BZDZ)* offer improvement that is often transitory and lacks published controlled data. The most frequent benzodiazepines are *clonazepam (CZP)* and *clobazam (CLB)*. CZP is easy to use because it presents as a solution and the doses can be fragmented during the day. But in infants its side effects may be devastating: drowsiness, hypotonia, ataxia, hypersialorrhea and upper respiratory tracts "drowning". *CLB* is more popular, but unavailable in solution. Its adverse effects, which often result in irritability and hyperexcitability, can be managed by reducing the dose.

Barbiturates have been largely given without clear improvement and their use is controversial. However, they can be useful in case of convulsive seizures and SE that is resistant to VPA and BZDZ.

Ethosuximide was used successfully in some patients suffering from countless myoclonic seizures. However it does not protect against convulsive seizures and its side effects can be unacceptable: loss of appetite and weight, withdrawal behavior.

Corticosteroids can be useful in cases of repeated SEs but do not have long-term efficacy.

Among the most recent AEDs, several open-label studies show that *Topiramate (TPM)* leads to relatively good control of convulsive and focal seizures[33–37] in spite of side effects. Seizure reduction of ≥50% occurred in 50–85% of patients, 16–18% were seizure-free for 11–13 months. Maximal daily dosages varied from 9 to 12 mg/kg, with 3 mg/kg being optimal. Slow titration facilitated better tolerance, but side effects were observed in approximately 15% of patients, consisting mainly of anorexia and weight loss but also behavior disturbances, emotional and language regression, and, more rarely, renal stones.

One recent study evaluated *Levetiracetam (LEV)* in a series of 28 patients, aged 3–23 years, of whom 16 carried one *SCN1A* mutation, who were then followed for 6–36 months (mean 16.2 ± 13.4).[38] In this open-label trial, in addition to a mean of 3.6 other AEDs, 64.3% of the patients were responders for one seizure type (GTCS) with three patients being seizure-free (11%), and 39.2% for two seizure types (GTCS and focal or myoclonic seizures) with two patients being seizure-free. Four of nine patients (44%) were responders for absences. Three patients had monthly bouts of repeated SE. The dosage varied from 750 to 3000 mg per day (mean 2016 mg per day) and the target dose was 50–60 mg/kg per day. Five patients (18%) stopped the trial because of side effects: irritability, cutaneous rash, worsening of myoclonic seizures, thrombocytopenia, but the drug was well tolerated in the others.

Two randomized placebo-controlled trials were performed for *Stiripentol (STP).*[39–41] STP is an inhibitor of CYP450 and increases the plasma concentrations of carbamazepine (CBZ) and VPA. Similar interactions have been demonstrated for CLB by Chiron et al.[39] The plasma concentrations of CLB and metabolites result from STP-induced inhibition by STP of the hydroxylation of the active metabolite norclobazam into hydroxyl norclobazam.

The efficacy of STP was demonstrated in this trial in association with VPA and CLB. However, a direct antiepileptic effect of STP is probable and new trials are needed to test this hypothesis. STP has recently been used apart from its association with VPA and CLB; good results were reported anecdotally by many parents. In the first study,[39] 41 patients with SMEI were included, 21 receiving placebo and 20 receiving the active drug. In the latter group, 15 (71%) were responders, including nine who became free from clonic and tonic clonic seizures, versus one (5%) in the placebo group where none became seizure-free. The mean daily dose of STP was 49.3 mg/kg/d. Plasma concentrations of CLB and norclobazam were significantly increased on STP compared with baseline whereas those of hydroxy norclobazam were significantly decreased. Moderate side effects occurred in all STP-treated patients (drowsiness, loss of appetite, loss of weight) versus five on placebo, but side effects disappeared when the doses of the comedication was decreased in 17 of the 21 cases.

These findings were confirmed by an Italian study 40, 41) according to the same protocol. The long-term effects of STP were reported in another study.[42] In 46 patients, seizure frequency and duration were significantly reduced as well as the number of convulsive SEs at a median follow up of three years. Ten patients (22%) were dramatically improved and SEs disappeared. Twenty (43%) were moderately improved, mainly by reduction of the seizure duration and of the number of convulsive SEs. Four (9%) had no response and efficacy was not supportive in 12, mainly because of adverse effects. Loss of appetite and weight did not permit an increase of the dose to 50 mg/kg per day in patients older than 12 years. On the whole, the STP has demonstrated its usefulness in decreasing the frequency of convulsive seizures, but mainly their duration and the number of SEs. It has not been evaluated for the other seizure types.

There is no data in Europe on *Zonisamide*. In Japan, it has been proven in the borderline form without myoclonia with a good result if started early.[43] The authors suggested that Zonisamide could prevent the appearance of myoclonia.

WHICH AEDs SHOULD BE AVOIDED?

In 1986[44] two patients with SMEI were reported among 49 children *aggravated by CBZ*. In 1992 we were aware of this risk and we did not use it. In 1996, Wakai et al[45] reported a worsening effect of CBZ in four patients among six with SMEI and no effect in the two others. They suggested the use of CBZ in the early phase of SMEI as a test to confirm the diagnosis. In the same way, Wang et al[46] used CBZ in nine patients, of whom two experienced an increase in myoclonic seizures, whereas two were well controlled with VPA+CBZ, and the others taking multiple medications with variable results.

An aggravating effect of *lamotrigine (LTG)* has been demonstrated by Guerrini et al.[47] LTG induced worsening of 17 of 21 patients (80%), no change in three, and improvement in one. Worsening was observed mainly in convulsive and myoclonic seizures. It appeared clearly within 3 months in most patients but occasionally had an insidious course. These findings were confirmed by Wallace.[48]

There is no study concerning *phenytoïn (PHT)* but its aggravating effect was reported anecdotally.

All three AEDs are not similar but share a mechanism of action that involves the use-dependent inhibition of sodium channels necessary for the "firing" of action potentials, responsible for convulsive seizures. This property could be the basis for an explanation of their ability to increase the seizures in sodium channelopathy epilepsy. However, this deleterious effect could be dependent on the age. In some older patients taking polytherapy including PHT, CBZ or LTG, attempts to stop them were followed by an aggravation.

In infants and children, *Vigabatrin* should be avoided because it increases the myoclonic seizures. But, in our older patients we observed an improvement in convulsive and focal seizures.

WHICH ALTERNATIVE TREATMENTS?

The ketogenic diet (KD) has been shown to be beneficial. In a series of seventeen patients treated by KD in Argentina,[49] nine achieved significant improvement; 75–100% seizure reduction in seven, 50–74% reduction in two. Only two patients did not tolerate the diet, which was interrupted (vomiting, diarrhea) at the outset, and six did not improve. In the responders, seizures remained controlled for more than one year and the other AEDs were lowered, allowing a better quality of life. Korff et al[50] reported good results in 4/6 patients. No similar study has been performed in Europe but the results obtained in anecdotal cases were not convincing.

Only one small study has focused on the immunologic aspects of SMEI without reaching a definite conclusion.[51] However, considering the sensibility to infections and their role in triggering seizures, we administered *immunoglobulins* to some patients with relative success. Our results are confirmed by Nieto-Barrera et al.[52]

WHEN TO START CONTINUOUS TREATMENT?

In an infant less than one year of age, rectal benzodiazepines are employed to abort new seizures. If two

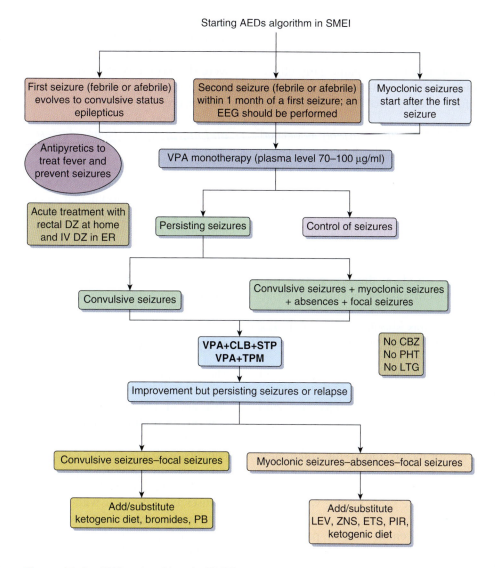

Figure 14–5. AEDs algorithm in SMEI.

additional seizures occur after a short interval without a temperature spike, it is reasonable to consider SMEI as a possible diagnosis, after the workup for symptomatic seizures is negative, and the patient fulfills the above-described criteria. Particular attention must be given to unilateral seizures, and a continuous treatment must be instituted. The same approach is required if one seizure either has evolved to SE or becomes resistant to rectal injection, and when the convulsive seizures are not repeated frequently at the onset but other seizure types (focal, myoclonic) or EEG abnormalities appear (Fig. 14–5).

Which AEDs?

Monotherapy with VPA (with control of the plasma levels) or TPM should be commenced. If seizures continue, it is recommended to introduce polytherapy with VPA, CLB or STP.

When STP is unavailable, the combination of VPA and TPM, and VPA and Br, or CZP and Br, can be efficacious. In reality, complete control is never reached in most of the patients and the good effect at the onset does not last more than weeks or months. Thus, successive changes in AEDs are necessary, using substitution rather than addition to avoid a heavy polytherapy. Some authors propose to limit the use of BZDZ, when possible, because of their side effects.[53]

Other Therapeutic Measures

The place of KD is difficult to define. It can be offered to patients with repeated bouts of SE. It requires full cooperation between family, neuropediatrician and dietician; commercially available dietetic preparations are available (see Chapter 53).

When *atypical absences and myoclonic seizures* are extremely frequent, ETS may be particularly efficacious. Punctual administration of BZDZ is also helpful. We have successfully used *Piracetam (PIR)* at high doses.

Photic and pattern sensitivities, variably associated with self-stimulation, are extremely drug-resistant and can produce long-lasting obtundation and myoclonic status, as well as clonic seizures. Wearing sunglasses is recommended but not sufficient. The Japanese[54] and Italian[55] studies suggest that, it is possible to control photosensitivity by wearing commercially available special blue lens. However, these lenses often have only partial efficacy for pattern sensitivity. Glasses masking one eye can be used, based on the observation that monocular light and pattern stimulation fails to provoke epileptic discharges.

Other triggering factors should be avoided: hot bathes, excess physical activity, emotional stress and other individual situations.

Given the deleterious consequences of prolonged convulsive seizures, it is necessary to avoid SE by *appropriate treatment and prophylaxis of infections and hyperthermia.* The use of rectal BZDZ can prevent the evolution of a long seizure into a status. This procedure remains the best one for infants and young children. It is difficult to apply in adolescents and adults and it has been recently assessed that the oral administration of BZDZ solution could give the same results, with midazolam, CZP[53] as well as DZP.

When SE occurs, intravenous BZDZ, particularly lorazepam and midazolam are indicated,[56] associated with chloral hydrate, and eventually followed by intravenous PHT. However, there is no controlled study in the literature and no recommendations may be proposed. In particular, the role of barbiturates is unclear. In Japan they seem to be the most efficacious[57] and in Canada two cases of children were successfully treated by pentobarbital on multiple occasions, through a subcutaneous permanent accessed central line.[58] Therefore, in SEs resistant to other drugs, they should be used with caution, with monitoring of the plasma levels, EKG, hepatic and renal functions, in order to avoid severe complications.[59]

Recommended immunizations can be performed in spite of the risk of the occurrence of one convulsive seizure. This risk is real[60] and caution is necessary including the need to not inject one vaccine when the child is ill or febrile, or give an antipyretic agent before and after the immunization, associated with additional BZDZ for one week. Many infants had their first seizure after immunization, but immunization is not responsible for the disease as has been recently demonstrated.[61] These investigators studied 14 patients for whom immunization (diphtheria–pertussis–tetanus,

diphtheria–pertussis–tetanus-inactivated polio–hemophilus) was alleged as the cause of the subsequent epileptic encephalopathy. They found that 11 patients were diagnosed as SMEI or SMEB and had one *SCN1A de novo* mutation. Thus, immunization only triggered a first seizure.

Attention should be paid to the risk of *orthopedic and nutritional problems* which sometimes need therapeutic intervention.

Besides treating epileptic events, *management of the developmental and behavioral aspects* of the children is mandatory. Developmental assessments should begin as early as possible and be repeated regularly. Early implementation of global therapies is essential: physical, occupational, speech, and social/play therapies. Socialization and learning are facilitated by early integration in schools with children with special needs. Both children and their parents benefit from a psychologist.

▶ OUTCOME

The outcome of Dravet syndrome has historically been unfavorable. Recently, two studies of outcome after age 20 years in 22[62] and 14 patients[63] respectively revealed concordant findings (Table 14–1), ultimately confirmed by Akiyama et al.[64] Convulsive seizures persisted in all patients, with a trend to localize later in the night. Myoclonic seizures may disappear or occur only before a convulsive seizure. CPS, atypical absences, and absence statuses become rarer with advancing age. Photosensitivity and pattern sensitivity are variable. Temperature sensitivity typically decreases; EEG findings vary by age. Generalized SWs often disappear, whereas focal and multifocal abnormalities persist, often activated by sleep. Background activity may deteriorate with frequent convulsive seizures and between ages five to 10 years. All patients are cognitively impaired, and 50% of patients in the second decade are severely retarded.

After the regression between ages 1–5 years, mental impairment remains more or less stable except in rare cases. Slowness, perseverations, and language impairment are prominent; motor difficulties and orthopedic problems are also common. Almost all patients ultimately become fully dependent and live at home or in an institution. However, the course may be variable in recently diagnosed patients and some reach elementary school or a higher level.[65] In the most recent study of a series of 37 patients followed up to a mean age of 16 years,[66] the authors hypothesize the cognitive outcome should be multifactorial, resulting from epilepsy course, genetic background, but also medical care, rehabilitation and social environment.

The mortality rate in this disorder is high, approximating 15.9–18%.[5] The cause of death is variable, including drowning, accident, seizure, SE, infection, and sudden unexpected death (SUDEP) which may occur in adulthood.

► **TABLE 14–1.** LONG-TERM OUTCOME IN TWO STUDIES

	Long-term Outcome	
	Jansen et al, 2006	**Dravet et al, 2009**
Patient number	14	24
Age at follow-up	18–47 yr (mean 26 yr)	18–46 yr (mean 30 yr)
Convulsive seizure	14 pts	22 pts
Myoclonic seizure	2 pts	2 pts
Absence seizure	4 pts	6 pts
Focal seizure	7 pts	1 pt
T° sensitivity	Not available	12 pts
Photosensitivity	2 pts	Not available
Generalized SWs	9 pts	6 pts
Focal–multifocal SWs	Not available	18 pts
Slow background	Not available	11 pts
Subnormal background	Not available	8 pts
Variable background	Not available	2 pts
Normal low IQ	1 pt	None
Mild delay	2 pts	None
Moderate–severe delay	11 pts	24 pts
Motor problems	10 pts	15 pts
Independent	2 pts	1 pt
Partially dependent	2 pts	8 pts
Dependent	10 pts	15 pts
AEDs current number	2–5	2–5
Death	1	5
SCN1A mutation	Present in 11/14 pts	Present in 6/11 pts
GABRG2 mutation	Present in 1/14 pts	Absent

Source: Dravet C, Daquin G, Battaglia D. Severe myoclonic epilepsy of infancy (Dravet syndrome). In: Nikanorova M, Genton P, Sabers A (eds), *Long-Term Evolution of Epileptic Encephalopathies.* Montrouge: John Libbey Eurotext, 2009; pp. 29–38; Jansen FE, et al. Severe myoclonic epilepsy of infancy (Dravet syndrome): recognition and diagnosis in adults. *Neurology* 2006;67:2224–2226.

► CONCLUSIONS

Early appropriate treatment is the best way to decrease not only the frequency but also the duration of the seizures and to avoid the status epilepticus. Early diagnosis of SMEI mandates the following: an infant without pathological history, with a normal physical and psychomotor development, who presents with convulsive seizures, with or without high temperature, before age one year should be considered as a possible SMEI disorder. Repeated and prolonged unilateral or predominantly unilateral seizures, and seizures shifting from one side to the other should raise suspicion of SMEI. At this stage chronic treatment with a combination of the most efficacious AEDs must be started, preferentially with STP. It is also important to ignore potentially worsening drugs (PHT, CBZ, OXC, LTG).

The appearance of myoclonic seizures strongly suggests the diagnosis, particularly if related to photic or pattern sensitivity. Therefore, it is important to try to control them by using VPA, ETS, TPM, BZDZ, and maybe ZNS, LEV, and PIR as well.

The diagnosis of SMEI is predominantly clinical. Genetic analysis should be performed early but one should not wait for the result to commence treatment.

As the disease evolves with age, it is essential to adapt the treatment according to these changes.

The treatment of the Dravet syndrome is challenging and cannot be left to the neuropediatrician alone. It requires the collaboration between a multidisciplinary team and the families. We must keep in mind that every child has his own characteristics and we do not know why the response to drug is not the same in all.

REFERENCES

1. Commission on Classification and Terminology of the International League Against Epilepsy. Proposal for revised classification of epilepsies and epileptic syndromes. *Epilepsia* 1989;30:289–299.
2. Engel J Jr. A proposed diagnostic scheme for people with epileptic seizures and with epilepsy: report of the ILAE Task Force on Classification and Terminology. International League Against Epilepsy (ILAE). *Epilepsia* 2001;42:796–803.
3. Claes L, et al. *De novo* mutations in the sodium-channel gene *SCN1A* cause severe myoclonic epilepsy of infancy. *Am J Hum Genet* 2001;68:1327–1332.
4. Hurst DL. Epidemiology of severe myoclonic epilepsy of infancy. *Epilepsia* 1990;31:397–400.

5. Dravet C, et al. Severe myoclonic epilepsy in infancy (Dravet syndrome). In: Roger J, Bureau M, Dravet C, Genton P, Tassinari CA, Wolf P (eds), *Epileptic Syndromes in Infancy, Childhood, and Adolescence*. London: John Libbey Eurotext Ltd, 2005; 4th edn: pp. 89–113.

6. Ogino T, et al. Severe myoclonic epilepsy beginning in infancy. *Folia Psychiatr Neurol Jpn* 1982;39:357–358.

7. Takahashi Y, et al. Photosensitive epilepsies and pathophysiologic mechanisms of the photoparoxysmal response. *Neurology* 1999;53:926–932.

8. Dalla Bernardina B, Capovilla G, Gattoni M. Epilepsie myoclonique grave de la première année. *Rev Electroencephalogr Neurophysiol Clin* 1982;12:21–25.

9. Cassé-Perrot C, Wolff M, Dravet C. Neuropsychological aspects of severe myoclonic epilepsy in infancy. In: Jambaqué I, Lassonde M, Dulac O (eds), *The Neuropsychology of Childhood Epilepsy*. New-York: Plenum Press/Kluwer Academic, 2001; pp. 131–140.

10. Wolff M, Cassé-Perrot C, Dravet C. Neuropsychological disorders in children with severe myoclonic epilepsy. *Epilepsia* 2006; 47(Suppl 2):61.

11. Battaglia D, et al. Neuropsychological features of eleven patients with severe myoclonic epilepsy (Dravet syndrome). *International Symposium on Febrile Seizures and Related Conditions (ISFS)*, Otsu, Japan, April 10–11, 2008 (abstract book).

12. Siegler Z, et al. Hippocampal sclerosis in severe myoclonic epilepsy in infancy: a retrospective MRI study. *Epilepsia* 2005;46:704–708.

13. Striano P, et al. Brain MRI findings in severe myoclonic epilepsy in infancy and genotype–phenotype correlations. *Epilepsia* 2007;48:1092–1096.

14. Caraballo RH, Fejerman N. Dravet syndrome: a study of 53 patients. *Epilepsy Res* 2006;70S:S231–S238.

15. Ogino T, et al. An investigation on the borderland of severe myoclonic epilepsy in infancy. *Jpn J Psychiatry Neurol* 1988;42:554–555.

16. Dravet C, et al. Severe myoclonic epilepsy in infancy. In: Roger J, Bureau M, Dravet C, Dreifuss FE, Perret A, Wolf P (eds), *Epileptic Syndromes in Infancy, Childhood and Adolescence*. London: John Libbey & Company Ltd, 1992; 2nd edn: pp. 75–88.

17. Fujiwara T, et al. Long-term course of childhood epilepsy with intractable grand mal seizures. *Jpn J Psychiatry Neurol* 1992;46:297–302.

18. Fujiwara T, et al. Mutations of sodium channel α subunit type 1 (*SCN1A*) in intractable childhood epilepsies with frequent generalized tonic clonic seizures. *Brain* 2003;126:531–546.

19. Doose H, et al. Severe idiopathic generalized epilepsy of infancy with generalized tonic–clonic seizures. *Neuropediatrics* 1998;29:229–238.

20. Marini C, et al. Idiopathic epilepsies with seizures precipitated by fever and *SCN1A* abnormalities. *Epilepsia* 2007;48:1678–1696.

21. Nabbout R, et al. Spectrum of *SCN1A* mutations in severe myoclonic epilepsy of infancy. *Neurology* 2003;60:1961–1967.

22. Oguni H, et al. Severe myoclonic epilepsy in infants. Typical and borderline groups in relation to *SCN1A* mutations. In: Delgado-Escueta V, Guerrini R, Medina MT, Genton P, Bureau M, Dravet C (eds), *Myoclonic Epilepsies (Advances in Neurology Series Volume 95)*. Philadelphia: Lippincott Williams & Wilkins, 2005; pp. 103–117.

23. Fukuma G, et al. Mutations of neuronal voltage-gated Na⁺ channel alpha 1 subunit gene *SCN1A* in core severe myoclonic epilepsy in infancy (SMEI) and in borderline SMEI (SMEB). *Epilepsia* 2004;45:140–148.

24. Gennaro E, et al. Familial severe myoclonic epilepsy of infancy: truncation of Nav1.1 and genetic heterogeneity. *Epileptic Disord* 2003;5:21–25.

25. Morimoto T, et al. *SCN1A* mutation mosaïcism in a family with severe myoclonic epilepsy in infancy. *Epilepsia* 2006; 47:1732–1736.

26. Gennaro E, et al. Somatic and germline mosaïcisms in severe myoclonic epilepsy of infancy. *Biochem Biophys Res Commun* 2006;341:489–493.

27. Depienne C, et al. Parental mosaïcism can cause recurrent transmission of *SCN1A* mutations associated with severe myoclonic epilepsy of infancy. *Hum Mutat* 2006;27:389.

28. Madia F, et al. Cryptic chromosome deletions involving *SCN1A* in severe myoclonic epilepsy of infancy. *Neurology* 2006;67:1230–1235.

29. Depienne C, et al. Sporadic infantile epileptic encephalopathy caused by mutations in *PCDH19* resembles Dravet syndrome but mainly affects females. *PLoS Genet* 2009; 5(2):e1000381.

30. Singh R, et al. Severe myoclonic epilepsy of infancy: extended spectrum of GEFS+? *Epilepsia* 2001;42:837–844.

31. Kassai B, et al. Severe myoclonic epilepsy in infancy: a systematic review and a meta-analysis of individual patient data. *Epilepsia* 2008;49:343–348.

32. Oguni H, et al. Treatment of severe myoclonic epilepsy in infants and its borderline variant with bromide. *Epilepsia* 1994;35:1140–1145.

33. Nieto-Barrera M, et al. Topiramate in the treatment of severe myoclonic epilepsy in infancy. *Seizure* 2000;8:590–594.

34. Coppola G, et al. Topiramate as add-on drug in severe myoclonic epilepsy in infancy: an Italian multicenter open trial. *Epilepsy Res* 2002;49:45–48.

35. Villeneuve N, et al. Topiramate (TPM) in severe myoclonic epilepsy in infancy (SMEI): study of 27 patients. *Epilepsia* 2002;43(Suppl 8):155.

36. Grosso S, et al. Efficacy and safety of topiramate in infants according to epilepsy syndromes. *Seizure* 2005;14:183–189.

37. Kroll-Seger J, et al. Topiramate in the treatment of highly refractory patients with Dravet syndrome. *Neuropediatrics* 2006;37:325–329.

38. Striano P, et al. An open-label trial of levetiracetam in severe myoclonic epilepsy of infancy. *Neurology* 2007; 69:250–254.

39. Chiron C, et al. Stiripentol in severe myoclonic epilepsy in infancy: a randomized placebo-controlled syndrome-dedicated trial. STICLO study group. *Lancet* 2000;356 (9242):1638–1642.

40. Guerrini R, Pons G. Comparative study of the efficacy of Stiripentol used in combination in severe myoclonic epilepsy in infancy (SMEI). A double-blind, multicenter, placebo-controlled phase III study. Università di Pisa-IRCCS Stella Maris, Via dei Giacinti, 256018 Calambrone (Pisa), Italy, 2000.

41. Guerrini R, et al. Stiripentol in severe myoclonic epilepsy in infancy (SMEI): a placebo-controlled trial. *Epilepsia* 2002;43(Suppl 9):S155.

42. Than TN, et al. Long-term efficacy and tolerance of Stiripentol in severe myoclonic epilepsy of infancy (Dravet's syndrome). *Arch Pediatr* 2002;9:1120–1127.

43. Kanazawa O, Shirane S. Can early zonizamide medication improve the prognosis in the core and peripheral types of severe myoclonic epilepsy in infants ? *Brain Dev* 1999; 21:503.

44. Horn CS, Ater SB, Hurst DL. Carbamazepine-exacerbated epilepsy in children and adolescents. *Pediatr Neurol* 1986; 2:340–345.

45. Wakai S, et al. Severe myoclonic epilepsy in infancy and carbamazepine. *Eur J Pediatr* 1996;155:724.

46. Wang PJ, et al. Severe myoclonic epilepsy in infancy: evolution of electroencephalographic and clinical features. *Zhonghua Min Guo Xiao Er Ke Yi Xue Hui Za Zhi* 1996;37:428–432.

47. Guerrini R, et al. Lamotrigine and seizure aggravation in severe myoclonic epilepsy. *Epilepsia* 1998;39:508–512.

48. Wallace SJ. Myoclonus and epilepsy in childhood: a review of treatment with valproate, ethosuximide, lamotrigine and zonizamide. *Epilepsy Res* 1998;29:147–154.

49. Fejerman N, Caraballo R, Cersosimo R. Ketogenic diet in patients with Dravet syndrome and myoclonic epilepsies in infancy and early childhood. In: Delgado-Escueta V, Guerrini R, Medina MT, Genton P, Bureau M, Dravet C (eds), *Myoclonic Epilepsies (Advances in Neurology Series Volume 95)*. Philadelphia: Lippincott Williams & Wilkins, 2005; pp. 299–305.

50. Korff C, et al. Dravet syndrome (severe myoclonic epilepsy in infancy): a retrospective study of 16 patients. *J Child Neurol* 2007;22:185–194.

51. Nieto-Barrera M, et al. Immunological study in patients with severe myoclonic epilepsy in childhood. *Rev Neurol* 2000;30:1–15.

52. Nieto-Barrera M, et al. Epilepsia mioclonica grave de la infancia. Tratamiento con gammaglobulina humana. *Rev Neurol* 1995;24:1250–1270.

53. Ceulemans B, et al. Severe myoclonic epilepsy in infancy: towards an optimal treatment. *J Child Neurol* 2004;19:516–521.

54. Takahashi Y, et al. Self-induced photogenic seizures in child with severe myoclonic epilepsy in infancy: optical investigations and treatments. *Epilepsia* 1995;36:728–732.

55. Capovilla G, et al. Suppressive efficacy by a commercially available blue lens on PPR in 610 photosensitive epilepsy patients. *Epilepsia* 2006;47:529–533.

56. Minakawa K. Effectiveness of intravenous midazolam for the treatment of status epilepticus in a child with severe myoclonic epilepsy in infancy. *No To Hattatsu* 1995; 27:498–500.

57. Tanabe T, et al. Management of and prophylaxis against status epilepticus in children with severe myoclonic epilepsy in infancy (SMEI; Dravet syndrome)—a nationwide questionnaire survey in Japan. *Brain Dev* 2008;30(10):629–635.

58. Dooley J, Camfield P, Gordon K. Severe polymorphic epilepsy of infancy. *J Child Neurol* 1995;10:339–340.

59. Chipaux M, et al. Unusual consequences of status epilepticus in Dravet syndrome. *Seizure* 2010;19:190–194.

60. Nieto-Barrera M, et al. Epilepsia mioclonica severa de la infancia. Estudio epidemiologico analitico. *Rev Neurol* 2000;30:620–624.

61. Berkovic SF, et al. De novo mutations of the sodium channel gene *SCN1A* in alleged vaccine encephalopathy: a retrospective study. *Lancet Neurol* 2006;5:488–492.

62. Dravet C, Daquin G, Battaglia D. Severe myoclonic epilepsy of infancy (Dravet syndrome). In: Nikanorova M, Genton P, Sabers A (eds), *Long-Term Evolution of Epileptic Encephalopathies*. Montrouge: John Libbey Eurotext, 2009; pp. 29–38.

63. Jansen FE, et al. Severe myoclonic epilepsy of infancy (Dravet syndrome): recognition and diagnosis in adults. *Neurology* 2006;67:2224–2226.

64. Akiyama M, Kobayashi K, Yoshinaga H, Ohtsuka Y. A long-term follow-up study of Dravet syndrome up to adulthood. *Epilepsia* 2010;51:1043–1052.

65. Buoni S, et al. *SCN1A* (2528delG) novel truncating mutation with benign outcome of severe myoclonic epilepsy of infancy. *Neurology* 2006;66:606.

66. Ragona F, et al. Dravet syndrome: early clinical manifestations and cognitive outcome in 37 Italian patients. *Brain Dev* 2010;32:71–77.

CHAPTER 15

Errors of Metabolism in the Neonatal Period

Nicole I. Wolf and Robert Surtees

▶ OVERVIEW

Seizures in the neonatal period are a frequent and ominous sign of a multitude of conditions. Quick and effective treatment is important to prevent late sequelae in cognitive development; treatment efficacy however depends on the underlying cause. It is also hampered by the sometimes-difficult recognition of seizures in the setting of a neonatal intensive care unit in often critically ill children, as neonatal seizures might be very subtle in their manifestation. Simultaneous video EEG studies are at times necessary to correctly identify all seizure events. They may present as focal clonic seizures, oral automatisms, grimacing, complex movements like pedaling, myoclonic seizures or tonic seizures, and rarely as apnea. The most important cause of neonatal seizures is birth asphyxia. Inborn errors of metabolism as a group are also important, and prompt recognition of the few treatable disorders is crucial for preserving the potential of normal development. In this chapter, we would like to present the inborn errors of metabolism presenting with neonatal seizures (see also Tables 15–1 and 15–2) and focus on treatable disorders, offering algorithms for treatment and the diagnostic approach.

APPROACH TO A NEONATE WITH SEIZURES

Diagnostic Approach

First-line diagnostic tests have to rule out easily recognizable and treatable conditions such as hypoglycemia, hypocalcemia or hypomagnesemia. Ammonia concentrations should also be measured, because neonatal seizures may be the first symptoms before hyperammonemic coma develops. Treatment with pyridoxine and pyridoxal phosphate is diagnostic as well as possibly therapeutic—if a neonate responds to pyridoxine, one can concentrate on proving this inborn error instead of running all possible tests. Full resuscitation equipment should be present when cofactors are given. Apnea in pyridoxine phosphate responsive seizures is also possible with oral administration of this vitamin.

The diagnostic approach should be stepwise (Fig. 15–1). First, common and treatable conditions should be sought for; the rare disorders such as GABA transami-

nase deficiency or the defect in glutamate transport are not among the disorders screened in first-line testing. If there is no response to cofactor treatment, lumbar puncture should be performed including analysis of glucose, cell count, protein, lactate, and amino acids. If possible, 1 or 2 mL of cerebrospinal fluid (CSF) should be stored for further investigations. Analysis of amine neurotransmitter metabolites may be helpful in pyridoxal phosphate-dependent seizures (pyridox(am)ine 5′-phosphate oxidase [PNPO] deficiency), but may also be normal in this condition.[12] Fibroblasts and DNA should be stored if there is no definitive diagnosis.

Cranial ultrasound should be performed promptly in all neonates with seizures. Hemorrhage or edema may be found, some malformations as agenesis of the corpus callosum or lissencephaly may be visible. Cranial MRI, if possible with ¹H-MR spectroscopy, should be done if seizures persist after treatment with cofactors and the child is sufficiently stable. It allows diagnosis of malformations, neonatal stroke, or asphyxia. In many of the inborn errors of metabolism, initial MR imaging is normal or shows nonspecific abnormalities, which may even imitate those of birth asphyxia.

Therapeutic Approach

Cofactors should be given as first-line treatment, even in neonates in whom asphyxia is strongly suspected. Figure 15–2 proposes a practical approach. Any underlying treatable metabolic disorder must be treated appropriately as soon as diagnosis has been made, if necessary, in a specialized centre. If cofactor treatment fails, seizures have to be treated with conventional antiepileptic drugs. Phenobarbital is still the medication of choice although there is concern about increasing nerve cell apoptosis. Phenytoin may be used if phenobarbital does not control seizures. The role of the newer antiepileptic drugs is not yet clear. If, as often is the case, initial treatment was with conventional antiepileptic drugs, cofactor treatment also has to be started. Each institution should have a protocol for treatment and diagnostic approach of neonates with seizures.

Problems

Most neonatal seizures are not due to metabolic disorders, but to birth asphyxia or neonatal stroke. Many

▶ **TABLE 15–1.** INBORN ERRORS OF METABOLISM PRESENTING WITH SEIZURES IN THE NEONATAL PERIOD

Disorder	OMIM Number	Diagnostic Test
Pyridoxine dependency	266100	Response to pyridoxine; elevated pipecolic acid (CSF, plasma) and α-aminoadipic semialdehyde (urine)
PNPO deficiency	610090	Response to pyridoxal 5-phosphate; elevated glycine, threonine, orthomethyldopa
Folinic acid dependency		Response to folinic acid; unknown peak in CSF HPLC
Phosphoserine aminotransferase deficiency	610936	Low CSF and plasma serine and glycine
Nonketotic hyperglycinemia	605899	Elevated CSF: plasma glycine ratio
Urea cycle defects		Hyperammonemia, plasma amino acids, urine orotic acid
Organic acidurias		Urinary organic acids, acylcarnitines
Maple syrup urine disease	248600	Plasma amino acids: elevation of leucine
Zellweger syndrome	214100	Elevated VLCFA
Neonatal adrenoleukodystrophy	202370	Elevated VLCFA
Holocarboxylase synthetase deficiency	253270	Organic acids
Molybdenum cofactor disease	252150	Sulphite test in fresh urine, fibroblast studies
Sulphite oxidase deficiency	272300	Sulphite test in fresh urine, fibroblast studies
Adenylosuccinate lyase deficiency	103050	Modified Bratton–Marshall test in urine
Respiratory chain disorders and PDHc deficiency		Lactate elevation, activity of respiratory chain enzymes and PDHc in muscle
Glutamate transporter deficiency	609302	Glutamate oxidation in fibroblasts, sequencing of *SLC25A22*
Congenital glutamine deficiency	610015	Extremely low glutamine in plasma, urine, and CSF
Neonatal form of neuronal ceroid lipofuscinosis	610127	Cathepsin D activity

Note: HPLC, high performance liquid chromatography; VLCFA, very long chain fatty acids; PDHc, pyruvate dehydrogenase.

neonatologists are therefore reluctant to run elaborate diagnostic tests including a spinal tap and trying vitamins to treat seizures. EEG or MRI are not always helpful in the differential diagnoses. In birth asphyxia, neonates typically recover from the initial crisis and can be extubated and weaned off antiepileptic medication. In contrast inborn errors of metabolism, do not improve without specific treatment, and often deteriorate over time. Still, a few metabolic disorders can imitate neonatal asphyxia and can develop into a residual state, which is easily mistaken for the sequelae of birth asphyxia. A pragmatic approach could be always to treat with cofactors, but to reserve further metabolic investigations for those infants without clear evidence of hypoxic–ischemic encephalopathy.

In many cases, a final diagnosis cannot be made. Here, one should always store skin fibroblasts of the patient and DNA, if possible, from all family members, in order to investigate for "new" metabolic or genetic disorders in the future.

▶ **TABLE 15–2.** METABOLIC DISORDERS PRESENTING WITH SEIZURES IN EARLY INFANCY, BUT ONLY EXCEPTIONALLY IN THE NEONATAL PERIOD

Disorder	OMIM Number	Diagnostic Test
GLUT1 deficiency syndrome	606777	Decreased CSF: serum glucose ratio
Serine biosynthesis defects	601815, 172480	Low serine in CSF amino acid analysis
Biotinidase deficiency	253260	Decreased biotinidase activity
Creatine synthesis defects (especially GAMT deficiency)	601240, 602360, 300352	Absent creatine peak in cerebral ^{1}H-MR spectroscopy; elevated guanidinoacetate; elevated creatine:creatinine ratio
Organic acidurias		Urinary organic acids, acylcarnitines
Aminoacidopathies		Plasma amino acids
Ganglioside synthesis deficiency	609056	Ganglioside analysis in plasma
Storage disorders		Enzyme analysis, demonstration of storage material
Menke's disease	309400	Serum copper and ceruloplasmin

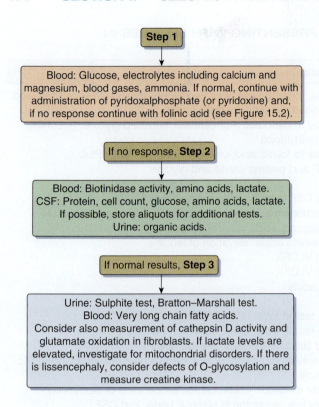

Figure 15–1. Stepwise diagnostic approach in unexplained neonatal seizures.

▶ TREATABLE DISORDERS WHICH CAUSE SEIZURES

HYPOGLYCEMIA

Diagnosis

Hypoglycemia is a frequent cause for neonatal seizures, and blood glucose should be immediately measured in every infant with seizures.

Treatment

In recurrent hypoglycemia, the underlying problem has to be actively sought for and appropriately treated. Prolonged untreated hypoglycemia is deleterious and leads to lasting injury of the parietal and occipital cortex and its underlying white matter.[1] Treatment with glucose is straightforward and stops the seizures (see below for more detail).

PYRIDOXINE DEPENDENT EPILEPSY

Etiology

Although pyridoxine dependent epilepsy (OMIM 266100) was first described in 1954;[2] the molecular basis was discovered only recently.[3] Mutations in the *ALDH7A1* gene catalyzing a step in the lysine degradation pathway lead

to elevation of Δ^1-piperideine-6-carboxylate (Fig. 15–3), which inactivates pyridoxal phosphate by a condensation reaction. Pipecolic acid, a metabolite in this pathway, has been found elevated in plasma, CSF, and urine of patients with pyridoxine dependent epilepsy.[4]

Diagnosis

Another metabolite, α-aminoadipic semialdehyde, is found elevated in urine and is diagnostic for pyridoxine dependent epilepsy.[3,5] Therefore it is no longer necessary to withdraw pyridoxine to confirm the diagnosis of pyridoxine-dependent epilepsy.[6] Still, one has to remember that not all cases of pyridoxine dependent epilepsy are caused by mutations in *ALDH7A1*, as there are patients who do not show linkage to this locus.[3,7] Negative biochemical testing thus does not preclude this diagnosis, and successful treatment should not be withdrawn because of negative metabolic or genetic testing.

Clinical Presentation

Seizures usually begin within the first 24–48 hours, but can manifest up to the age of two or even three years. Prenatal seizures are also described.[8] Seizures may be preceded by an encephalopathic phase, and neonates may demonstrate abdominal distension, vomiting or signs of septicemia. In these situations, seizure recognition is often difficult, and seizures may be wrongly attributed to another cause. Seizure semiology is sometimes characteristic with bizarre, spasm-like convulsions, multifocal myoclonus and grimacing—several seizure types can be seen in one infant. The same is true for the EEG: whilst there is no pathognomonic pattern, abnormalities may be highly variable in one single child. Burst-suppression pattern and continuous, high-voltage delta activity can be found.[9]

Treatment

Seizures respond promptly to the administration of 100 mg pyridoxine. In some cases, the dose necessary to stop seizures is higher, and it has been suggested to give up to 500 mg pyridoxine in single doses of 100 mg each. The response might be delayed or not unequivocal in a critically ill neonate. The intravenous administration of pyridoxine can lead to central depression in around a fifth of patients. Though usually resulting in hypotonia and sleepiness, apnea, coma and cardiovascular instability can occur, and ventilation may become necessary. The same is true for oral administration. Optimally, pyridoxine is given during an EEG recording and after urine and plasma (and CSF) have been taken for metabolic investigations. However, because of the risk of central depression, it is safer to give pyridoxine on a ward with full resuscitation facilities than in a neurophysiology department. This should, however, never delay pyridoxine administration.

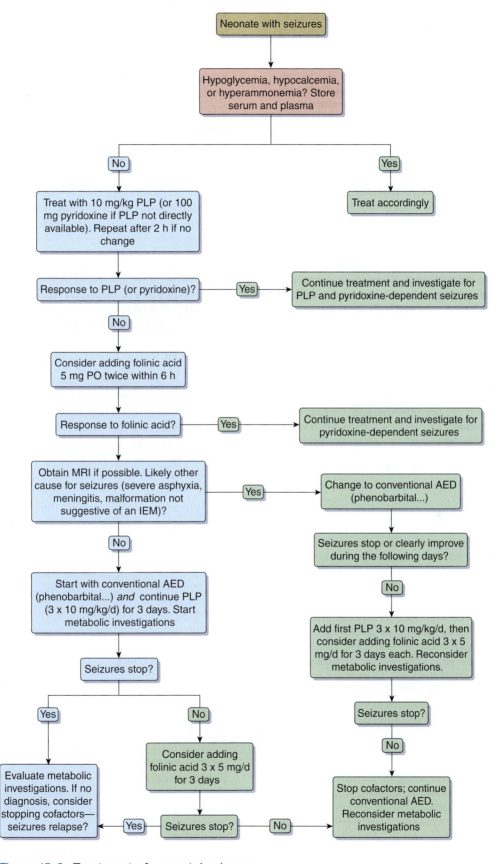

Figure 15–2. Treatment of neonatal seizures.

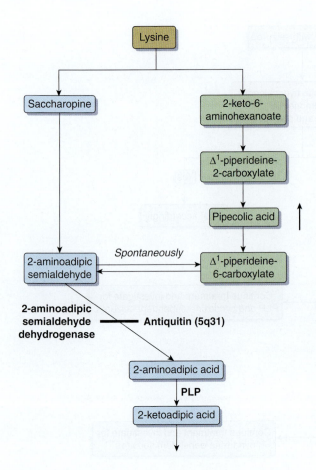

Figure 15–3. Pyridoxine-dependent seizures: metabolic basis.

Folinic acid responsive seizures were long thought to represent a separate entity, also causing otherwise refractory neonatal seizures. Response to small doses of folinic acid (3 to 5 mg/kg per day) was discovered serendipitously. Affected infants showed characteristic, but hitherto unidentified peaks on CSF monoamine analysis.[10] Recently it could be demonstrated that this disorder is identical to pyridoxine-dependent epilepsy— affected patients harbor mutations in the *ALDH7A1* gene. α-aminoadipic semialdehyde is elevated in CSF of these children.[11] Whether treatment with folinic acid in addition to pyridoxine therapy is beneficial in patients with pyridoxine-dependent seizures is unknown but should be considered in patients with otherwise refractory seizures.

PYRIDOXAL-PHOSPHATE RESPONSIVE SEIZURES (PYRIDOX(AM)INE PHOSPHATE OXIDASE DEFICIENCY)

Etiology

Pyridoxal 5-phosphate responsive seizures (OMIM 610090) were only recently described in several infants;[12,13] the molecular basis was solved shortly after the recognition of this syndrome. This disorder is caused by mutations in the gene encoding pyridox(am)ine 5′-phosphate oxidase (PNPO), an enzyme catalyzing the phosphorylation of pyridoxine and pyridoxamine to pyridoxal 5-phosphate, the active essential cofactor for over one hundred enzymes, among them aromatic amino acid decarboxylase, the glycine cleavage system, glutamate decarboxylase and threonine dehydratase (Fig. 15–4).[14]

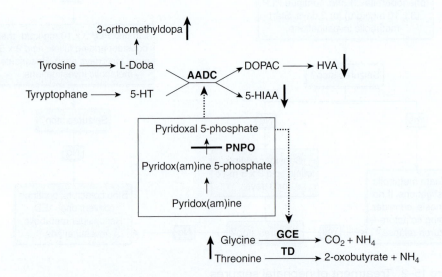

Figure 15–4. Pyridoxal-5-phosphate-dependent seizures (PNPO deficiency): metabolic basis.

Diagnosis

Glycine and threonine can be elevated in body fluids, and CSF findings may mimic aromatic amino acid decarboxylase deficiency, but not necessarily so.[12,15]

Treatment

In pyridox(am)ine phosphate oxidase deficiency administration of pyridoxine is not successful, because it cannot be converted to pyridoxal 5-phosphate. Most affected children die within the first months of life if pyridoxal 5-phosphate is not given. If started early in the neonatal period, development can be normal.[15] In one child, the diagnosis was made only at the age of 3 years, and therapy was introduced at that time. The severe epilepsy that had proved resistant to all therapy greatly improved with pyridoxal 5-phosphate, and the condition of the severely affected child stabilized but there were no additional benefits for his development. Seizure semiology has not been well described. Affected newborns are said to resemble neonates with pyridoxine dependency. EEG shows a discontinuous pattern with bursts of epileptic activity.

The therapeutic dose of pyridoxal 5-phosphate is around 30–50 mg/kg per day. One should start with 3 × 10 mg/kg daily. The response is quick and EEG may show complete resolution after the first dose. Seizures might restart shortly before the next dose is due, and can be prevented by increasing the amount of doses given per day.[15] The optimal dose and dosage interval probably differ from child to child.

As pyridoxal 5-phosphate successfully stops both pyridoxal 5-phosphate dependent seizures and pyridoxine dependent epilepsy, it should be used as first-line treatment in every neonate with seizures. Results of diagnostic tests or EEG should not be awaited, as timely treatment is of utmost importance for the cognitive outcome. Asphyxia, preterm birth, or sepsis-like illness are not arguments against a metabolic disorder, as in both conditions children with signs and symptoms of all these have been described.[12,15] The difficult question is how and when to stop and/or start with conventional antiepileptic drugs. There is no consensus yet. Neonatologists often omit a cofactor trial and administer conventional antiepileptic drugs. If they fail, the decision to give cofactors a trial is an easy one. Vice versa, it is more difficult. Still, as most infants respond quickly to pyridoxal 5-phosphate, a short trial before starting antiepileptic medication is warranted. If pyridoxal 5-phosphate is not available quickly in the neonatal intensive care unit, pyridoxine should be given instead. If seizures do not respond, pyridoxal 5-phosphate should be evaluated as soon as possible regardless of the results of metabolic investigations.

HOLOCARBOXYLASE SYNTHETASE AND BIOTINIDASE DEFICIENCY

Clinical Presentation and Diagnosis

In holocarboxylase synthetase deficiency, a rare inborn error of metabolism, affected neonates develop symptoms shortly after birth. Seizures are not obligate, occurring in 25–50% of all children. Lactic acidosis is common.

Prognosis

In biotinidase deficiency, endogenous biotin cannot be recycled, and activity of the biotin-dependent carboxylases is reduced. Different metabolites accumulate in urine, and lactic acidosis is frequent. Epilepsy is also frequent. However, the epilepsy does not normally start during the neonatal period, but usually begins after the first 3 or 4 months of life, often as infantile spasms; optic atrophy and hearing loss are frequent. General clinical features suggesting biotinidase deficiency are stridor, alopecia, conjunctivitis, and perioral, nasal, and ocular dermatitis. The otherwise refractory seizures promptly respond to small doses of biotin, usually 5–20 mg per day. Biotinidase deficiency is part of the neonatal screening in several countries. If treated early, development is normal.[16]

Treatment

Biotin controls all symptoms and leads also to normalization of metabolic abnormalities. It is usually effective at similar doses as in biotinidase deficiency, and only a few children require higher doses.

AMINOACIDOPATHIES, ORGANIC ACIDURIAS, AND UREA CYCLE DEFECTS

Clinical Presentation

The neonatal form of maple syrup urine disease presents with seizures in a critically ill neonate. Additional symptoms (vomiting, abnormal movements) are frequent.

Diagnosis

The EEG shows a peculiar comb-like rhythm, reminiscent of the delta-brush pattern in preterm infants.[17] Measuring plasma amino acids readily diagnoses this condition, and treatment must be started immediately, usually with dialysis to lower the toxic branched-chain amino acids and appropriate diet.

Most other amino acidopathies present later. Some defects in serine biosynthesis (3-phosphoglycerate dehydrogenase deficiency) have a prenatal onset and affected infants are born microcephalic. However, seizures usually start later in infancy, not in the neonatal period.[18]

Treatment

Treatment with serine improves epilepsy; if started prenatally, it can prevent symptoms altogether. Other defects in serine biosynthesis (phosphoserine aminotransferase deficiency) can present with neonatal seizures, and early treatment with serine can lead to a normal outcome.[19] Phenylketonuria leads almost invariably to epilepsy (West syndrome) in infancy if left untreated, but does not present in the neonatal period.

Methylmalonic aciduria and propionic aciduria often present acutely during the neonatal period. Seizures may occur during acute decompensation, but are not a leading symptom. Diagnosis is straightforward with analysis of urinary organic acids or acylcarnitine esters.

In urea cycle defects with neonatal presentation, seizures may precede hyperammonemic coma, but are usually not prominent. The clinical state rapidly deteriorates until the neonate is in a deep coma. EEG shows a severely disturbed, slow background activity. Timely diagnosis and treatment are crucial to minimize central nervous system damage.

▶ DISORDERS PRESENTING WITH SEIZURES THAT ARE NOT AMENABLE TO TREATMENT

NONKETOTIC HYPERGLYCINEMIA

Clinical Presentation

The most frequent form of this disorder characterized by deficient degradation glycine starts within the first days of life. Early signs and symptoms are lethargy, hypotonia, hiccups (mothers may report them already during pregnancy), ophthalmoplegia, and disturbance of other vegetative functions of the brain stem. The infant's condition deteriorates with apnea leading to intubation and frequent segmental myoclonic jerks. If the child survives, severe refractory epilepsy, which needs treatment by conventional antiepileptic drugs and tetraplegia, develops over the ensuing months. Initially, the EEG shows a burst–suppression pattern, changing to high-voltage slow activity and finally to hypsarrhythmia.[20]

Diagnosis

Diagnosis is usually straightforward by demonstrating an increased glycine concentration in plasma, CSF and urine. CSF to plasma glycine ratio (>0.08) is elevated. Decreased activity of the hepatic glycine cleavage system and positive mutation analysis proves this disorder.

MISCELLANEOUS

Deficiency of *GABA transaminase* is an extremely rare disease; only three patients have been reported.[21] Seizures may be present from birth. The diagnosis is made by demonstrating elevated GABA levels in CSF and plasma. In two patients, growth was accelerated. There is no treatment for this disorder.

Sulphite oxidase and *molybdenum cofactor deficiency* are rare disorders presenting in neonates with intractable seizures. Lens dislocation may follow. MRI shows cystic changes and severe atrophy, but may mimic the changes of hypoxic–ischemic encephalopathy early in the disease.[22] A simple urine dipstick test, which has to be done with fresh urine, helps in diagnosing this group of disorders. The exact enzyme deficiency can be established in fibroblast cultures. A child with molybdenum cofactor deficiency type A was successfully treated with cyclic pyranopterin monophosphate (cPMP)—seizures subsided, and the child showed reasonable, albeit delayed, psychomotor development in an otherwise lethal disease. Whether early treatment with cPMP can lead to normal development, is not known.[23]

Mitochondrial encephalopathies and *pyruvate dehydrogenase deficiency* may present early in the neonatal period with lactic acidosis and neonatal seizures. This group of disorders is heterogeneous and may be mistaken for birth asphyxia. Other organs may also be involved. If a mitochondrial disorder presents that early, prognosis is usually extremely poor. Treatment with cofactors (especially thiamine and carnitine) should be tried, but are without success in most cases. The exact diagnosis is difficult, and a muscle biopsy should be done whenever possible in addition to fibroblast cultures in order to pinpoint the respiratory chain defect. Inheritance is usually autosomal recessive, but maternal inheritance is possible. Pyruvate dehydrogenase deficiency is X-linked. Genetic counseling is often very difficult and prenatal diagnosis is not always possible.

Deficiency of one the two *mitochondrial glutamate transporters* were recently demonstrated in a single family where four of eight children developed early myoclonic epileptic encephalopathy. Myoclonic seizures started within the very first hours of life and persisted together with a burst-suppression pattern in the EEG. MRI showed later unspecific atrophy. There were no metabolic abnormalities. The defect was found by a genetic approach in this consanguineous family; impaired glutamate oxidation in fibroblasts could be demonstrated and might be a reliable biochemical test for this condition.[24]

Peroxisomal disorders (*Zellweger syndrome* or *neonatal adrenoleukodystrophy*) can present early in the neonatal period. Myoclonic and focal motor seizures dominate the clinical picture, the latter reflecting the frequent brain malformations in Zellweger syndrome.[25]

Disorders of *purine and pyrimidine metabolism* may lead to seizures. The only defect associated with seizures in the neonatal period is *adenylosuccinate lyase* deficiency in its severe form. Seizure types and EEG features are not well described, but do not respond to treatment. Affected infants are microcephalic and may present with other abnormalities (e.g., arthrogryposis). Prognosis is poor.[26]

Defects of *O-glycosylation,* such as the Walker–Warburg syndrome, lead to abnormal cortical development and thus often to seizures usually starting in infancy. In a few children, these seizures may already be manifest in the neonatal period.

Congenital glutamine deficiency secondary to mutations in the gene coding for glutamine synthetase has recently been described in two newborns. Both had seizures; MRI showed agyria or pachygyria and hyperintense white matter. Both infants died within the newborn period.[27]

The neonatal form of the neuronal ceroid lipofuscinosis (CLN10) has recently been shown to be caused by mutations in the gene coding for cathepsin D, a lysosomal protease. Affected infants are born microcephalic, develop seizures from birth and die within the first few days of life.[28]

INBORN ERRORS OF METABOLISM LEADING TO SEIZURES IN INFANCY

There are many more inborn errors of metabolism associated with epilepsy starting in infancy, although generally not during the neonatal period.[25,29] In these disorders, neonatal seizures are the exception. This is true for Menkes disease, glucose transporter 1 deficiency, the disorders of creatine transport and synthesis, the recently described defect in ganglioside synthesis, or storage disorders. Also biotinidase deficiency and the defects in serine synthesis usually present with seizures during infancy although in some serine synthesis disorders, microcephaly is present already *in utero.*[17] Diagnosis in the latter two disorders and in the disorders of creatine synthesis is important because there is effective treatment available.

▶ CONCLUSIONS

Neonatal seizures are an emergency and have to be investigated and treated appropriately. Although inborn errors of metabolism are rare, they must be included in the differential diagnosis. As timely treatment is important, all neonates with seizures should have a trial with pyridoxal phosphate initially, even before diagnostic testing or EEG recording have started. If pyridoxal phosphate, which cures pyridoxine-dependent epilepsy as well as pyridoxal phosphate-dependent seizures, is not immediately available, pyridoxine can be given instead; but pyridoxal phosphate has to be tested if seizures persist, as well as additional treatment with folinic acid. If all these are not successful, the differential diagnosis is broad and extensive investigation needs to be initiated.

REFERENCES

1. Barkovich AJ, Ali FA, Rowley HA, Bass N. Imaging patterns of neonatal hypoglycemia. *AJNR Am J Neuroradiol* 1998; 19:523–528.
2. Hunt AD Jr, Stokes J Jr, McCrory WW, Stroud HH. Pyridoxine dependency: report of a case of intractable convulsions in an infant controlled by pyridoxine. *Pediatrics* 1954;13:140– 145.
3. Mills PB, et al. Mutations in antiquitin in individuals with pyridoxine-dependent seizures. *Nat Med* 2006;12:307–309.
4. Plecko B, Stockler-Ipsiroglu S, Paschke E, Erwa W, Struys EA, Jakobs C. Pipecolic acid elevation in plasma and cerebrospinal fluid of two patients with pyridoxine-dependent epilepsy. *Ann Neurol* 2000;48:121–125.
5. Bok LA, Struys E, Willemsen MA, Been JV, Jakobs C. Pyridoxine-dependent seizures in Dutch patients: diagnosis by elevated urinary alpha-aminoadipic semialdehyde levels. *Arch Dis Child* 2007;92:687–689.
6. Baxter P, Griffiths P, Kelly T, Gardner-Medwin D. Pyridoxine-dependent seizures: demographic, clinical, MRI and psychometric features, and effect of dose on intelligence quotient. *Dev Med Child Neurol* 1996;38:998– 1006.
7. Cormier-Daire V, et al. A gene for pyridoxine-dependent epilepsy maps to chromosome 5q31. *Am J Hum Genet* 2000;67:991–993.
8. Baxter P. Pyridoxine-dependent and pyridoxine-responsive seizures. *Dev Med Child Neurol* 2001;43:416–420.
9. Nabbout R, Soufflet C, Plouin P, Dulac O. Pyridoxine dependent epilepsy: a suggestive electroclinical pattern. *Arch Dis Child Fetal Neonatal Ed* 1999;81:F125–F129.
10. Torres OA, Miller VS, Buist NM, Hyland K. Folinic acid-responsive neonatal seizures. *J Child Neurol* 1999;14:529– 532.
11. Gallagher RC, et al. Folinic acid-responsive seizures are identical to pyridoxine-dependent epilepsy. *Ann Neurol* 2009;65:550–556.
12. Clayton PT, Surtees RA, DeVile C, Hyland K, Heales SJ. Neonatal epileptic encephalopathy. *Lancet* 2003;361:1614.
13. Kuo MF, Wang HS. Pyridoxal phosphate-responsive epilepsy with resistance to pyridoxine. *Pediatr Neurol* 2002;26: 146–147.
14. Mills PB, et al. Neonatal epileptic encephalopathy caused by mutations in the PNPO gene encoding pyridox(am)ine 5′-phosphate oxidase. *Hum Mol Genet* 2005;14:1077–1086.
15. Hoffmann GF, et al. Pyridoxal 5′-phosphate may be curative in early-onset epileptic encephalopathy. *J Inherit Metab Dis* 2007;30:96–99.
16. Wolf B. Clinical issues and frequent questions about biotinidase deficiency. *Mol Genet Metab* 2010;100:6–13.
17. Tharp BR. Unique EEG pattern (comb-like rhythm) in neonatal maple syrup urine disease. *Pediatr Neurol* 1992; 8:65–68.
18. de Koning TJ, Klomp LW. Serine-deficiency syndromes. *Curr Opin Neurol* 2004;17:197–204.

19. Hart CE, et al. Phosphoserine aminotransferase deficiency: a novel disorder of the serine biosynthesis pathway. *Am J Human Genet* 2007;80:931–937.

20. Applegarth DA, Toone JR. Glycine encephalopathy (nonketotic hyperglycinaemia): review and update. *J Inherit Metab Dis* 2004;27:417–422.

21. Jaeken J. Genetic disorders of gamma-aminobutyric acid, glycine, and serine as causes of epilepsy. *J Child Neurol* 2002;17(Suppl 3):3S84–3S87; discussion 3S8.

22. Hobson EE, Thomas S, Crofton PM, Murray AD, Dean JC, Lloyd D. Isolated sulphite oxidase deficiency mimics the features of hypoxic ischaemic encephalopathy. *Eur J Pediatr* 2005;164:655–659.

23. Veldman A, et al. Successful treatment of molybdenum cofactor deficiency type A with cPMP. *Pediatrics* 2010;125: e1249–e1254.

24. Molinari F, et al. Impaired mitochondrial glutamate transport in autosomal recessive neonatal myoclonic epilepsy. *Am J Hum Genet* 2005;76:334–339.

25. Wolf NI, Bast T, Surtees R. Epilepsy in inborn errors of metabolism. *Epileptic Disord* 2005;7:67–81.

26. Mouchegh K, et al. Lethal fetal and early neonatal presentation of adenylosuccinate lyase deficiency: observation of 6 patients in 4 families. *J Pediatr* 2007;150:57–61. e2.

27. Haberle J, et al. Congenital glutamine deficiency with glutamine synthetase mutations. *N Engl J Med* 2005; 353:1926–1233.

28. Siintola E, et al. Cathepsin D deficiency underlies congenital human neuronal ceroid-lipofuscinosis. *Brain* 2006;129:1438–1445.

29. Bahi-Buisson N, et al. Neonatal epilepsy and inborn errors of metabolism. *Arch Pediatr* 2006;13:284–292.

CHAPTER 16

Episodes in Neonates, Infants, and Toddlers Mimicking Epilepsy

John BP Stephenson

▶ OVERVIEW

The misdiagnosis of epilepsy is common in infancy and childhood,[1–4] This book is devoted to epilepsy treatment, but if therapy is given for epilepsy that does not exist, then the result may be deleterious to the patient. This chapter outlines the conditions in neonates, infants, and toddlers that may beguile the physician (and even the surgeon) into misdiagnosis.

DEFINITIONS OF EPILEPSY

Past the neonatal period, the definition of an epileptic seizure is fairly straightforward, with the presumption that were an EEG recorded in a seizure, paroxysmal ictal discharges would be evident. Epilepsy is defined as repeated unprovoked epileptic seizures. However, in neonates and very young infants the epileptic "discharge" may appear as a suppression or attenuation of the EEG[5] and the epileptic discharge must be inferred by the observer.

TIME LINE OF PAROXYSMAL PHENOMENA EMERGENCE

For this chapter, the disorders or phenomena are arranged according to median age of first appearance to the parent or the doctor. With notable exceptions,[6–9] median age of onset (MA) is seldom specified in the literature. Episodic events that are liable to be misdiagnosed as epilepsy with a MA of up to age 2 years will be reviewed.

▶ HYPEREKPLEXIA (MA DAY 1)

The MA of 1 day does not take into account the onset of symptoms in fetal life (aside from hyperekplexia, "convulsive" fetal movements are best known in pyridoxine dependency but are also seen in cerebral malformations, and other rarer causes of epilepsy). Those with dominantly inherited hyperekplexia due to a mutation in a glycine receptor subunit, especially *GLRA1*, are stiff infants or neonates, and while they may be at risk of apnea and sudden death they are not usually misdiagnosed as having epilepsy. However, in "sporadic" cases[10–17] and in those with mutations in the glycine transporter gene[18] prominent nonepileptic neonatal seizures are an important feature.

Vigevano et al[10] and Bernardina et al[11] gave the first detailed clinical descriptions of the nonepileptic seizures in neonatal hyperekplexia. Aside from massive myoclonic jerks, symptoms were marked by diffuse muscle stiffness, extension of all limbs, and intense cyanosis with bradycardia. The attacks were resistant to intravenous diazepam and oral phenobarbitone, nitrazepam and clonazepam.[10] Spontaneous and induced generalized attacks with "sudden massive stiffness and shaking of the limbs lasting one to several minutes, and the mimicked generalized clonic or myoclonic fits" might induce severe bradycardia necessitating cardiac massage.[11] A published polygraphic recording[11] of one of these attacks that was tonic and vibratory revealed high-voltage repetitive muscle potentials in the upper and lower limb muscles, on most of the EEG channels and on the ECG channel. This polygraphic appearance consisting of bursts of EMG "spikes" is pathognomonic of neonatal hyperekplexia[12] (Figs. 16–1 and 16–2).

Pascotto and Coppola[13] noted that attacks occurred when the infant was asleep, lasting 20 seconds to several minutes. Polygraphy recorded rhythmic 12 Hz myoclonus from both deltoid muscles. Bernardina et al[11] previously emphasized that while the frequent massive and violent jerks that occurred spontaneously or in response to unexpected stimuli disappeared during sleep, the generalized attacks characterized by massive generalized stiffness with violent shaking of the limbs, apnea, cyanosis, and tachycardia followed by bradycardia, could occur spontaneously while asleep.

Misdiagnosis of epilepsy is common from the neonatal period until adult life. A typical example was the reported case of a girl with "fits" from birth, who was diagnosed with myoclonic epilepsy by neurologists when she was 16 years old.[20]

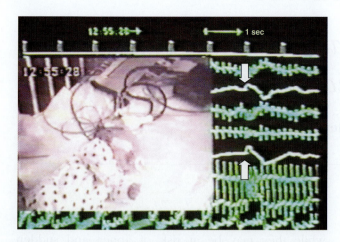

Figure 16–1. Neonatal hyperekplexia. A still from the video of an episode of profound syncope is superimposed on the simultaneous EEG and ECG (recorded with Oxford Medical Systems), with 8 seconds of the trace displayed. The infant is stiff and apneic. The EEG is isoelectric but shows a slow "artefact" (duration less than 1 sec) indicated by the white arrows, clinically associated with a (nonepileptic) anoxic spasm. The ECG shows gross bradycardia with atrioventricular dissociation (junctional rhythm). Superimposed on all but two of the EEG channels and on the ECG channel are very high-voltage compound muscle action potentials (CMAP). For most of the visible recording, the CMAPs are rhythmic at about 7 Hz, but at the time of the arrowed spasm the CMAP rate is around 22 Hz (see Fig. 16–2 for further detail). The two EEG channels that do not show these repetitive CMAPs are from the sagittal midline and over bone rather than over muscle. The clinical history was that he developed severe convulsions at age 40 hours, up to 6 per day, most often precipitated by bathing.[18,19] He seemed "normal" and not stiff in between episodes of twitching, but after immersion in warm water he had rapid quivering of his limbs, an interrupted cry with fast grunting, and then silence with intense stiffening in a semiflexed posture leading to deep cyanosis. Nose tap was positive but the response gradually waned, such that in due course he was able to play club rugby football. In due course, he was found to have a pathogenic mutation in the GlyT2 gene *SLC6A5* ([16]—patient 6) (www.stars.org.uk. or www.stars-us.org).

A simple diagnostic maneuver for hyperekplexia is the nose-tap test. Kurczynski[21] first proposed the nose-tap response as a characteristic feature, noting: "A prominent startle response consisting of eye blinking and a flexor spasm of the trunk could be elicited easily and repetitively by tapping the *tip* of the nose but no other part of the nose, forehead, or face" and "This response seemed to show no habituation. Sudden unexpected loud noises could also elicit a similar startle response."

It has been known since the first description of hyperekplexia that extremely strong brain stem reflexes

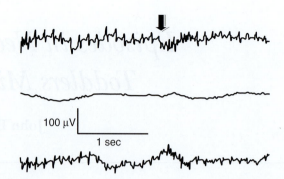

Figure 16–2. This figure shows an extract from the EEG of the same infant with neonatal hyperekplexia due to a mutation in the gene for the presynaptic glycine transporter GlyT2 that was introduced in Figure 16–1 ([16]—patient 6). The middle trace is virtually isoelectric in keeping with the profound syncope. The first and third channels show superimposed the high-voltage CMAPs mainly at about 8 per second that are typical of neonatal hyperekplexia. In addition, at the solid black arrow, there is a slow deflection of duration about 500 ms with irregular CMAPs superimposed at about 24 Hz. This is the EEG/EMG signature of a nonepileptic anoxic spasm (www.stars.org.uk. or www.stars-us.org).

are a constant feature.[22] It is thus important to emphasize that the response to nose tap (percussing the *tip* of the nose) in hyperekplexia is not simply a startle (with trunk flexion) but involves prominent head retraction.[22–24] In this regard, Shahar's description[23] is instructive: "nose tapping was followed by extension of the head accompanied by a brief episode of generalized myoclonic jerking, which recurred with repeated taps." These two aspects—startle and head retraction reflex—have been confused or conflated in the literature. For instance, Nigro and Lim[24] referred to the "hyperekplexic startle response" to nose tapping, and published photographs of an infant showing "startle with sudden adduction of the arms and extension of the head following nose tap."

Aside from avoiding the misdiagnosis of neonatal epileptic seizures, management includes genetic testing, especially for mutations affecting the GlyT2 gene,[18] cardiorespiratory monitoring, and use of the Vigevano maneuver,[10] and oral clonazepam for several months[18] or if need be for life.

▶ PAROXYSMAL EXTREME PAIN DISORDER (MA DAY 2)

Formerly known as familial rectal pain syndrome,[25,26] this rare disorder was once thought to be a form of reflex epilepsy[27] and responds to some extent to carbamazepine[26–28] because of the properties of the mutated sodium channel *SCN9A*.[29]

Episodes are provoked by maneuvers such as perineal stimulation and consist of flushing—usually with the harlequin phenomenon, such as the right side of the face red with tonic posturing. The "distant" look in the neonate's eyes is likely a result of extreme pain. Tachycardia is followed by extreme bradycardia or asystole and often profound syncope.[26] Severe cyanotic breath-holding[28] is not an uncommon manifestation.

▶ BENIGN NEONATAL SLEEP MYOCLONUS (MA DAY 3)

The main importance of benign neonatal sleep myoclonus (BNSM)[9] is for it to be recognized by observation. BNSM begins in otherwise completely normal neonates but is very easily mistaken for epilepsy,[9,30–34] including status epilepticus.[33] Rhythmic myoclonus noted only in sleep may affect one or more limbs, and facial muscles are occasionally involved.[31,35,36] Although jerking may continue for 90 minutes,[37] polygraphy (and on video) reveals a series of very short bursts of 4–5 per second jerking.[31] Perhaps the best way to ensure a correct diagnosis is for all neonatal caretakers to view symptoms on video recordings of BNSM.[31] It has been reported that rocking the crib of the infant will reproduce BNSM,[38] but otherwise it is helpful to show the mother a video of another baby with BNSM.[31,39] Antiepileptic medications may worsen BNSM;[30] oversedated infants have been admitted to neonatal intensive care units for ventilator support.[40]

It is now clear that BNSM is overrepresented after maternal opioid drug use in pregnancy.[41]

▶ JITTERINESS (MA "NEONATE")

Jitteriness is said to occur in 50% of normal-term newborns, but occurs in abnormal neonates as well. Pediatricians and neonatologists do not have problems recognizing this tremor-like phenomenon in the waking state, and it should therefore not prove a diagnostic problem, even when it persists.[42]

▶ UNCLASSIFIED NEONATAL BEHAVIOURS (MA "NEONATE")

When neonatal seizures have no EEG correlates, they are assumed to be nonepileptic.[43] Behaviors such as pedaling come into this category.

It is most important to note that some neonatal behaviors, notably a combination of multifocal myoclonus with no EEG change, and peculiar eye movements and grimacing may indicate the beginnings of

pyridoxine dependent (or pyridoxal phosphate responsive) epilepsy.[44]

Whether or not the opsoclonus-like eye movements and the apneas that may indicate the start of GLUT1 deficiency are epileptic in mechanism is not clear, but it is also important to think of this treatable disorder in that context[45–47] and indeed in any unexplained paroxysmal movement disorder in later infancy and childhood.[47]

The peculiar eye movements (such as monocular nystagmus) that herald alternating hemiplegia of childhood (AHC) commonly begin in the newborn period,[8] but this condition is discussed later under MA 3 months.

▶ TONIC REFLEX SEIZURES OF EARLY INFANCY (MA 1–2 MONTHS)

Vigevano and Lispi[48] described 13 infants aged between 1 and 3 months with nonepileptic seizures characterized by tonic stiffening with apnea and cyanosis in response to tactile stimulation and almost exclusively when the infants were held in a vertical position. The description is reminiscent of the "awake apnea of Spitzer"[49] in which gastroesophageal reflux is the mechanism, but the Italian patients are not reported to have had such reflux. Spontaneous remission within 2 months was the rule.[48]

▶ IMPOSED UPPER AIRWAYS OBSTRUCTION (MA ~3 MONTHS)

Repeated intentional suffocation of an infant by the mother is a potentially serious medical condition[40,50–55] that may masquerade as infantile epilepsy. In this disorder, only the mother sees the onset of an episode, but shows the limp-shocked infant to family or medical staff before effecting resuscitation. It is hazardous for the doctor to make such a diagnosis, but may be fatal if the diagnosis is not made. Experts called on the mother's behalf will argue that the attacks were a type of reflex infantile syncope, especially cyanotic breath-holding spells, Table 16–1 lists factors clarifying this diagnosis.

▶ ALTERNATING HEMIPLEGIA OF CHILDHOOD (MA 3 MONTHS, BUT WIDE RANGE)

Many infants with AHC were formerly misdiagnosed with epilepsy, but the clinical picture is now well known.[8,56–58] In as many as a third of cases, the first symptoms begin in the neonatal period, with eye movement disturbances

▶ **TABLE 16–1.** DIFFERENTIAL DIAGNOSIS OF SEVERE BLUE SYNCOPES

Feature	IUAO	CBHS/PEA	Epileptic Apnea	Obstructive Sleep Apnea	Apnea in CMS
Clinical features					
Characteristic provocation	No (that is, not known to doctors)	Yes	No	No	No, or often not obvious
Onset of events seen by doctors	No (except on covert video)	Often	Often	Maybe	Often
Grunting cry heard or reported	?	Often	?	Maybe	Maybe
Some events in sleep	Often	No	Often	Yes	Maybe
Events continue after diagnosis	No	Yes	Yes (unless treated)	Yes (unless treated)	Yes (unless treated)
Monitoring characteristics					
Rapid onset EEG slowing	No	Yes	No	Maybe	?
Rapid onset flat EEG	No	Often	No	Maybe	?
EEG discharges (spikes etc.) during	No	No	Yes	No	No
Long duration of bradycardia	Yes	No	Often	Variable	?
Prolonged movement in event	Yes	No	Often	Yes	?
Delayed activation of event marker or calling for aid	Yes	No	No	Not if parent witnesses	No

CBHS, cyanotic breath-holding spell (same as PEA); CMS, congenital myasthenic syndrome(s); IUAO, imposed upper airways obstruction; PEA, prolonged expiratory apnea; ?, insufficient information.

(especially nystagmus, including monocular nystagmus), and respiratory irregularities including apneas.[8] By contrast, the age of onset of hemiplegic (or quadriplegic) episodes and dystonic attacks was 6 months.

Episodes of AHC may be precipitated by domestic bathing[8,19,59,60] and the misdiagnosis of bathing (epileptic) seizures[59] may be made.[60]

Choreoathetosis and other neurodevelopmental impairments often add to the child's difficulties. The explanation for the pathogenesis of AHC has advanced little following the recognition of the beneficial effect of the calcium-channel blocker flunarazine.[61] There has been one report of the beneficial effect of the dopaminergic NMDA-receptor antagonist amantadine,[62] but this was not mentioned in a recent large review.[8]

In AHC episodes of alternating or double hemiplegia only appear in the waking state and always disappear with sleep, so that the child is never paralyzed on awakening. By contrast, in the very rare condition benign familial nocturnal AHC[63] attacks of alternating or bilateral hemiplegia arise exclusively out of sleep.

▶ **BENIGN NONEPILEPTIC INFANTILE SPASMS (MA 6 MONTHS)**

This close mimicker of epileptic infantile spasms was first described as benign myoclonus of early infancy[64] and subsequent authors have used this terminology.[65–67]

Vigevano[66] supports the continued use of "benign myoclonus of early infancy" but Dravet and coworkers[65] suggest that the better term is benign nonepileptic spasms (les spasmes infantiles bénins nonépileptiques). There are two reasons for keeping spasms in the term. First, the condition is a convincing clinical imitator of West syndrome.[67] Second, it helps to distinguish myoclonic episodes from spasms and tonic episodes,[40] the duration of each movement being the important criterion. Hence, spasms are intermediate between brief myoclonic jerks and longer tonic contractions.[68]

There is no unanimity as to whether benign nonepileptic infantile spasms can be distinguished clinically from the epileptic infantile spasms of West syndrome. In the original description[64] the spasms, sometimes described as jerky tremors, were in extension or flexion, with more involvement of the neck muscles—sometimes with facial grimacing and nodding—and of the upper limbs more than the lower. Dravet et al[65] studied smaller numbers of patients with ictal polygraphy and did not find this difference. They concluded that the absence of EEG correlates was the only way to distinguish patients from West syndrome.

Epileptic spasms in clusters without hypsarrhythmia[69] are distinguished by ictal EEG changes, and it would seem prudent to attempt to obtain ictal recordings on any infant with serial spasms.

In a recent study of 102 infants with benign nonepileptic infantile spasms, the movements were described as myoclonus, spasms, shuddering, negative myoclonus, and combinations of two or more of these.[33] Following this report, Benardina[70] suggested that the condition be renamed Fejerman syndrome. Later, side-to-side shaking attacks, different from Fejerman syndrome but with the same MA of 6 months, were described by Capovilla.[71]

▶ SHUDDERING (MA ~6–12 MONTHS)

Shuddering spells were first emphasized as a reaction to monosodium glutamate,[72] but subsequent investigations have provided no confirmation. The Montreal group[73] thought they were a precursor to essential tremor, but this appears unlikely, although features of tremor may be observed.[74] Kanazawa[75] considers shuddering and benign infantile myoclonus/benign infantile nonepileptic spasms to be a single disorder, and Dravet et al[65] wrote that the "description of these shuddering attacks is not so far from that of spasms: 'shuddering movements, posture consisting of flexion of the head, elbows, trunk and knees, and the abduction of the elbows and knees.'"

So-called stool-withholding nonepileptic seizures[76] are likely in the same class of benign events as shuddering and benign nonepileptic infantile spasms.

▶ INFANTILE MASTURBATION (MA 10 MONTHS)

Parents may prefer the name gratification disorder or even benign infantile dyskinesia[6] for infantile masturbation, but it is certainly an important differential diagnosis of early onset epilepsy[6,77] and movement disorders.[78] In the largest published study to date,[6] 21 of 31 patients were referred for evaluation of possible epileptic seizures and two had previously been diagnosed with and managed as definite epilepsy. Diagnostic uncertainty was increased by the frequent absence of direct stimulation of the genitalia.[6] Dystonic posturing was a major component[6,78] and episodes tended to occur in particular settings, especially in a car seat.[6] Other features included grunting noises, rocking, and sweating.[6] Cessation with[78] and annoyance at[6] distraction were characteristic, the interruption being temporary. Review of home video was helpful in making the diagnosis.[6,78]

▶ REFLEX INFANTILE SYNCOPE (MA ~12 MONTHS)

The terms used for these reflex syncopes vary with the age and stage of development of the child and between doctors of different specialties and geographical origin. Doubtless some of this multiplicity of terms results from uncertainty about what are the mechanisms involved. Another reason may be the constraints on the vocabulary used by pediatricians when speaking to parents about their children's attacks.

In North America such episodes are called breath-holding spells,[79] cyanotic, and pallid,[80,81] whereas in the United Kingdom they may be termed respectively prolonged expiratory apnea[82,83] and reflex anoxic seizures[84,85] where RAS also stands for reflex asystolic syncope.

These confusions do not matter too much provided a clinical history is taken that includes discovering the setting and situation, and the provocations, precipitants, stimuli or triggers that may induce the episodes. Most syncopes occur in certain situations and most have provocations. If a bump on the head precedes the event, then what follows is a syncope with a high probability.[84,85]

Families with an affected infant or child may wish to contact **S**yncope **T**rust **A**nd **R**eflex **A**noxic **S**eizures (STARS), the syncope support group on www.stars.org.uk or www.stars-us.org.

▶ REPETITIVE SLEEP STARTS (MA ~13 MONTHS)

The importance of recognizing nonepileptic sleep starts[86] in young children who also have or have had epilepsy is to prevent toxicity from unnecessarily increasing antiepileptic medication. The "starts" occur in runs or clusters[86] and often have the duration of spasms. Overnight EEG with coregistration of the "sleep starts" will confirm the diagnosis.

▶ ANOXIC–EPILEPTIC SEIZURES (MA 17 MONTHS)

The usual convulsive syncope is a pure anoxic seizure,[40] but occasionally syncopes induce epileptic seizures, making what is known as an anoxic–epileptic seizure.[7,87] Children with anoxic–epileptic seizures do not have epilepsy in the usual sense insofar as they do not also have unprovoked epileptic seizures.

▶ EPISODES IN THE NEURODEVELOPMENTALLY IMPAIRED PATIENT

Many of the described paroxysmal events may be seen in neurodevelopmentally abnormal as well as normal infants. It is important to be particularly careful in this situation, as epileptic seizures are often expected to arise from the "abnormal brain," whether awake or asleep. As in the situation of sleep starts, discussed earlier, diagnosis is even more difficult when there is epilepsy as well. It is worth remembering that patients with cerebral palsy and multiple spike discharges on EEG may also experience infantile syncope.[40,88]

► MISCELLANEOUS PAROXYSMAL DISORDERS

Many paroxysmal disorders have not been discussed in this chapter, either because it should be obvious that these are not epileptic in mechanism—such as benign infantile torticollis and Sandifer's syndrome—or because the MA seems to be over 2 years—such as the Ward-Romano prolonged QT syndrome and benign paroxysmal vertigo of childhood. Only some of the known transient movement disorders[89] have been mentioned and it is likely that more will be described. Further, not all paroxysmal episodes are "disorders"[1,2,90] and some such as infantile masturbation, we only call a disorder[6] because of the easy danger of misdiagnosing epilepsy.

REFERENCES

1. Beach R, Reading R. The importance of acknowledging clinical uncertainty in the diagnosis of epilepsy and non-epileptic events. *Arch Dis Child* 2005;90:1219–1222.
2. Hindley D, Ali A, Robson C. Diagnoses made in a secondary care "fits, faints, and funny turns" clinic. *Arch Dis Child* 2006;91:214–218.
3. Uldall P, Alving J, Hansen LK, Kibaek M, Buchholt J. The misdiagnosis of epilepsy in children admitted to a tertiary epilepsy centre with paroxysmal events. *Arch Dis Child* 2006;91:219–221.
4. Ferrie CD. Preventing misdiagnosis of epilepsy. *Arch Dis Child* 2006;91:206–209.
5. Helmers S, Weiss MJ, Holmes GL. Seizures presenting as apnea in infancy. *J Epilepsy* 1992;4:173–180.
6. Nechay A, Ross LM, Stephenson JBP, O'Regan M. Gratification disorder ("infantile masturbation"): a review. *Arch Dis Child* 2004;89:225–226.
7. Horrocks IA, Nechay A, Stephenson JBP, Zuberi SM. Anoxic-epileptic seizures: observational study of epileptic seizures induced by syncope. *Archives of Dis Child* 2005;90:1283–1287.
8. Sweney MT, et al. Alternating hemiplegia of childhood: early characteristics and evolution of a neurodevelopmental syndrome. *Pediatrics* 2009;123:e534–e541.
9. Paro-Panjan D, Neubauer D. Benign neonatal sleep myoclonus: experience from the study of 38 infants. *Eur J Paediatr Neurol* 2008;12:14–18.
10. Vigevano F, Di Capua M, Dalla Bernardina B. Startle disease: an avoidable cause of sudden infant death. *Lancet* 1989;1:216.
11. Dalla Bernardina B, et al. Neonatal hyperexplexia. In: Beaumanoir A, Gastaut H, Naquet R (eds), *Reflex Seizures and Reflex Epilepsy.* Geneve: Editions Medicine & Hygiene, 1989:409–414.
12. King MD, Stephenson JBP. *A Handbook of Neurological Investigations in Children.* London: Mac Keith Press, 2009.
13. Pascotto A, Coppola G. Neonatal hyperekplexia: a case report. *Epilepsia* 1992;33:817–820.
14. Gherpelli JLDG, et al. Hyperekplexia, a cause of neonatal apnea: a case report. *Brain Dev* 1995;17:114–116.
15. McMaster P, Cadzow S, Vince J, Appleton B. Hyperekplexia: a rare differential of neonatal fits described in a developing country. *Ann Trop Paediatr* 1999;19:345–358.
16. Elkay M, Incecik F, Herguner MO, Leblebisatan G, Altunbasak S. Startle disease—two sibling cases. *Turk J Pediatr* 2005;47:275–278.
17. Rivera S, et al. Congenital hyperekplexia: five sporadic cases. *Eur J Pediatr* 2006;165:104–107.
18. Rees MI, et al. Mutations in the gene encoding GlyT2 (SLC6A5) define a presynaptic component of human startle disease. *Nat Genet* 2006;38:801–806.
19. Nechay A, Stephenson JBP. Bath-induced paroxysmal disorders in infancy. *Eur J Paediatr Neurol* 2009;13:203–208.
20. Rees MI, Andrew M, Jawad S, Owen MJ. Evidence for recessive as well as dominant forms of startle disease (hyperekplexia) caused by mutations in the alpha 1 subunit of the inhibitory glycine receptor. *Hum Mol Genet* 1994;3:2175–2179.
21. Kurczynski TW. Hyperekplexia. *Arch Neurol* 1983;40:246–248.
22. Kok O, Bruyn GW. An unidentified hereditary disease. *Lancet* 1962;1:1359.
23. Shahar E, Brand N, Uziel Y, Barak Y. Nose tapping test inducing a generalized flexor spasm: a hallmark of hyperexplexia. *Acta Paediatr Scand* 1991;80:1073–1077.
24. Nigro MA, Lim HC. Hyperekplexia and sudden neonatal death. *Pediatr Neurol* 1992;l8:221–225.
25. Fertleman CR, Ferrie CD. What's in a name—familial rectal pain syndrome becomes paroxysmal extreme pain disorder. *J Neurol Neurosurg Psychiatry* 2006;77:1294–1295.
26. Fertleman CR, et al. Paroxysmal extreme pain disorder (previously familial rectal pain syndrome). *Neurology* 2007;69:586–595.
27. Schubert R, Cracco JB. Familial rectal pain: a type of reflex epilepsy. *Ann Neurol* 1992;32:824–826.
28. Bednarek N, Arbues AS, Motte J, Sabouraud P, Plouin P, Morville P. Familial rectal pain: a familial autonomic disorder as a cause of paroxysmal attacks in the newborn baby. *Epileptic Disord* 2005;7:360–362.
29. Fertleman CR, et al. *SCN9A* mutations in paroxysmal extreme pain disorder: allelic variants underlie distinct channel defects and phenotypes. *Neuron* 2006;52:767–774.
30. Daoust-Roy J, Seshia SS. Benign neonatal sleep myoclonus. A differential diagnosis of neonatal seizures. *Am J Dis Child* 1992;146:1236–1241.
31. Di Capua M, Fusco L, Ricci S, Vigevano F. Benign neonatal sleep myoclonus: clinical features and video-polygraphic recordings. *Mov Disord* 1993;8:191–194.
32. Egger J, Grossmann G, Auchterlonie IA. Benign sleep myoclonus in infancy mistaken for epilepsy. *BMJ* 2003;326 (7396):975–976.
33. Turanli G, Senbil N, Altunbasak S, Topcu M. Benign neonatal sleep myoclonus mimicking status epilepticus. *J Child Neurol* 2004;19:62–63.

34. Ramelli GP, Sozzo AB, Vella S, Bianchetti MG. Benign neonatal sleep myoclonus: an under-recognized, non-epileptic condition. *Acta Paediatr* 2005;94:962–963.

35. Caraballo RH, Capovilla G, Vigevano F, Beccaria F, Specchio N, Fejerman N. The spectrum of benign myoclonus of early infancy: clinical and neurophysiologic features in 102 patients. *Epilepsia* 2009;50:1176–1183.

36. Kaddurah AK, Holmes GL. Benign neonatal sleep myoclonus: history and semiology. *Pediatr Neurol* 2009; 40:343–346.

37. Blennow G. Benign infantile nocturnal myoclonus. *Acta Paediatr Scand* 1985;74:505–507.

38. Alfonso I, Papazian O, Aicardi J, Jeffries HE. A simple maneuver to provoke benign neonatal sleep myoclonus. *Pediatrics* 1995;96:1161–1163.

39. Stephenson JBP, Whitehouse W, Zuberi SM. Paroxysmal non-epileptic disorders: differential diagnosis of epilepsy. In Wallace SJ, Farrell K (eds), *Epilepsy in Children*. London: Arnold, 2004; pp. 4–20.

40. Stephenson JBP. *Fits and Faints*. London: Mac Keith Press, 1990.

41. Held-Egli K, Rüegger C, Das-Kundu S, Schmitt B, Bucher HU. Benign neonatal sleep myoclonus in newborn infants of opioid dependent mothers. *Acta Paediatr* 2009;98:69–73.

42. Shuper A, Zalzberg J, Weitz R, Mimouni MR. Jitteriness beyond the neonatal period: a benign pattern of movement in infancy. *J Child Neurol* 1991;6:243–245.

43. Mizrahi EM, Kellaway P. Characterization and classification of neonatal seizures. *Neurology* 1987;37:1837–1844.

44. Schmitt B, et al. Seizures and paroxysmal events: symptoms pointing to the diagnosis of pyridoxine-dependent epilepsy and pyridoxine phosphate oxidase deficiency. *Dev Med Child Neurol* 2010;52:e133–e142.

45. De Vivo DC, Leary L, Wang D. Glucose transporter 1 deficiency syndrome and other glycolytic defects. *J Child Neurol* 2002;17(Suppl 3):3S15–3S23.

46. Wang D, et al. GLUT-1 deficiency syndrome: clinical, genetic, and therapeutic aspects. *Ann Neurol* 2005;57:111–118.

47. Leen WG, et al. Glucose transporter-1 deficiency syndrome: the expanding clinical and genetic spectrum of a treatable disorder. *Brain* 2010;133:655–670.

48. Vigevano F, Lispi ML. Tonic reflex seizures of early infancy: an age-related non-epileptic paroxysmal disorder. *Epileptic Disord* 2001;3:133–136.

49. Spitzer AR, Boyle JT, Tuchman DN, Fox WW. Awake apnea associated with gastroesophageal reflux: a specific clinical syndrome. *J Pediatr* 1984;104:200–205.

50. Rosen CL, Frost JD Jr, Bricker T, Tarnow JD, Gillette PC, Dunlavy S. Two siblings with recurrent cardiorespiratory arrest: Munchausen syndrome by proxy or child abuse? *Pediatrics* 1983;71:715–720.

51. Rosen CL, Frost JD Jr, Glaze DG. Child abuse and recurrent infant apnea. *J Pediatr* 1986;109:1065–1067.

52. Southall DP, Stebbens VA, Rees SV, Lang MH, Warner JO, Shinebourne EA. Apnoeic episodes induced by smothering: two cases identified by covert video surveillance. *Br Med J (Clin Res Ed)* 1987;294(6588):1637–1641.

53. Meadow R. Suffocation, recurrent apnea, and sudden infant death. *J Pediatr* 1990;117:351–357.

54. Samuels MP, McClaughlin W, Jacobson RR, Poets CF, Southall DP. Fourteen cases of imposed upper airway obstruction. *Arch Dis Child* 1992;67:162–170.

55. Southall DP, Plunkett MC, Banks MW, Falkov AF, Samuels MP. Covert video recordings of life-threatening child abuse: lessons for child protection. *Pediatrics* 1997;100:735–760.

56. Silver K, Andermann F. Alternating hemiplegia of childhood: a study of 10 patients and results of flunarizine treatment. *Neurology* 1993;43:36–41.

57. Bourgeois M, Aicardi J, Goutieres F. Alternating hemiplegia of childhood. *J Pediatr* 1993;122:673–679.

58. Mikati MA, Kramer U, Zupanc ML, Shanahan RJ. Alternating hemiplegia of childhood: clinical manifestations and long-term outcome. *Pediatr Neurol* 2000;23:134–141.

59. Incorpora G, et al. Neonatal onset of hot water reflex seizures in monozygotic twins subsequently manifesting episodes of alternating hemiplegia. *Epilepsy Res* 2008;78: 225–231.

60. Incorpora G, Pavone P, Cocuzza M, Privitera M, Pavone L, Ruggieri M. Neonatal onset of bath-induced alternating hemiplegia of childhood. *Eur J Paediatr Neurol* 2010;14: 192–193.

61. Casaer P. Flunarizine in alternating hemiplegia in childhood. An international study in 12 children. *Neuropediatrics* 1987;18:191–195.

62. Sone K, Oguni H, Katsumori H, Funatsuka M, Tanaka T, Osawa M. Successful trial of amantadine hydrochloride for two patients with alternating hemiplegia of childhood. *Neuropediatrics* 2000;31:307–309.

63. Andermann E, Andermann F, Silver K, Levin S, Arnold D. Benign familial nocturnal alternating hemiplegia of childhood. *Neurology* 1994;44:1812–1814.

64. Lombroso CT, Fejerman N. Benign myoclonus of early infancy. *Ann Neurol* 1977;1:138–143.

65. Dravet C, Giraud N, Bureau M, Gobbi G, Dalla Bernardina B. Benign myoclonus of early infancy or benign non-epileptic infantile spasms. *Neuropediatrics* 1986;17:33–38.

66. Pachatz C, Fusco L, Vigevano F. Benign myoclonus of early infancy. *Epileptic Disord* 1999;1:57–61.

67. Maydell BV, Berenson F, Rothner AD, Wyllie E, Kotagal P. Benign myoclonus of early infancy: an imitator of West's syndrome. *J Child Neurol* 2001;16:109–112.

68. Vigevano F, Fusco L, Pachatz C. Neurophysiology of spasms. *Brain Dev* 2001;23:467–472.

69. Caraballo RH, et al. Epileptic spasms in clusters without hypsarrhythmia in infancy. *Epileptic Disord* 2003;5:109–113.

70. Dalla Bernardina B. Benign myoclonus of early infancy or Fejerman syndrome. *Epilepsia* 2009;50:1290–1292.

71. Capovilla G. Shaking body attacks: a new type of benign non-epileptic attack in infancy. *Epileptic Disord* 2011;13:140–144.

72. Reif-Lehrer L, Stemmermann MG. Monosodium glutamate intolerance in children. *N Engl J Med* 1975;293(23):1204–1205.

73. Vanasse M, Bedard P, Andermann F. Shuddering attacks in children: an early clinical manifestation of essential tremor. *Neurology* 1976;26:1027–1030.

74. Holmes GL, Russman BS. Shuddering attacks. Evaluation using electroencephalographic frequency modulation

radiotelemetry and videotape monitoring. *Am J Dis Child* 1986;140:72–73.

75. Kanazawa O. Shuddering attacks—report of four children. *Pediatr Neurol* 2000;23:421–424.

76. Cohn A. Stool withholding presenting as a cause of non-epileptic seizures. *Dev Med Child Neurol* 2005;47:703–705.

77. Fleisher DR, Morrison A. Masturbation mimicking abdominal pain or seizures in young girls. *J Pediatr* 1990;116:810–814.

78. Yang ML, Fullwood E, Goldstein J, Mink JW. Masturbation in infancy and early childhood presenting as a movement disorder: 12 cases and a review of the literature. *Pediatrics* 2005;116:1427–1432.

79. Breningstall GN. Breath-holding spells. *Pediatr Neurol* 1996;14:91–97.

80. Lombroso CT, Lerman P. Breath-holding spells (cyanotic and pallid infantile syncope). *Pediatrics* 1967;39:563–581.

81. DiMario FJ Jr. Prospective study of children with cyanotic and pallid breath-holding spells. *Pediatrics* 2001;107:265–269.

82. Southall DP, et al. Prolonged expiratory apnoea: a disorder resulting in episodes of severe arterial hypoxaemia in infants and young children. *Lancet* 1985;2(8455):571–577.

83. Southall DP, Samuels MP, Talbert DG. Recurrent cyanotic episodes with severe arterial hypoxaemia and intrapulmonary shunting: a mechanism for sudden death. *Arch Dis Child* 1990;65:953–961.

84. Stephenson JBP. Reflex anoxic seizures ('white breath-holding'): nonepileptic vagal attacks. *Arch Dis Child* 1978;53:193–200.

85. Stephenson JBP, McLeod KA. Reflex anoxic seizures. In: David TJ (ed), *Recent Advances in Paediatrics, Vol. 18.* Edinburgh: Churchill Livingstone, 2000:1–17.

86. Fusco L, Pachatz C, Cusmai R, Vigevano F. Repetitive sleep starts in neurologically impaired children: an unusual non-epileptic manifestation in otherwise epileptic subjects. *Epileptic Disord* 1999;1:63–67.

87. Stephenson J, et al. Anoxic-epileptic seizures: home video recordings of epileptic seizures induced by syncope. *Epileptic Disord* 2004;6:15–19.

88. Stephenson JBP. Cerebral palsy. In Engel J, Pedley TA (eds), *Epilepsy: A Comprehensive Textbook.* Philadelphia: Lippincott Williams & Wilkins, 2008; 2nd edn: pp. 2631–2636.

89. Fernandez-Alvarez E. Transient movement disorders in children. *J Neurol* 1998;245:1–5.

90. Gall J. "Binkie flutter," an apparently voluntary behavior of infants, possibly related to vibratory jaw movements in dogs: report of 4 cases. *Pediatrics* 2005;115:e367–e369.

SECTION III
Seizures in Childhood

CHAPTER 17

Febrile Seizures

Joshua Mendelson, Sandra Helmers, and Andrew Escayg

▶ CLINICAL OVERVIEW

Febrile seizures (FS) are the most common type of convulsion among pediatric patients. The prevalence of FS varies between different populations, affecting, for example, an estimated 2%–5% of European and North American children and 6%–9% of children from Japan. In a large registry-based study of febrile seizures in children born in Denmark between 1977 and 2004, 50% experienced their first febrile seizure between 6 and 18 months of age, and 93% before the age of 48 months.[1]

Febrile seizures are classified as either simple or complex in nature. Simple FS are defined as short (<15 minutes), generalized tonic, clonic, or tonic–clonic seizures that occur during the course of a febrile illness[2–4]; approximately 80%–90% of FS are simple febrile convulsions.[5] Complex FS consist of either focal or generalized seizures that are prolonged (>15 minutes) or recurrent over a 24-hour period. Febrile seizures that persist for longer than 30 minutes or that involve multiple shorter seizures without return to a baseline level of consciousness are termed febrile status epilepticus.[6]

▶ RISK FACTORS

Febrile seizures, whether simple or complex, generally occur in the context of an illness that causes a fever of at least 38.0°C.[3] FS tend to be seen in conjunction with common infections, such as upper respiratory tract infections, otitis media, and gastrointestinal disorders; however, there is no specific infectious agent connected to febrile seizures. FS associated with fevers secondary to immunizations are also common. In this setting, the seizure typically occurs within 48 hours after adminis-

tration of the immunization.[7] Most often, both simple and complex FS occur early in the course of an illness or during the initial rise in body temperature, but the seizure may also precede the onset of fever.

In addition to fever, FS are precipitated by other environmental and/or genetic factors that remain largely unidentified. Vestergaard and Christensen[1] observed that low birth weight and short gestational ages were significant risk factors for FS; however, there was no association between birth weight, birth order, or 1- or 5-minute Apgar scores and an increased risk for FS in a study of disease-discordant twins.[8] Moreover, prenatal exposure to other common insults, such as maternal smoking, alcohol or coffee consumption, and stress, appear to have little to no effect on the incidence of FS.[1]

Twin and family studies reveal that genetic factors play an important role in FS, and that there are different modes of inheritance. Large pedigrees with recurrent FS are often consistent with a model of autosomal dominant inheritance with reduced penetrance, although the majority of cases are likely due to more complex, polygenic inheritance. Genetic linkage analysis of FS families points to at least 10 loci that are suspected of harboring FS genes (reviewed in[9]), yet there has been little progress toward identifying the actual disease-causing genes.

Ion channels play an important role in the regulation of neuronal excitability, and altered ion channel function is responsible for a range of epilepsy subtypes, several of which include FS. Over 600 mutations in the voltage-gated sodium channel (VGSC) gene *SCN1A*[10,11] have been linked to disorders such as genetic (generalized) epilepsy with febrile seizures plus (GEFS+)[12–14] and Dravet syndrome (DS),[15–17] in which FS are common. A *SCN1A* mutation was also found in a large, multigenerational pedigree affected by simple FS,[18] raising the possibility that altered *SCN1A* function may be responsible for some isolated cases of simple FS, as well. Interestingly, mice with *SCN1A* mutations are more susceptible to FS.[19,20]

GEFS+ is also caused by mutations in the sodium channel β1 subunit, *SCN1B*[21,22] and two GABAA receptor genes, *GABRG2* and *GABRD*,[23–26] suggesting that these genes, too, may contribute to some cases of simple FS. Notably, mutations in the VGSC gene, *SCN9A*, which is traditionally considered a peripheral sodium channel, were recently found in 5 out of 92 unrelated FS patients.[27]

▶ MECHANISMS

The rate of temperature increase used to be considered a causative factor in febrile seizure generation, but this is no longer believed to be true. Although the etiology of FS is not fully understood, there are several known contributing factors. Fever is known to cause an immune response mediated by the release of proinflammatory cytokines, such as interleukin (IL)1β, which can enhance neuronal excitability, in part by augmenting glutamate receptor function.[28] Mice that lack the IL-1β receptor exhibit increased thresholds to experimentally induced FS, supporting a role for IL-1β in seizure generation.[29] Proinflammatory cytokines, which include IL-1β, IL-6, IL-10, and tumor necrosis factor alpha, are also elevated in patients with febrile seizures.[30] Febrile seizure induction experiments in immature rat pups also reveal a link between hyperthermia-induced hyperventilation and alkalosis in febrile seizure generation (reviewed in[31]); however, whether this holds true for human FS remains unclear.

▶ EVALUATION (FIG. 17–1)

The evaluation and treatment of a febrile seizure depends largely on the patient's history and clinical presentation. The first steps in evaluating a child with a febrile seizure are obtaining a detailed history and performing a physical examination. The American Academy of Pediatrics has established guidelines for children presenting with their first febrile seizure. As detailed in Table 17–1, the recommendation for a child 18 months or older who presents with a simple febrile seizure and is clinically stable, with no focal abnormalities, is that extensive diagnostic investigations, including routine electroencephalogram and neuroimaging, are unnecessary. Furthermore, patients with a single, simple febrile seizure do not require hospital admission.[2] Children younger than 18 months who present with a febrile

seizure, on the other hand, should be observed for 24 hours and may require a lumbar puncture (LP), as the signs and symptoms of meningitis may not be obvious in this population.[32]

A child who presents with a complex febrile seizure demands a more rigorous evaluation. The American Academy of Pediatrics recommends routine laboratory investigations and neuroimaging with computed tomography or magnetic resonance imaging for patients presenting with a complex febrile seizure. A LP should also be performed to evaluate the cerebrospinal fluid for evidence of meningitis.

It is important to note that EEG abnormalities are quite common in patients with complex FS, with the incidence of abnormalities on the electroencephalogram ranging from 2% to 86%.[33] Therefore, routine EEG is not indicated in patients with either simple or complex febrile seizures, since EEG abnormalities found in the setting of a febrile seizure may not be predictive of the development of epilepsy later in life.

Finally, the differential diagnosis should always include the possibility of a chronic epilepsy syndrome. Patients who present with an atypical course, such as febrile status epilepticus or frequent recurrent febrile and afebrile seizures, will require a more detailed workup. Depending upon the clinical presentation and family history, these patients may require genetic screening for GEFS+ or Dravet syndrome.

▶ TREATMENT (FIG. 17–2)

The treatment of FS is focused largely on controlling the fever and treating the underlying illness. Antipyretics along with other methods, such as a tepid bath, should be used to reduce fever. Furthermore, if there is an underlying bacterial infection, it must be treated with the appropriate antibiotics.[5]

Literature on the use of antiepileptic medications for FS focuses on their efficacy in the prevention of recurrent febrile seizures. For example, phenobarbital is known to be effective at preventing future FS.[34,35] In a study of 79 children with FS, Camfield and colleagues[35] observed that just 5% of those who were treated with daily phenobarbital had another febrile seizure, whereas 25% of the untreated patients had a recurrence. However, Wolf and colleagues[34] found that 20%–40% of children treated with phenobarbital developed side effects that included hyperactivity, irritability, lethargy, and sleep disturbances. Treatment with phenobarbital has also been shown to affect cognitive function. In one study, 217 children, 8–36 months old, with at least one febrile seizure had their cognitive function assessed after being placed on phenobarbital; the mean intelligence quotient of patients treated with phenobarbital was seven points lower than the placebo group after 2 years.[36]

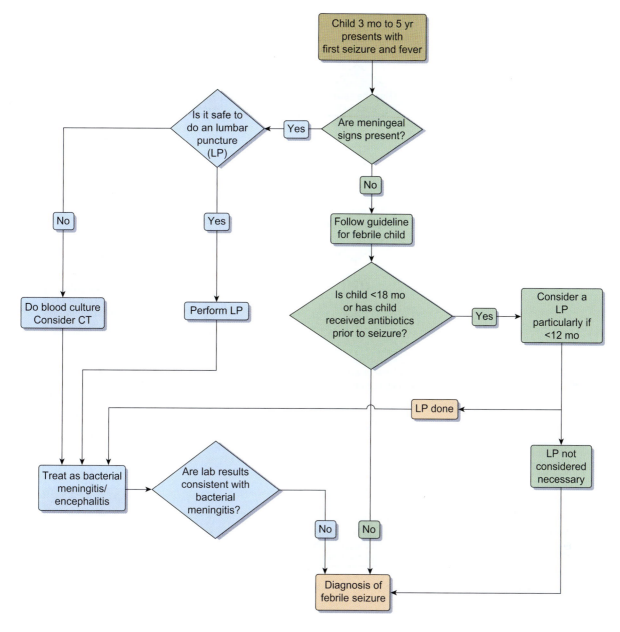

Figure 17–1. How to diagnose a febrile seizure. (© Kevin Farrell, MD.)

▶ **TABLE 17–1. DIAGNOSTIC AND TREATMENT PARADIGM FOR FEBRILE SEIZURES**

	Simple Febrile Seizure	Simple Febrile Seizure	Complex Febrile Seizure
Age	<18 mo	>18 mo	Any age
Neuroimaging	Recommended	Not recommended	Recommended
CSF studies	Recommended	Not recommended	Recommended
EEG	Not recommended	Not recommended	Not recommended
Treatment	Antipyretics treat underlying infection	Antipyretics treat underlying infection	Antipyretics treat underlying infection
AED	Not recommended	Not recommended	May be indicated, depending on the patient's risk factors for developing afebrile seizures

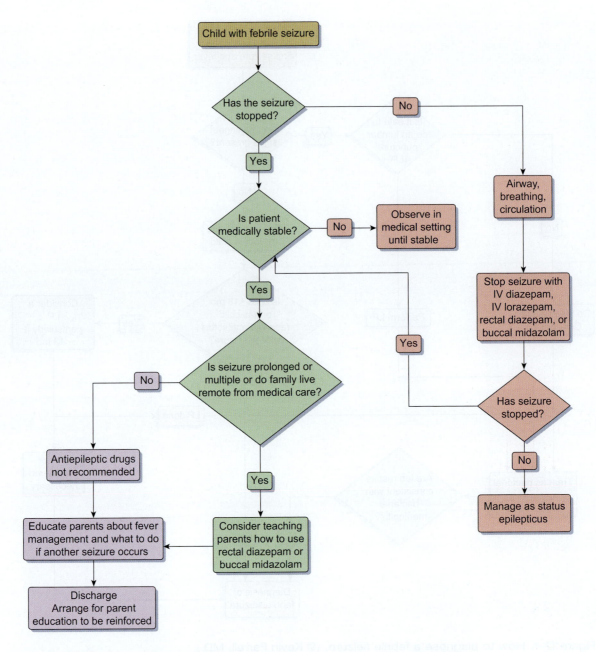

Figure 17-2. How to treat a child with febrile seizure. (© Kevin Farrell, MD.)

Valproic acid is also known to be effective in the prevention of recurrent FS. Lee and Melchoir[37] randomized 90 children with FS to treatment with phenobarbital, valproic acid, or placebo. They found that valproic acid was as effective as phenobarbital in preventing febrile seizure recurrence and more effective than placebo. In another study, Ngwane and Bower[38] looked at children between the ages of 6 and 18 months who had experienced a prior febrile seizure. They randomized the patients into groups who were treated with phenobarbital, valproic acid, or placebo

and found that both valproic acid and phenobarbital prevented recurrent FS compared with placebo. However, valproic acid is associated with serious side effects, such as hepatotoxicity, thrombocytopenia, weight gain, gastrointestinal disturbances, and pancreatitis, particularly in young children.

Carbamazepine and phenytoin have been looked at as possible treatments for FS, as well, but neither was effective at preventing febrile seizure recurrence.[39,40] Diazepam administered rectally, intravenously, nasally, or orally can be used for the immediate termination of prolonged or recurrent seizures,[41] and many studies have evaluated whether or not treatment with diazepam can prevent recurrent febrile seizures. Rosman and colleagues[42] found that oral diazepam given every 8 hours during the course of a febrile illness effectively reduced febrile seizure recurrence. Others have examined intermittent diazepam dosing during a febrile illness and found that it does not prevent febrile seizures.[43] Although the efficacy of prophylactic diazepam remains debated, we do know its use is not without risk, as diazepam may cause sedation, hyperactivity, and respiratory depression.

The current recommendation from the American Academy of Pediatrics is that no antiepileptic medications be given to a child who has had one or more simple FS, and antipyretics along with appropriate management of the underlying illness should be the mainstay of treatment. The risks associated with the deleterious side effects of antiepileptic drugs are worse than the risks of experiencing future febrile seizures. Nevertheless, the use of antiepileptic medications in the appropriate clinical setting may be considered for a patient with febrile status epilepticus or complex febrile seizures to prevent further FS. Notably, though, the prevention of future FS, whether simple or complex, may not alter the risk of developing afebrile seizures later in life.

▶ RISK OF RECURRENCE

Most patients (60%–70%) who experience a febrile seizure will not have another. But approximately 33% will go on to have more, and children with a history of two FS, have a 50% risk of experiencing further FS.[44] A number of factors put a patient at higher risk of developing recurrent FS, among them a young age at onset (<6 months), a complex febrile seizure at presentation, and febrile seizures in first-degree relatives.[6] Note that children with an abnormal neurodevelopmental history are at no greater risk of febrile seizure recurrence.[44]

▶ RISK OF DEVELOPING EPILEPSY

Prospective studies on children who experience short or simple FS suggest that there is no significant impact on neuronal function or on the likelihood of developing epilepsy.[45] The consequences of prolonged or complex focal FS, on the other hand, remain unclear.[46–48] Known risk factors for children with FS to develop epilepsy later in life include a first-degree relative with afebrile seizures, abnormal development prior to the first febrile seizure, and a complex febrile seizure. The likelihood of developing afebrile seizures later in life depends on the number of risk factors a patient has. A child with a simple febrile seizure and no additional risk factors has a 0.9% chance of developing epilepsy by age seven,[49] whereas those with one risk factor have a 2.4% risk of developing a seizure disorder by the age of 25.[50] Patients with multiple risk factors have a proportionally greater chance of developing epilepsy later in life.[6]

The mechanism by which FS can cause epilepsy later in life is unclear. Studies exploring the effect of FS in rodent models have uncovered a host of molecular changes,[47] although the relevance of most of these changes to human epilepsy has not been established. In humans, there is a relationship between febrile seizures and the development of hippocampal sclerosis and temporal lobe epilepsy.[51] Right-sided hippocampal sclerosis is seen more commonly in patients with a history of FS; however, the pathophysiology behind this relationship is not well understood, either. Prolonged FS may cause an increase in metabolic demand that is greater than the arterial blood supply, resulting in ischemia.[52] On the other hand, Bower and colleagues[53] retrospectively evaluated patients with hippocampal sclerosis and found no relationship between febrile seizures and hippocampal volume reduction. The relationship between FS and the development of temporal lobe epilepsy and hippocampal sclerosis remains controversial.

▶ SUMMARY

Febrile seizures are common in the pediatric population, and the vast majority of FS are both simple in nature and self-limited. A detailed history and physical examination are paramount in determining the nature of the FS. The diagnostic evaluation will depend on the type of FS and age of the patient. The mainstay of treatment for FS, whether simple or complex, is antipyretics and management of the underlying infection. Complex febrile seizures carry a higher risk of developing epilepsy later in life, especially in a child who has a family history of epilepsy and neurodevelopmental delay. These children may require antiepileptic medications to prevent further seizures; however, it is important to understand that treatment with antiepileptics may not alter the risk of developing epilepsy.

REFERENCES

1. Vestergaard M, Christensen J. Register-based studies on febrile seizures in Denmark. *Brain Dev* 2009;31:372–377.
2. American Academy of Pediatrics. Practice parameter: the neurodiagnostic evaluation of the child with a first simple febrile seizure. Provisional Committee on Quality Improvement, Subcommittee on Febrile Seizures. *Pediatrics* 1996;97:769–772; discussion 73–75.
3. Fukuyama Y, Seki T, Ohtsuka C, Miura H, Hara M. Practical guidelines for physicians in the management of febrile seizures. *Brain Dev* 1996;18:479–484.

4. American Academy of Pediatrics. Practice parameter: long-term treatment of the child with simple febrile seizures. Committee on Quality Improvement, Subcommittee on Febrile Seizures. *Pediatrics* 1999;103:1307–1309.

5. Verity CM, Butler NR, Golding J. Febrile convulsions in a national cohort followed up from birth. I—Prevalence and recurrence in the first five years of life. *Br Med J (Clin Res Ed)* 1985;290:1307–1310.

6. Knudsen FU. Febrile seizures: treatment and prognosis. *Epilepsia* 2000;41:2–9.

7. Hirtz DG, Lee YJ, Ellenberg JH, Nelson KB. Survey on the management of febrile seizures. *Am J Dis Child* 1986;140:909–914.

8. Helbig I, Scheffer IE, Mulley JC, Berkovic SF. Navigating the channels and beyond: unravelling the genetics of the epilepsies. *Lancet Neurol* 2008;7:231–245.

9. Nakayama J. Progress in searching for the febrile seizure susceptibility genes. *Brain Dev* 2009;31:359–365.

10. Lossin C. A catalog of SCN1A variants. *Brain Dev* 2009;31:114–130.

11. Claes LR, et al. The SCN1A variant database: a novel research and diagnostic tool. *Hum Mutat* 2009;30:E904–E920.

12. Escayg A, Heils A, MacDonald BT, Haug K, Sander T, Meisler MH. A novel SCN1A mutation associated with generalized epilepsy with febrile seizures plus—and prevalence of variants in patients with epilepsy. *Am J Hum Genet* 2001;68:866–873.

13. Escayg A, et al. Mutations of SCN1A, encoding a neuronal sodium channel, in two families with GEFS+2. *Nat Genet* 2000;24:343–345.

14. Wallace RH, et al. Neuronal sodium-channel alpha1-subunit mutations in generalized epilepsy with febrile seizures plus. *Am J Hum Genet* 2001;68:859–865.

15. Claes L, Del-Favero J, Ceulemans B, Lagae L, Van Broeckhoven C, De Jonghe P. De novo mutations in the sodium-channel gene SCN1A cause severe myoclonic epilepsy of infancy. *Am J Hum Genet* 2001;68:1327–1332.

16. Mulley JC, Scheffer IE, Petrou S, Dibbens LM, Berkovic SF, Harkin LA. SCN1A mutations and epilepsy. *Hum Mutat* 2005;25:535–542.

17. Fujiwara T. Clinical spectrum of mutations in SCN1A gene: severe myoclonic epilepsy in infancy and related epilepsies. *Epilepsy Res* 2006;70(Suppl 1):S223–S230.

18. Mantegazza M, et al. Identification of an Nav1.1 sodium channel (SCN1A) loss-of-function mutation associated with familial simple febrile seizures. *Proc Natl Acad Sci USA* 2005;102:18177–18182.

19. Martin MS, et al. Altered function of the SCN1A voltage-gated sodium channel leads to GABAergic interneuron abnormalities. *J Biol Chem* 2010;285:9823–9834.

20. Oakley JC, Kalume F, Yu FH, Scheuer T, Catterall WA. Temperature- and age-dependent seizures in a mouse model of severe myoclonic epilepsy in infancy. *Proc Natl Acad Sci USA* 2009;106:3994–3999.

21. Wallace RH, et al. Generalized epilepsy with febrile seizures plus: mutation of the sodium channel subunit SCN1B. *Neurology* 2002;58:1426–1429.

22. Wallace RH, et al. Febrile seizures and generalized epilepsy associated with a mutation in the Na$^+$-channel beta1 subunit gene SCN1B. *Nat Genet* 1998;19:366–370.

23. Baulac S, et al. First genetic evidence of GABA(A) receptor dysfunction in epilepsy: a mutation in the gamma2-subunit gene. *Nat Genet* 2001;28:46–48.

24. Dibbens LM, et al. GABRD encoding a protein for extra- or peri-synaptic GABAA receptors is a susceptibility locus for generalized epilepsies. *Hum Mol Genet* 2004;13:1315–1319.

25. Harkin LA, et al. Truncation of the GABA(A)-receptor gamma2 subunit in a family with generalized epilepsy with febrile seizures plus. *Am J Hum Genet* 2002;70:530–536.

26. Wallace RH, et al. Mutant GABA(A) receptor gamma2-subunit in childhood absence epilepsy and febrile seizures. *Nat Genet* 2001;28:49–52.

27. Singh NA, et al. A role of SCN9A in human epilepsies, as a cause of febrile seizures and as a potential modifier of Dravet syndrome. *PLoS Genet* 2009;5:e1000649.

28. Vezzani A, Granata T. Brain inflammation in epilepsy: experimental and clinical evidence. *Epilepsia* 2005;46:1724–1743.

29. Dube C, Vezzani A, Behrens M, Bartfai T, Baram TZ. Interleukin-1β contributes to the generation of experimental febrile seizures. *Ann Neurol* 2005;57:152–155.

30. Virta M, Hurme M, Helminen M. Increased plasma levels of pro- and anti-inflammatory cytokines in patients with febrile seizures. *Epilepsia* 2002;43:920–923.

31. Schuchmann S, Vanhatalo S, Kaila K. Neurobiological and physiological mechanisms of fever-related epileptiform syndromes. *Brain Dev* 2009;31:378–382.

32. Carroll W, Brookfield D. Lumbar puncture following febrile convulsion. *Arch Dis Child* 2002;87:238–240.

33. Yucel O, Aka S, Yazicioglu L, Ceran O. Role of early EEG and neuroimaging in determination of prognosis in children with complex febrile seizure. *Pediatr Int* 2004;46:463–467.

34. Wolf SM, Forsythe A. Behavior disturbance, phenobarbital, and febrile seizures. *Pediatrics* 1978;61:728–731.

35. Camfield PR, Camfield CS, Shapiro SH, Cummings C. The first febrile seizure—antipyretic instruction plus either phenobarbital or placebo to prevent recurrence. *J Pediatr* 1980;97:16–21.

36. Farwell JR, Lee YJ, Hirtz DG, Sulzbacher SI, Ellenberg JH, Nelson KB. Phenobarbital for febrile seizures–effects on intelligence and on seizure recurrence. *N Engl J Med* 1990;322:364–369.

37. Lee K, Melchior JC. Sodium valproate versus phenobarbital in the prophylactic treatment of febrile convulsions in childhood. *Eur J Pediatr* 1981;137:151–153.

38. Ngwane E, Bower B. Continuous sodium valproate or phenobarbitone in the prevention of 'simple' febrile convulsions. Comparison by a double-blind trial. *Arch Dis Child* 1980;55:171–174.

39. Antony JH, Hawke SH. Phenobarbital compared with carbamazepine in prevention of recurrent febrile convulsions. A double-blind study. *Am J Dis Child* 1983;137:892–895.

40. Bacon CJ, Hierons AM, Mucklow JC, Webb JK, Rawlins MD, Weightman D. Placebo-controlled study of phenobarbitone and phenytoin in the prophylaxis of febrile convulsions. *Lancet* 1981;2:600–604.

41. Kriel RL, Cloyd JC, Hadsall RS, Carlson AM, Floren KL, Jones-Saete CM. Home use of rectal diazepam for cluster and prolonged seizures: efficacy, adverse reactions, quality of life, and cost analysis. *Pediatr Neurol* 1991;7:13–17.

42. Rosman NP, et al. A controlled trial of diazepam administered during febrile illnesses to prevent recurrence of febrile seizures. *N Engl J Med* 1993;329:79–84.

43. Autret-Leca E, Ployet JL, Jonville-Bera AP. Treatment of febrile convulsions. *Arch Pediatr* 2002;9:91–95.

44. Berg AT, et al. A prospective study of recurrent febrile seizures. *N Engl J Med* 1992;327:1122–1127.

45. Shinnar S, Glauser TA. Febrile seizures. *J Child Neurol* 2002;17(Suppl 1):S44–S52.

46. Dube CM, Brewster AL, Baram TZ. Febrile seizures: mechanisms and relationship to epilepsy. *Brain Dev* 2009; 31:366–371.

47. Dube CM, Brewster AL, Richichi C, Zha Q, Baram TZ. Fever, febrile seizures and epilepsy. *Trends Neurosci* 2007; 30:490–496.

48. Reid AY, Galic MA, Teskey GC, Pittman QJ. Febrile seizures: current views and investigations. *Can J Neurol Sci* 2009;36:679–686.

49. Nelson KB, Ellenberg JH. Predictors of epilepsy in children who have experienced febrile seizures. *N Engl J Med* 1976;295:1029–1033.

50. Annegers JF, Hauser WA, Elveback LR, Kurland LT. The risk of epilepsy following febrile convulsions. *Neurology* 1979;29:297–303.

51. Koepp MJ. Hippocampal sclerosis: cause or consequence of febrile seizures. *J Neurol Neurosurg Psychiatry* 2000; 69:716–717.

52. Falconer MA. Febrile convulsions in early childhood. *Br Med J* 1972;3:292.

53. Bower SP, Kilpatrick CJ, Vogrin SJ, Morris K, Cook MJ. Degree of hippocampal atrophy is not related to a history of febrile seizures in patients with proved hippocampal sclerosis. *J Neurol Neurosurg Psychiatry* 2000;69:733–738.

CHAPTER 18

Focal Seizures in Early Childhood

J. Helen Cross

Several studies have demonstrated that seizure manifestations evolve according to developmental age. Although myelination is largely complete by two years of age, clinical seizure manifestations continue to evolve beyond this age (probably reflecting the caudorostral pattern of brain development), with an adult pattern of semiology unlikely before age 6 years. A high index of suspicion is therefore required when evaluating the clinical description of events for focality. The assessment will have obvious management implications, particularly for the diagnosis of an epilepsy syndrome. Most studies evaluating seizure semiology have been performed in surgical cohorts, where documentation of seizure type is made with video EEG telemetry and confirmed by seizure freedom after removal of the suspect area.

One study examined the localizing and lateralizing value of behavior change in focal seizures in childhood and found it was much more likely at seizure onset for children under age 6 years, occurring in 46% (25/56) compared to only 8/53 in the older group.[1] Behavioral change was far more likely to be of an affective type (agitation, fearful expression, looking for shelter) than an arrest type. Both could represent an aura that could not be verbalized by children in this age group.

In another study of autonomic symptoms (respiratory, gastrointestinal, cutaneous, papillary, urinary) in children age 10 months to 12 years with temporal and extratemporal focal epilepsy, 60/100 patients produced at least one autonomic symptom during their seizures: 43 (70%) of 61 with temporal lobe epilepsy and 17 (44%) of 39 with extratemporal epilepsy. Apnea/bradycardia were more frequent in children <3 years[2] with temporal lobe onset. Only twelve reported an epigastric aura, the youngest presenting at age 5.3 years reported as abdominal pain or discomfort. It was most frequently associated with temporal lobe onset, and was not lateralizing.

Age dependence has also been demonstrated in ictal automatisms, lateralizing signs and secondary generalization in studies of children with temporal lobe onset seizures.[3] However emotional expressions and autonomic signs did not show age dependent manifestation. Emotional expressions (fear, crying, smile, pain, happiness, and laughing) appear more frequently in extratemporal (49%) than temporal (26%) lobe seizures.[4] Positive emotional expressions were more frequently associated with right sided seizure onset.

Frontal lobe semiology under the age of 7 years is characterized by high seizure frequency (up to 40 per day), approximately half of whom show a tendency to cluster. In a study of 111 seizures in 14 patients, 47% attacks arose from sleep and were of short duration; no correlation was seen between age and duration.[5] Auras were infrequent. Motor manifestations were most common. All had motor seizures; in fact, only 6 of 11 analyzed attacks displayed no motor signs at all. Besides tonic seizures, clonic components and epileptic spasms were the leading manifestations. Epileptic spasms typically began from age 2 to 16 months, and persisted well beyond infancy. Psychomotor seizures were rare. Behavior change however was seen frequently, with 36% showing some form of vocalization (crying, moaning, and grunting).

A study of children with frontal lobe epilepsy (FLE) and others with seizures arising from the posterior cortex showed little difference in seizure frequency, but revealed a nocturnal predominance in those with FLE.[6] Visual aura, nystagmus and versive seizures were observed exclusively in the posterior onset group, whereas somatosensory aura and hypermotor seizures appeared only in FLE but less frequently than adults. Tonic seizures were more frequent in FLE. Both groups showed myoclonic seizures, epileptic spasms, psychomotor and atonic seizures, oral and manual automatisms as well as vocalization and eye deviation. Characteristic features of focal onset seizures described in adults with extratemporal epilepsy are frequently missing during childhood, especially infants and school children. In contrast to adults, secondarily generalized seizures are rare.

▶ SYNDROME DIAGNOSIS

There are few syndromes with focal seizures as a prominent feature that present at this age. *Panayiotopolous syndrome* is regarded as a common childhood onset epilepsy involving a prominence of autonomic seizures. Peak age of onset is between 4–5 years; presentation with a single episode of status epilepticus is common. Seizures manifest with a constellation of behavior change, vomiting, color change, and other more typical ictal manifestations. Formerly thought to have an occipital onset, autonomic symptoms are more prominent and therefore it is now more preferably considered an autonomic epilepsy. However although the prognosis for seizure remission in this particular type of epilepsy is extremely good, a low threshold should be maintained for detailed neuroimaging in view of overlap with some of the semiology with that presenting from occipital structural abnormalities (see Chapter 26).

Benign epilepsy with centrotemporal spikes (BECTS) has a peak onset between 5 and 8 years. The seizures are characterized by focal motor involvement of the face and upper limb although secondarily generalized tonic clonic seizures may occur from sleep. This typical pattern of presentation, along with recognized centrotemporal spikes on the waking or sleep EEG facilitates the diagnosis. However the presence of atypical features should prompt the need to obtain brain imaging. The prognosis for seizure remission is extremely good, and discussion often centers on the need for treatment rather than which medication (see Chapter).

Late onset childhood occipital epilepsy of Gastaut type is characterized by focal seizures commonly involving elementary visual hallucinations. The consistency and stereotyped nature of the hallucinations often enables the child to draw them. Ictal blindness is also common and either occurs de novo or follows the hallucinations. Consciousness is not impaired but may be impaired or lost during the later stages of the seizure that often progresses to hemi or bilateral convulsions. Onset is from 3–15 years with a mean of 8 years. Prognosis for seizure control is good with remission within 2–4 years from onset in about 50–60% cases (see Chapter). The differential diagnosis includes migraine in view of the high frequency of postictal headache.

Ring chromosome 20 is now a recognized electroclinical syndrome characterized by focal onset seizures of likely frontal origin, involving fear, visual symptoms and hallucinations and episodes of nonconvulsive status epilepticus.[7] The typical EEG pattern is characterized by runs of long-lasting bilateral paroxysmal high voltage slow waves with occasional spikes over the frontal lobes. Increasing cognitive difficulty is noted with increasing age and problematic behavior including poor attention and concentration, impulsivity, disinhibition, obsessive behaviors, and aggressive outbursts are highly characteristic (see Chapter).

▶ INVESTIGATION

The interictal EEG recording may reveal abnormalities consistent with focal epilepsy, although in this age group may not provide useful localizing information. The sleep EEG may be more revealing (see Fig. 18–1), although may still be nonlocalizing. Ictal EEG recording may be required to characterize seizure type and likely region of onset. Ictal recording may also help with epilepsy syndrome diagnosis. Magnetic resonance imaging is imperative to determine whether there is a responsible structural area of abnormality (see Fig. 18–2).[8] If there are other neurological manifestations particularly regression, focal seizures may be the initial manifestation of a mitochondrial disorder, particularly Polymerase gamma (POLG).[9] Assessment for Ring chromosome 20 should be considered in children presenting with lesion-negative frontal lobe seizures, especially if there is a history of nonconvulsive status epilepticus (see above).

▶ MANAGEMENT (SEE FIG. 10–1)

Accurate diagnosis is required with particular consideration given to the more common epilepsy syndromes. Choice of medication depends on the presence or absence of an underlying cause as well as syndrome diagnosis (see Table 18–1).

There is insufficient data in children to support a particular monotherapy. A recent study compared newer AEDs against carbamazepine and sodium valproate.[10,11] Physicians were asked to choose between carbamazepine and sodium valproate for the clinical presentation, and if carbamazepine was selected, individuals were randomized to topiramate, gabapentin, lamotrigine, or oxcarbazepine (levetiracetam was not a comparator). Although study design did not base choice of drug on seizure type, the majority of individuals in the carbamazepine arm of the study had focal seizures. Using time to treatment failure whether due to seizure occurrence or side effects, lamotrigine was significantly better than carbamazepine gabapentin and topiramate, with a nonsignificant advantage over oxcarbazepine.[10] However, the relevance to childhood onset epilepsy has been questioned as although the study inclusion criteria included children down to the age of 4 years, in practice few children were recruited with a mean age of those included of 39 years. Further, very few individuals with idiopathic syndromes were included although most would consider similar AEDs in first line management to other types of focal seizure. The European Medicines Agency recently suggested that focal epilepsies in children older than 4 years are likely to have a similar clinical expression to focal epilepsies in adults and adolescents and the results of efficacy trials in adults for focal epilepsy could be extrapolated to children provided the correct dose is established (European Medicines Agency, http://www.ema.europa.eu).

A randomized controlled trial of sulthiame compared to placebo in the treatment of Benign Epilepsy

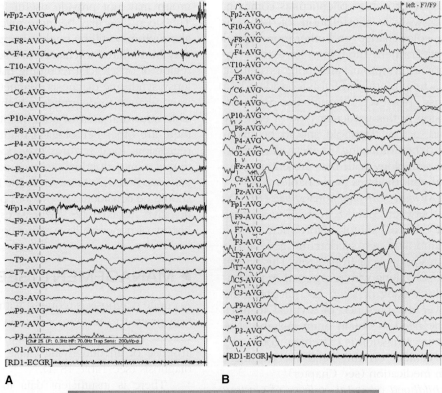

A   **B**

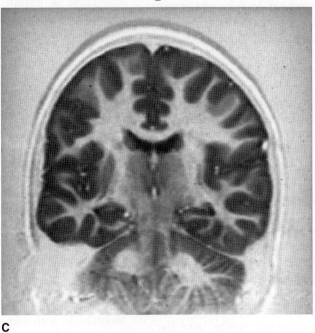

C

Figure 18–1. Wake (**A**) and sleep (**B**) EEG of a seven-year-old girl with a left mesiotemporal sclerosis (**C**). Wake EEG showed subtle left temporal spikes; these were enhanced in sleep.

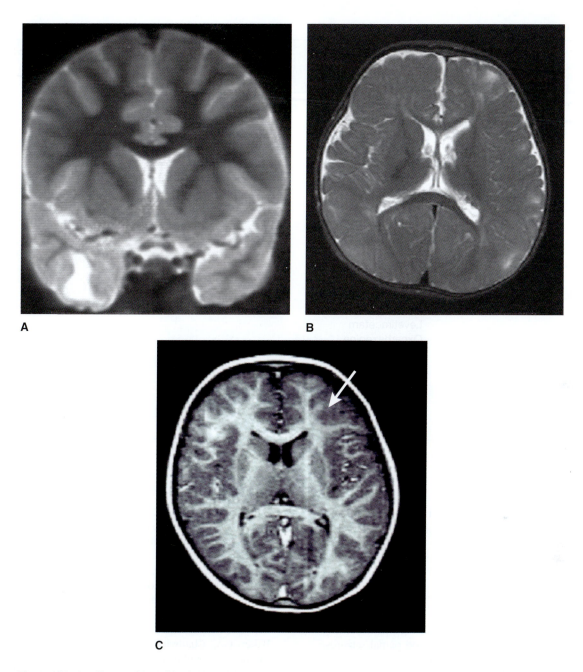

Figure 18–2. Examples of lesions that can cause focal seizures in early childhood. (**A**) Right temporal dysembryoplastic neuroepithelial tumor. (**B**) Tuberous sclerosis. (**C**) Left frontal cortical dysplasia.

▶ **TABLE 18–1. TREATMENT OF FOCAL SEIZURES**

	First Line	Second Line	Further Medication to be Considered as Add-on Therapy
Focal seizures	Carbamazepine Lamotrigine Levetiracetam Oxcarbazepine Sodium valproate	Carbamazepine Clobazam Gabapentin Lamotrigine Levetiracetam Oxcarbazepine Sodium valproate Topiramate	Eslicarbazepine acetate Lacosamide Phenobarbital Phenytoin Pregabalin Tiagabine Vigabatrin Zonisamide
BECTS	Carbamazepine Lamotrigine Levetiracetam Oxcarbazepine Sulthiame		
Panyiotopolous syndrome	Carbamazepine Lamotrigine Levetiracetam Oxcarbazepine Sodium valproate		
Late-onset occipital epilepsy Gastaut type	Carbamazepine Lamotrigine Levetiracetam Oxcarbazepine Sodium valproate		

with Centrotemporal spikes demonstrated significant benefit for seizure control and resolution of EEG discharges.[12,13] The ketogenic diet may be useful in resistant nonidiopathic cases.[14]

REFERENCES

1. Fogarasi A, Janszky J, Tuxhorn I. Localising and lateralising value of behavioral change in childhood partial seizures. *Epilepsia* 2007;48:196–200.
2. Fogarasi A, Janszky J, Tuxhorn I. Autonomic symptoms during childhood partial epileptic seizures. *Epilepsia* 2006; 47:584–588.
3. Fogarasi A, Tuxhorn I, Janszky J, Janszky I, Rasonyi G, Kelemen A, Halasz P. Age-dependent seizure semiology in temporal lobe epilepsy. *Epilepsia* 2007;48:1697–1702.
4. Fogarasi A, Janszky J, Tuxhorn I. Ictal emotional expressions of children with partial epilepsy. *Epilepsia* 2007;48:120–123.
5. Fogarasi A, Janszky J, Faveret E, Pieper T, Tuxhorn I. A detailed analysis of frontal lobe seizure semiology in children younger than 7 years. *Epilepsia* 2011;42:80–85.
6. Fogarasi A, Tuxhorn I, Hegyi M, Janszky J. Predictive clinical factors for the differential diagnosis of childhood extratemporal seizures. *Epilepsia* 2005;46:1280–1285.
7. Augustijn PB, Parra J, Wouters CH, Joosten P, Lindhout D. Ring chromosome 20 epilepsy syndrome in children: electroclinical features. *Neurology* 2001;57:1108–1111.
8. Gaillard WD, Chiron C, Cross JH, Harvey AS, Kuzniecky R, Hertz-Pannier L, Gilbert VL. Guidelines for imaging infants and children with recent-onset epilepsy. *Epilepsia* 2009;50:2147–2153.
9. Engelsen BA, Tzoulis C, Karlsen B, Lillebe A, Laegreid LM, Aasly J, Zeviani M, Bindoff LA. POLGI mutations cause a syndromic epilepsy with occpital lobe predilection. *Brain* 2008;131:818–828.
10. Marson AG, Al-Kharusi AM, Alwaidh M, Appleton R, Baker GA, Chadwick DW, Cramp C, Cockerell OC, Cooper P, Doughty J, Eaton B, Gamble C, Goulding PJ, Howell SJL, Hughes A, Jackson M, Jacoby A, Kellett M, Lawson GR, Leach JP, Nicolaides P, Roberts R, Shackley P, Shen J, Smith DF, Smith PE, Smith CT, Vanoli A, Williamson PR; SANAD Study Group. The SANAD study of effectiveness of carbamazepine, gabapentin, lamotrigine, oxcarbazepine, or topiramate for treatment of partial epilepsy: an unblinded randomised controlled trial. *Lancet* 2007;369:1000–1015.
11. Marson AG, Al-Kharusi AM, Alwaidh M, Appleton R, Baker GA, Chadwick DW, Cramp C, Cockerell OC, Cooper P, Doughty J, Eaton B, Gamble C, Goulding PJ, Howell SJL, Hughes A, Jackson M, Jacoby A, Kellett M, Lawson GR, Leach JP, Nicolaides P, Roberts R, Shackley P, Shen J, Smith DF, Smith PE, Tudor Smith C, Vandi A, Williamson PR, SANAD Study Group. The SANAD study of effectiveness of valproate, lamotrigine, or topiramate for generlaised and unclassifiable epilepsy:

an unblinded randomised controlled trial. *Lancet* 2007;369:1016–1026.

12. Rating D, Wolf C, Bast T. Sulthiame as monotherapy in children with benign childhood epilepsy with centrotemporal spikes: a 6-month randomized, double blind, placebo-controlled study. Sulthiame Study Group. *Epilepsia* 2000;41:1284–1288.

13. Bast T, et al. The influence of sulthiame on EEG in children with benign childhood epilepsy with centrotemporal spikes (BECTS). *Epilepsia* 2003;44:215–220.

14. Kossoff EH, et al. Optimal clinical management of children receiving the ketogenic diet: recommendations of the international ketogenic diet study group. *Epilepsia* 2008;47:1–14.

CHAPTER 19

Focal Seizures in Older Childhood and Adolescence

J. Helen Cross

Focal seizures in the older child and adolescent are usually similar in presentation to the adult. However, children with profound developmental delay may still display an immature seizure semiology. Stereotyped seizure patterns suggesting focal origin apart from benign epilepsy syndromes should prompt a search for a structural lesion. If seizures persist despite aggressive AED treatment, referral for presurgical evaluation is appropriate.[1]

▶ CLINICAL EVALUATION

In this age group, semiology can be informative not only with regard to lobe of seizure origin but also as in the case of the frontal lobe, the particular region of involvement (see Table 19–1). The seizure semiology may also indicate lateralization (see Table 19–2). Frontal lobe seizures are typically brief (<30 seconds), and rapid in onset and offset with almost immediate recovery. They typically occur in clusters, and often occur out of sleep. Seizures arising from rolandic and primary motor cortex typically involve clonic movement of one side of the body. Supplementary motor area seizures involve sudden onset of an asymmetric "fencing" posture of the upper limbs. Hypermotor activity and ictal hallucinations are reported in orbitofrontal seizures, and fear/laughter in seizures arising from the cingulate gyrus. Mesial temporal lobe seizures classically present with an aura, most commonly of fear or epigastric sensation (rising feeling from the abdomen). Some degree of behavioural arrest may follow with or without impaired awareness, or confusion with ictal or postictal dysphasia. Automatisms, most commonly oroalimentary (e.g., swallowing, lip smacking) or motor (picking) may also occur. Seizures typically last 60–90 seconds, followed by a period of recovery, with or without confusion. Lateral or posterior temporal onset seizures often have similar characteristics, although the aura typically differs, for example, auditory or complex visual changes.

Occipital seizures present with an aura of an elementary visual hallucination that can often be described in detail (see Fig. 19–1). The aura is then variably followed by contralateral eye deviation. Ictal vomiting or retching (ictus emeticus) may or may not be prominent. Ictal nystagmus is observed more commonly with involvement of the temporal parietal occipital junction. Aurae are reported in 80%–90% of children with occipital or temporal lobe seizure onset. Parietal seizure onset is associated with nonspecific features. Sensory aura may be apparent, but other features such as atonic attacks result from rapid spread to motor cortex.

▶ SYNDROME DIAGNOSIS

AUTOSOMAL DOMINANT NOCTURNAL FRONTAL LOBE EPILEPSY (ADNFLE)

This relatively recently recognized syndrome involves recurrent nocturnal seizures, usually brief and with a consistent and unusual semiology. They are characterized by onset shortly after falling asleep, with a nonspecific aura such as a shiver or fear. Attacks have prominent motor features, occur in clusters and individuals often retain awareness.[7] An autosomal dominant form is recognized with a mean age of onset of 11 years, with some families showing linkage to a mutation in the ci4 subunit of the ligand-gated neuronal nicotinic acetylcholine receptor (nAChR).[7] However, a familial occurrence of attacks in individuals with nocturnal frontal lobe seizures occurs in only 25%.[8] Most affected individuals are cognitively normal, and interference in life style from sleep disruption is seen more often in the families rather than the individuals themselves (see Chapter 27).

Autosomal dominant epilepsy with auditory features is a familial epilepsy syndrome with a relatively later onset of likely lateral temporal lobe origin. The age of onset may occur between ages 1 and 60 years, with a mean of 18 years.[9] The syndrome is characterized by focal seizures and secondarily generalized tonic–clonic seizures. Auditory aurae are reported in 64%, and include psychic, complex visual, autonomic, vertiginous, and

▶ **TABLE 19–1.** SEMIOLOGICAL CHARACTERISTICS OF SEIZURES ARISING FROM DIFFERENT AREAS OF THE BRAIN

Frontal lobe seizures	Sudden offset/onset, short duration, nocturnal, clusters, brief or absent postictal confusion[2,3]
Opercular	Profuse salivation, oral facial apraxia, and possibly some focal facial clonic activity
Orbitofrontal	Autonomic changes and heightened motor activity (hypermotor seizures)
Perirolandic	Typically motor with unilateral clonic jerking contralateral face and limbs
Supplementary motor area	Speech arrest and "fencing" posture, with asymmetric motor movements and contralateral head and eye version
Dorsolateral frontal	Contralateral head and eye tonic elevation and contralateral clonic movements arms and face
Cingulate gyrus	Intense fright, facial expression of fear, incomplete loss of awareness
Temporal lobe seizures	Aura, longer duration, postictal confusion
Mesial	Abdominal aura or fear, oroalimentary/motor automatisms
Lateral neocortical	Auditory, vertiginous and complex visual aurae, early contralateral dystonic posturing in the absence of oral alimentary automatisms, early loss of contact, shorter seizure duration
Posterior basal	Behavioral arrest followed by motor manifestations (mainly contralateral head version and contralateral arm tonic stiffening)[4]
Parietal lobe seizures	Somatosensory aura, or relatively silent until anterior propagation[5]
Occipital lobe seizures	Elementary visual hallucinations, ictal amaurosis, rapid eye blinking, sensations of eye movement[6]

more rarely other sensory aurae. The interictal EEG reveals temporal lobe abnormalities in 47%.[9] Mutations in the leucine-rich glioma inactivated 1 (*LGI1*) gene occurs in 50% of affected individuals; there is no reported phenotypic difference in pedigrees with and without the mutation. Sporadic nonfamilial cases share a similar phenotype and have a mean age of seizure onset of 19 years. Focal seizures with prominent auditory aurae, a high rate of secondarily generalized tonic–clonic seizures, a good response to medication, and unrevealing EEG and MRI are typical features.[10]

▶ **TABLE 19–2.** LATERALISING FEATURES

Contralateral signs
• *Unilateral dystonic posturing*
• *Unilateral forced head turning*
• *Unilateral clonus*
• *Eye deviation at secondary generalization*
• *Ictal hemiparesis*
• *Postical paresis or visual field defects*

Ipsilateral signs
• *Unilateral motor automatisms*
• *Unforced early head turning*
• *Unilateral eye blinking*

Dominant hemisphere
• *Postictal dysphasia/aphasia*

Nondominant hemisphere
• *Ictal speech*
• *Ictal vomiting*

RASMUSSEN SYNDROME

Rasmussen encephalitis is an acquired progressive encephalitis of one cerebral hemisphere. Children typically present between ages 5 and 10 years with focal seizures, often focal motor seizures, associated with progressive atrophy of the contralateral hemisphere.[11] Epilepsia partialis continua is described in about half of affected individuals and is typically associated with progressive hemiparesis, hemianopia, and cognitive deterioration. Immunopathological studies suggest that this is likely to be an autoimmune process with a prominent role played by cytotoxic T lymphocytes. Although treatments targeted at the immune system appear to slow the disease, hemidiconnection remains the only definitive cure of seizures (with the inevitable functional deficit).[12] Early referral to a surgical unit is imperative, as careful planning will need to be undertaken as to the timing of surgery (see Chapter).

▶ INVESTIGATION

All children and young adults with a history of focal seizures should undergo EEG recording, preferably with a segment of sleep. Abnormalities may be apparent supportive of the clinical diagnosis (Fig. 19–2). In the absence of a diagnosis of benign syndrome, an MRI should be performed to identify a structural etiology. Ictal EEG recording is useful, but frontal lobe seizures may have EEG changes masked by movement artefact (Fig. 19–3), or fail to demonstrate any changes. The

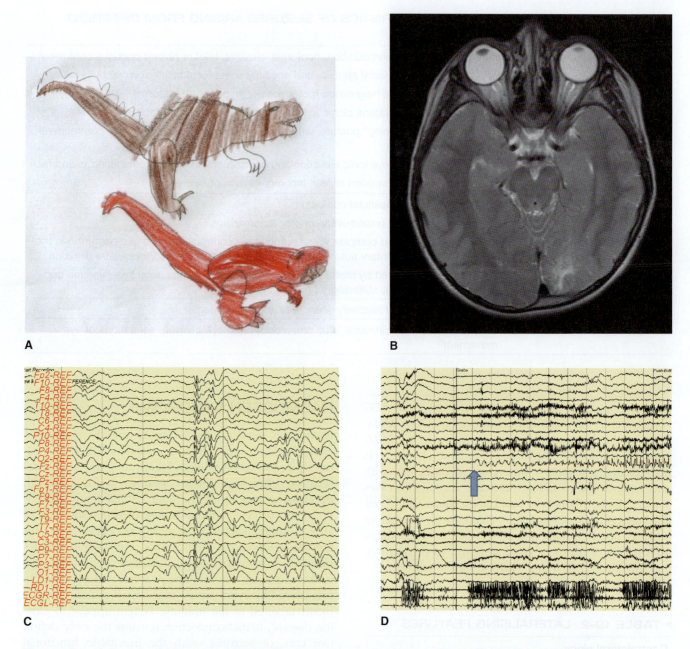

Figure 19–1. A 6-year-old boy presented with stereotyped seizures involving a well-formed visual aura ("dinosaurs" so drawn [**A**]). MRI showed a left occipital malformation (**B**). Although a continuous interictal abnormality is demonstrated over this area on interictal recording (**C**), the ictal recording suggests onset over the right (**D**).

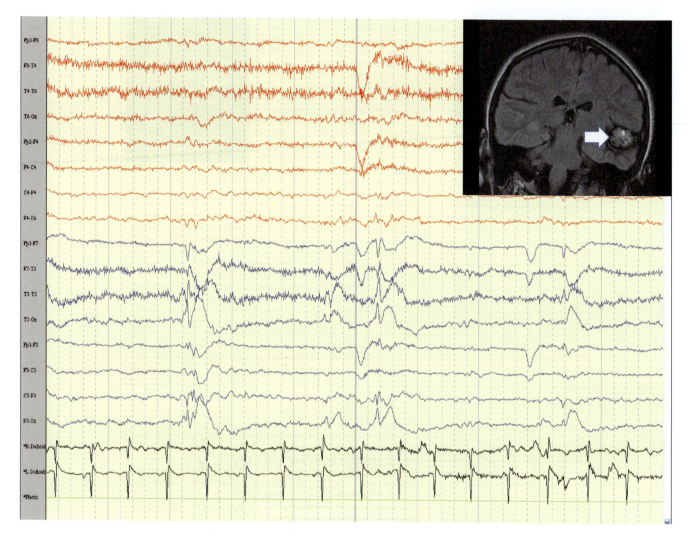

Figure 19–2. Temporal sharp and slow wave activity in a child with temporal lobe onset seizures arising from a lateral temporal cavernoma.

diagnosis of pseudoseizures may be challenging and relies heavily on clinical experience. Seizure semiology, family history, and the EEG characteristics may all be used to determine whether a familial epilepsy syndrome is likely. Genetic studies will further guide these findings.

▶ MANAGEMENT (SEE FIGURE 10–1)

Following the diagnosis of focal seizures, consideration must be given to starting antiepileptic drug treatment. The algorithm outlined in Chapter 10 can be followed in the management of this age group. In the majority, children presenting with at least two epileptic seizures are unlikely to have a self-limited epilepsy syndrome. As outlined in Chapter 18, although RCT data inclusive of children alone is sparse, data from adult studies for the treatment of focal seizures are likely to be relevant. Guidelines for childhood onset focal seizures are therefore common to adult focal seizures. Carbamazepine or lamotrigine are considered first-line agents. In this age group particularly where lifelong treatment may be required, careful consideration should be given prior to prescribing sodium valproate to girls/women in view of the possible teratogenic effects. Levetiracetam remains an alternate choice. Thereafter where add on treatment is required, most approved medications have demonstrable benefit in the treatment of focal seizures.

General management principles would include trial of sequential monotherapy, with add-on therapy should monotherapy fail. A maximum of two AEDs should be considered at any time. Where a lesion is identified on MRI, as with other age groups, referral for consideration of surgery should be made early in the natural history (see Chapter 55); Persistent stereotyped focal seizures

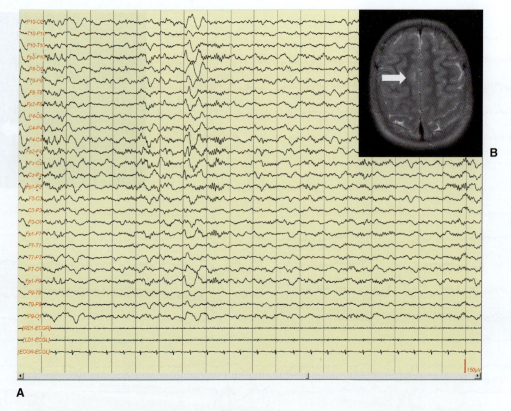

A

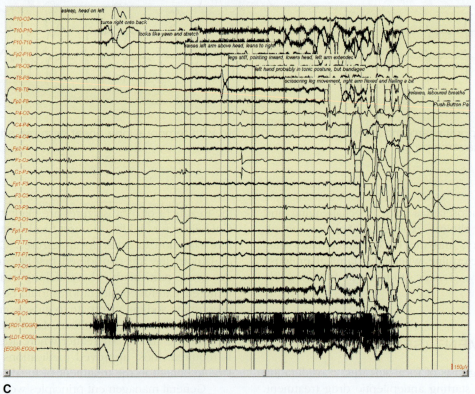

C

Figure 19–3. Interictal (**A**) and ictal (**B**) EEG recording of a 12-year-old girl with seizures arising from an area of probable cortical dysplasia in the right frontal lobe (**C**). Interictal sleep recording shows isolated right frontal sharp waves; the ictal recording shows generalized attenuation with subsequent movement artefact.

despite trial of two AEDs in MRI-negative individuals should also prompt referral to a specialist epilepsy center for consideration of surgery. Compliance with the ketogenic diet (KD) is often challenging in this age group, although more tolerable alternatives have been suggested.[13–16]

REFERENCES

1. Cross JH, et al. Proposed criteria for referral and evaluation of children for epilepsy surgery: recommendations of the Subcommission for Paediatric Epilepsy Surgery. *Epilepsia* 2006;47:952–959.
2. Williamson PD, Spencer DD, Spencer SS, Novelly RA, Mattson RH. Complex partial seizures of frontal lobe origin. *Ann Neurol* 1985;18:497–504.
3. Williamson PD. Frontal lobe seizures. Problems of diagnosis and classification. *Adv Neurol* 1992;57:289–309.
4. Duchowny M, Jayakar P, Resnick T, Levin B, Alvarez L. Posterior temporal epilepsy: electroclinical features. *Ann Neurol* 1994;35:427–431.
5. Williamson PD, et al. Parietal lobe epilepsy: diagnostic considerations and results of surgery. *Ann Neurol* 1992; 31:193–201.
6. Williamson PD, Thadani VM, Darcey TM, Spencer DD, Spencer SS, Mattson RH. Occipital lobe epilepsy: clinical characteristics, seizure spread patterns, and results of surgery. *Ann Neurol* 1992;31:3–13.
7. Scheffer IE. Autosomal dominant nocturnal frontal lobe epilepsy. *Epilepsia* 2000;41:1059–1060.
8. Provina F, Plazzi G, Tinuper P, Vandi S, Lugaresi E, Montagna P. Nocturnal frontal lobe epilepsy: a clinical and polygraphic overview of 100 consecutive cases. *Brain* 1999;122:1017–1031.
9. Michelucci R, Pasini E, Nobile C. Lateral temporal lobe epilepsies: clinical and genetic features. *Epilepsia* 2009; 50:52–54.
10. Bisulli F, et al. Idiopathic partial epilepsy with auditory features (IPEAF): a clinical and genetic study of 53 sporadic cases. *Brain* 2004;127:1343–1352.
11. Bien CG, et al. Pathogenesis, diagnosis and treatment of Rasmussen encephalitis. *Brain* 2005;128:454–471.
12. Bien CG, Schramm J. Treatment of Rasmussen encephalitis half a century after its initial description: promising prospects and a dilemma. *Epilepsy Res* 2009;86:101–112.
13. Muzykewicz DA, Lyczkowski DA, Memon N, Conant KD, Pfeifer HH, Thiele EA. Efficacy, safety, and tolerability of the low glycemic index treatment in pediatric epilepsy. *Epilepsia* 2009;50(5):1118–1126.
14. Kossoff EH, McGrogan JR, Bluml RM, Pillas DJ, Rubenstein JE, Vining EPG. Modified Atkins diet is effective for the treatment of intractable pediatric epilepsy. *Epilepsia* 2006; 47:421–424.
15. Kossoff EH, et al. Optimal clinical management of children receiving the ketogenic diet: recommendations of the international ketogenic diet study group. *Epilepsia* 2008;47:1–14.
16. Kossoff EH, Rowley H, Sinha SR, Vining EPG. A prospective study of the modified Atkins diet for intractable epilepsy in adults. *Epilepsia* 2008;49:316–319.

CHAPTER 20

Generalized Seizures in Childhood and Adolescence

Raj D. Sheth

▶ OVERVIEW

Management of epilepsy in childhood and adolescents requires accurate characterization of seizures and epilepsy syndrome. The inability to do so may result in the selection of inappropriate treatment options. As an example, diagnosing absence epilepsy for staring in the context of complex partial epilepsy may result in the choice of carbamazepine instead of an antiabsence seizure agent. Carbamazepine is well known to exacerbate absence seizures and is rarely associated with spike-wave stupor. Failure to accurately classify epilepsy syndromes may also limit the ability to prognosticate and limit decisions regarding medication withdrawal.

The types of generalized seizures include: typical absence, atypical absence, myoclonic, generalized tonic–clonic, tonic and atonic seizures. Generalized seizures often have an age-dependent presentation. The spectrum of generalized seizures as a function of age of onset is shown in Figure 20–1.

The generalized epilepsy syndromes encompass generalized seizure types associated with specific clinical accompaniments, age, EEG, and the presence or absence of neurological deficits and imaging findings.[1] Generalized seizures occurring in the context of a normal neurological and cognitive examination and in the context of normal cerebral imaging typically indicate one of the idiopathic generalized epilepsies. Examples include childhood absence, juvenile absence, and juvenile myoclonic epilepsy. In contrast generalized seizures occurring in the context of cognitive impairment, neurological deficits and/or imaging lesions suggest one of the symptomatic generalized epilepsies. An intermediate group referred to as the cryptogenic generalized epilepsies may have normal imaging and laboratory investigations but are associated with developmental, cognitive, and neurological deficits. Examples of symptomatic or cryptogenic epilepsy include West and Lennox–Gastaut syndromes.

Generalized seizures can occur in the context of any of these three broad categories. Differentiating between them carries important therapeutic and prognostic information.

The putative mechanism of the generalized epilepsies involves activation of the thalamic relay system, reticular neurons, and cortical pyramidal neurons. Thalamic relay neurons activate cortical pyramidal neurons in either a tonic or burst mode. T-type calcium channels underlie the burst mode. Drugs, such as ethosuximide, that are effective in controlling absence seizures affect the T-type calcium currents.

▶ DIFFERENTIATING GENERALIZED FROM PARTIAL SEIZURES

A generalized seizure implies that the entire cerebrum is electrically involved at seizure onset (Fig. 20–1). Generalized seizures typically manifest clinically at the onset of the electrographic discharge. In contrast, partial seizures evolve to start in one cerebral hemisphere and propagate to involve expanding areas of brain until clinical manifestations become obvious. Epilepsia partialis continua seizures present with continuous recurrent clonic motor manifestations that are focal and associated with repetitive electrographic discharges.

Generalized seizures may present in several distinct presentations: as a convulsive seizure involving all extremities at onset (generalized tonic–clonic seizures), as sudden brief whole-body jerk (myoclonic seizures), as sudden whole-body stiffening (tonic seizures), as a staring spell (absence seizures), as a "slump" (atonic seizures), or as a body jerk that if severe can cause the patient to fall to the ground (myoclonic seizures). Consciousness is typically impaired at seizure onset but returns instantaneously at seizure offset. Exceptions include prolonged generalized convulsions where there is typically a period of postictal unresponsiveness.

TYPICAL ABSENCE SEIZURES

Approximately 5%–10% of all childhood epilepsy presents with absence seizures. Typical absence seizures produce impaired consciousness that is associated with a 2.5–4 Hz generalized spike-wave discharges. Impaired consciousness may be quite subtle and only be demonstrable on special testing. A blank stare is often associated with automatisms, eyelid myoclonia, and autonomic disturbances. Absence seizures are typically activated by hyperventilation, a useful finding

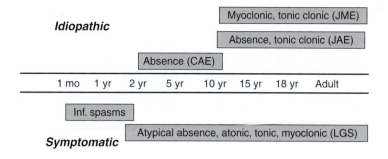

Figure 20–1. Generalized seizures across childhood and adolescents showing age overlap of idiopathic and symptomatic seizures and ages at which they typically appear and disappear. CAE, childhood absence epilepsy; JAE, juvenile absence epilepsy; JME, juvenile myoclonic epilepsy; LGS, Lennox–Gastaut syndrome.

allowing them to be easily elicited in the clinic by having the patient blow on a pinwheel.

Differentiating absence seizures from complex partial seizures and nonepileptic day-dreaming spells may be challenging; guidelines for a differential diagnosis are given in Table 20–1.

Epilepsy syndromes with typical absences include the idiopathic generalized epilepsies: childhood absence epilepsy, juvenile absence epilepsy, and juvenile myoclonic epilepsy. Myoclonic absence epilepsy is a component of the cryptogenic/symptomatic generalized epilepsies.

ATYPICAL ABSENCE SEIZURES

Atypical absence seizures are much less common than typical absence seizures. They are often observed in patients with the Lennox–Gastaut syndrome where they accompany atonic and tonic seizures. Atypical absence seizures are often associated with developmental delay or mental retardation whereas mental function in typical absence epilepsy is normal. The EEG differentiates atypical from typical absence seizures by the characteristic finding of diffuse slow (<2.5 Hz) spike-wave discharges; in addition the EEG background is usually slow and disorganized.

GENERALIZED TONIC–CLONIC SEIZURES

Generalized convulsions in childhood are much more likely to occur as secondarily generalized seizures due to propagation of localized partial seizure activity. In contrast, primary generalized convulsions begin in both cerebral hemispheres simultaneously and are much less common

The sequelae of generalized convulsions include oral and head trauma, stress fractures during the tonic phase, aspiration pneumonia, pulmonary edema, and sudden unexpected death in epilepsy (SUDEP).

The interictal EEGs reveal either a normal background or runs of occipital delta activity and may show either fragmented spike-wave, polyspike-wave, or frank generalized spike-wave discharges. EEG findings at ictal onset include high-amplitude anteriorly dominant generalized spike-wave discharges followed by low-amplitude diffuse fast frequencies that evolve to generalized spike-wave or polyspike-wave discharges. Once the seizure is clinically manifest, muscle activity often precludes accurate seizure localization. The postictal EEG typically demonstrates diffuse slowing and slow spike-wave discharges.

▶ **TABLE 20–1.** DIFFERENTIATING COMPLEX PARTIAL SEIZURES, ABSENCE AND DAY-DREAMING SPELLS AT THE BEDSIDE

Features	Complex Partial Seizures	Absence	Day-Dreaming Spells
Onset	May have simple partial onset	Abrupt	Variable
Duration	Usually >30 s	Usually <30 s	Variable
Automatisms	Present	Duration dependent	None
Awareness	No	No	Partial
Ending	Gradual postictal	Abrupt	Variable
State	Active or passive	Active or passive	Always in passive state

MYOCLONUS AND MYOCLONIC SEIZURES

Myoclonus, a sudden involuntary brief shock-like muscle contraction activated within the central nervous system, is a nonepileptic phenomenon unassociated with epileptiform discharges. In contrast, myoclonic seizures are associated with epileptiform discharges (often fast polyspike-wave discharge) that arise from the cerebral cortex. Consciousness is typically impaired but may appear preserved due to the short duration of the myoclonic seizure. Myoclonic seizures may precede generalized motor convulsions.

If the neurological examination and neuroimaging findings are normal, myoclonic seizures in the adolescent strongly suggest a diagnosis—juvenile myoclonic epilepsy. In younger children, myoclonic seizures may accompany the Lennox–Gastaut syndrome or myoclonic–astatic epilepsy of Doose. Myoclonic seizures can be distinguished from sleep myoclonus as the seizures often occur with awakening or randomly throughout the day.

TONIC AND ATONIC SEIZURES

Both tonic and atonic seizure typically occur in patients with symptomatic generalized epilepsies and have been reported in up to 90% of patients with the Lennox–Gastaut syndrome. They characteristically induce a drop attack, as muscle tone is compromised and the patient is either propelled to the ground (tonic seizures), or slumps to the ground (atonic seizures). Both seizures types are usually brief lasting under 1 minute in duration and may be associated with autonomic changes, including facial flushing, tachycardia, hypertension, and papillary changes. The EEG typically demonstrates sudden interruption of the slow background for the duration of the seizures (see EEG patterns elsewhere). This activity resembles the electrodecremental response seen on the EEG in infantile spasms.

▶ TREATMENT

While there are several treatment options for generalized seizures, certain medications should be avoided. Phenytoin, gabapentin, and carbamazepine are ineffective for absence seizures; exacerbation of the absences with carbamazepine are well documented. Myoclonic seizures also do not typically respond to phenytoin, carbamazepine, or lamotrigine. While ineffective for absence and myoclonic seizures, these medications are useful for the treatment of other forms of generalized convulsive seizures.

▶ TREATMENT ALGORITHM

There is a paucity of well-designed, randomized clinical trials for patients with generalized seizures. American Academy of Neurology has issued broad recommendations for the treatment of generalized seizures. Generally, wherever possible monotherapy is preferable.[2]

A treatment algorithm for generalized seizures is presented (Fig. 20–2). A starting point in the treatment algorithm is an EEG that is essential to appropriately classify seizures, including avoiding the misidentification of secondarily generalized seizures as being primarily generalized seizures. The EEG may show focal spikes in which case the diagnosis of a true generalized epilepsy is questionable. The EEG in generalized seizure is often abnormal, although, its diagnostic power is dependent on length of recording and the use of activation procedures. Should seizures relapse on therapy video-EEG and MRI may be indicated. If video-EEG demonstration of generalized spike-wave discharges, confirms the diagnosis and allows treatment to commence. If video-EEG recording (including sleep) fails to show epileptiform discharges, the diagnosis must remain questionable; an empiric antiepileptic medication trial may be considered.

The EEG also serves to differentiate juvenile myoclonic epilepsy with generalized polyspike-waves of 4–6 Hz frequencies, from either childhood or juvenile absence epilepsy and its characteristic 3-Hz generalized spike-waves. Similarly, the slow spike-wave discharges (usually <2.5 Hz of symptomatic Lennox–Gastaut syndrome) are easily distinguished. In infants, the EEG may demonstrate hypsarrythmia, a finding diagnostic of infantile spasms and West syndrome.

Cerebral imaging is rarely indicated in patients with idiopathic generalized epilepsy. MRI may be considered in the presence of focal epileptiform EEG discharges, atypical clinical features, or in the absence of a definitive epilepsy syndrome diagnosis. The presence of either cognitive deficits or focal deficits may also lead to diagnostic imaging studies.

First-line agents for the treatment of generalized epilepsy, especially those associated with generalized spike-wave, polyspike-wave, and slow spike-wave, include levetiracetam, lamotrigine, and sodium valproate. Valproate is the most effective agent for the spectrum of generalized seizures. Its potential for neural tube defects should be considered in treating women of child-bearing age. Second-line agents include clonazepam, topiramate, and zonisamide. Medications to be avoided include carbamazepine, phenytoin, or oxcarbazepine.

Childhood absence is rarely associated with convulsive seizures, making ethosuximide a first-line agent. However, juvenile absence epilepsy is associated with an increased risk of generalized convulsive seizures against which ethosuximide has not been shown to be effective.

The presence of hypsarrythmia suggests the diagnosis of West syndrome. Effective agents include ACTH and vigabatrin.[3]

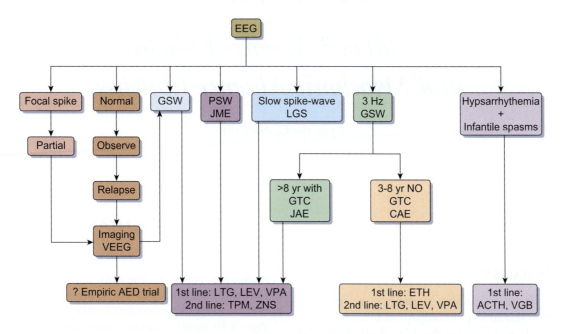

Figure 20–2. Diagnostic and treatment algorithm for generalized seizures. GSW, generalized spike-wave; PSW, polyspike-wave; JME, juvenile myoclonic epilepsy; JAE, juvenile absence epilepsy; CAE, childhood absence epilepsy; LGS, Lennox–Gastaut syndrome; ETH, ethosuximide; LTG, lamotrigine; LEV, levetiracetam; VPA, valproate; TPM, topiramate; VGB, vigabatrin; ZNS, zonisamide.

The American Academy of Neurology has published a position statement suggesting the use of vigabatrin as a first-line therapy for the treatment of infantile spasms. This provides an added option to the long-established use of ACTH. ACTH has many adverse effects including weight increase, hyperglycemia, hypertension, and the possible associated cerebral atrophy. Vigabatrin has been reported to constrict visual fields and because reversible MRI white matter changes.[4,5]

Felbamate has a broad spectrum of activity in generalized seizures, but rare reports of fatal aplastic anemia, and hepatic failure limit its use to a third-line agent when other treatment alternative have failed.

▶ PROGNOSIS AND OUTCOME

The prognosis for the idiopathic generalized epilepsies is generally favorable with regard to mental development. The majority of children with typical childhood-onset absence epilepsy can expect to outgrow their seizures by mid-adolescence, although 10%–15% may experience persistent medically resistant seizures. In contrast, juvenile myoclonic epilepsy and juvenile absence epilepsy rarely remit and therefore are lifelong conditions, whereas childhood absence epilepsy usually ceases by age 10 years. The symptomatic generalized epilepsies, particularly syndromes of epileptic encephalopathy share a much poorer long-term prognosis. It is not unusual

for West syndrome to transition to Lennox–Gastaut syndrome with increasing age.

The EEG can help guide treatment as the EEG is usually normal when seizures are clinically controlled. Not uncommonly, however, EEG abnormalities persist long after clinical seizure activity has ceased.

REFERENCES

1. Duchowny M, Harvey AS. Pediatric epilepsy syndromes: an update and critical review. *Epilepsia* 1996;37(Suppl 1): S26–S40.
2. Mackay MT, Weiss SK, Adams-Webber T, Ashwal S, Stephens D, Ballaban-Gill K, Baram TZ, Duchowny M, Hirtz D, Pellock JM, Shields WD, Shinnar S, Wyllie E, Snead OC 3rd, American Academy of Neurology, Child Neurology Society. Practice parameter: medical treatment of infantile spasms: Report of the American Academy of Neurology and the Child Neurology Society. *Neurology* 2004;62(10):1668–1681.
3. Lerner JT, Salamon N, Sankar R. Clinical profile of vigabatrin as monotherapy for treatment of infantile spasms. *Neuropsychiatr Dis Treat* 2010;6:731–740.
4. Dracopoulos A, Widjaja E, Raybaud C, Westall CA, Snead OC 3rd. Vigabatrin-associated reversible MRI signal changes in patients with infantile spasms. *Epilepsia* 2010;51(7): 1297–1304.
5. Gidal BE, Privitera MD, Sheth RD, Gilman JT. Vigabatrin: a novel therapy for seizure disorders. *Ann Pharmacother* 1999;33(12):1277–1286.

CHAPTER 21

Childhood Absence Epilepsy
and Myoclonic Absence Epilepsy

Lynette G. Sadleir

► CHILDHOOD ABSENCE EPILEPSY (CAE)

EPIDEMIOLOGY

Childhood absence epilepsy is defined as frequent daily absence seizures (pyknolepsy) in normal school age children. It accounts for 8%–15% of all childhood epilepsies[1] with an annual incidence of 4.7–8.0 per 100,000 children between the ages of 1 and 15 years. The average age at presentation is 6 years (range 2–10 years) with previous febrile seizures reported in 11%.[2]

PATHOPHYSIOLOGY

This syndrome is likely due to complex inheritance involving several genes.[3] High concordance rates for absence seizures in monozygotic twins confirm that genes play a major role. However, as the concordance rate is not 100%, nongenetic factors are also involved. Most of the genes known to be associated with CAE encode calcium channel and GABA receptor subunits. Some of these mutations may have major effect but do not explain the phenotypic heterogeneity within families nor are they found commonly in CAE. Mutations in *SLC2A1*, the gene encoding glucose transporter type 1 (GLUT1), have recently been reported in children with CAE.[4] Most of these children also had paroxysmal exertional dyskinesia but this was subtle and not diagnosed until a molecular diagnosis was made. GLUT 1 deficiency should be considered in children with family histories suggestive of dominant inheritance of genetic generalized epilepsy (GGE)[4] as this may have therapeutic implications particularly if the epilepsy is intractable. Microdeletions in 15q13.13 are found in 1%–2% of children with GGE and are felt to behave as a susceptibility component in a polygenic model where a combination of susceptibility alleles contribute to the phenotype in any one patient.[3] The presence of this copy number variation increases a person's risk of developing GGE from 1 in 200 to 1 in 3.[3]

CLINICAL PRESENTATION

Seizures

Absence seizures are the only seizure at presentation[2,5] occurring up to thousands of times per day. They are enhanced by hyperventilation (HV) in over 90% of children with many clinicians suggesting this is essential to the diagnosis.[2] The clinical and EEG features of absence seizures are influenced by a number of factors which result in variation from seizure to seizure both between and within individual children. Some of these factors are inherent to the child, such as age, while others, such as state (awake, drowsy, asleep) or provocation (HV, intermittent photic stimulation (IPS)), reflect a changing environment in which the seizures occur.

The mean duration of the absence seizure in CAE is 10 seconds (range 1–44 seconds) with 75% lasting 4–20 seconds.[2] If response testing is performed most seizures reveal a clinical change.[2] Children usually arrest or alter their activity if performing a task.[2] Abnormal eyelid movements are common, with 3-Hz eyelid movements seen in 40% of seizures.[2] Eye opening occurs in 70% of seizures in which the eyes were initially closed and just over half of children open their eyes in every seizure. Staring is one of the cardinal features occurring in up to 94% of seizures. Occasionally (10% of children) mild myoclonic rhythmic movements of the face and limbs occur during the seizure. Automatisms occur in approximately 22% of spontaneous seizures but occur frequently during seizures recorded in HV. Children who are response tested during a seizure are usually (75%) completely unaware (no response to testing and no memory of event) but occasionally they may show some degree of responsiveness particularly at the end of the seizure.[2]

DIAGNOSIS

EEG

The EEG in CAE shows interictal fragments of generalized spike and wave (GSW) in 92% of sleep-deprived EEGs (41% while awake, 100% in sleep).[2,6] These fragments have the morphology of GSW but may not have a generalized distribution. Truly focal epileptiform discharges are seen in 15% of children predominantly in the central area.[2] Interictal polyspikes are seen in 43% of sleep deprived EEGs but only when drowsy or asleep.[6] Rhythmic posterior bilateral delta activity (PBDA) is seen in 32% of children and varies in frequency between 2.5 and 4 Hz (Fig. 21–1). It is enhanced by hyperventilation and not seen in sleep.[2] It is notched in 40% of cases and almost always either bilateral or seen independently on both sides.[2] A photoparoxysmal response (PPR) has been reported in 13%–18% of children with CAE although some investigators consider CAE with photosensitivity a separate electroclinical syndrome.[2,7]

The ictal discharge is often not generalized for the first second (Fig. 21–1).[2] The initial morphology may consist of single or multiple spikes, disorganized or organized spike and wave and is most often in the bifrontal or biooccipital areas.[2] Although occasionally a unilateral onset can be seen, these children generally also have seizures starting from the other hemisphere as well as seizures which have a generalized onset.[2] The majority (87%) of seizures have one or two spikes per wave. More than two spikes per wave are most commonly seen in children with a PPR. Eighty percent of seizures consist of organized discharges with complexes of uniform morphology repeated throughout the discharge. However, 20% of the seizures in a sleep deprived EEG show some degree of disorganization, which is more often seen during IPS, drowsiness, and sleep. The frequency of the GSW in CAE ranges from 2.5 to 5 Hz but is usually close to 3 Hz and may be faster in the first second.[2]

Diagnostic criteria are listed in Table 21–1.

Imaging Studies

Neuroimaging is not necessary in a child who presents with features consistent with the diagnosis of CAE.[8] If there are atypical findings such as consistent focality on EEG or lack of response to therapy then an MRI should be considered.

Differential Diagnosis

Other epilepsies that present in normal children with only absence seizures include: juvenile absence epilepsy (JAE), eyelid myoclonia with absences, and myoclonic absence epilepsy. JAE is differentiated from CAE by its age of presentation (>10 years) and the frequency of the absence seizures (infrequent and usually not daily). The absences are clinically and electrographically similar to those of CAE although the frequency of the GSW may be slightly faster.[6] These children may present with generalized tonic clonic seizures (GTCS) with the absences only recognized in retrospect or on the EEG.

Seventy-five percent of children develop GTCS, which present at the same time as the absence seizures. This is in contrast to CAE, where if GTCS occur, they usually present after the absence seizures are outgrown.

The rare epilepsy syndrome eyelid myoclonia with absences, or Jeavons syndrome, is not as yet recognized by the International League Against Epilepsy (ILAE). The absence seizures are different to those in CAE in that they are brief and associated with eyelid myoclonia, which consists of 4–6-Hz myoclonic jerks of the eyelids with simultaneous upward deviation of the eyes. These seizures occur mainly on eye closure and absences without eyelid myoclonia do not occur. Children present in early childhood and are photosensitive.[7] The EEG consists of brief (3–6 seconds) bursts of GSW and polyspikes with a normal background.

TREATMENT

Criteria for Starting Treatment

Children with CAE have significantly more absence seizures per day than are recognized. These frequent seizures, usually with severe loss of awareness, contribute to learning and behavior difficulties as well as accidents.[9,10] Treatment with antiepileptic drugs (AEDs) results in beneficial effects on cognitive functioning in these children and is therefore recommended after an EEG confirms the diagnosis. There is little information in the literature regarding the outcome of untreated CAE as all children are generally treated in the modern era. Older studies before the availability of effective medications lack consistency and certainty of diagnosis as they were prior to both EEG and diagnostic classification schemes. Adie reported in 1924 that children with pyknolepsy aged 4–10 years were not effectively treated with available therapies at that time but that after weeks to years the seizures stopped and there were no residual problems. There is some evidence that longer periods of uncontrolled seizures prior to therapy is associated with more learning and behavioral difficulties. However, it is unclear whether therapy alters prognosis or whether children with CAE that is likely to remit have absence seizures that are easier to treat.

Optimal Treatment Regimen (Fig. 21–2)

Psychosocial difficulties as young adults are common following CAE, even in those who outgrow their epilepsy and have discontinued AEDs.[9] Changes in parenting and expectations may contribute to this. Parents and teachers should be encouraged not to alter the way they interact with their child simply because of the epilepsy. Extra precautions may be necessary due to seizures but the child should not be limited unnecessarily.

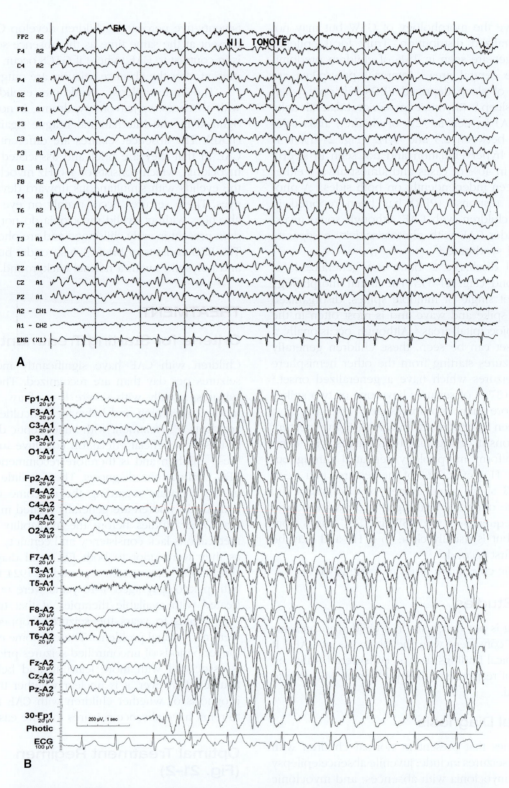

Figure 21-1. Examples of EEG features of CAE. (**A**) Posterior bilateral delta activity recorded during HV in a 6-year-old girl with CAE. The delta activity was seen intermittently in the awake and drowsy portions of the recording but was attenuated with eye opening and disappeared in sleep. (**B**) Ictal recording of the beginning of a 12-second absence seizure in an 8-year-old boy with CAE. The discharge is initially seen in the bianterior quadrants before becoming regular organized GSW.

▶ **TABLE 21–1. DIAGNOSTIC CRITERIA FOR CHILDHOOD ABSENCE EPILEPSY AND MYOCLONIC ABSENCE EPILEPSY**

Syndrome		Criteria
Childhood absence epilepsy	Inclusion	Presentation at 2–12 yr of age
		Cognition and development within the normal range
		Daily frequent absence seizures
		EEG shows normal background apart from posterior bilateral delta activity
		Ictal EEG shows GSW of at least 2.5 Hz
	Exclusion	Absence seizures with eyelid myoclonia
		Myoclonic absences
		Other seizure types at presentation
Myoclonic absence epilepsy	Inclusion	Presentation in childhood
		Frequent daily seizures
		Myoclonic absence seizures
		EEG shows normal background
		Ictal EEG shows rhythmic symmetrical GSW around 3 Hz

Recommended First-Line AEDs—Ethosuximide, Sodium Valproate, and Lamotrigine. Ethosuximide (ETX), sodium valproate (VPA), and lamotrigine (LTG) are all used as first-line medication in CAE.[11] The first-line AED used for an individual child should consider efficacy, side-effect profile, and titration schedule of the AED, as well as patient comorbidities (headaches, weight, etc.). The ideal initial AED for one patient may not be ideal for another.

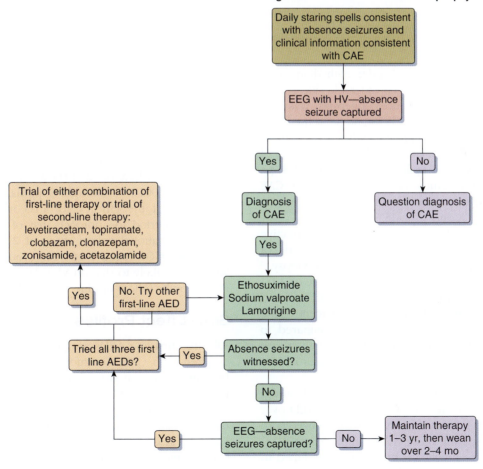

Figure 21–2. Treatment algorithm.

▶ **TABLE 21–2. RANDOMIZED CONTROLLED TRIALS OF AEDS IN CAE**

Study	Type of Study	N	Patient Characteristics	Duration of FU	Successful Treatment (Mean Effective Dose)			Success Criteria
					Ethosuximide	Valproic Acid	Lamotrigine	
Glauser, et al (2010)[10]	Double-blind, randomized, controlled	453	New-onset CAE: 2.5–13 yr	16–20 wk	53% (34 mg/kg/d)	58% (35 mg/kg/d)	29% (9.7 mg/kg/d)	Clinical + 1-h video-EEG seizure free with no GTCS + no intolerable adverse effects
Coppola, et al (2004)[15]	Randomized, open-label, parallel	38	New-onset CAE + JAE: 3–13 yr	1 mo, 3 mo, 12 mo		53%, 63%, 68%, (25 mg/kg/d)	5%, 37%, 52%, (8 mg/kg/d)	Clinical + 24-h ambulatory EEG + 30-min video-EEG with HV
Martinovic (1983)[17]	Randomized, open–label, parallel	20	New-onset absences: 5–8 yr	12–48 mo	80%	70%		Clinical + EEG seizure free
Sato, et al (1982)[12]	Double-blind response-conditional crossover	45	GGE patients with absences: 4–18 yr Drug naive,[15] intractable[29]	12 wk	50%, 38%	75%, 37%		Clinical + 12-h EEG seizure free
Callaghan, et al (1982)[14]	Randomized, open-label, parallel	28	New-onset GGE: 5–15 yr	18–48 mo	57%	40%		Clinical + 6-h EEG

N, number of children; GGE, genetic generalized epilepsy; CAE, childhood absence epilepsy; JAE, juvenile absence epilepsy; FU, follow-up; yr, years; mo, months; wk, weeks; h, hours; N/A, not applicable.

Efficacy

Prior to the 1950s, phenobarbital and trimethadione were used with varying success and considerable side effects. Reasonable efficacy for absence epilepsies was first reported with ethosuximide in 1958 and subsequently a decade later with sodium valproate. Early studies of these drugs included small populations with varying severity of mixed seizure types and epilepsy syndromes.[12] A large observational cohort study of 75 children with CAE reported a positive response to initial monotherapy in 60% (31/50) for ETX and 75% (15/20) for VPA.[12]

Lamotrigine has been shown to be more effective than placebo in a responder enriched open label trial of children (age 2–16) with new onset absence epilepsy.[13] Twenty-eight children who became seizure free on LTG were subsequently randomized to be blindly weaned to placebo or remain on LTG. Sixty-two percent of the children on LTG remained seizure free compared to 22% of those weaned to placebo.[13] Subsequently a case series showed LTG eliminated absence seizures in 55% of 20 children with new onset CAE.

Until recently, there has been a lack of strong evidence to support the use of one first-line AED over another in CAE as there were only four randomized controlled trials comparing these AEDs (Table 21–2).[12,14–17] These trials had relatively small numbers and failed to show a significant difference between therapies; however, the confidence intervals were wide and important

differences could not be excluded.[12,14,15,17,18] In 2010, a large multicenter double-blind, randomized, controlled trial compared ETX, VPA and LTG in 453 children with CAE.[10] After 16–20 weeks of therapy, VPA and ETX were found to have similar efficacy and be superior to LTG (Table 21–2). The odds ratio with VPA versus ETX was 1.26 (95% confidence interval (CI), 0.8–1.98, $p = 0.35$), VPA versus LTG was 3.34 (95% CI 2.06–5.45, $p = 0.001$) and ETX versus LTG was 2.66 (95% CI 1.65–4.28, $p = 0.001$).[10] Although Coppola and colleagues reported that the efficacy for LTG increased over a 12-month period to approach that of VPA,[15] a recent large observational cohort study of 214 children with new onset GGE (aged 4–16 years) found that children were more likely to stay on VPA (89%) than LTG (69%) at 12 months follow-up due to lack of efficacy of LTG.[19]

Side-Effect Profiles

All three first-line AEDs are generally well tolerated in children with CAE. Common adverse effects reported by patients are often mild and do not require discontinuation[10,12,13,15,18] (Table 21–3). There was no significant difference in intolerable adverse effects requiring discontinuation of therapy between ethosuximide, valproic acid and lamotrigine in 453 children with CAE (Table 21–4).[10] Important differences have been reported in attentional effects of these drugs. Neuropsychiatric testing after 4 months of randomized therapy of

▶ **TABLE 21-3.** COMMON ADVERSE EFFECTS OF FIRST-LINE AEDS REPORTED IN 5% OR MORE OF CHILDREN WITH CAE

	Gastrointestinal	Neurological
Ethosuximide	Nausea, vomiting, stomach upset, poor appetite	Fatigue, somnolence, headache, hyperactivity, sleep disturbance, dizziness
Valproic acid	Nausea, vomiting, increased appetite, weight gain, stomach upset	Fatigue, hostility, personality change, sleep disturbance, hyperactivity, decrease in concentration, attentional difficulties, depression, memory problems headache
Lamotrigine	Increased appetite	Fatigue, headache, hyperactivity, hostility, personality change

Source: From Glauser TA, et al. Ethosuximide, valproic acid, and lamotrigine in childhood absence epilepsy. *N Engl J Med* 2010;362:790–799.

ethosuximide, valproate or lamotrigine in 453 children with CAE found significantly higher rates of attentional dysfunction in the children on valproic acid (49%) than those taking ethosuximide (33%) or lamotrigine (24%).[10]

Gastrointestinal effects of VPA are reduced by enteric-coated formulations and those children who are overweight at initiation of therapy are most likely to gain excess weight with this drug. Expert consensus has suggested that a fall in platelet count is not a reason to withdraw Valproate unless bruising or coagulation disorders are present. If the platelet count falls below 90,000 then close monitoring is recommended. There is concern regarding the teratogenetic potential and cognitive impact of fetal exposure to VPA. As the majority of the girls with CAE will have outgrown their epilepsy and be off AEDs prior to becoming sexually active this is less of an issue when making an AED choice in CAE than in the other GGEs.

Second-Line Therapeutic Options

If the initial AED is not effective a trial of another first-line AED should be made.[20] Replacing LTG with VPA or adding VPA to LTG can be difficult due to the complex interaction between VPA and LTG which can result in toxic levels of LTG. The degree of inhibition of the LTG clearance is independent of the dose of VPA. One option is to reduce the LTG by 50% as soon as VPA is introduced and then continue to decrease the LTG as

the VPA is increased. This scheme can still result in drug toxicity in some individuals. An alternative scheme is to abruptly discontinue LTG when VPA is initiated and to make quick increases over the next three days.

When monotherapy with LTG, VPA, or ETX is not effective, small case series have shown efficacy for combinations of VPA and ETX or VPA and LTG. Other therapeutic options for intractable CAE include newer AEDs that have shown effect in anecdotal reports. A small open label series of 5 children with CAE treated with topiramate reported some efficacy. Levetiracetam has been found to be effective at reducing absence seizures and GSW in animals, adults and children although these are uncontrolled reports with small numbers. A larger multicenter prospective open label study of 21 children with new onset CAE or JAE found that 52% of children were seizure free with no clinically significant adverse effects at 6 months of levetiracetam monotherapy.[21] A retrospective series reported seizure freedom in 51% of children with intractable absence seizures when treated with zonisamide.

Uncontrolled trials found acetazolamide effective in intractable CAE but tolerance and toxicity limit its use. Small studies, including an early placebo controlled clinical trial, reported clonazepam both as monotherapy or combined with VPA controlled absence seizures in both intractable and naïve patients however over 50% had side effects. There is little published data assessing clobazam in the treatment of absences. It has

▶ **TABLE 21-4.** INTOLERABLE ADVERSE EFFECTS RESULTING IN DISCONTINUATION OF AED IN CHILDREN WITH CAE

	Total (%)	Nervous System, Behavioral or Psychological	Digestive Disorders	Rash	Fatigue	Headache	Weight Increase	Laboratory Abnormality	Other
Ethosuximide (*N* = 154)	24	8	6	4	2	2	0	1	3
Valproic acid (*N* = 146)	24	14	4	1	3	1	3	1	3
Lamotrigine (*N* = 146)	17	6	2	3	1	2	1	1	3

Source: From Glauser TA, et al. Ethosuximide, valproic acid, and lamotrigine in childhood absence epilepsy. *N Engl J Med* 2010;362:790–799.

been recommended as it has a better side-effect profile and less tolerability than clonazepam.[8]

AEDs to Avoid

A double blind placebo controlled multicenter study showed gabapentin is not effective in CAE. Carbamazepine, phenytoin, vigabatrin and gabapentin have been associated with the development of absence status. There is evidence that carbamazepine, oxcarbazepine, phenytoin, and tiagabine are not effective in the GGEs and when used are a common reason why these epilepsies may appear intractable.

EEGs in Monitoring Therapy

As GSW impairs awareness and concentration and persisting absence seizures are associated with a poor prognosis,[9] many experts arrange a repeat EEG when the family report no seizures. An EEG with 5 minutes of HV is more reliable at detecting absence seizures and GSW than 6 hours of routine recording, so it is an effective way to assess control. In areas with insufficient resources for this, physicians can take comfort in that only 5% of children whom are seizure free by parental/teacher assessment and trials of office HV have persistent absence seizures on EEG.

Treatment Duration

There is also little evidence regarding duration of therapy in CAE. A prospective study of uncomplicated epilepsy found that persistent 3-Hz GSW after 6 months of therapy or irregular GSW at 1 year was associated with a higher relapse rate after discontinuation of therapy at 1 year in children with absence seizures. In another study of CAE, 45% relapsed when treated for 1 year compared to 27% treated for 3 years. Anecdotal reports suggest a high rate of successful AED discontinuation after 1 year of seizure freedom in children with CAE and good prognostic factors.[8] Therapy should probably be continued for 1–3 years depending on prognostic factors and EEG findings at 6 and 12 months.

The ideal method of tapering therapy has not been established. Expert opinions range from 6 weeks to 6 months with most feeling that 6 weeks is adequate for uncomplicated CAE with good prognostic indications. Some experts recommend an EEG 6 weeks after AED discontinuation looking for frequent spike-and-wave discharges.[8]

Referral Guidelines

The timing of referral to a pediatric neurologist will depend on the available resources. In some areas a child with simple CAE may see a pediatric neurologist at presentation. Children should be referred to a pediatric neurologist when: (1) the diagnosis is in doubt, (2) the seizures are not controlled by the first two medication trials, and (3) the child is not seizure free after 1 year.

PROGNOSIS AND OUTCOME

Children with CAE have a good prognosis. Most (65%) become and remain seizure free by 12 years of age (range 4–24 years), with the mean duration of epilepsy being 3.6 years.[1,5] A small proportion (7%–9%) have persistent absence seizures,[1,5,7] 13%–30% develop GTCS and 15% develop myoclonic seizures.[1,5] GTCS occur at a mean age of 20 years (range 10–30 years).[5] Prognostic factors are listed in Table 21–5. When recently proposed stricter criteria are used to define CAE,[7] higher terminal remission (82% vs. 51%) occurs. As these criteria exclude the majority of children presently diagnosed with CAE, they are perhaps more useful in selecting a good prognostic group rather than as diagnostic criteria.[2]

Children with CAE are in the normal cognitive range, but when compared to matched controls without epilepsy, have significantly lower full IQ scores.[22] Attentional problems are noted at presentation in a significant number of children and persist in children despite seizure cessation.[10,22] Compared to controls, children with CAE are significantly more likely to have linguistic difficulties (43%) and a psychiatric diagnosis (61%), particularly

▶ **TABLE 21–5.** FACTORS ASSOCIATED WITH PROGNOSIS FOR CAE

Outcome	Good Prognostic Factor	Poor Prognostic Factor
Remission	Age of onset <5 years[5]	GTCS[5]
	Response to first AED[15]	Myoclonic seizures[5]
	Response to AED within a year[1,5]	Cognitive difficulties at onset[5]
	Absence seizure duration >10 s	Absence status
		Generalized seizures in first degree relative[5]
		Polyspikes
Develop GTCS	Absence seizure duration >10 s	Age of onset >8 years[5]
	Posterior bilateral delta activity	Irregular spike and wave while awake

ADHD and anxiety disorders.[22] Longer duration of illness and seizure frequency were significantly associated with the presence of a psychiatric diagnosis in 69 children with CAE.[22] Children with CAE can also be left with long-term psychosocial difficulties.[9,22] This is often, but not exclusively seen in patients with persistent seizures and includes repeating school years, not completing high school, not going to university, heavy alcohol use, criminal convictions, unplanned pregnancies, and difficulties with relationships.[9]

► MYOCLONIC ABSENCE EPILEPSY (EMA)

EPIDEMIOLOGY

This rare syndrome is found in 0.5%–1% of children with epilepsy in a tertiary centre[23] and is defined by the presence of the characteristic seizure type of myoclonic absence seizures (MA). It was first described by Tassinari and colleagues in 1969. There have been several subsequent series but Bureau and Tassinari's 2005[23] follow-up of 53 children is the largest.

CLINICAL PRESENTATION

The onset of this syndrome is usually around 7 years of age (1–12 years).[23] The myoclonic absence seizures occur many times a day and are often precipitated by HV and awakening. IPS induces myoclonic absence seizures in 14% of cases.[23] Other seizure types occur in 66% of cases.[23] In one-third of cases these begin before the onset of myoclonic absence seizures and consist of rare GTCS and absence seizures without myoclonic jerks.[23] The other third of cases develop GTCS (45%), absences without myoclonic limb jerks (occasionally with mild eyelid movements) (4%), drops (33%), and absence status without myoclonias (17%) after the presentation of myoclonic absence seizures.[23] The vast majority of children only have two seizure types.

Just under half of affected children present with mental retardation prior to the seizures.[23] Potential etiological factors exist in 35% of cases at presentation and include prematurity, perinatal brain damage, and chromosomal abnormalities.[23] Mild diffuse cerebral atrophy is seen on MRI in 17%. A genetic component to the etiology is suggested as there is a family history of epilepsy (usually generalized) in 20%.[23]

Seizures

Myoclonic absence seizures are distinct from absence seizures in other GGEs. The main differentiating feature is the myoclonic jerks of the shoulders and arms. These prominent repetitive jerks are rhythmic and often associated with tonic contractions of the upper

arms resulting in the distinguishing progressive lifting of the arms during the seizure.[23] They are typically bilateral but may be unilateral or asymmetric[23] and are sometimes overlooked due to the tonic contraction or treatment decreasing the intensity. The mild repetitive myoclonic jerks of the eyelids seen in CAE are absent but perioral myoclonias and rhythmic jerks of the head and legs may occur. The degree of loss of awareness is variable but is often complete.[23] Seizures have an abrupt onset and offset as seen in the absence seizures in the other GGEs but are longer lasting from 10–60 seconds.

EEG

The EEG reveals normal background activity.[23] Interictally occasional GSW and polyspike and wave are seen and rarely focal or multifocal spike and wave.[23] These fragments of GSW are enhanced by sleep.[23] PBDA is not seen.[23] The ictal EEG shows rhythmic organized regular symmetrical 3-Hz GSW similar to that observed in CAE with generally abrupt onset and offset.[23,24] EMG recordings from the upper arm show a constant relationship between the bilateral myoclonia and the spike wave with a latency of 15–40 ms for the proximal muscles and 50–70 ms for the more distal muscles. This begins about 1 second after the initial spike. The shoulder and deltoid muscle then demonstrate tonic contractions.[23]

Differential Diagnosis

Differentiating EMA from other epilepsies can be challenging when: (1) the seizures clinically mimic the semiology of myoclonic absences such as seen in some chromosomal abnormalities and nonspecific epileptic encephalopathies, (2) the characteristic myoclonic aspects of the absences are overlooked and CAE or other GGE is mistakenly diagnosed, or (3) absences of other GGEs have mild clonic components. In these cases, video-EEG with simultaneous EMG recordings enables the diagnosis to be made.[23]

The diagnostic criteria for EMA is shown in Table 21–1.

TREATMENT

Criteria for Starting Treatment

Treatment is usually recommended as soon as the diagnosis is confirmed with EEG.

Optimal Treatment Regimen

No trials are available to guide therapy decisions. Standard first-line therapy used for absence seizures in CAE is only effective in 25% of cases.[24] Monotherapy with either VPA or ETX has not been found to be very effective in this syndrome. However, a report of six cases of early onset EMA found VPA monotherapy effective in 66% of cases. Anecdotal case reports and small series suggest that combinations of high dose VPA and ETX are most effective. It has been recommended that VPA plasma levels of 550–900 µmol/L and ETX at 500–770 µmol/L are necessary. Children with only MA and no other seizure types are most likely to respond to this combination.[23]

Early reports found that children with GTCS required the addition of high dose Phenobarbital or benzodiazepine but these therapies may have contributed to the poor cognitive outcome of these groups.[25] LTG has been reported to show benefit in some children[24] and does not seem to aggravate the myoclonias in this syndrome.[25]

A suggested therapeutic approach is to start VPA monotherapy, followed by the addition of ETX or LTG. Other combinations of these drugs should be the next option. If these do not work then other AEDs effective for absence seizures should be trialed (topiramate, levetiracetam, benzodiazepams, or zonisamide). Drugs that exacerbate absence seizures should be avoided and phenobarbital should only be used as a last treatment option.[25]

PROGNOSIS AND OUTCOME

Prognosis is often poor with resistance to therapy, mental deterioration and evolution to Lennox–Gastaut syndrome (13%).[25] Long-term follow-up of children with this syndrome (mean 13 years range 3–29 years) found that 38% of the children outgrew their epilepsy after a mean period of 5.5 years. This is more likely to occur if the child develops no other seizure type other than myoclonic absences plus or minus simple absence seizures (80% remission vs. 40% with other seizure types). A family history of epilepsy and other etiological factors are seen in both children who remit and those with a poor outcome.[23] Mental retardation develops in 25% of children, resulting in 70% of children eventually having mental retardation. Mental retardation is severer and more common in children in whom the epilepsy does not remit.[23] Previously it had been felt that adequate therapy with VPA and ETX while avoiding AEDs which exacerbate absence seizures predicted good prognosis however this has not been confirmed on further follow-up.[23] Cognitive function is always preserved in children in whom the myoclonic absences resolve quickly.

REFERENCES

1. Callenbach PM, et al. Long-term outcome of childhood absence epilepsy: Dutch study of epilepsy in childhood. *Epilepsy Research* 2009;83:249–256.
2. Sadleir LG, Farrell K, Smith S, Connolly MB, Scheffer IE. Electroclinical features of absence seizures in childhood absence epilepsy. *Neurology* 2006;67:413–418.
3. Dibbens LM, et al. Familial and sporadic 15q13.3 microdeletions in idiopathic generalized epilepsy: precedent for disorders with complex inheritance. *Human Molecular Genetics* 2009;18:3626–3631.
4. Mullen SA, Suls A, De Jonghe P, Berkovic SF, Scheffer IE. Absence epilepsies with widely variable onset are a key feature of familial GLUT1 deficiency. *Neurology* 2010;75:432–440.
5. Wirrell EC, Camfield CS, Camfield PR, Gordon KE, Dooley JM. Long-term prognosis of typical childhood absence epilepsy: remission or progression to juvenile myoclonic epilepsy. *Neurology* 1996;47:912–918.
6. Sadleir LG, Scheffer IE, Smith S, Carstensen B, Farrell K, Connolly MB. EEG features of absence seizures in idiopathic generalized epilepsy: impact of syndrome, age, and state. *Epilepsia* 2009;50:1572–1578.
7. Loiseau P, Duche B. Childhood absence epilepsy. In: Duncan JS, Panayiotopoulos CP (eds), *Typical Absences and Related Epileptic Syndromes.* London: Churchill Livingstone, 1995:152–160.
8. Camfield C, Camfield P. Management guidelines for children with idiopathic generalized epilepsy. *Epilepsia* 2005;46:112–116.
9. Wirrell EC, Camfield CS, Camfield PR, Dooley JM, Gordon KE, Smith B. Long-term psychosocial outcome in typical absence epilepsy: sometimes a wolf in sheeps' clothing. *Arch Pediatr Adolesc Med* 1997;151:152–158.
10. Glauser TA, et al. Ethosuximide, valproic acid, and lamotrigine in childhood absence epilepsy. *N Engl J Med* 2010;362:790–799.
11. Coppola G, Licciardi F, Sciscio N, Russo F, Carotenuto M, Pascotto A. Lamotrigine as first-line drug in childhood absence epilepsy: a clinical and neurophysiological study. *Brain Dev* 2004;26:26–29.
12. Sato S, White BG, Penry JK, Driefuss FE, Sackellares JC, Kupferberg HJ. Valproic acid versus ethosuximide in treatment of absence seizures. *Neurology* 1982;32:157–163.
13. Frank LM, et al. Lamictal (lamotrigine) monotherapy for typical absence seizures in children. *Epilepsia* 1999;40:973–979.
14. Callaghan N, O'Hare J, O'Driscoll D, O'Neill B, Daly M. Comparative study of ethosuximide and sodium valproate in the treatment of typical absence seizures (petit mal). *Dev Med Child Neurology* 1982;24:830–836.
15. Coppola G, Auricchio G, Federico R, Carotenuto M, Pascotto A. Lamotrigine versus valproic acid as first-line monotherapy in newly diagnosed typical absence seizures: an open-label, randomized, parallel-group study. *Epilepsia* 2004;45:1049–1053.
16. Glauser T, et al. ILAE treatment guidelines: Evidence-based analysis of antiepileptic drug efficacy and effectiveness as initial monotherapy for epileptic seizures and syndromes. *Epilepsia* 2006;47:1094–1120.
17. Martinovic Z. Comparison of ethosuximide and sodium valproate as monotherapies of absence seizures. In: Parsonage M, Grant RHE, Craig AG, Ward AW Jr (eds), *Advances in Epileptology: The XIVth Epilepsy International Symposium.* New York: Raven Press, 1983:301–305.
18. Posner EB, Mohamed K, Marson AG. A systematic review of treatment of typical absence seizures in children and

adolescents with ethosuximide, sodium valproate or lamotrigine. *Seizure* 2005;14:117–122.

19. Mazurkiewicz-Beldzińska M, Szmuda M, Matheisel A. Long-term efficacy of valproate versus lamotrigine in treatment of idiopathic generalized epilepsies in children and adolescents. *Seizure* 2010;19:195–197.

20. Wirrell E, Camfield C, Camfield P, Dooley J. Prognostic significance of failure of the initial antiepileptic drug in children with absence epilepsy. *Epilepsia* 2001;42:760–763.

21. Verrotti A, et al. Levetiracetam in absence epilepsy. *Dev Med Child Neurol* 2008;50:850–853.

22. Caplan R, et al. Childhood absence epilepsy: Behavioural, cognitive and linguistic comorbidities. *Epilepsia* 2008;49:1838–1846.

23. Bureau M, Tassinari CA. The syndrome of myoclonic absences. In: Roger J, Bureau M, Dravet C, Genton P, Tassinari CA, Wolf P (eds), *Epilepstic Syndromes in Infancy, Childhood and Adolecence*. Montrouge: John Libbey Eurotext Ltd., 2005; 4th edn: pp. 337–344.

24. Manonmani V, Wallace SJ. Epilepsy with myoclonic absences. *Arch Dis Child* 1994;70:288–290.

25. Genton P, Bureau M. Epilepsy with myoclonic absences. *CNS Drugs* 2006;20:911–916.

CHAPTER 22

Episodic Events Mimicking Seizures in Childhood and Adolescence

Lawrence W. Brown

▶ INTRODUCTION

Epilepsy has often been described as the great imitator with protean paroxysmal manifestations from sudden arousals out of sleep, to confusional states, to stiffening only when the individual arises and turns to one side and not the other. However, each of the behaviors listed previously (and many, many others) can be equally well explained in many individuals by nonepileptic mechanisms. According to the International League Against Epilepsy, imitators of epileptic seizures are defined not by the presentation but by the absence of abnormal and excessive neuronal discharges. The International League Against Epilepsy (ILAE) subdivides nonepileptic events into physiological disturbances with a non-epileptic mechanism such as syncope, sleep disorders, paroxysmal movements, transient global amnesia, and migraine as well as nonepileptic events of psychogenic origin (which may occur in the same patient with documented epileptic seizures).[1]

There is an expression in medicine that "all that wheezes is not asthma." Yet many parents and primary care physicians still assume that all paroxysmal events are epileptic in origin. This becomes even more problematic in high-risk individuals such as developmentally delayed toddlers with nocturnal arousals, academically challenged children who "zone out," or adolescents with syncope. It often comes as a shock to many observers that so many individuals admitted to an epilepsy-monitoring unit (EMU), even those with undisputed epilepsy, have a nonepileptic basis for the event in question. A recent series of 223 children referred to a specialized epilepsy center in Denmark found that 39% did not have epilepsy.[2] Even in a selected group from the Danish study where the referring physician was certain about the diagnosis of seizure disorder, fully 35% did not have epilepsy. It has also been demonstrated that there were occasional children diagnosed with medically refractory epilepsy who had a nonepileptic basis for their entire clinical syndrome.

The value of electroencephalographic (EEG) is indisputable, but nonspecific abnormalities or unrelated epileptiform features like rolandic spikes may be wrongly interpreted to explain confusional episodes, headaches, or attention deficit disorder. A positive response to clinical trials or antiepileptic medication may not always provide a definitive answer to the challenge of the etiology of paroxysmal behavior such as aggression, headache, or movement disorders. Certainly there are many antiepileptic drugs such as lamotrigine, carbamazepine, and oxcarbazepine that are used (off-label) for mood stabilization, and topiramate and valproate have been approved for migraine prophylaxis. While it has long been recognized that carbamazepine can induce tics, there are recent reports demonstrating the value of topiramate and levetiracetam for controlling symptoms of Tourette syndrome.

It is difficult to organize the imitators of epilepsy into a pathophysiologically based or clinically relevant schema. One could choose syndromes that occur primarily in sleep versus waking, disorders of early childhood or older childhood into adolescence, or paroxysmal disorders with presenting symptoms such as unusual movements or altered awareness, respiratory abnormalities, perceptual changes, or sudden behavioral alterations. This chapter will review the major imitators of epileptic seizures in children and try to combine and synthesize all of these approaches starting with sleep disturbances at different ages followed by movement disorders during the day, breathing abnormalities, and acute behavioral changes.

▶ MOVEMENT DISORDERS IN SLEEP

SLEEP MYOCLONUS

Sleep starts, also called massive hypnogogic myoclonus, is a normal phenomenon at the transition from wakefulness to sleep.[3] This is almost always unrecognized by the individual but commonly reported by parents or bed partners. It is unusual to have single hypnic jerks come to medical attention, but occasionally one sees repetitive, prominent jerking, or rarely injury from falling out of bed. The myoclonic jerks are of subcortical origin, and can be brought out by marked fatigue, stress, interaction with caffeine, or other stimulants. Reassurance that it is a normal phenomenon is all that is necessary, and no specific treatment is indicated beyond avoidance of known precipitants.

More persistent migratory myoclonus is also reported during light stages of non-rapid eye movement (non-REM) sleep, and it typically abates after the first hour as sleep staging descends into N3 (deep non-REM sleep). Asymmetric and asynchronous movements of the facial muscles, trunk, or extremities are more common with narcolepsy and periodic limb-movement disorder.

RLs AND PLMs

Restless legs (RLs) syndrome is an unusual phenomenon in children probably because it requires subjective reporting, but the associated objective finding of periodic limb movements (PLMs) can be found in children. PLMs have actually become a fairly common finding now that surface limb electromyography (EMG) electrodes have become a standard feature of pediatric polysomnography.

RLs syndrome is a common complaint in adults and is characterized by an uncomfortable, sometimes painful sensation in the extremities, usually more pronounced in the legs; it typically gets worse as the day progresses and peaks at night. Affected individuals report the inability to get comfortable and may walk around in an effort to relax. Often, the uncomfortable sensation and need to move around interferes with the ability to fall asleep or to achieve consolidated sleep. While uncommon in children, a detailed history can sometimes elicit the same complaint. Often it is attributed to "growing pains."

Most affected individuals have associated PLMs, especially children and adolescents.[4] PLMs are clusters of brief (0.5–5 seconds) movements of the extremities recurring every 10–60 seconds. These are usually subtle in children and rarely produce full awakening, but brief minor arousals are common and may contribute to sleep fragmentation with resultant daytime irritability and impaired concentration mimicking attention deficit hyperactivity disorder (ADHD).

While the pathophysiology of PLMs and RLs are incompletely understood, they may relate to dopaminergic dysfunction. Treatment usually consistent of repletion of low iron stores if found (dopamine hydroxylase requires an iron-containing cofactor). Dopaminergic agonists have become the first-line treatment otherwise, but benzodiazepines at bedtime can be used symptomatically, presumably working by decreasing arousability.

RHYTHMIC MOVEMENTS OF SLEEP

Rhythmic movements of sleep used be called *jactatio capitis nocturna* in recognition of the prominence of head banging, but legs or trunk are involved in many cases. It is felt to be a form of self-soothing that is most common in infants and typically disappears by 2–4 years of age. Typically starting in drowsiness, it may continue into light non-REM sleep.[5]

Rhythmic movement disorder of sleep is rarely confused with epilepsy. However, it becomes a problem when the motor symptoms are primarily described in the arousals from sleep rather than the typical self-soothing behaviors noted during drowsiness. It can also be quite challenging when rhythmic movements are found in children with developmental delay. Not only is the behavior more common in the disabled population but also it is often more severe and persists longer in the cognitively impaired population where the index of suspicion is already higher for epilepsy. Only in these situations have there been reports of serious injuries including subdural hematomas and even blindness.

NON-REM PARASOMNIAS

Most non-REM parasomnias occur during the first third of the night predominately, but not exclusively, during transition from the first or second cycle of deep non-REM (N3) sleep, and cluster between 1 and 3 hours after sleep onset. Typical presentations include sleep talking (somniloquoy), sleep walking (somnambulism), agitated arousals, and full-blown night terrors (*pavor nocturnus*).[6] Sleep talking is rarely confused with epilepsy, but sleep walking with complex automatic activity such as fidgeting and shuffling gait may be misinterpreted as a complex partial seizure, especially when it ends with return to sleep that mimics postictal unresponsiveness. Night terrors with agitated thrashing and screaming can look just like a partial seizure of frontal lobe origin, especially when there are no definable surface EEG abnormalities due to movement and muscle artifact or deep subcortical localization. All of the nonepileptic paradoxical arousals share a misperception and relative unresponsiveness to the environment, automatic behavior, and a variable degree of amnesia for the event. The EEG is characterized by muscle and motor artifact with persistence of slow (delta) activity of deep sleep or by a mixture of frequencies without features of full arousal.

Occasional confusional arousals are seen in the majority of normal preschoolers. Night terrors affect up to 6% of prepubertal children with a peak incidence of 5–7 years, while sleepwalking peaks at an older age (8–12 years).[7] Many children have a family history of similar events and support a hypothesis of genetic predisposition, although environmental factors from febrile illness, to emotional stress, sleep deprivation, or medications are often reported.[8] Anything that produces arousal at a vulnerable point in the sleep cycle can trigger typical motor patterns from forced awakenings to obstructive sleep,

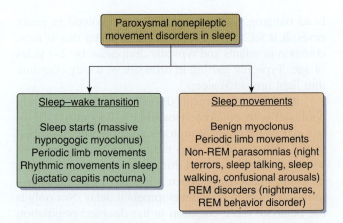

Figure 22–1. Paroxysmal nonepileptic movement disorders in sleep.

and conversely treating the underlying sleep disorder can make parasomnias disappear.[9] As with any behavior that can be caused by different etiologies, it is important to consider the rare possibility of refractory night terrors proven to have an epileptic mechanism.[10]

REM behavior disorder (RBD) is an unusual parasomnia in childhood, except in the few recognized cases associated with narcolepsy or brain stem pathology such as pontine gliomas.[11] In this condition, the usual muscular paralysis of REM is lost, and patients literally act out their dreams. RBD may be misinterpreted as hypermotor epileptic seizures. Pointing toward RBD is the presence of dream content, the lack of stereotyped movements, and any report of typical generalized tonic–clonic seizures.

Because seizures are always in the differential diagnosis, it is important to recognize the differences and similarities between seizures and parasomnias.[12]

While video-EEG is clearly the only way to definitively distinguish epileptic seizures from other "things that go bump in the night," there are certain features that can be helpful. Nocturnal seizures are usually stereotypic, are not limited to the first third of the night, occur most often out of lighter stages of non-REM sleep, and are usually associated with epileptiform EEG abnormalities (Fig. 22–1).

▶ NONEPILEPTIC PAROXYSMAL MOVEMENT DISORDERS

Nonepileptic paroxysmal movement disorders during wakefulness are a diagnostic challenge that can mimic seizures, and conversely there are epileptic seizures that are misinterpreted as movement's disorders. Abrupt paroxysmal, involuntary movements including chorea, athetosis, dystonia, and tics can be confused with seizures as well as disorders of impaired coordination such as tremor and paroxysmal ataxia.

PAROXYSMAL DYKINESIAS

Affected children have movement-induced attacks of brief dystonia, chorea, or ballismus, often brought out under stressful conditions.[13,14] Paroxysmal dystonic choreoathetosis (Mount Reback syndrome) often starts very early in infancy; it is usually an autosomal dominant disorder with relative brief attacks lasting a few minutes that can be brought out by fatigue, hunger, stress, caffeine, or alcohol. Paroxysmal kinesigenic choreoathetosis typically presents in childhood and often includes a brief sensory prodrome with paresthesias and dizziness. Attempts to swing a bat or to write on the blackboard in front of the class can cause the bat or the chalk to fly out of the child's hand. Events occur frequently, sometimes many times per day. Most cases are sporadic although occasionally it occurs in families or in the context of a prior neurological insult. These very brief events, usually lasting seconds, typically respond to sodium channel drugs like carbamazepine or phenytoin even though the EEG is always normal during the event. Recently, there have been genetic breakthroughs.

Paroxysmal nonkinesigenic dystonia may look similar, except that the episodes come on without apparent precipitation by movement and events last much longer (usually 10 minutes to 2 hours); most are autosomal dominant. Both types present more often with fatigue, stress, alcohol, and fatigue, Paroxysmal nonkinesigenic dystonia is harder to treat. It does not respond to the sodium channel drugs and there is only minimal success with benzodiazepines.

MYOCLONUS

Myoclonus is characterized by rapid, forceful, usually isolated, and nonrhythmic jerking movements. It is considered nonepileptic when the paroxysmal movements occur in the absence of an ictal EEG pattern and the patient has no other neurological signs and follows a benign course.

Nonepileptic myoclonus in older children can be a diagnostic challenge since it may occur in situations where epilepsy is also found. This includes following acute encephalopathies and in progressive degenerative disorders. When the movements are of cortical origin they can be considered myoclonic seizures, and the EEG will demonstrate spike or polyspike slow activity. Both cortical and subcortical myoclonus may respond to GABAergic drugs such as benzodiazepines or valproate.

TICS

Motor tics are stereotyped, repetitive movements of one or more muscle groups usually involving head, eyes, face, or neck.[15] Most children are fully alert and many are aware of the mannerisms. Unlike seizures, it is usually

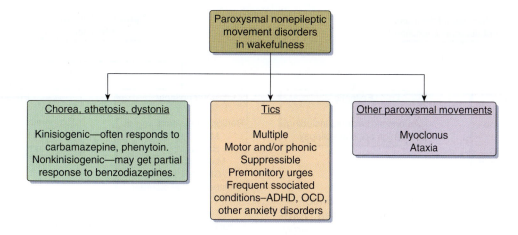

Figure 22–2. Paroxysmal nonepileptic movement disorders in wakefulness.

possibly to voluntarily inhibit tics, at least for brief periods of time. They are not often confused unless the mannerisms overlap with features more typical for seizures such as eye blinking with apparent loss of awareness to suggest nonconvulsive status epilepticus or prolonged unilateral twitching of an extremity to be confused with *epilepsia partialis continua.* A pediatric epilepsy monitoring unit will see the occasional child referred for such repetitive, stereotyped movements that "seize" the child and leave him without the ability to suppress the rapid blinking, motor activity, or "automatisms" and leave him exhausted as in a postictal stupor.

A history of waxing and waning pleomorphic mannerisms that evolve over time, associated ADHD symptoms that typically precede the tics (seen in more than 60%), anxiety disorders including obsessive compulsive disorder and a family history of tics and related neuropsychiatric disorders point strongly away from epilepsy and toward a developmental disorder of basal ganglia and its connections. However, there are children who will have both typical tics and evidence for epilepsy. For example, both tics and seizures are frequent in autistic spectrum disorders. Under these circumstances, one might well consider treatment with topiramate or levetiracetam, both of which have some support for efficacy in treating tics as well as being broad-spectrum antiseizure medications (Fig. 22–2).

► CYCLIC VOMITING, PAROXYSMAL VERTIGO, AND MOTION SICKNESS

These disorders of balance and autonomic function are usually straightforward in appearance and easy to diagnose. However, pediatric neurologists must be aware of the rare child whose symptoms are the presentations of autonomic seizures.

Cyclic vomiting is a disorder of clusters of vomiting, usually of unknown etiology that is most often seen in children 3–9 years of age. It usually starts in sleep or upon awakening, and it is associated with other signs of autonomic distress including abdominal pain, pallor, nausea, drooling, diarrhea, and lethargy. The diagnosis of cyclic vomiting is one of exclusion because many neurological, endocrine, metabolic, renal, and even surgical causes can produce the same features.

The most common neurological cause of repetitive nocturnal vomiting with autonomic features is Panyiotopoulos syndrome, or benign occipital epilepsy.[16] Migraine may be considered due to nonspecific headaches associated with light and sound sensitivity, but visual disturbances are rare. Cyclic vomiting looks very much like abdominal migraine, although other neurologically based mechanisms have been raised including mitochondrial disorders, channelopathies affecting critical brain regions for control of emesis such as the area postrema, deficits in intrinsic pathways involving the opioid system that can modulate brain stem vomiting control.

Treatment is symptomatic. Although neurologists are often asked to evaluate these children for possible abdominal epilepsy, a recent review of the literature was only able to find few documented cases who fulfill all criteria of otherwise unexplained gastrointestinal complaints (including laboratory tests, imaging, and endoscopy) symptoms of a central nervous system disturbance, abnormal EEG, and sustained improvement on antiseizure medication.[17]

Benign paroxysmal vertigo is the most common cause of true vertigo in children. It typically presents between 1 and 5 years of age with acute attacks of nausea, vomiting, pallor, diaphoresis, and nystagmus. The cause is unknown, but possibly related to either a predisposition for migraine or an imbalance in cochlear input since cold caloric testing often produces an uneven response.[18]

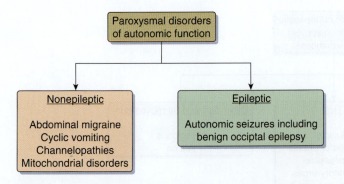

Figure 22–3. Paroxysmal disorders of autonomic function. Symptoms may include pallor, nausea, vomiting, drooling, diarrhea, pain, confusion, and lethargy.

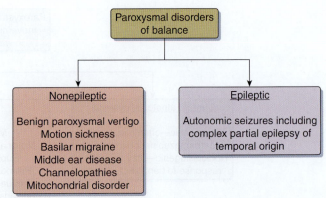

Figure 22–4. Paroxysmal disorders of balance. Symptoms may include pallor, nausea, vomiting, drooling, nystagmus, confusion, and lethargy.

Motion sickness is a response to the perception of movement, and it is more common in the absence of confirmatory visual input. While it can occur at any age, it is most common in young children age 4–10 years. In its typical presentation, there is abdominal distress, increased salivation, eructation, and the symptoms then progress to nausea, vomiting, pallor, and diaphoresis. It is more easily confused with seizures when the GI features are minimal and the clinical disturbance emphasizes initial generalized distress followed by sudden drowsiness, headache, and altered awareness (Fig. 22–3).

▶ MIGRAINE VERSUS OCCIPITAL EPILEPSY

Migraine and epilepsy are both common disorders of childhood with protean manifestations that can overlap with each other and cause confusion in diagnosis.[19] In addition, it is known that seizures can be precipitated by migraine in the susceptible individual in addition to vascular compromise from any cause including stroke. Also, headache may be part of the acute seizure or more often as a component of the postictal state. However, as similar as the two syndromes can appear, the mechanisms and treatment are distinctly different.

Occipital seizures can be confused with migraine if the manifestations include a combination of elementary visual hallucinations, ictal blindness, and headache. Visual phenomena with colored patterns or simple shapes that appear abruptly and last for only a few minutes or less indicate an epileptic etiology. This is the case even if the seizure semiology includes severe headache and vomiting. Occipital epilepsy also tends to occur frequently, sometimes, daily, while migraine is characterized by longer episodes lasting at least 30 minutes in children (and 1 hour in adults) and longer interval between attacks.

Basilar migraine of Bickerstaff presents in early childhood with frightening but transient symptoms of acute dizziness, vertigo, ataxia, diplopia, dysarthria, and other features pointing to brainstem or occipital disturbance. Visual symptoms are reported from flashing lights to "Alice in Wonderland" distortions of shape to tunnel vision, hemianopsia, or complete amaurosis.[20] These symptoms typically develop over a few minutes and can last up to 1 hour. Impaired consciousness is common, but unlike any acute seizure or postictal state, it builds up slowly and is rarely as profound. The child often has momentary alertness upon stimulation. Basilar migraine is generally infrequent, and the natural history is to disappear by school age or to evolve into typical pediatric migraine (Fig. 22–4).

▶ SYNCOPE

Syncope is a loss of postural tone or consciousness caused by transient decreased cerebral perfusion with spontaneous recovery.[21] Symptoms from loss of postural tone to unconsciousness, pallor, diaphoresis, and stiffening or myoclonic jerks can occur within seconds of inadequate blood flow to the brain. This can be caused by vascular or direct cardiac pathology, but most etiologies of syncope in childhood are neurally mediated. The presentation of syncope is mostly confused with drop attacks caused by atonic or tonic seizures, but prolonged syncope can also lead to clonic jerking that mimics generalized tonic–clonic seizures.

NEURALLY MEDIATED SYNCOPE

Vasovagal syncope, or simple faint, is seen when a susceptible child stands up too quickly or after prolonged standing, especially under conditions predisposing to peripheral vasodilatation like hot, enclosed, crowded situations such as church, following drug, or alcohol exposure, or under circumstances encouraging marked vagal tone with strong emotion, pain, or exposure to blood. Other features pointing to syncope include vagal stimuli such as micturition.

Distinguishing syncope from epileptic seizures may be challenging as urinary incontinence may be seen in approximately 10% and convulsive jerks in 50% of proven syncope.[13] Even an aura of epigastric rising, visual, or somatosensory sensations can be seen with syncope.[22] An EEG with interictal epileptiform features would point to epileptic mechanism while an electrocardiography (EKG) with arrhythmia or prolonged QT or a positive tilt test would indicate syncope as the correct etiology. Vagovagal syncope can be triggered by vomiting or repetitive swallowing, and prolonged bradycardia or asystole can produce similar convulsive twitching.

In the immediate period before syncope, children may report dizziness, anxiety, light headedness, weakness, yawning, and dimming of vision. During the full syndrome there is often a relatively slow fall. The presyncope syndrome can also alert the individual so he can usually get a position where injury can be avoided. Pallor, diaphoresis, and brief clonic twitching are common. However, this is "convulsive syncope" and not related to epilepsy; there are no epileptiform discharges of a cerebral seizure, and simultaneous EEG of an event will demonstrate only diffuse slowing. Even without benefit of video-EEG in the EMU, convulsive syncope can be strongly suspected by the consistent environmental circumstances precipitating the event, the dimming of vision as the only aura and the slow fall.

Vasovagal syncope is the most common presentation of neurally mediated syncope. It results from the combination of excess vagal tone, abnormal response to stress, venous pooling in the upright position, and impaired cardiac filling. Reflex bradycardia, a drop in blood pressure, or both leads to symptoms. When it begins in infancy, it is known as pallid breath holding, but the condition can occur at any age. Typical provoking causes include trivial head trauma, sudden scares, anticipation of pain, or the sight of blood. Any of these events can lead to bradycardia (even asystole) with consequent syncope. Pallid breath holding can occur in any position, and it is not whether the child is sitting or supine but rather the circumstance of venipuncture that is most important. This condition needs to be distinguished from cyanotic breath holding that is neither syncopal nor epileptic, but rather prolonged expiratory apnea most commonly brought about by anger or frustration.[23]

ORTHOSTATIC HYPOTENSION

Although position may not be important in pallid breathholding and an uncommon cause of syncope in children, chronic orthostatic intolerance is a common cause of symptoms in adolescents. Positional orthostatic tachycardia syndrome (POTS) has only recently been recognized; it can cause fatigue, exercise intoler-ance, dizziness and lightheadedness, palpitations, and true syncope.[24] There are also rare causes of primary autonomic failure of which familial dysautonomia is the most often encountered. It should be considered in all severe cases, even when there is no history of Ashkenazic Jewish background, but affected children almost always have a history of developmental delay, hypotonia, recurrent pneumonias, and frequent febrile illnesses.[25]

Other neurally mediated syncope can be caused by coughing, urination, or carotid sinus pressure. It is not uncommon for syncope to be produced by voluntary valsalva maneuver; this forceful exhalation against a closed glottis leads to increased vagal tone with bradycardia and reduced cardiac output. Particularly common in girls with Rett syndrome, this can be confused with seizures.[26]

CARDIOGENIC SYNCOPE

Syncope in a child with structural heart disease or other rhythm disorder, causing tachycardia or bradycardia, is a serious and confusing problem. Palpitations, shortness of breath, chest pain, and fatigue are rare in other etiologies for syncope. Cardiac-induced syncope can occur at any time of day including sleep, but is most common with strong emotion or physical exertion. Both tachy- and brady-arrhythmias can lead to syncope. Rapid heart rate can lead to inadequate ventricular filling and slow rates can lead to inadequate cardiac output. Causes of cardiogenic syncope included complete heart block, supraventricular tachycardia, fibrillation, mitral valve prolapse, aortic stenosis, and cardiac myopathy.

Long QT syndrome is an especially important cause of cardiogenic syncope that can closely mimic convulsive seizures.[27] The mechanism is ventricular tachyarrhythmia, often *torsade de pointes,* which is usually precipitated by strong emotion during exercise or during sleep. Several genetic syndromes involving potassium or sodium channels have been identified, and many drugs, particularly psychopharmacological agents such as the atypical neuroleptics can prolong the QT interval. Although an EKG rhythm strip is a routine part of most EEG recordings, a single-channel EKG is inadequate to diagnose many cases of potentially life-threatening syncope (Fig. 22–5).

▶ BORDERLAND

Although it is usually possible to make a definitive distinction between syncope and epilepsy, neurally mediated syncope can occasionally induce an EEG-proven clinical-electrographic generalized clonic seizure. This mechanism is different from a nonepileptic reflex anoxic seizure in which a few seconds of generalized clonic twitching corresponds to EEG slowing.

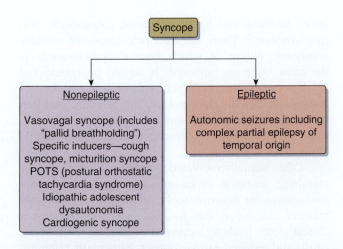

Figure 22–5. Syncope. Symptoms include pallor, diaphoresis, dizziness, and visual dimming, and may be associated with myoclonic jerks, stiffening, and clonic jerking. Workup includes EEG (normal except for ictal slowing, may show bradycardia or ictal asystole); EKG (may show arrhythmia or prolonged QTc); and positive tilt test. Triggers may include postural change, vomiting, or repetitive swallowing.

▶ PSYCHOGENIC NONEPILEPTIC SEIZURES

Children and adolescents with nonepileptic seizures (NESs) form a very challenging set of problems for neurologists. Conversion reactions are not immediately obvious, and the frightening presentation that mimics a prolonged generalized tonic–clonic seizure often leads to treatment with intravenous benzodiazepines whose sedative properties confirm the effectiveness of the approach to treat status epilepticus. Many children are given the diagnosis of epilepsy, and the underlying psychological issues may take a back seat to management with antiepileptic medications. Half of all cases in children in one report were on anticonvulsants when the proper diagnosis of NESs was made.[28]

It is nearly impossible to absolutely distinguish epileptic from nonepileptic convulsive seizures without simultaneous EEG. Clever and sophisticated patients may correctly surmise the convincing diagnostic criteria, especially after being questioned by multiple examiners. It is not hard to voluntarily bite one's tongue or to urinate at will. No clinician is so convinced of his powers as a medical detective to dismiss an otherwise obvious case of NES under such circumstances. One study of children found that focal CT or MRI abnormalities were seen in 37% of cases of NESs.[29] A family history of epilepsy, proven coexistence of epileptic seizures and EEG abnormalities have all been reported in patients with nonepileptic events with surprising frequency.[30–32]

Short of capturing typical events in the EMU, there are a number of clues that should raise concern for NESs from the circumstances precipitating the event to the variable semiology to the nonphysiological ictal examination.

NESs are typically found in stressful conditions such as fighting with parents or breaking up with a boyfriend or girlfriend. This is a weak criterion because stress can also precipitate epileptic events.

It is often possible to induce a NES.[33] While no longer considered ethical to inject colored saline to bring on an event and then to stop it with a different colored placebo, some children can be safely induced to have an event initiated and then terminated by simple suggestion while being monitored in the EMU. The combination of the circumstances, noncharacteristic movements, and preservation of normal EEG background is absolute proof of a nonepileptic basis.

It is most common for a NES to occur during wakefulness in the presence of witnesses. While it is not uncommon in epilepsy for seizures to be observed, it is more typical of NESs for events to begin as soon as someone enters the room and stop as soon as the witness departs.

There is often no stereotypic course of events in NESs, and one can sometimes see it wax and wane with attention and intervention, while the typical epileptic seizure is the same each time it occurs. Atypical characteristics such as asynchronous, asymmetric, and variable movements are not seen in epileptic seizures unless they occur during sleep (nocturnal partial seizures of frontal origin). Nocturnal seizures are usually very brief and last less than 30 seconds. Pelvic thrusting, flailing movements, and shifting laterality that last for minutes during wakefulness are only seen in NESs. True epileptic seizures almost always have eyes open with staring, supraversion, or deviation of gaze to one side; eyes are often closed in NES, and there may be resistance to passive eye opening. Indeed, it has been suggested that closed eyes during a convulsive event with loss of consciousness is "almost a certainty" of a nonepileptic basis.[34]

"Give way" weakness is common on examination in NES. Reactivity is often counterintuitive to what is expected in typical epileptic events. Responsiveness during active convulsive movements or marked variability in alertness in the immediate postictal period is not seen with cerebral seizures. In NESs one may see full awareness throughout, marked agitation with directed aggression or bizarre reactions such as whispered responses or wild movements. Occasionally one encounters a lack of concern (*la belle* indifference) in the interictal state as opposed to the hyperemotional reaction during and immediately following the attack.

Management of psychogenic NESs requires extreme sensitivity and tact. There may well be significant underlying emotional issues, although a history of physical

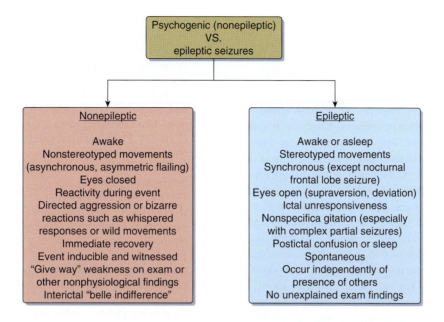

Figure 22–6. Psychogenic (nonepileptic) versus epileptic seizures. Beware: no definitive distinctions and may occur simultaneously in same patient.

or sexual trauma is far less reported in children than in adults. Many children have been treated for years with antiseizure drugs, and have lived with a diagnosis of refractory epilepsy; some have no evidence for actual epileptic seizures while others with dual pathology need to learn to distinguish events that have an electrocortical basis from those that are nonepileptic. A multidisciplinary approach including psychiatry and psychology as well as neurology is best prepared to successfully help a child and his family to deal with the diagnosis. Fortunately, experience has demonstrated that the prognosis of NESs in childhood can be quite positive when handled sensitively[28] (Fig. 22–6).

▶ CONFUSIONAL ATTACKS

Prolonged confusional episodes can be caused by nonconvulsive status epilepticus, but alternative etiologies are far more common, even in hospitalized children with acute encephalopathies. It is not possible to detail all of the causes of altered awareness from hypoglycemia to diabetic ketoacidosis, renal or hepatic failure, head trauma, infections from sepsis to meningoencephalitis, hypertensive encephalopathy, drug intoxication, etc. However, with the growing acceptance of long-term monitoring in the intensive care units, there has been new recognition of the role of nonconvulsive status epilepticus in medically complex children with any of the previously mentioned disorders as well as any patient whose neurological status compromises or cannot be evaluated due to treatment with sedatives or paralytic agents.[35]

▶ FUGUE STATES

This is a purely psychogenic state in which there is an acute traumatic origin of sudden loss of awareness, sometimes with substitution of an alternative identity. It is a diagnosis of exclusion after elimination of other causes of amnesia. While it may suggest willful malingering, there is a consensus that it is most often a form of dissociative state that results from overwhelming stress. This loss of awareness is usually relatively brief and followed by rapid improvement.[36]

▶ TRANSIENT GLOBAL AMNESIA

Transient global amnesia presents with sudden profound loss of both anterograde as well as frequent retrograde memory in the absence of other focal neurological abnormalities.[37] While uncommon in children, it may be more common if considered as an overlap between hemiplegic and basilar migraine. It was originally described in children with acute confusional states associated with agitation and aphasia, and attributed to migraine. It is more common in males who are agitated, restless, disorientated, or combative for minutes to hours. Following return to baseline, patients may be confused, disoriented, and unable to remember a preceding headache. There is often a strong family history of migraine. However, transient global amnesia is a diagnosis of exclusion, and encephalitis, drug intoxication, vasculitis, metabolic encephalopathies, and other etiologies must be eliminated before making the diagnosis in a child with an acute confusional state.[38]

▶ ZONING-OUT SPELLS

Although many children experience staring spells or periods of relative unresponsiveness, they are usually overlooked unless there are other questions raised about neurological or behavioral function. Almost all parents of a child with ADHD will admit to episodes where there is no response (earth to Johnny), he has to be called several times, and occasionally will not even answer if a hand is waved in front of his eyes or his shoulders are shaken.[39] Many children with autistic spectrum disorders will have such significant preoccupations with internal thoughts that they do not immediately respond. This can be even more likely to be confused with epilepsy when the unresponsiveness is associated with autistic stereotypies. Anxious children may withdraw into themselves with fears and concerns and go into "shutdown mode." Any child may become overwhelmed, bored, or drowsy.

What connects all of these events in distinction to an absence seizure or complex partial seizure is voluntary removal from social interaction or involuntary internal preoccupation or normal sleep. If lucky, one can get the child to describe what is going on in his head while apparently unaware, such as a child with Asperger syndrome who admits that he imagines planning cities because "it is more interesting than what the teacher is saying." Often the circumstances are obvious like a linkage to a specific challenging class or on days following a particularly poor night's sleep. There is no aura, associated eye flutter, myoclonus, or automatisms, and postictal headache or confusion is not reported. Long-term monitoring may be very helpful in the differential diagnosis of this type of spell.[40,41]

▶ CONCLUSIONS

It is essential to differentiate the basis of paroxysmal events in children. The same appearance of convulsive events, movement disorders, syncope, sleep disruption, and many other sudden episodes can be produced by epileptic or other mechanisms. It is critically important to avoid mislabeling nonepileptic events, and conversely it is equally important to recognize potentially life-threatening nonepileptic events such as one of the prolonged QT syndromes.

REFERENCES

1. ILAE Commission Report. The epidemiology of the epilepsies: future directions. International League Against Epilepsy. *Epilepsia* 1997;38:614–618.

2. Stroink H, et al. The accuracy of the diagnosis of paroxysmal events in children. *Neurology* 2003;60:979–982.

3. Tinuper P, et al. Movement disorders in sleep: guidelines for differentiating epileptic from non-epileptic motor phenomena arising from sleep. *Sleep Med Rev* 2007;11:255–267.

4. Simikajornboon M, Kheirandish-Gozal L, Gozal D. Diagnosis and management of restless legs syndrome in children. *Sleep Med Rev* 2009;13:149–156.

5. Hoban TF. Rhythmic movement disorders in children. *CNS Spectrums* 2003;8:135–138.

6. Mahowald MW, Borneman MC, Schenck CH. Parasomnias. *Semin Neurol* 2004;24:283–292.

7. Ohayon MM, Guilleminault C, Priest RG. Night terrors, sleep walking and confusional arousals in the general population: their frequency and relationship to other sleep and mental disorders. *J Clin Psychiatry* 1999;60: 268–276.

8. Hublin C, Kaprio J. Genetic aspects and genetic epidemiology of parasomnias. *Sleep Med Rev* 2003;7:413–421.

9. Guilleminault C, et al. Sleepwalking and sleep terrors in prepubertal children: what triggers them? *Pediatrics* 2003; 111:17–25.

10. Lombroso CT. Pavor nocturnus of proven epileptic origin. *Epilepsia* 2000;41:1221–1226.

11. Stores G. Rapid eye movement sleep behaviour disorder in children and adolescents. *Dev Med Child Neurol* 2008; 50:728–732.

12. Sheldon SH, Jacobsen J. REM–sleep motor disorder in children. *J Child Neurol* 1998;13:257–260.

13. Obeid M, Mikati MA. Expanding spectrum of paroxysmal events in children: potential mimickers of epilepsy. *Pediatr Neurol* 2007;37:309–316.

14. Zorzi G, et al. Paroxysmal dyskinesias in childhood. *Pediatr Neurol* 2003;28:168–172.

15. Brown LW. Tourette syndrome. In: Burg FD, Ingelfinger JR, Polin RA, Gershon A (eds), *Current Pediatric Therapy 18.* Philadelphia: WB Saunders Co., 2006.

16. Covanis A. Panyiotopoulos syndrome: a benign childhood autonomic epilepsy frequently imitating encephalitis, syncope, migraine, sleep disorder or gastroenteritis. *Pediatrics* 2006;118:e1237–e1243.

17. Zinkin NT, Peppercorn MA. Abdominal epilepsy. *Best Pract Res Clin Gastroenterol* 2005;19:263–274.

18. Calder J. Benign paroxysmal vertigo of childhood: a long-term follow-up. *Cephalgia* 1994;14:395.

19. Panayiotopoulis CP. Visual phenomena and headache in occipital epilepsy: a review, a systematic study and differentiatijn from migraine. *Epileptic Disord* 1999;1:206–216.

20. Evans RW, Rolak LA. The alice in wonderland syndrome. *Headache* 2004;44:624–625.

21. Kapoor WN. Syncope. *N Engl J Med* 2000;343:1856–1862.

22. Benke T, Hochleitner M, Bauer G. Aura phenomena during syncope. *Eur Neurol* 1997;37:28–32.

23. Stephenson JBP. Episodes in neonates, infants and toddlers mimicking epilepsy (in this book)

24. Medow MS, Stewart JM. The postural tachycardia syndrome. *Cardiol Rev* 2007;15:67–75.

25. Gold-von Simson G, Axelrod FB. Familial dysautonomia: update and recent advances. *Curr Probl Pediatr Adolesc Health Care* 2006;36:218–237.

26. Glaze DG, Schultz RJ, Frost JD. Rett syndrome: characterization of seizures versus non-seizures. *Electroencephalogr Clin Neurophysiol* 1998;106:79–83.

27. Friedman MJ, Mull CC, Sharieff GQ, Tsarouhas N. Prolonged QT syndrome in children: an uncommon but potentially fatal entity. *J Emerg Med* 2003;24:173–179.

28. Lancman ME, et al. Psychogenic seizures in children: long-term analysis of 43 cases. *J Child Neurl* 1994;9:404–407.

29. Metrick ME, et al. Nonepileptic events in childhood. *Epilepsia* 1991;32:322–328.

30. Guberman A. Psychogenic pseudoseizures in non-epileptic patients. *Am J Psychiatry* 1982;27:401–404.

31. Devinsky O, et al. Clinical profile of patients with epileptic and nonepileptic seizures. *Neurology* 1996;46:1530–1533.

32. Reuber M, et al. Interictal EEG abnormalities in patients with psychogenic nonepileptic seizures. *Epilepsia* 2002;43:1013–1020.

33. Devinsky O, Fisher R. Ethical use of placebos and provocative testing in diagnosing non-epileptic seizures. *Neurology* 1996;47:866–870.

34. Panayiotopolous CP. Imitators of epileptic seizures. In: *A Clinical Guide to Epileptic Syndromes and their Treatment, Second edition.* London: Springer-Verlag, 2007; pp. 79–117.

35. Jette N, Claassen J, Emerson RG, Hirsch LJ. Frequency and predictors of non-convulsive seizures during continuous electroencephalographic monitoring in critically ill children. *Arch Neurol* 2006;63:1750–1755.

36. Kopelman MD, Panayiotopolous CP, Lewis P. Transient epileptic amnesia differentiated from psychogenic "fugue" neuropsychological, EEG and PET findings. *J Neurol Neurosurg Psychiatry* 1994;57:1002–1004.

37. Quinette P, et al. What does transient global amnesia really mean? Review of the literature and thorough study of 142 cases. *Brain* 2006;129:1640–1658.

38. Amit R. Acute confusional state in childhood. *Child Nerv Syst* 1988;4:255.

39. Schubert R. Attention deficit disorder and epilepsy. *Pediatr Neurol* 2005;32:1–10.

40. Carmant L, et al. Differential diagnosis of staring spells in children: a video-EEG study. *Pediatr Neurol* 1996;14:199–202.

41. Kotagal P, Costa M, Wylie E, Wolgamuth B. Paroxysmal nonepileptic events in children and adolescents. *Pediatrics* 2002;110:e46(1–5).

SECTION IV

Seizures in Adolescence

CHAPTER 23

Juvenile Myoclonic Epilepsy

Beatriz G. Giráldez, Ainhoa Marinas, and Jose M. Serratosa

▶ OVERVIEW

Juvenile myoclonic epilepsy (JME) is a common epilepsy syndrome classified as a type of idiopathic generalized epilepsy (IGE).[1] The syndrome is also known as *impulsiv petit mal* or the syndrome of Janz.[2] JME represents approximately 10% of all epilepsies. Seizures typically begin in early adolescence, most often between the ages of 12 and 18 years, with a mean age of onset of 14 years.

The main characteristic symptom is sudden, mild to moderate myoclonic jerks that appear more frequently in shoulders and arms, although they can also affect neck or legs. They typically occur early after awakening. Consciousness is either not impaired or very briefly and mildly affected. Myoclonic jerks are the only seizure type in 5% of JME patients. More than 90% of patients have generalized tonic–clonic or clonic–tonic–clonic seizures,[3] and a third also have absences.[3,4] Myoclonic jerks precede the onset of generalized tonic–clonic seizures in almost half the patients. Common precipitating factors for seizures are sleep deprivation, alcohol intake, and fatigue.

Although results of treatment in JME are often excellent, recurrence of seizures occurs in up to 90% of the patients after withdrawal of antiepileptic drugs (AEDs).[4,5] Therefore, JME is considered a lifelong disorder and discontinuation of therapy is generally not recommended, even after long seizure-free periods.

▶ DIAGNOSTIC CRITERIA

The diagnosis of JME is made from the clinical history and electroencephalographic (EEG) findings. A detailed clinical history can suggest the diagnosis of JME. The interview should focus on the presence of myoclonic jerks, specifically whether they result in dropping or throwing things in the morning, soon after awakening. A detailed and careful family history should also be obtained in order to reveal any history of myoclonic jerks or the presence of any IGE syndrome.

The neurologic examination in JME is normal. This feature helps to distinguish JME from the progressive myoclonus epilepsies because of the lack of progressive neurologic deterioration, dementia, and ataxia.[6] Patients with JME have been found to be somewhat immature, emotionally unstable, and disinhibited.[7,8] Neuropsychological studies reveal that JME patients have serious impairments in frontal functions, meaning deficits in cognitive processes involved in planning, concept formation, elaborating strategies for the attainment of immediate or future goals, and verbal fluidity.[9] Psychiatric disorders have been described in 47% of the JME patients at any time of life and the substantially increased number of personality disorders might be attributed to frontal lobe deficits.[10]

Routine magnetic resonance imaging (MRI) studies are normal in JME and therefore rarely indicated. Quantitative MRI studies reveal cortical gray matter atrophy in the frontal and temporal lobes as well as subcortical gray matter volume increases in the superior mesiofrontal regions and progressive thalamic atrophy. These findings support the pathophysiological concept of JME as a disorder of thalamocortical circuits.[11,12]

The EEG is the most valuable test in the diagnosis of JME. An EEG performed in the morning in comparison with an afternoon session[13] or an EEG record after

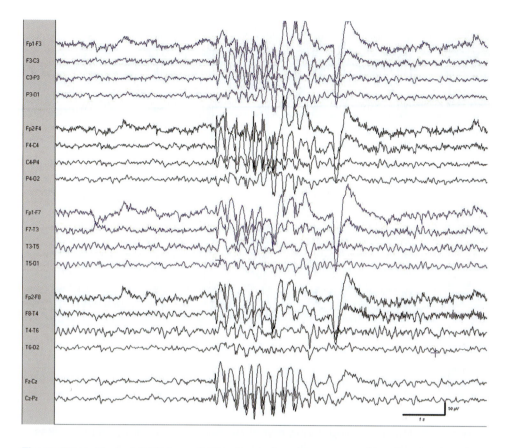

Figure 23–1. Typical EEG in a JME patient showing a normal background and a bilateral, symmetric and synchronous, 4-Hz polyspike-wave discharge.

sleep deprivation will yield a higher rate of abnormalities. However, continuous video-EEG monitoring provides definitive diagnosis. The characteristic interictal EEG pattern of JME consists of bilateral, symmetric, and synchronous discharges of 3.5–6-Hz polyspike-wave complexes (Fig. 23–1). The resting awake EEG background activity is uniformly normal with a well-developed alpha rhythm of 10–11 Hz.

The EEG correlate of the myoclonic jerks is a burst of medium to high amplitude 10–16-Hz polyspikes followed by irregular 1–3-Hz slow waves of different amplitude (Fig. 23–2). The bilateral symmetric polyspikes have maximum amplitude in frontal and central regions and are much less synchronized and regular than the classic 3-Hz spike-wave complexes seen in childhood absence epilepsy. A diffuse discharge of irregular 2–5-Hz spike-wave complexes may precede the multispike discharge.[4] The usual EEG pattern of 1–10 seconds may last longer than the clinical seizure. Photosensitivity or the precipitation of bilaterally synchronous spike-wave patterns by intermittent photic stimulation is common in JME.[14] Intermittent photic stimulation may also induce myoclonic jerks. Focal EEG abnormalities are described in as many as 30%–50% of the JME patients[15,16] (Fig. 23–3).

JME should be distinguished from the progressive myoclonus epilepsies, other primary generalized epilepsies, such as epilepsy with myoclonic absences, epilepsy with grand mal seizures on awakening, and partial epilepsies with focal motor seizures.

Not infrequently, JME, childhood absence epilepsy, and epilepsy with grand mal seizures on awakening occur in the same patient at different times in life. For example, childhood absence epilepsy may evolve to JME during adolescence.

► WHEN TO START TREATMENT

JME carries an excellent prognosis as treatment with AEDs will control seizures in the majority of patients. The condition should be treated as soon as a diagnosis is made unless the only symptom is rare or stimuli-related myoclonic seizures. In this case, avoiding precipitants and careful followup may be appropriate.

► OPTIMAL TREATMENT REGIMEN

Optimal management of the patient with JME should include not only selection of an appropriate AED but

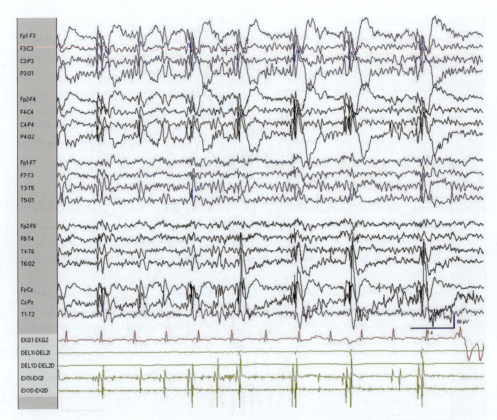

Figure 23–2. Ictal recording during myoclonic seizures: generalized polyspikes synchronous with muscle contractions are followed by a slow wave.

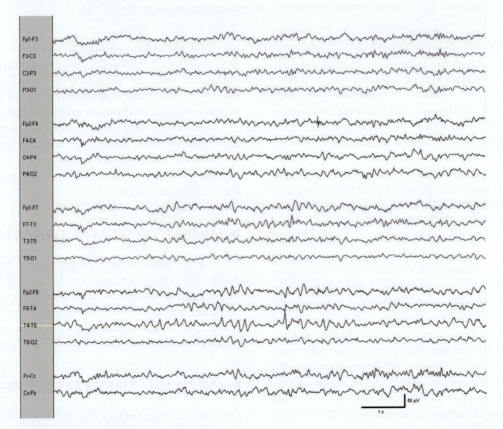

Figure 23–3. Focal abnormalities in JME: right temporal sharp wave abnormality during stage I sleep.

also control of precipitating factors and prevention of accidents and injuries in case of generalized tonic–clonic seizures. Patients with JME should be encouraged to establish regular sleep–wake cycles and avoid precipitating factors such as alcohol or illegal drugs and excessive fatigue. Patients with seizures precipitated by visual stimuli should avoid flickering lights or similar stimuli. Patients should be informed about the need for drug compliance and the risks of recurrence after drug withdrawal so that expectations will be realistic.

▶ PHARMACOLOGIC TREATMENT

The selection of a particular AED to start treatment in a patient with JME is challenging (Fig. 23–4). The final decision relies on finding a balance between the best efficacy and the least-adverse effects expectation. The latter needs to take into consideration not only the known adverse effects of the chosen drug but also the gender and comorbidities of the patient (i.e., migraine, obesity, or mood disorders).

Since most of the evidence of the effectiveness of the classic AEDs in JME comes from case series and retrospective studies, the selection of a specific AED to start treatment has largely relied on personal experience and preferences of the treating physician. To date, a few randomized clinical trials (RCTs) have studied the efficacy of the newer AED in specific types of generalized seizures, thus including heterogeneous groups of patients, some of them with JME (Table 23–1). However, data from RCTs, specifically designed to study the efficacy of AEDs in a selective population of JME patients, are still lacking.

VALPROIC ACID

Valproic acid is effective in 86%–90% of JME patients.[4,17] It continues to be the drug of choice for treating the generalized epilepsies[18] effectively controlling several seizure types as myoclonic, tonic–clonic, clonic–tonic–clonic, and absence seizures.

Therapeutic doses range from 20 to 30 mg/kg per day, but lower doses of 500 mg per day with extended-release valproic acid may also be effective.[19] Patients on valproic acid monotherapy usually require a lower dose than those on polytherapy. At present a dose–response or concentration–response relationship has not been established. In one study, the authors found that increasing dosages from 1000 to 2000 mg per day did not improve seizure control.[20]

Valproic acid is generally well tolerated. However, some of its adverse effects are of great concern when considering that patients are mostly adolescents and individuals in their early twenties. Weight gain, tremor,

hair loss, menstrual irregularities, polycystic ovarian syndrome, or risk of teratogenicity in childbearing aged women are typically drug use-limiting adverse effects. Doses of valproic acid should not exceed 1000 mg per day in women of childbearing age. Recently, Meador et al.[21] reported that in utero exposure to valproate, as compared with other commonly used antiepileptic drugs, is associated with an increased risk of impaired cognitive function at 3 years of age. This effect appears to be dose related.

LAMOTRIGINE

In monotherapy, lamotrigine is not superior to valproic acid to control seizures in the generalized epilepsies.[5,18] However, given its better tolerance and low risk of teratogenicity it may be a good alternative, particularly in young women. It has shown efficacy to control primary generalized tonic–clonic seizures as add-on therapy[22] and data from retrospective studies suggest that the combination of valproic acid and lamotrigine helps control seizures in some refractory patients.[5,23] Concerns about rash and the possibility of aggravating myoclonic seizures in some patients may limit the use of lamotrigine in JME.[24] Lamotrigine levels are largely diminished during pregnancy resulting in an increased risk for breakthrough seizures and a need for continuous dose adjustments to maintain seizure control during pregnancy.

TOPIRAMATE

Topiramate may have a role in treating JME although it seems to be more effective in controlling primary generalized tonic–clonic seizures and has a low effect in controlling absences or myoclonic jerks.[25–27] However, side effects associated with topiramate may preclude its use reserving it for drug-resistant patients.[18,28]

LEVETIRACETAM

Levetiracetam has been shown to be as effective as adjunctive therapy in controlling both primary generalized tonic–clonic and myoclonic seizures in patients with uncontrolled IGE.[29,30] Evidence from open-label trials supports the efficacy of levetiracetam monotherapy both in newly diagnosed patients[31] and in patients with a previous suboptimal control with valproic acid.[32] Levetiracetam has also been shown to be effective in decreasing epileptiform EEG abnormalities and suppressing the photoparoxysmal response (PPR) in JME patients.[33] Increasing accumulated experience on the efficacy and safety profile of levetiracetam in children and adults makes it an attractive alternative to valproic acid as a first-line option for the treatment of JME.

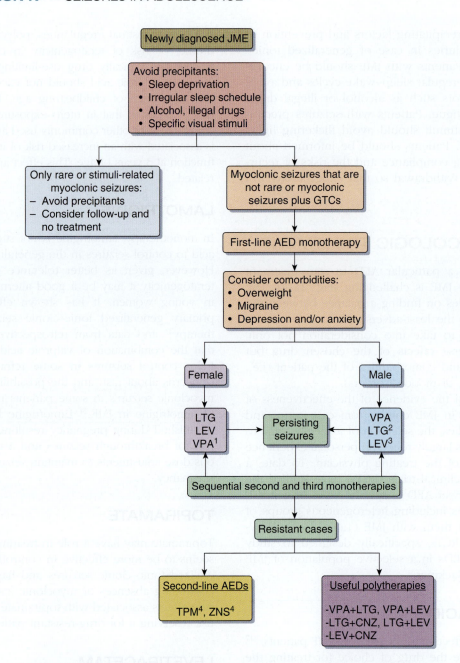

Figure 23–4. Management algorithm. AEDs, antiepileptic drugs; CNZ, clonazepam; GTCS, generalized tonic–clonic seizure; LEV, levetiracetam; LTG, lamotrigine; TPM, topiramate; VPA, valproic acid; ZNS, zonisamide. [1]Risk of teratogenicity and cognitive impairment in utero-exposed infants. Consider after other first-line AEDs failure. [2]May worsen myoclonic seizures. [3]May worsen psychiatric comorbidities. [4]May be beneficial for patients with migraine and/or overweight.

ZONISAMIDE

Despite the lack of controlled studies and experience with zonisamide in Europe, data from open-label studies and experience with zonisamide in Japan indicate that this broad-spectrum antiepileptic drug may be effective in JME.[34,35]

CLONAZEPAM

In patients with uncontrolled jerks, clonazepam can be added to valproic acid or other first-line AED. Clonazepam alone is not effective, as it controls only the myoclonic jerks and not the generalized tonic–clonic seizures.[36] If used alone, it may suppress the jerks that

▶ **TABLE 23-1.** RCTs OF NEW AEDS IN GENERALIZED SEIZURES

AED	Trial Design	Age (years)	Epilepsy Syndrome	Seizure Type	Number of Patients[2]	Number of JME Patients	References
LTG	Adjunctive RCT[1]	2–55	Idiopathic Generalized epilepsy	GTCS	117	[b]	Biton et al, 2005 (22)
TPM	Adjunctive RCT[1]	3–59	Idiopathic Generalized epilepsy	GTCS	80	[b]	Biton et al, 1999 (25)
LEV	Adjunctive RCT[1]	4–65	Idiopathic Generalized epilepsy	GTCS	164	[b]	Berkovic et al, 2007 (29)
	Adjunctive RCT[1]	12–65	Idiopathic Generalized epilepsy with myoclonic seizures	Myoclonic seizures	120	120[a]	Noachtar et al, 2008 (30)
VPA, LTG, TPM	Monotherapy RCT Unblinded	>5	Idiopathic Generalized epilepsy Unclassified epilepsy	[b]	716	129	Marson et al, 2007 (18)

AEDs, antiepileptic drugs; GTC, generalized tonic–clonic seizure; LTG, lamotrigine; LEV, levetiracetam; VPA, valproic acid; TPM, topiramate; RCT, randomized controlled trial.
[1]Double-blinded, controlled with placebo clinical trials.
[2]Only randomized patients are indicated.
[a]Eight patients originally diagnosed as Juvenile absence epilepsy.
[b]Data not provided in the study.

herald a generalized tonic–clonic seizure and may not allow the patient to prepare himself for this type of attack.

OTHER DRUGS

Ethosuximide may be added to valproic acid in JME patients with uncontrolled absences. Acetazolamide has been favored by some authors in patients with JME and refractory generalized tonic–clonic seizures or tolerability problems.[37] According to these authors, acetazolamide does not control myoclonic jerks as well as valproic acid, but does effectively control generalized tonic–clonic seizures and is a useful adjunct to valproic acid in resistant cases.

Phenytoin, phenobarbital, or primidone, when added to valproic acid may be useful in resistant cases. When used in monotherapy, control rates are much less than with valproic acid. Before valproic acid was in the market, primidone as a single drug was the drug of choice for treating JME.

Carbamazepine, vigabatrin, tiagabine, and gabapentin[38,39] have all been associated with absence and myoclonic status epilepticus in patients with idiopathic generalized epilepsies and should be avoided in JME patients.

NONPHARMACOLOGICAL TREATMENT

The value of vagus nerve stimulation (VNS) for treating patients with drug-resistant IGE is not well doc-

umented. However, preliminary data from case series and small open-label studies indicate that adjunctive VNS therapy may be a favorable treatment option in refractory idiopathic generalized epilepsies, including JME. Kostov et al[40] reported a total seizure reduction of 61% in 12 patients with drug-resistant generalized seizures after adjunct VNS. Maximal efficacy was achieved in generalized tonic–clonic seizures with a 62% reduction with respect to the preimplantation period, but significant reduction in absences and myoclonic seizures was also found (58% and 40%, respectively). Adverse effects were mild and generally transient.

REFERENCES

1. Commission on Classification and Terminology of the International League against Epilepsy. Proposal for revised classification of epilepsies and epileptic syndromes. *Epilepsia* 1989;30:389–99.
2. Janz D. *Die Epilepsien.* Stuttgart: Georg Thieme; 1969.
3. Salas Puig J, Tuñón A, Vidal JA, Mateos V, Guisasola LM, Lahoz CH. Janz's juvenile myoclonic epilepsy: a little-known frequent syndrome. A study of 85 patients. *Med Clin (Barc)* 1994;103(18):684–689.
4. Delgado-Escueta AV, Enrile-Bacsal F. Juvenile myoclonic epilepsy of Janz. *Neurology* 1984;34:285–294.
5. Nicolson A, Appelton RE, Chadwick DW, Smith DF. The relationship between treatment with valproate, lamotrigine, and topiramate and the prognosis of the idiopathic generalised epilepsies. *J Neurol Neurosurg Psychiatry* 2004;71:75–79.
6. Berkovic SF, Andermann F, Carpenter S, Wolfe LS. Progressive myoclonus epilepsies: specific causes and diagnosis. *N Engl J Med* 1986;315:296–305.

7. Janz D. Epilepsy with impulsive petit mal (juvenile myoclonic epilepsy). *Acta Neurol Scand* 1985;72(5):449–459.

8. Hommet C, Sauerwein HC, De Toffol B, Lassonde M. Idiopathic epileptic syndromes and cognition. *Neurosci Biobehav Rev* 2006;30(1):85–96.

9. Piazzini A, Turner K, Vignoli A, Canger R, Canevini MP. Frontal cognitive dysfunction in juvenile myoclonic epilepsy. *Epilepsia* 2008;49(4):657–662.

10. Trinka E. Psychiatric comorbidity in juvenile myoclonic epilepsy. *Epilepsia* 2006;47(12):2086–2091.

11. Tae WS, et al. Cortical thickness abnormality in juvenile myoclonic epilepsy. *J Neurol* 2008;255(4):561–566.

12. Kim JH, Lee JK, Koh SB, Lee SA, Lee JM, Kim SI, Kang JK. Regional grey matter abnormalities in juvenile myoclonic epilepsy: a voxel-based morphometry study. *Neuroimage* 2007;37(4):1132–1137.

13. Labate A, Ambrosio R, Gambardella A, Sturniolo M, Pucci F, Quattrone A. Usefulness of a morning routine EEG recording in patients with juvenile myoclonicepilepsy. *Epilepsy Res* 2007;77(1):17–21.

14. Janz D. Juvenile myoclonic epilepsy. In: Dam M, Gram L (eds), *Comprehensive Epileptology*. New York: Raven Press, 1990; pp. 171–185.

15. Lombroso C. Consistent EEG focalities detected in subjects with primary generalized epilepsies monitored for two decades. *Epilepsia* 1997;38:797–812.

16. Aliberti V, Grunewald RA, Panayiotopoulos CP, Chroni E. Focal electroencephalographic abnormalities in juvenile myoclonic epilepsy. *Epilepsia* 1994;35:287–301.

17. Penry JK, Dean JC, Riela AR. Juvenile myoclonic epilepsy: long-term response to therapy. *Epilepsia* 1989;30(Suppl 4):S19–S23.

18. Marson AG. The SANAD study of effectiveness of valproate, lamotrigine, or topiramate for generalised and unclassifiable epilepsy: an unblinded randomised controlled trial. *Lancet* 2007;369:1016–1026.

19. Karlovassitou-Koniari A, et al. Low dose of sodium valproate in the treatment of juvenile myoclonic epilepsy. *J Neurol* 2002;249(4):396–399.

20. Sundqvist A, Tomson T, Lundkvist B. Valproate as monotherapy for juvenile myoclonic epilepsy: dose-effect study. *Ther Drug Monit* 1998;20(2):149–157.

21. Meador KJ, et al. Cognitive function at 3 years of age after fetal exposure to antiepileptic drugs. *N Engl J Med* 2009;360:1597–1605.

22. Biton V, et al. Double-blind, placebo-controlled study of lamotrigine in primary generalized tonic-clonic seizures. *Neurology* 2005;65:1737–1743.

23. Buchanan N. The use of lamotrigine in juvenile myoclonic epilepsy. *Seizure* 1996;5:149–151.

24. Carrazana EJ, Wheeler SD. Exacerbation of juvenile myoclonic epilepsy with lamotrigine. *Neurology* 2001;56:1424–1425.

25. Biton V, et al. A randomized, placebo-controlled study of topiramate in primary generalized tonic–clonic seizures. *Neurology* 1999;52:1330–1337.

26. Prasad A, et al. Evolving antiepileptic drugs in juvenile myoclonic epilepsy. *Arch Neurol* 2003;60(8):1100–1105.

27. Biton V, Bourgeois BF, YTC/YTCE Study Investigators. Topiramate in patients with juvenile myoclonic epilepsy. *Arch Neurol* 2005;62:1705–1708.

28. Kellet MW, Smith DF, Stockton PA, Chadwick DW. Topiramate in clinical practice: first year's postlicensing experience in a specialist clinic. *J Neurol Neurosurg Psychiatry* 1999;66:759–763.

29. Berkovic SF, Knowlton RC, Leroy RF, Schiemann J, Falter U. Placebo-controlled study of Levetiracetam in idiopathic generalized epilepsy. Levetiracetam N01057 study group. *Neurology* 2007;69:1751–1760.

30. Noachtar S, Andermann E, Meyvisch P, Andermann F, Gough WB, Schiemann-Delgado J. Levetiracetam for the treatment of idiopathic generalized epilepsy with myoclonic seizures. *Neurology* 2008;70:607–616.

31. Verrotti A, et al. Levetiracetam in juvenile myoclonic epilepsy: long-term efficacy in newly diagnosed adolescents. *Dev Med Child Neurology* 2008;50:29–32.

32. Sharpe DV, Patel AD, Abou-Khalil B, Fenichel GM. Levetiracetam monotherapy in juvenile myoclonic epilepsy. *Seizure* 2008;17:64–68.

33. Specchio N, et al. Effects of levetiracetam on EEG abnormalities in juvenile myoclonic epilepsy. *Epilepsia* 2008;49(4):663–669.

34. Kothare SV, Valencia I, Khurana DS, Hardison H, Melvin JJ, Legido A. Efficacy and tolerability of zonisamide in juvenile myoclonic epilepsy. *Epileptic Disord* 2004;6:267–270.

35. Marinas A, Villanueva V, Giráldez BG, Molins A, Salas-Puig J, Serratosa JM. Efficacy and tolerability of zonisamide in idiopathic generalized epilepsy. *Epileptic Disord* 2009;11:61–66.

36. Obeid T, Panayiotopoulos CP. Clonazepam in juvenile myoclonic epilepsy. *Epilepsia* 1989;30:603–606.

37. Resor SR Jr, Resor LD. Chronic acetazolamide monotherapy in the treatment of juvenile myoclonic epilepsy. *Neurology* 1990;40:1677–1681.

38. Knake S, Hamer HM, Schomburg U, Oertel WH, Rosenow F. Tiagabine-induced absence status in idiopathic generalized epilepsy. *Seizure* 1999;8:314–317.

39. Thomas P, Valton L, Genton P. Absence and myoclonic status epilepticus precipitated by antiepileptic drugs in idiopathic generalized epilepsy. *Brain* 2006;129:1281–1292.

40. Kostov H, Larsson PG, Roster GK. Is vagus nerve stimulation a treatment option for patients with drug-resistant IGE? *Acta Neurol Scand* 2007;115(Suppl 187):55–58.

CHAPTER 24

Generalized Tonic–Clonic Seizures on Awakening

Bruno Maton

▶ OVERVIEW

Generalized tonic–clonic seizures (GTCS) or "grand-mal seizures" are easily recognizable and their selective occurrence during early morning in some patients has been identified for many years (Gowers, 1885). Epilepsy with GTCS on awakening (EGTCSA) was identified early as part of idiopathic generalized epilepsy (Janz, 1953),[1] and abundant literature is available for review (Wolf, 2002). In contrast, little attention has been dedicated to the epilepsies with GTCS occurring during sleep or at random.

Clinical and electroencephalographic (EEG) characteristics of the EGTCSA were defined in the 1989 ILAE classification of seizures and epilepsy as a *"Syndrome with onset mostly on the second decade of life. The generalized tonic–clonic seizures occur exclusively or predominantly (>90 per cent of the time) shortly after awakening or around a second peak in the evening period of relaxation. Absence or myoclonic seizures may occur. Seizures may be precipitated by sleep deprivation. The EEG shows one of the patterns of idiopathic generalized epilepsy. The patient may be photosensitive."*

EGTCSA is no longer an isolated syndrome in the new proposed diagnostic scheme from the ILAE[2] but is part of "Epilepsy With Generalized Tonic–Clonic Seizures Only." It is unclear if the patients with associated absences and/or myoclonic seizures are included. "Epilepsy With Generalized Tonic–Clonic Seizures Only" implies inclusion of only those patients with GTC alone as recommended by some authors.[3] Others consider the epilepsies with GTCS only as a broader category rather than a syndrome and include also patients with mild absences, myoclonic jerks, or both.[4]

EGTCSA is a diagnosis currently used by many groups that emphasize specific management issues including the importance of precipitating factors and the difficulties of pharmacological control in some cases.[5] In most of the literature available for review, the presence or the absence of minor seizures is not established.

▶ ETIOLOGY–NOSOLOGY

EGTCSA is part of the idiopathic generalized epilepsies (IGEs); well-defined partial epilepsies that closely mimic the EEG and clinical features of EGTCSA[6] are excluded. EGTCSA is genetically determined.[7] Between 3.3% and 26% of patients with EGTCSA have a positive family history[5,7] and good concordance is noted within the syndrome.[5]

EGTCSA has a complex mode of inheritance and, like other IGE syndromes, probably results from the interaction of multiple genes and environmental factors.[8,9]

Multiple susceptibility factors for IGE have been identified. Interestingly, some are common to Juvenile myoclonic epilepsy (JME) and EGTCSA suggesting a closely shared genetic background. EJM1, for example, is a locus of susceptibility for JME on chromosome 6 that is also noted in patients with EGTCSA but not in patients with sporadic GTCS.[8] Another group using genome-wide linkage scans has determined recently that susceptibility loci on 5q34, 6p12, and 19q13 confer susceptibility to both myoclonic and GTCSA as predominant seizure types.[10] Rare channelopathies with Mendelian transmission have been identified in generalized epilepsies. Among them, mutations in voltage-gated channel CLCN2 are described in patients with idiopathic generalized epilepsy with and without GTCSA.[11]

▶ CLINICAL OVERVIEW

PREVALENCE

Janz reported EGTCSA in 10% of patients having GTCS without and 17% with additional minor seizures.[12] The percentage of epilepsy with pure GTCS is low if seizures are studied with prolonged video-EEG.[13]

All syndromes of IGE characterized by minor seizures starting during childhood and adolescence may be associated with GTCS usually of the awakening type.[7] When GTCS occur, they are of the GTCSA type in 96% of cases of childhood absence epilepsy and 90% of cases in JME.[7]

SEX DISTRIBUTION

EGTCSA shows a male preponderance that is more pronounced in pure EGTCSA than in GTCA associated with minor seizures.[7] Differences between sexes regarding alcohol exposure and sleep habits are proposed to explain these differences.[4]

AGE AT ONSET

Age at onset varies from 6 to 47 years with a peak in the second decade of life.[7] More than two-third of the patients experience their first attack before the age of 19 years. The onset of seizures coincided with menarche in one-third of female patients.

SEIZURES

All patients have GTCS, which occur within 1–2 hours after awakening either from nocturnal or diurnal sleep. A second peak is noted during the period of rest in the evening. Minor seizures when present are also activated upon awakening and patients may report prolonged confusional episodes during this period.

CHRONOBIOLOGY AND BIORHYTHMICITY

GTCS can be classified into three groups according to their relationship with the sleep–wake cycle:[14] GTCS on awakening (16%–38%), GTCS during sleep (28%–33%), and diffuse or random GTCS in both sleep and wakefulness.

If seizures are not controlled, modifications in the time distribution of seizures may appear during the evolution and the initial history is key.[1,14] For Janz,[14] 17% of the cases starting as EGTCSA diffused. None of the cases that started during the sleep or at random showed evolution toward EGCTSA supporting the identity of EGTCSA.

PRECIPITATING FACTORS

Sleep deprivation, fatigue, and excessive alcohol intake are the main precipitating factors. Shift work and changes in sleep habits, particularly during holidays and celebrations, predispose to GTCS on awakening.

CLINICAL EXAMINATION

By definition, seizures of IGE occur in persons without neurological or mental disturbances. Neurological and cognitive examinations are normal.

Janz[7] suggested that seizures in patients with GTCSA were associated with psychological traits such as hedonism, passivity, and a tendency to live a disorderly life. These findings remain controversial and likely biased as these patients are more prone to be exposed to precipitating factors and seizures.

EEG

The routine EEG typically reveals generalized spike-wave discharges and/or polyspike-waves in 41%–50% of patients with EGTCSA.[7] A sleep-deprived afternoon nap shows generalized discharges in 70% of patients with a normal routine EEG.[15] A photoparoxysmal response in the EEG occurs in 13% of patients.[4] Generalized discharges are more likely to occur after awakening in patients with EGTCSA. GTCS are rarely recorded and are often precipitated by an imposed awakening and preceded by long runs of spike-wave discharges of as illustrated in Fig. 24–1.

NEUROIMAGING FINDINGS

Head computed tomography (CT) and conventional brain magnetic resonance imaging (MRI) studies are normal in patients with EGTCSA. Nonspecific findings[16] and subtle structural abnormalities[17] are reported.

DIFFERENTIAL DIAGNOSIS

Partial epilepsy with secondary generalized seizures may mimic closely the electroclinical findings of EGTCSA.[6] Conversely, EGTCSA can be misdiagnosed as partial epilepsy. Activation of minor seizures after awakening is frequently associated with a prolonged confusional state prior to the convulsion and may be misinterpreted as complex partial seizures. A clear description of the GTCSA is rarely available or may be misleading. Auras may be reported and the initial motor phase can be asymmetric with apparent version or circling.[18]

GTCSA may be preceded or accompanied by absences or myoclonic seizures that are nor reported or noted by patients.[19] In addition, GTCSA can be the first seizure type in up to 30% of patients with JME, with myoclonic jerks reported later.[13]

NATURAL COURSE

Similar to other types of IGE with onset in the second decade, EGTCSA is associated with a lifelong predisposition for seizures. Maximum seizure activity occurs during the second decade and the young–adult periods. For Janz, the duration of the active period of the epilepsy with EGTCSA with only one peak in the morning was 10 years in mean while it was 12.2 years when bimodal.[14]

▶ DIAGNOSTIC CRITERIA

EGTCA requires that more than 90% of GTCS occur during the first 2 hours after awakening or during the period of rest in the evening. No specifics are indicated regarding the necessary number of seizures in the 1989 ILAE definition. Janz[7] requires six GTC before being able to confirm the chronobiology and the diagnosis. In contrast, other authors consider one GTCS sufficient for

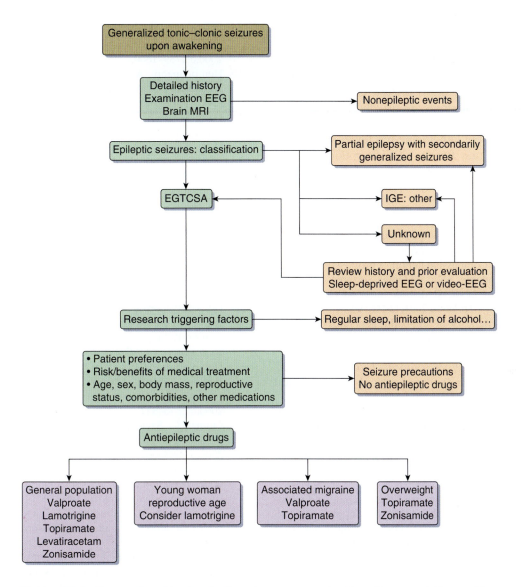

Figure 24–1. Generalized tonic–clonic seizures recorded in a 9-year–old boy with EGTCSA. The tonic contraction is preceded by a long discharge of generalized spikes, polyspikes, and slow waves.

the diagnosis if prolonged EEG recording demonstrates activation of abnormalities during awakening.[5] The chronobiology should be assessed at seizure onset as the distribution of the GTCS may become less obvious after a few years.

Neurological examination and all neuroimaging tests other than EEG are also normal or represent incidental findings. A normal routine EEG should prompt a sleep-deprived EEG or a video-EEG evaluation performed in sleep and on awakening. Myoclonic jerks or brief absences will often be revealed. Focal EEG abnormalities in the absence of generalized discharge are rare.

Atypical clinical and/or EEG features should prompt MRI evaluation.

▶ CRITERIA FOR STARTING TREATMENT

Recommendations regarding the need for regular sleep and limiting alcohol exposure should be emphasized after the first seizure; they are a key element to prevent seizure recurrence. In selected cases, when the seizure follows a prolonged sleepless period, proper sleep may be sufficient to prevent further seizures. These simple recommendations are often ignored by adolescents and young adults. Pharmacological treatment of the first GTCS does not affect long-term remission of epilepsy.[20]

After a second seizure, antiepileptic drugs would start in most cases but proper life habits are essential for seizure control.

► OPTIMAL TREATMENT REGIMEN

The prevention of precipitants such as sleep deprivation and alcohol intake play a key role in controlling the seizures. It may achieve seizure control in some cases but antiepileptic drugs are usually necessary.

Monotherapy with valproate is often recommended as the first choice but lamotrigine has fewer side effects particularly in young females. Other options include topiramate, levatiracetam, and zonisamide.

REFERENCES

1. Loiseau P. Crises epileptiques survenant au reveil et epilepsie du reveil. *Sud Med Chir* 1964;99:11492–11502.
2. Engel J Jr. ILAE Commission Report. A proposed diagnostic scheme for people with epileptic seizures and with epilepsy: report of the ILAE task force on classification and terminology. *Epilepsia* 2001;42:796–803.
3. Andermann F, Berkovic SF. Idiopathic generalized epilepsy with generalized and other seizures in adolescence. *Epilepsia* 2001;42:317–320.
4. Panayiotopoulos CP. *A Clinical Guide to Epileptic Syndromes and Their Treatment*. Oxford: Bladon Medical Publishing, 2002.
5. Unterberger I, et al. Idiopathic generalized epilepsies with pure grand mal: clinical data and genetics. *Epilepsy Res* 2001;44:19–25.
6. Roger J, Bureau M. Distinctive characteristics of frontal lobe versus idiopathic generalized epilepsy. *Adv Neurol* 1992;57:399–410.
7. Janz D. Epilepsy with grand mal on awakening and sleep-waking cycle. *Clin Neurophysiol* 2000;111(Suppl 2):103–110.
8. Greenberg DA, et al. The genetics of idiopathic generalized epilepsies of adolescent onset: differences between juvenile myoclonic epilepsy and epilepsy with random grand mal and with awakening grand mal. *Neurology* 1995;45:942–946.
9. Ferraro TN, Dlgos DJ, Buono RJ. Role of genetics in the diagnosis and treatment of epilepsy. *Expert Rev Neurother* 2006;6:1789–1800.
10. Hempelmann A, et al. Exploration of the genetic architecture of idiopathic generalized epilepsies. *Epilepsia* 2006;47:1682–1690.
11. Haug K, et al. Mutations in CLCN2 encoding a voltage-gated chloride channel are associated with idiopathic generalized epilepsies. *Nat Genet* 2003;33:527–532.
12. Janz D. Pitfalls in the diagnosis of grand mal on awakening. In: Wolf P (ed), *Epileptic Seizures and Syndromes*. London: John Libbey & Company Ltd, 1994; pp. 213–220.
13. Delgado-Escueta AV, et al. Gene mapping in the idiopathic generalized epilepsies. Juvenile myoclonic epilepsy, childhood absence epilepsy, epilepsy with grand mal seizures and early childhood myoclonic epilepsy. *Epilepsia* 1990;31(Suppl 3):19–29.
14. Janz D. The grand-mal epilepsies and the sleeping-waking cycle. *Epilepsia* 1962;3:69–109.
15. Genton P, Gonzalez-Sanchez M, Thomas P. Epilepsy with grand mal on awakening. In: Roger J, Bureau M, Dravet C, Genton P, Tassinari CA, Wolf P (eds), *Epileptic Syndromes in Infancy, Childhood and Adolescence*. London: John Libbey Eurotext Ltd, 2005; pp. 389–394.
16. Betting LE, et al. MRI reveals structural abnormalities in patients with idiopathic generalized epilepsy. *Neurology* 2006;67:848–852.
17. Ciumas C, Savic I. Structural changes in patients with primary generalized tonic and clonic seizures. *Neurology* 2006;67:683–686.
18. Gastaut H, Aguglia U, Tinuper P. Benign versive or circling epilepsy with bilateral 3-cps spike-and-wave discharges in late childhood. *Ann Neurol* 1986;19:301–303.
19. Jain S, Padm M, Maheshwari MC. Occurrence of only myoclonic jerks in juvenile myoclonic epilepsy. *Acta Neurol Scand* 1997;95:263–267.
20. Leone M, Solari A, Beghi E (FIRST group). Treatment of the first tonic–clonic seizure does not affect long-term remission of epilepsy. *Neurology* 2006;67:2227–2229.

SECTION V
Epilepsy Syndromes

CHAPTER 25

Benign Epilepsy with Centrotemporal Spikes (BECTS)

Natalio Fejerman, Giuseppe Gobbi, and Salvatore Grosso

► CLINICAL OVERVIEW

Benign childhood epilepsy with centrotemporal spikes (BCECTS) is among the most frequent benign focal epilepsies in childhood and accounts for about 15%–25% of all epileptic syndromes in children with ages between 4 and 12 years.[1] The annual incidence ranges between 7.1 and 21 per 100,000 in children under the age of 15 years[2] with a slight male predominance.[3] Absence of neurological and intellectual deficits are part of the definition, even though BCECTS has also been reported in patients with neuroradiologically documented cerebral lesions.[4,5] Genetic factors play an important etiological role, as corroborated by the higher incidence of positive family history for epilepsy and focal electroencephalographic (EEG) abnormalities in BCECTS patients.[6] Linkage to chromosome 15q14 was pointed out,[7] but not confirmed in several studies.[8]

Age at onset ranges between 4 and 10 years in 90% of patients, with a peak around 7 years. Seizures occur during sleep in 80%–90% of patients, and only while awake in less than 10%. Seizure frequency is usually low with 10% of patients experiencing one seizure only.[1] Duration of seizures commonly ranges from 30 seconds up to no more than 2–3 minutes. Major clinical findings include: (i) o*rofacial motor signs*, specially tonic or clonic contractions of one side of the face with a predilection for the labial commissure (contralateral to centrotemporal spikes); (ii) *speech arrest*; (iii) s*ialorrhea*, a characteristic ictal symptom which may not be related to increased salivation, swallowing disturbance, or both; (iv) s*omatosensory symptoms*, represented by unilateral numbness or paresthesias of the tongue, lips, gums, and inner cheek. Less-frequent ictal manifestations include: (i) generalized seizures which are not infrequently observed in younger children and probably related to rapid generalization of focal seizures and (ii) postictal paresis.[9]

The benign character of Rolandic spikes was recognized in the 1950s.[10,11] Several long-term follow-up studies confirmed the good prognosis,[12–15] and over 90% of cases will achieve remission by age 12 years.[16] The prognosis is favorable even for patients whose seizures are difficult to control, and seizures almost always remit spontaneously in adolescence. No differences in seizure frequency, seizure relapse rate, duration of active period of epilepsy, and social adjustments have been found between BCECTS patients receiving an antiepileptic drug (AED) and untreated patients.[17] The only predictor of short-term prognosis is the age at BETCS onset: the earlier the onset of seizures, the longer the active period. The occurrence of GTCS seizures after recovery from BCECTS is a rare event, involving approximately 2% of subjects, similar to the incidence in partial seizures.[18]

EEG PATTERNS

The cornerstone of BCECTS diagnosis is the characteristic interictal EEG pattern. *Background EEG activity* is normal both during wakefulness and sleep. *Interictal epileptic discharges and location of spikes* include typical sharp/spike-waves located in centrotemporal or Rolandic areas (CTSW). CTSW are broad, diphasic, high-voltage (100–300 microvolts) sharps, with a horizontal dipole, and are often followed by a slow wave. Spikes may be isolated or in clusters,[18] and focal rhythmic slow activity is occasionally observed in the same region as the spikes.[19] The spikes may occur in one or both hemispheres. Bilateral synchronous discharges or independent CTSW appear in wakefulness or sleep in about one-third of cases[20] and the characteristic dipolar pattern in the EEG has been emphasized.[21] *Enhancement of discharges* is observed in drowsiness and in all stages of sleep. In about one-third of children, spikes appear only in sleep.[22] *Spikes in other areas, multifocal paroxysms, and spike-wave discharges* at the onset or during evolution may also appear.[23] In some cases, multifocal paroxysms are especially evident during sleep. Generalized spike-wave discharges are rarely seen in the waking state, but may be frequent during drowsiness and sleep.[24,25] *Ictal EEG patterns* are generally characterized by a sequence of rhythmic spikes remaining monomorphous throughout the sequence.

Atypical Features in Patients with BCECTS

Children with BCECTS are classically considered free of neuropsychological impairments.[26] However, learning, language, and behavioural disabilities are present in many affected patients,[27] but are less frequent compared to other forms of childhood epilepsy. We have reviewed a large list of transient neuropsychological impairments in children with atypical features of BCECTS.[28] In a study investigating the influence of cognition on quality of life of 30 children with BCECTS, parental emotional impact was the major independent predictor of quality of life.[29] However, even when children with BCECTS show some learning difficulties, the intellectual abilities or behavior disorders did not differ from healthy children,[30] and a vast majority of the patients attend normal schools. In adolescents and young adults in complete remission from BCECTS there were no significant differences with controls in cognitive functions. It has recently been noted that all attentional networks (alerting, orienting, and executive attention networks) are impaired in children with active centrotemporal spikes and that these impairments resolve upon EEG remission.[31] By contrast, qualitative analysis suggested a different organizational pattern for cerebral language.[32]

These transient sectorial cognitive impairments tend to occur in the active phase of the disease, and appear more correlated to the ongoing epileptiform activity in the awake state and, in particular, during NON-REM sleep than to seizure frequency.[33–35] More frequently, visual perception, short-term memory, memory, phonologic awareness, reading, spatial perception, including spatial orientation, numeracy and/or spelling abilities are significantly delayed.[36–38]

Six distinct interictal EEG patterns are hallmarks of BCECTS patients who, after complete seizure remission and normalization of the EEG, evidenced serious cognitive difficulties and impaired quality of life at home and at school.[39]

In a study with combination of EEG, magnetoencephalography and MRI, BCECTS children with lower language test scores had left perisylvian spikes, while children with right perisylvian location performed within normal ranges in all parts of the tests.[40]

It is important to employ appropriate neuropsychological tests patients in BCECTS. In a study of 21 children with BCECTS compared to controls, tests measuring phonemic fluency, verbal reelaboration of semantic knowledge, and lexical comprehension showed mild language defects that correlated with a high spike frequency in wakefulness, multifocal location, and temporal prominence of EEG spike-wave discharges.[41]

A significantly higher percentage of learning and behavioral disabilities are reported in BCECTS patients with atypical features. No patient developed status epilepticus, Landau Kleffner syndrome, or CSWSS syndrome.[42]

Gobbi et al[43] suggested that these conditions be termed BCECTS "plus" disorders to differentiate them from the other Rolandic epilepsy-related disorders such as ABPE/pseudo Lennox syndrome, CSWS, acquired epileptic frontal syndrome, LKS ± CSWS, and the early development dysphasia ± CSWS (or LKS variant) (Table 25–1). A differentiation between "malignant" and "nonmalignant" forms of atypical presentations of BCECTS was also proposed.[44]

Atypical BCECTS

The term "atypical BCECTS" is used to describe a subset of patients with severe epileptic manifestations and marked language, and cognitive or behavioral impairments. Aicardi and Chevrie[45] first described this condition in seven children with BCECTS during periods of new types of seizures, mainly atonic and myoclonic, associated with continuous spike-wave discharges in slow wave sleep (CSWS/ESES [electrical status epilepticus during sleep]), and transient deterioration in school performance. They used the term "atypical benign partial epilepsy of childhood" (ABPE) and commented that the majority had been previously diagnosed as Lennox-Gastaut syndrome. In fact, in the German literature this condition was named "Pseudo Lennox Syndrome."[46] As BCECTS may occur in patients with brain lesions, ABPE (or Pseudo Lenox Syndrome) may be both idiopathic and symptomatic in origin.

ABPE can be a particularly severe with respect to its cognitive consequences. In a recent prospective study of 44 children that included 28 with typical BCECTS, and 16 with ABPE, patients from the latter group had significantly lower full scale and verbal intelligence quotient scores. Abnormalities were also noted in performance tasks.

Neuropsychological impairments may precede the onset of the disorder, and persist consistently during the

▶ **TABLE 25-1. ROLANDIC EPILEPSY SPECTRUM DISORDERS**

(A) Typical benign Rolandic epilepsy (BCECTS)
   a. Clinical features: age of onset between 4 and 10 years. Seizures related to sleep, brief, starting with orofacial motor signs.
   b. EEG features: normal background with interictal spikes in centrotemporal (Rolandic) areas. Discharges increased during sleep.

(B) Atypical features in BCECTS
   a. Clinical features: early onset of seizures (below 4 years), day-time only seizures, prolonged seizures, Todd's paresis, status epilepticus (status of BCECTS), transient cognitive impairment.
   b. EEG features: more frequent spikes discharges, atypical spike morphologies, slow-wave focus, generalized 3 Hz spike-wave discharges.

(C) Atypical BCECTS and atypical evolutions of Rolandic epilepsies
   a. Atypical benign partial epilepsy (ABPE)
   b. Status of Rolandic epilepsy (status of BCECTS with ESES)
   c. Landau–Kleffner syndrome (LKS)
   d. Continuous spike-waves during slow sleep syndrome (CSWSS)
      (All have in common the presence of ESES.)
      • ABPE and status of BCECTS with ESES usually remit with adequate treatment with cognitive sequelae in some of the patients.
      • Children with idiopathic LKS and CSWSS may remain with residual linguistic deficits and mental impairment.

clinical course. Long-term follow-up reveals persistent verbal deficits in all ABPE patients after remission, and the longer the duration of ESES pattern the more severe are permanent cognitive impairments.[47] However, in the experience of one of us (NF), seizures remitted in all 16 patients with ABPE and the EEG normalized; none resented significant neurocognitive sequelae.[48]

CSWS/ESES has also been reported in some patients with the so-called "status of BCECTS." Status of BCECTS, or status epilepticus of benign partial epilepsy in children, which may last days or weeks, has been described by Fejerman and Di Blasi in 1987, and Colamaria et al in 1991.[49,50] *Clinical semiology* consists of focal motor seizures such as anarthria, dysarthria, sialorrhea, drooling, oromotor dyspraxia, swallowing difficulties, hemifacial contraction, and atonic head nods. Focal atonic events (epileptic negative myoclonus) may be so frequent to cause limb difficulties. The *ictal EEG* is characterized by continuous bilateral or diffuse spike discharges that predominate in the Rolandic regions, may be synchronous with hemifacial twitching and inhibited by voluntary mouth and tongue movements. *Interictal awake EEG*

shows bilateral sharp- and sharp-slow wave complexes with higher amplitude in the Rolandic area, which increases during sleep and bilateral synchronization. Continuous spike-waves during slow sleep may also occur in some patients (see Section "Atypical BCECTS").

In a minority of patients, BCECTS may evolve into Landau-Kleffner syndrome (LKS) and the continuous spike-and-wave during slow sleep syndrome (CSWSS), and *vice versa*.[48,51–54] It remains to be defined whether these conditions—ABPE (or pseudo lenox syndrome), LKS (and LKS variant), CSWSS (including the acquired epileptic frontal syndrome)—are independent syndromes or syndromes related to BCECTS as part of a continuum. In this context, the atypical evolution in a minority of patients with BCECTS may possibly be considered as "system epilepsy."[55]

DIAGNOSTIC CRITERIA

Criteria for diagnosis include typical Rolandic seizures especially during sleep, normal psychomotor and mental development, normal neurological examination, and the characteristic awake and sleep EEG patterns. Therefore, awake and sleep EEG recording is mandatory for diagnosis. A comprehensive neuropsychological assessment should be performed at the onset of the disorder. In fact, any sign of neuropsychological impairments or of learning disorders may suggest atypical features of BCECTS or atypical BCECTS.

Structural neuroimaging studies, when the clinical and EEG features are typical should be avoided.[56] Hippocampal asymmetries and white matter abnormalities in MRI have been reported in 33% of 18 children with BCECTS, although their etiology was considered unclear.[57] Cases with electroclinical phenotypes of BCECTS associated with brain malformations such as cortical dysplasia[17,58] or heterotopia[51,53] and with nonevolutive clastic brain lesions[4] have also been described. Therefore, it is reasonable to suggest an MRI if there is suspicion of associated abnormalities.

Karyotype analysis is needed to exclude chromosomal disorders which may have an EEG pattern similar to BCECTS including fragile X (FRAXA) syndrome, deletion of chromosome 7,[59] inv-dup15 (GG, personal observation), and Klinefelter syndrome.[60]

Differential diagnosis requires special attention (Tables 25–2 and 25–3). The differential diagnosis should consider other benign idiopathic childhood focal epilepsies as the morphology of their EEG abnormalities may overlap with BCECTS, and their localization may change with advancing age. Although rare, autosomal dominant Rolandic epilepsy with speech dyspraxia,[61,62] should also be considered in the differential diagnosis. Difficulties in diagnosis accompany signs or symptoms from Rolandic–Sylvian areas. In the so-called "malignant Rolandic–Sylvian epilepsy" secondary to neuronal

▶ **TABLE 25–2. DIAGNOSIS OF BCECTS IN CHILDREN WITH CEREBRAL PATHOLOGY**

- Occasional associations of BCECTS with nonevolutive cerebral lesions
- BCECTS "phenotype" and unilateral focal heterotopia
- BCECTS in children with cerebral palsy
  - As a fortuitous association
  - As a peculiar syndrome (not so benign) in children with unilateral polymicrogyria

migration disorders and gliosis, clinical and EEG features may be similar to BCECTS and magnetoencephalography has been advocated to assist in diagnosis.[63]

CRITERIA FOR STARTING TREATMENT

When facing the decision to treat or not BCECTS, the natural course of the disease should be weighed against the efficacy and risks of treatment.[64] Unfortunately, data available on the natural course of BCECTS are scarce. The active seizure period is less than 1 year in 50% of patients but more than 6 years in 9.5% of subjects.[15] Seizures are difficult to control in only a small number of cases,[14,65] and are frequent in only 6% of patients.[15] For these reasons, many authors suggest that drug treatment is not necessary.[1,3,66]

Possible predictive factors of seizure frequency and duration of antiepileptic treatment in patients with BCECTS have also been emphasized. Ambrosetto and Tassinari[17] retrospectively compared patients with two to six seizures with those who had six or more seizures. Patients with fewer than six seizures were significantly more likely to have a longer interval between first and second seizures

▶ **TABLE 25–3. DIFFERENTIAL DIAGNOSIS BETWEEN BCECTS AND OTHER EPILEPSY SYNDROMES**

- With symptomatic or probably symptomatic epilepsies
  - Mesial temporal lobe epilepsy
  - Symptomatic lateral temporal lobe epilepsy
  - Other focal epilepsies with seizures arising from neocortical areas
  - Symptomatic epilepsies arising from Rolandic–Sylvian areas
- With other idiopathic epilepsy syndromes
  - Benign infantile focal epilepsy with midline spikes and waves during sleep
  - Panayiotopoulos syndrome
  - Late-onset occipital lobe epilepsy (Gastaut type)
  - Other proposed benign focal epilepsy syndromes
  - Autosomal dominant partial epilepsy with auditory features
  - Autosomal dominant Rolandic epilepsy with speech dyspraxia

(7.8 vs. 3.5 months), and a shorter total duration of disease (1.5 vs. 4.5 years). On that basis, the authors suggested that it may be appropriate to delay treatment until after the third seizure. Alternatively, Loiseau and Duche[18] advocated medication in approximately half of the patients. The presence of neuropsychological impairments, either transitory or persistent may influence the decision to treat.

We believe that decisions about initiation of treatment or withholding therapy must be individualized. Parents' opinion about treatment must also be taken into account as the ictal events are disruptive to the patient or family.[53]

Factors favoring treatment include (i) a short interval between the first three seizures; (ii) younger age at seizure onset; (iii) generalized convulsive seizures; (iv) daytime seizures;[64] and (v) evident transient cognitive dysfunctions (Fig. 25–1).

OPTIMAL TREATMENT REGIMEN

There is no definitive data supporting specific choice of drug therapy (Table 25–4). Although carbamazepine (CBZ) has historically been the drug of choice,[54] class I and class II randomized controlled trials (RCTs) for children with BCECTS are lacking. Based on available efficacy and effectiveness evidence alone for children with newly diagnosed BCECTS, CBZ, and valproate (VPA) are equally suitable for initial monotherapy.[67] Therefore, the selection of first-line AED therapy requires consideration of patient-specific, AED-specific, and nation-specific variables that affect overall response to therapy.[67]

Class III RCT evidence of effectiveness for BCECTS is available for gabapentin (GBP) and sulthiame (STM). A placebo-controlled double-blind trial included 225 children with BCECTS randomized to GBP ($n = 113$), 30 mg/kg per day or placebo ($n = 112$). Previous medications were tapered and patients remained in the study for 36 weeks. The analysis indicated significant superiority of GBP over placebo ($p = 0.0254$).[68]

A placebo-controlled double-blind trial involved 66 children with BCECTS randomized to either STM ($n = 31$) or placebo ($n = 35$). STM showed superior effectiveness compared with placebo ($p = 0.00002$) in patients completing 6 months without a treatment-failure event.[69] Other trials confirmed the effectiveness of STM in BCECTS,[70] resulting as effective as CBZ.[46] Doose et al[71] treated 56 BCECTS patients with STM, 4–6 mg/kg per day. Seizure control was obtained in 82% of patients who had experienced three to five seizures before treatment, and in 89% of those who had had more than five seizures before treatment. EEG normalization was observed in 51 patients soon after starting STM. Seizures relapsed in approximately 25% of patients.

A meta-analysis of 13 cohorts, comprising 794 patients with long-term retrospective follow-up, showed

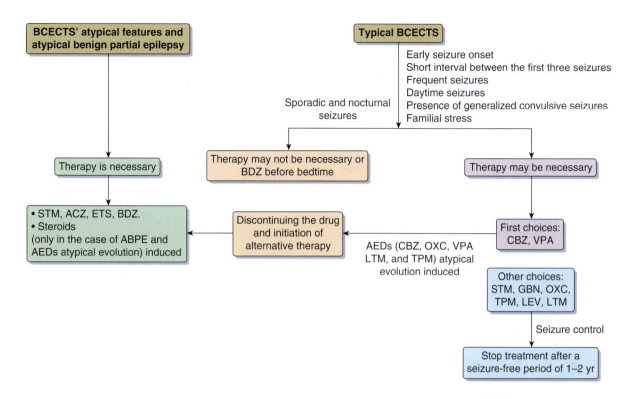

Figure 25–1. Management Algorhythm.

that PHT, PB, VPA, CBZ, and clonazepam (CZP) provided similar efficacy.[72] However PHT and PB are contraindicated due to their adverse effect profiles. Short or prolonged period of treatment with benzodiazepines (BZDs) has also been recommended.[73] In comparison

▶ **TABLE 25–4. BCECTS TREATMENT**

(1) Typical benign Rolandic epilepsy (BCECTS)
   a. BDZ low doses before bedtime
   b. CBZ 15–20 mg/kg per day
   c. VPA 15–20 mg/kg per day
   d. LEV 10–30 mg/kg per day
   e. STM 4–6 mg/kg per day
   f. XC 20–30 mg/kg per day
   g. TPM 3–9 mg/kg per day
   h. LTM 2–8 mg/kg per day
   i. GBN 30 mg/kg per day
(2) Atypical features in BCECTS
   a. ETS 15–20 mg/kg per day
   b. STM 5–15 mg/kg per day
   c. ACZ 16 mg/kg per day
   d. BDZ
     i. Clobazam 0.5–1 mg/kg per day
     ii. Clonazepam 0.1 mg/kg per day
(3) ABPE, status of BCECTS and LKS with ESES), and AEDs-induced atypical evolution
   a. Discontinuing the previously used AED and initiating an alternative therapy
   b. The treatment is the same as in atypical features of BCECTS, with possible treatment with steroids.

with VPA and CBZ, CZP was more effective in controlling Rolandic epileptiform discharges after 4 weeks of treatment.[74] At present, the use of BZD, especially clobazam, at night is considered a possible first choice in children who only have seizures during sleep and does not interfere with day time activities.

Almost all of the newer AEDs have been used, at least anecdotally, to treat children with BCECTS. Oxcarbazepine (OXC) monotherapy, in newly diagnosed patients with BCECTS followed for 18 months was considered effective in preventing seizures, normalizing the EEGs and preserving cognitive and behavioral functions.[75,76] There are no large series of patients with BCECTS treated with lamotrigine (LTM) or topiramate (TPM).

Two studies explored the efficacy of levetiracetam (LEV) in BCECTS. Coppola et al[77] compared LEV with OXC in 39 children with BCECTS randomly allocated to one of these drugs. Preliminary findings suggested that both were effective. In a recent uncontrolled study of 21 children with BCECTS, LEV monotherapy at doses ranging from 1000 to 2500 mg was effective and well tolerated.[42]

Specific duration of therapy is also unsupported by clear evidence.[64] Most physicians discontinue treatment before age 16 years. Medications should be discontinued in patients who are seizure-free for at least 1–2 years, even though the relapse rate following AED discontinuation is approximately 14%.[72] Normalization of the EEG may not be required for medication discontinuation in school age patients.

Worsening of BCECTS and Paradoxical Reactions

Worsening of BCECTS may occur due to drug-induced deterioration. It is defined as an increase in seizure frequency or the development of a new seizure type such as atypical absences with atonic components, associated with speech disturbance, decreased school performance and, continuous diffuse spike-wave EEG discharges during slow sleep.[78] The incidence of paradoxical drug reactions in BCECTS is small.[79] Predictive factors include the presence of diffuse interictal sharp and slow-wave discharges, and/or central spike-and-wave activity rather than Rolandic sharp diphasic waves.[79] EEGs obtained soon after initiation of AEDS, CBZ in particular, in young children may help identify patients at increased risk of seizure exacerbation. The susceptibility of some BCECTS patients to atypical evolution may not be purely drug related as underlying biologic factors may contribute. Although CBZ is the primary agent identified with triggering a paradoxical reaction in BCECTS patients,[48,80,81] aggravation of the electroclinical findings has also reported in patients taking PB, PHT,[52,79,82] and VPA.[83] OXC was considered responsible of atypical evolutions in three patients with BCECTS who already had some atypical features[84] and LTM[85,86] and TPM[87] induced seizure aggravation and negative myoclonus.

When a paradoxical reaction occurs, discontinuing the drug and initiating alternative therapy resolves the exacerbation in all cases. Anecdotical reports suggest that STM, BZD, and acetazolamide (ACZ) are effective therapeutic alternatives in patients with a paradoxical drug reaction and atypical BCECTS ([88], authors' personal experience).

REFERENCES

1. Dalla Bernardina B, Sgro V, Fejerman N. Epilepsy with centrotemporal spikes and related syndromes. In: Roger J, Bureau M, Dravet Ch, Genton P, Tassinari CA, Wolf P (eds), *Epileptic Syndromes in Infancy, Childhood and Adolescence*, 4th ed. London: John Libbey, 2005, p. 203.

2. Heijbel J, Blom S, Bergfors PG. Benign epilepsy of children with centrotemporal EEG foci. Study of incidence rate in outpatient care. *Epilepsia* 1975;16:657.

3. Panayiotopoulos CP. *Benign Childhood Partial Seizures and Related Epileptic Syndromes*. London: John Libbey, 1999.

4. Santanelli P, et al. Benign partial epilepsy with centrotemporal (or rolandic) spikes and brain lesion. *Epilepsia* 1989;30:182.

5. Degen R, et al. Benign discharges in patients with lesional partial epilepsies. *Pediatr Neurol* 1999;20:354.

6. Bray PF, Wiser WC. Evidence for a genetic etiology of temporal central abnormalities in focal epilepsy. *N Engl J Med* 1964;271:926.

7. Neubauer BA, et al. Centrotemporal spikes in families with rolandic epilepsy: linkage to chromosome 15q14. *Neurology* 1998;51:1608.

8. Pruna D, et al. Lack of association with the 15q14 candidate region for benign epilepsy of childhood with centro-temporal spikes in a Sardinian population. *Epilepsia* 2000;41:164.

9. Dai AI, Weinstock A. Post-ictal paresis in children with benign rolandic epilepsy. *J Child Neurol* 2005;20:834.

10. Bancaud J, Colomb D, Dell, MB. Les pointes rolandiques: un symtôme EEG propre à l'enfant. *Rev Neurol (Paris)* 1958;99:206.

11. Nayrac P, Beaussart M. Les pointes-ondes prerolandiques: expression EEG tres particuliere. Etude electroclinique de 21 cas. *Rev Neurol (Paris)* 1958;99:201.

12. Beaussart M. Benign epilepsy of children with rolandic (centrotemporal) paroxysmal foci. *Epilepsia* 1972;13:795.

13. Lerman P, Kivity S. Benign focal epilepsy of childhood. A follow-up study of 100 recovered patients. *Arch Neurol* 1975;32:261.

14. Beaussart M, Faou. Evolution of epilepsy with rolandic paroxysmal foci: a study of 324 cases. *Epilepsia* 1978;19:337.

15. Loiseau P, et al. Prognosis of benign childhood epilepsy with centrotemporal spikes. A follow-up study of 168 patients. *Epilepsia* 1988;29:229.

16. Watanabe K. Benign partial epilepsies. In: Wallace SJ, Farrell K (eds), *Epilepsy in Children*, 2nd ed. London: Arnold, 2004, p. 199.

17. Ambrosetto G, Tassinari CA. Antiepileptic drug treatment of benign childhood epilepsy with rolandic spikes: is it necessary? *Epilepsia* 1990;31:802.

18. Loiseau P, Duche B. Benign childhood epilepsy with centrotemporal spikes. *Cleve Clin J Med* 1989;56:17.

19. Mitsudome A, et al. Rhythmic slow activity in benign childhood epilepsy with centrotemporal spikes. *Clin Electroencephalogr* 1997;28:44.

20. Engel J, Fejerman N. Benign childhood epilepsy with centrotemporal spikes. In: Engel J, Fejerman N (eds), *MedLink Neurology (Section of Epilepsy)*. San Diego: MedLink Corporation, Available at www.medlink.com, 1999–2011.

21. Gregory DL, Wong PK. Topographical analysis of the centrotemporal discharges in benign Rolandic epilepsy of childhood. *Epilepsia* 1984;25:705.

22. Lombroso CT. Sylvian seizures and midtemporal spike foci in children. *Arch Neurol* 1967;17:52.

23. Dalla Bernardina B, Sgro V, Caraballo R. Sleep and benign partial epilepsies of childhood: EEG and evoked potential study. In: Degen R, Rodin EA (eds), *Epilepsy, Sleep and Sleep Deprivation*. Amsterdam: Elsevier, 1991, p. 83.

24. Fejerman N, Medina CS. *Convulsiones en la Infancia*. Buenos Aires: Editorial El Ateneo, 1986; 2nd edn: p. 166.

25. Beydoun A, Garofalo EA, Drury I. Generalized spike-waves, multiple loci, and clinical course in children with EEG features of benign epilepsy of childhood with centrotemporal spikes. *Epilepsia* 1992;33:1091.

26. Lerman P. Benign childhood epilepsy with centrotemporal spikes. In: Engel J, Pedly TA (eds), *Epilepsy: A Comprehensive Textbook*. Philadelphia: Lippincott-Raven, 1998, p. 2307.

27. Yung WY, et al. Cognitive and behavioural problems in children with Centrotemporal spikes. *Pediatr Neurol* 2000; 23:391.

28. Fejerman N. Atypical rolandic epilepsy. *Epilepsia* 2009; 50:9.

29. Connolly AM, et al. Quality of life of children with benign rolandic epilepsy. *Pediatr Neurol* 2006;35:240.

30. Croona C, et al. Neuropsychological findings in children with benign childhood epilepsy with centro-temporal spikes. *Dev Med Child Neurol* 1999;41:813.

31. Kavros PM, et al. Attention impairment in rolandic epilepsy: systematic review. *Epilepsia* 2008;49:1570.

32. Hommet C, et al. Cognitive function in adolescents and young adults in complete remission from benign childhood epilepsy with centro-temporal spikes. *Epileptic Disord* 2001;3:207.

33. Deonna T. Rolandic epilepsy: neuropsychology of the active epilepsy phase. *Epileptic Disord* 2000;2:59.

34. Baglietto MG, et al. Neuropsychological disorders related to interictal epileptic discharges during sleep in benign epilepsy of childhood with centrotemporal spikes. *Dev Med Child Neurol* 2001;43:407.

35. Dubois CM, et al. Acquired epileptic dysgraphia: a longitudinal study. *Dev Med Child Neurol* 2003;45:807.

36. Weglage J, et al. Neuropsychological, intellectual, and behavioral findings in patients with centrotemporal spikes with and without seizures. *Dev Med Child Neurol* 1997;39:646.

37. Pinton F, et al. Cognitive functions in children with benign childhood epilepsy with centrotemporal spikes (BCECTS). *Epileptic Disord* 2006;8:11.

38. Volkl-Kernstock S, Willinger U, Feucht M. Spacial perception and spatial memory in children with benign childhood epilepsy with centro-temporal spikes (BCECTS). *Epilepsy Res* 2006;72:39.

39. Massa R. EEG criteria predictive of complicated evolution in idiopathic Rolandic epilepsy. *Neurology* 2006;57:1071.

40. Wolff M, et al. Benign partial epilepsy in childhood: selective cognitive deficits are related to the location of local spikes determined by combined EEG/MEG. *Epilepsia* 2005;46:1661.

41. Riva D, et al. Intellectual and language findings and their relationship to EEG characteristics in benign childhood epilepsy with centrotemporal spikes. *Epilepsy Behav* 2007;10:278.

42. Verrotti A, et al. Levetiracetam monotherapy for children and adolescents with benign Rolandic seizures. *Seizure* 2007;16:271.

43. Gobbi G, Boni A, Filippini M. The spectrum of idiopathic rolandic epilepsy syndromes and occipital epilepsies: from the benign to the disabling. *Epilepsia* 2006;47:62.

44. Kramer U. Atypical presentations of benign childhood epilepsy with centrotemporal spikes: a review. *J Child Neurol* 2008;23:785–790.

45. Aicardi J, Chevrie JJ. Atypical benign partial epilepsy of childhood. *Dev Med Child Neurol* 1982;24:281.

46. Hahn A, Fischenbeck A, Stephani U. Induction of epileptic negative myoclonus by oxcarbazepine in symptomatic epilepsy. *Epileptic Disord* 2004;6:271.

47. Metz-Lutz MN, Filippini M. Neuropsychological findings in rolandic epilepsy and Landau-Kleffner syndrome. *Epilepsia* 2006;47:71.

48. Fejerman N, Caraballo RH, Dalla Bernardina B. Benign childhood epilepsy with centrotemporal spikes. In: Fejerman N, Caraballo RH (eds), *Benign Focal Epilepsies in Infancy, Childhood and Adolescence.* London: John Libbey, 2007; p. 77–113.

49. Fejerman N, Di Blasi AM. Status epilepticus of benign partial epilepsies in children: report of two cases. *Epilepsia* 1987;28:351.

50. Colamaria V, et al. Status epileptics in benign Rolandic epilepsy manifesting as anterior operculum syndrome. *Epilepsia* 1991;32:329.

51. Fejerman N. Atypical evolutions of benign partial epilepsies in children. *Int Pediatr* 1996;11:351.

52. Fejerman N, Caraballo R, Tenembaum SN. Atypical evolutions of benign localization-related epilepsies in children: are they predictable? *Epilepsia* 2000;41:380.

53. Fejerman N. Benign focal epilepsies in infancy, childhood and adolescence. *Rev Neurol* 2002;34:7.

54. Fejerman N. Benign childhood epilepsy with centrotemporal spikes. In: Engel J, Pedley TA (eds), *Epilepsy: A Comprehensive Textbook.* Philadelphia: Lippincott, Williams & Wilkins, 2008; 2nd ed: pp. 2369–2378.

55. Capovilla G, et al. Conceptual dichotomies in classifying epilepsies: partial versus generalized and idiopathic versus symptomatic. *Epilepsia* 2009;50:1645.

56. Arzimanoglou A, Guerrini R, Aicardi J. Epilepsies characterized by partial seizures. In: Arzimanoglou A, Guerrini R, Aicardi J (eds), *Aicardi´s Epilepsy in Children.* Philadelphia: Lippincott Williams & Wilkins, 2004; 3rd ed: p. 114.

57. Lundberg S, et al. Hippocampal assimetries and white matter abnormalities on MRI in benign childhood epilepsy with centrotemporal spikes. *Epilepsia* 1999;40:1808.

58. Sheth RD, Gutierrez AR, Riggs JE. Rolandic epilepsy and cortical dysplasia: MRI correlation of epileptiform discharges. *Pediatr Neurol* 1997;17:177.

59. Burke MS, Carroll JE, Burket RC. Benign Rolandic epilepsy and chromosome 7q deletion. *J Child Neurol* 1997;12:148.

60. Cassetti A. *Boll Lega It Epil* 2002;118:81. [Italian].

61. Scheffer IE, et al. Autosomal dominant Rolandic epilepsy and speech dyspraxia: a new syndrome with anticipation. *Ann Neurol* 1995;38:633.

62. Scheffer IE. Autosomal dominant rolandic epilepsy with speech dyspraxia. *Epileptic Disord* 2000;2:19.

63. Otsubo H, et al. Malignant rolandic-sylvian epilepsy in children: diagnosis, treatment, and outcomes. *Neurology* 2000;57:590.

64. Bourgeois BF. Drug treatment of benign focal epilepsies of childhood. *Epilepsia* 2000;41:1057.

65. Blom S, Heijbel J. Benign epilepsy of children with centrotemporal EEG foci: a follow-up study in adulthood of patients initially studied as children. *Epilepsia* 1982;23:629.

66. Galanopoulou A, et al. The spectrum of neuropsychiatric abnormalities associated with electrical status epilepticus in sleep. *Brain Dev* 2000;22:279.

67. Glauser TA, Double-blind placebo-controlled trial of adjunctive levetiracetam in pediatric partial seizures. *Neurology* 2000;66:1654.

68. Bourgeois B, et al. Gabapentin (neurontin) monotherapy in children with benign childhood epilepsy with centro-temporal spikes (BCECTS): a 36-week, double-blind, placebo-controlled study. *Epilepsia* 1998;39:163.

69. Rating D, Wolf C, Bast T. Sulthiame as monotherapy in children with benign childhood epilepsy with centrotemporal spikes: a 6-month randomized, double-blind, placebo-controlled study. Sulthiame Study Group. *Epilepsia* 2000;41:1284.

70. Engler F, et al. Treatment with sulthiame (Ospolot) in benign partial epilepsy of childhood and related syndromes: an open clinical and EEG study. *Neuropediatrics* 2003;34:105.

71. Doose H, et al. Benign partial epilepsy: treatment with sulthiame. *Dev Med Child Neurol* 1988;30:683.

72. Bouma PA, et al. The course of benign partial epilepsy of childhood with centrotemporal spikes: a meta-analysis. *Neurology* 1997;48:430.

73. De Negri M, Baglietto MG, Gaggero R. Benzodiazepine (BDZ) treatment of benign childhood epilepsy with centrotemporal spikes. *Brain Dev* 1997;19:506.

74. Mitsudome A, et al. The effectiveness of clonazepam on the rolandic discharges. *Brain Dev* 1997;19:274.

75. Tzitiridou M, et al. Oxcarbazepine monotherapy in benign childhood epilepsy with centrotemporal spikes: a clinical and cognitive evaluation. *Epilepsy Behav* 2005;7:458.

76. Donati F, et al. On behalf of The Oxcarbazepine Cognitive Study Group. The cognitive effects of oxcarbazepine versus carbamazepine or valproate in newly diagnosed children with partial seizures. *Seizure* 2007;16:670.

77. Coppola G, et al. Levetiracetam or oxcarbazepine as monotherapy in newly diagnosed benign epilepsy of childhood with centrotemporal spikes (BCECTS): an open-label, parallel group trial. *Brain Dev* 2007;29:281.

78. Perucca E, et al. Antiepileptic drugs as a cause of worsening seizures. *Epilepsia* 1998;39:5.

79. Guerrini R, et al. Exacerbation of epileptic negative myoclonus by carbamazepine or phenobarbital in children with atypical benign rolandic epilepsy. *Epilepsia* 1995; 36:65.

80. Caraballo R, et al. CBZ inducing atypical absences, drop-spells and continuous spike and waves during slow sleep (CSWS). *Boll Lega It Epil* 1989;66/67:379.

81. Guerrini R, et al. Epileptic negative myoclonus. *Neurology* 1993;43:1078.

82. Saltik S, et al. A clinical EEG study on idiopathic partial epilepsies with evolution into ESES spectrum disorders. *Epilepsia* 2005;46:524.

83. Prats JM, et al. Antiepileptic drugs and atypical evolution of idiopathic partial epilepsy. *Pediatr Neurol* 1998;18:402.

84. Grosso S, et al. Oxcarbazepine and atypical evolution of benign idiopathic focal epilepsy of childhood. *Eur J Neurol* 2003;13:1142.

85. Catania S, et al. Paradoxic reaction to lamotrigine in a child with benign focal epilepsy of childhood with centrotemporal spikes. *Epilepsia* 1999;40:1657.

86. Cerminara C, et al. Lamotrigine-induced seizure aggravation and negative myoclonus in idiopathic rolandic epilepsy. *Neurology* 2004;63:373.

87. Montenegro MA, Guerreiro MM. Electrical status epilepticus of sleep in association with Topiramate. *Epilepsia* 2002;43:1436.

88. Ben-Zeev B, et al. Sulthiame in childhood epilepsy. *Pediatr Int* 2004;46:521.

CHAPTER 26

Benign Occipital Epilepsies

Roberto H. Caraballo

▶ OVERVIEW

Gastaut presented a series of 36 patients with seizures suggesting occipital lobe origin, associated migraine-like symptoms, and occipital paroxysms of spike-waves, and proposed this condition as a new epileptic syndrome in childhood.[1] The 1989 International League Against Epilepsy (ILAE) Commission named this syndrome "childhood epilepsy with occipital paroxysms" and included it in the group of localization-related idiopathic epilepsies together with benign childhood epilepsy with centrotemporal spikes (BCECTSs).[2] In 1989, two studies by Panayiotopoulos based on a long follow-up of his patients called attention to a specific cluster of symptoms present in what he called "benign nocturnal childhood occipital epilepsy (COE)."[3,4] Vomiting as an ictal symptom and "cerebral insult-like" partial status epilepticus including autonomic symptoms were the most striking clinical manifestations.[3,4] Thereafter, several authors preferred the eponymic nomenclature of "Panayiotopoulos syndrome" (PS) in order to include patients with and without occipital spikes or occipital ictal origins.[5–7]

Our group proposed designating the first syndrome as "Gastaut type of benign childhood occipital epilepsy" in order to distinguish it from the "Panayiotopoulos type of benign childhood occipital epilepsy" or PS, which also manifests with occipital paroxysms.[5,6,8–10] These criteria were adopted by the Task Force on Classification and Terminology of the ILAE.[11]

In this chapter, we consider the therapeutic management of benign occipital epilepsies recognized in the Classification and Terminology of ILAE[11] that include, early-onset benign COE "Panayiotopoulos type" (PS) and late-onset childhood occipital epilepsy "Gastaut type" (COE of Gastaut).

▶ PANAYIOTOPOULOS SYNDROME

PS is a clearly recognized syndrome and the second-most frequent benign focal epilepsy syndrome in childhood after BCECTSs. PS is four to eight times more frequent than COE of Gastaut.[8]

Seventy-five percent of patients experience their first seizure between the ages of 3 and 6 years. PS affects boys and girls equally and in two-thirds of patients seizures occur only in sleep. Seizures may occur while awake and onset may be inconspicuous with pallor, agitation, nausea, and vomiting.[8]

The duration of the seizures is usually long, commonly lasting for more than 5 minutes, and in approximately 40% of cases lasts more than 30 minutes, constituting in those cases a focal or secondarily generalized status epilepticus. Three groups of symptoms are the most important in PS.[5–7,12–14]

▶ CLINICAL FEATURES

CORE CLINICAL FEATURES

Ictal Emetic Symptoms and Other Autonomic Manifestations

Ictal vomiting, which is relatively unusual in other epilepsies, occurs in approximately 80% of cases of PS. In seizures from wakefulness, other symptoms from the emetic spectrum such as nausea or retching occur during or before the vomiting.[15] Pallor is the most frequent autonomic manifestation.

Eye Deviation

Versive deviation of the eyes is as common as vomiting and occurs in approximately 80% of patients. Eye deviation is frequently accompanied by head deviation.

Impairment of Consciousness

Consciousness is usually intact at seizure onset but becomes impaired in 80%–90% of cases as the seizures progress.

FREQUENT FEATURES OF SEIZURES

Unilateral Clonic or Tonic–Clonic Seizures

Unilateral clonic or tonic–clonic seizures at onset or following vomiting and eye deviation occur in 25%–30% of cases.

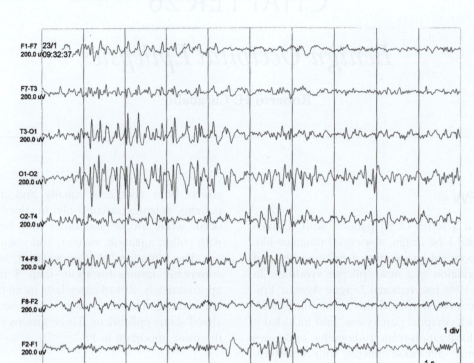

Figure 26–1. Five-year-old girl. Sleep EEG recording shows left occipital spikes and right temporal spikes independently.

Secondarily Generalized Tonic–Clonic Seizures

Secondarily generalized tonic–clonic seizures usually follow seizures starting with focal motor manifestations. In one series of patients, this course was seen in nearly 40% of the cases.[5]

Status Epilepticus

Status epilepticus is usually nonconvulsive, lasts more than 30 minutes, and occurs in approximately 30% of cases in all series.[5-7,13]

LESS FREQUENT (BUT NOT RARE) SYMPTOMS

Visual Symptoms

- Migraine-like headaches
- Incontinence of urine and faeces may occur when consciousness is impaired.
- Syncope-like manifestations

EEG FEATURES

Electroencephalographic Findings

The most useful laboratory test is the electroencephalographic (EEG). Occipital spikes are bilateral and synchronous, often with voltage asymmetry, or unilateral (Fig. 26–1). In the awake EEG, occipital paroxysms of high amplitude with sharp- and slow-wave complexes that occur immediately after closing the eyes are typically registered. These paroxysms are eliminated, or markedly attenuated, when the eyes are opened, a phenomenon due to fixation of sensitivity.[12] It has been emphasized that extraoccipital spikes (centrotemporal, frontal, or parietal) may also occur in children with PS.[5,6,12,16] According to a recent consensus report, normal EEGs during sleep are exceptional.[7]

ETIOLOGY

As an idiopathic epilepsy syndrome, PS is by definition not linked to a remote symptomatic or acute symptomatic etiology. It is most likely genetically determined, although no gene or chromosomic locus has been found. Affected siblings with PS have been reported.[5]

There is a high prevalence of febrile seizures, ranging from 16% to 45%, in children with PS.[5,8,16] A family history of epilepsy is reported in 30.3% of the cases.[5] The occurrence of several children with PS and Rolandic seizures and centrotemporal spikes typical of BCECTS,[17] as well as siblings having either Rolandic epilepsy or PS favors a genetic link between these syndromes, perhaps expressed as a reversible functional derangement of the brain cortical maturation.[3,5,15,17]

Recently, a family with atypical PS has been reported with an SCN1A missense mutation in the proband[18] that was not found in either her brother with febrile seizures or her parents. Two siblings with relatively early onset of seizures, prolonged time over which many seizures have occurred and strong association with febrile precipitants even after the age of 5 years.[19] These data indicate that SCN1A mutations when found contribute to a more severe clinical phenotype of PS.

PATHOPHYSIOLOGY

The basic mechanisms and pathophysiology of PS are largely unknown. The clinical findings suggest diffuse maturation-related cortical hyperexcitability.[7,16] While the majority of cases exhibit occipital EEG spikes, a significant number have spikes in other areas and spikes may appear in two brain areas at the same time or in the course of time in patients with PS and BCECTS.[15,17] In addition, the high frequency of ictal vomiting and other autonomic manifestations suggests that epileptic activity occurs in various cortical locations.

DIAGNOSTIC WORKUP

Neuroimaging and Other Laboratory Examinations

As in other idiopathic epilepsy syndromes, the neurological and neuropsychological evaluations of children with PS are normal. Vomiting and other autonomic symptoms are occasionally misleading and lead to excessive laboratory examinations. Cardiologic consultation is required if syncope-like manifestations occur. Brain imaging studies are typically normal but the unique ictal features and high frequency of status epilepticus may mandate magnetic resonance imaging (MRI) to rule out brain disorders that provoke focal, unilateral, or generalized seizures.

PROGNOSIS AND LONG-TERM OUTCOMES

Despite the high incidence of prolonged seizures and status epilepticus, PS is a remarkably benign epilepsy syndrome.[5,12,14,16] One-third of patients experience only a single seizure and most present no more than a total of two to five seizures. Remission usually occurs 1 or 2 years after seizure onset, and there is no data showing a significant difference in cases treated with antiepileptic drugs (AEDs).

In one series, 5 of 192 patients developed an atypical evolution characterized by negative myoclonus, absences, and frequent simple focal seizures associated with frequent or continuous bilateral spike-waves during slow wave sleep.[6] All presented transient neuropsychological impairment. Two cases were previously reported,[20] one

presented Rolandic seizures and ictal vomiting followed by eye deviation and impaired consciousness before atypical seizure onset. Four had a favorable evolution, but one was cognitively impaired at follow-up at 17 years of age.

TREATMENT

There is no consensus regarding treatment of PS. Since one-third of patients have only one seizure, either brief or prolonged, many authors recommend no AED treatment.[12,16] However, it is difficult to advise nontreatment after a prolonged seizure. We advocate treatment after a first prolonged seizure. Carbamazepine or Valproic acid is the drug of choice, with the latter preferred if the EEG shows spike-wave discharges. As seen in BCECTS, carbamazepine may also induce seizure exacerbation in PS.[6]

In patients with isolated seizures and seizures only at night during sleep, we recommend single nightly doses of Clobazam.

Levetiracetam is well tolerated by children as adjunctive treatment in pediatric partial seizures,[21] and is suggested as useful to treat the spectrum of continuous spikes and waves during slow sleep.[22] If confirmed, levetiracetam is another useful treatment alternative for benign focal epilepsies in childhood. However, we recently reported a case with cryptogenic focal epilepsy with continuous spikes and waves during slow sleep induced by levetiracetam.[23] Clear instructions should also be given to parents regarding the use of rectal diazepam immediately after the onset of a new seizure.

The prevention recommendations and therapeutic strategies to manage atypical evolutions in patients with PS are similar to the recommendations for BCECTS.[8]

An algorithm for treatment of PS is presented in Fig. 26–2.

▶ CHILDHOOD OCCIPITAL EPILEPSY OF GASTAUT

COE of Gastaut is a rare condition with a prevalence approximating 0.2%–0.9% of all epilepsies, and 2%–7% of benign childhood focal seizures.[16] It is estimated to account for 0.15% of all focal epilepsies in childhood.[24]

CLINICAL FEATURES

The seizures of COE of Gastaut are always of occipital lobe onset and primarily manifest with visual seizures, which are the most typical and usually the first ictal symptom. The main types of seizures recognized in patients with COE of Gastaut are visual manifestations, motor seizures, migraine-like symptoms, and less-frequent autonomic manifestations.[1,9,10,12,16,25,26]

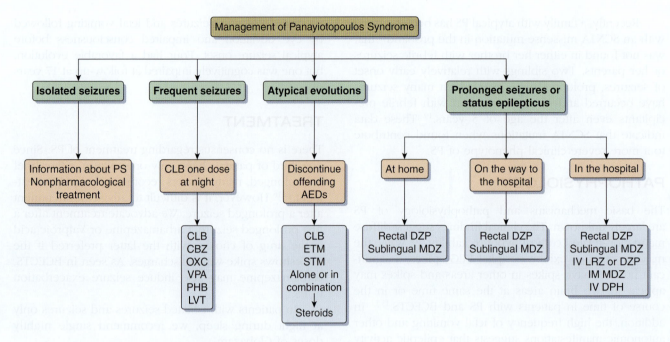

Figure 26–2. Management of Panayiotopoulos syndrome.

Visual Seizures

Visual seizures occur predominantly during the day at no particular time, but may also appear during sleep causing patients to awaken. They consist of elementary and complex visual hallucinations, visual illusions, blindness or partial visual loss, and sensory hallucinations.

The elementary visual hallucinations occur as an initial seizure symptom in the majority of the patients. These hallucinations are brief, seldom exceeding 1–2 minutes. The hallucinations are always stereotyped, and usually multicolored and circular, appearing either in the periphery of a hemifield or centrally. They may be the only ictal manifestation or they may progress to other seizures symptoms.

Complex visual hallucinations are less frequent. The patient may see a face or figures that often have the same location and movement sequence as that of the elementary visual hallucinations.

Ictal visual illusions, such as micropsia, metamorphopsia, palinopsia, and polyopia, are probably generated from the nondominant parietal regions.[10,16]

Acute transient blindness is the second-most common ictal symptom. It often occurs alone and may be the only ictal symptom in patients who experience visual hallucinations without blindness.[10,16]

Motor Seizures and Other Types of Seizures

Deviation of the eyes, often associated with ipsilateral head version, is the most common nonvisual symptom, occurring in approximately 70% of patients. Forced eyelid closure and blinking—an interesting ictal clinical symptom of occipital seizures—occurs in approximately 10% of patients.

Elementary visual hallucinations or other ictal symptoms may evolve into hemi- or generalized seizures.

Ictal vomiting is extremely rare in COE of Gastaut and probably represents overlapping between the PS syndrome and COE of Gastaut.[9]

Migraine-like Symptoms

Ictal or postictal headache occurs in 30%–50% of patients. As in classical migraine, the onset of the headache occurs immediately or within 5–10 minutes of the end of the visual hallucinations. The headache is often mild to moderate in severity and diffuse, but may be severe, pulsating, and associated with nausea, vomiting, photophobia, and phonophobia that may make it indistinguishable from migraine.[8,12,26]

EEG FEATURES

The EEG shows occipital paroxysms that, in routine recordings, occur when the eyes are closed and disappear or attenuate upon eye opening, reflecting fixation-off sensitivity (Fig. 26–3). EEGs with random occipital spikes, sometimes occurring only during sleep, are frequent.

A small number of patients with COE of Gastaut have rare occipital spikes and consistently normal EEGs.[26]

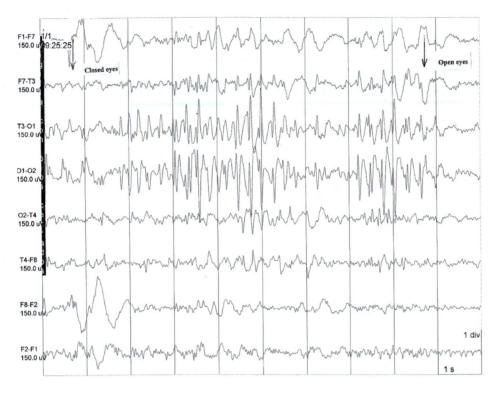

Figure 26–3. Eight-year-old boy. EEG recording while awake shows onset of occipital spike-wave discharges after eye closure and spike-wave discharges disappear after eye opening.

Centrotemporal, frontal, and giant somatosensory spikes are much less frequent than in PS.[8]

ETIOLOGY

A family history of epilepsy is found in 20%–30% of cases and a family history of migraine in 15%.[9,25] A history of febrile seizures is reported in 14% of patients.[9] Recently, two families with two members with COE of Gastaut were described by Grosso et al.[27]

In a genetic study of patients with PS and COE of Gastaut analyzing twin and multiplex families, Taylor et al[28] found a single concordant monozygotic and dizygotic twin pair suggesting that genetic factors play an important role.

Overlap between PS and COE of Gastaut has been observed infrequently[7,9,26,28] suggesting that the two epileptic syndromes might be a continuum related to a process of brain maturation.

Patients with PS, COE of Gastaut, and BCECTS have EEG features in common with idiopathic generalized epilepsies. For example, generalized spike-waves have been reported in PS, COE of Gastaut, and BCECTS.[8,26] We have observed patients with childhood absence epilepsy and focal EEG abnormalities with or without clinical manifestations.[29] The overlap between

idiopathic generalized and idiopathic focal epilepsies occurs at a number of levels, both within individuals and in relatives. It is probably due to the complex inheritance that underlies the common idiopathic epilepsies where a number of genes as well as environmental factors contribute to the etiology.

PATHOPHYSIOLOGY

Scalp and deep ictal EEG recordings clearly reveal that elementary visual hallucinations arise from the visual cortex.

DIAGNOSTIC WORKUP

Consistent with an idiopathic syndrome, neurological examination, mental status, and high-resolution MRI are normal. However, because of the high incidence of symptomatic occipital epilepsies with similar clinical and EEG manifestations, all patients should undergo high resolution MRI to rule out a static or progressive occipital disorder.

Although we have already described the EEG features in COE of Gastaut, it is important to underscore the need to check for changes in the EEG after eye opening in order to detect the peculiar phenomenon of

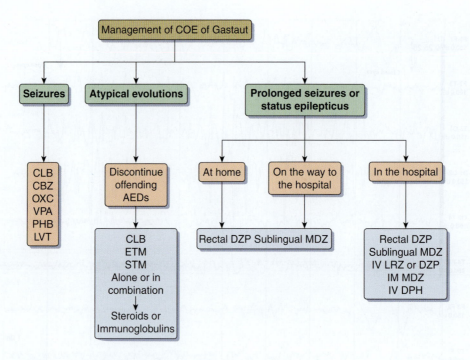

Figure 26–4. Management of COE of Gastaut.

disappearance of the occipital spike-wave discharges, even when it is not pathognomic of this syndrome.

PROGNOSIS AND LONG-TERM EVOLUTION

Some controversies in the diagnosis of idiopathic occipital epilepsies in childhood and adolescence may also shed doubts on its prognosis and long-term evolution.[8] Therefore, the prognosis of COE of Gastaut is less clear than PS. Available data indicate that remission occurs in 50%–60% of patients within 2–4 years after onset.[16,25] Seizures show a fairly good response to AEDs in more than 90% of patients.

Cases of symptomatic occipital epilepsy may present the same clinical and EEG features and probably bias the prognosis of patients with COE of Gastaut.

Two cases with COE of Gastaut have presented with atypical evolutions. Both had severe cognitive deterioration associated with continuous spike-waves during slow-wave sleep. One had a good response to intravenous γ-globulin and experienced an excellent evolution of cognitive abilities; the other child did not respond to AEDs or intravenous γ-globulin and evidenced persistent and severe cognitive impairment.[8] These atypical evolutions are similar to atypical patients with Rolandic epilepsy and PS.[20,30] Also, children with COE of Gastaut may rarely exhibit typical absence seizures which usually appear after the onset of occipital seizures.[31]

TREATMENT

Patients with COE of Gastaut often suffer from frequent seizures and medical treatment is mandatory. There is a lack of controlled data to indicate the drug of choice although it has been stated that seizures usually stop or are dramatically reduced within days after appropriate treatment with carbamazepine.[8,12,16] We have used valproic acid in cases with clear spike-wave activities in occipital areas with good results. However, we believe that carbamazepine, oxcarbazepine, valproic acid, levetiracetam, and other AEDs are equally effective.

A slow reduction in the dose of medication 2–3 years after the last visual or other minor or major seizure is advisable, but treatment should be reinitiated if visual seizures reappear.

The prevention recommendations and therapeutic strategies to manage the atypical evolutions in patients with COE of Gastaut are similar to the ones that should be considered in patients with BCECTS.[8] We show an algorithm for the treatment of PS (Fig. 26–4).

▶ SUMMARY

Recognition of benign epilepsies with occipital seizures is crucial to select the best treatment option. In a patient with PS who only had one seizure, pharmacological treatment may be avoided, but in patients with prolonged and recurrent seizures, AEDs are indicated. Instructions on the use of diazepam are useful for the parents, particularly when the child has prolonged seizures at home. However, the therapeutic approach should be individualized for each patient. In patients with COE of Gastaut, pharmacologic treatment should always be considered.

Patients with both types of occipital epilepsies may develop an atypical evolution and prevention recommendations and treatment strategies of this particular electroclinical picture should be managed accordingly.

REFERENCES

1. Gastaut H. A new type of epilepsy: benign partial epilepsy of childhood with occipital spike-waves. *Clin Electroencephalog* 1982;13:13–22.

2. Commission on Classification and Terminology of the International League Against Epilepsy. Proposal for revised classification of epilepsies and epileptic syndromes. *Epilepsia* 1989;30:389–399.

3. Panayiotopoulos CP. Benign nocturnal childhood occipital epilepsy: a new syndrome with nocturnal seizures, tonic deviation of the eyes, and vomiting. *J Child Neurol* 1989a; 4:43–49

4. Panayiotopoulos CP. Benign childhood epilepsy with occipital paroxysms: a 15-year prospective study. *Annal Neurol* 1989b;26:51–56.

5. Caraballo R, Cersosimo R, Medina C, Fejerman N. Panayiotopoulos-type benign childhood occipital epilepsy: a prospective study. *Neurology* 2000;55:1096–1100.

6. Caraballo R, Cersósimo R, Fejerman N. Panayiotopoulos syndrome: a prospective study of 192 patients. *Epilepsia* 2007;48(6):1054–1061.

7. Ferrie CD, et al. Panayiotopoulos syndrome: a consensus view. *Develop Med Child Neurol* 2006;48(3):236–240.

8. Fejerman N, Caraballo R. *Benign Focal Epilepsies in Infancy, Childhood and Adolescence.* London: John Libbey Eurotext, 2007.

9. Caraballo RH, Cersosimo RO, Medina CS, Tenembaum S, Fejerman N. Epilepsias parciales idiopáticas con paroxismos occipitales. *Revista de Neurologia* 1997;25:1052–1058.

10. Caraballo R, Fejerman N. Late-onset childhood occipital epilepsy (Gastaut type). In: Fejerman N, Caraballo R, (eds), *Benign Focal Epilepsies in Infancy, Childhood and Adolescence.* London: John Libbey Eurotext, 2007; pp 145–167.

11. Engel J Jr. A proposed diagnostic scheme for people with epileptic seizures and with epilepsy: Report of the ILAE Task Force on Classification and Terminology. *Epilepsia* 2001;42(6):796–803.

12. Panayiotopoulos CP. *Benign Childhood Partial Seizures and Related Epileptic Syndromes.* London: John Libbey, 1999.

13. Ferrie CD, et al. Autonomic status epilepticus in Panayiotopoulos síndrome and other childhood and adult epilepsias: a consensos view. *Epilepsia* 2007;48:1165–1172.

14. Specchio N, Trivisano M, Balestri M, Cappelletti S, Di Ciommo V, Gentile S, Masciarelli G, Silvestri D, Volkov J, Fusco L, Vigevano F. 2010a. Panayiotopoulos syndrome: a clinical, EEG and neuropsychological study of 93 consecutive patients. *Epilepsia* 2010;51:2098-2107.

15. Covanis A, Lada C, Skiadas K. Children with Rolandic spikes and ictus emeticus: rolandic epilepsy or Panayiotopoulos syndrome? *Epileptic Disorders* 2003;5:139–143.

16. Covanis A, et al. Panayiotopoulos syndrome and Gastaut type idiopathic childhood occipital epilepsy. In: Roger J, Bureau M, Dravet CH, et al. (eds), *Epileptic Syndromes in Infancy, Childhood and Adolescence.* London: John Libbey Eurotext, 2005; 4th edn: pp. 227–253.

17. Caraballo R, Cersosimo R, Fejerman N. Idiopathic partial epilepsies with rolandic and occipital sikes appearing in the same children. *J Epilepsy* 1998;11:261–264.

18. Grosso S, et al. SCN1A mutation associated with atypical Panayiotopoulos syndrome. *Neurology* 2007;69:609–611.

19. Livinstong JH, Cross JH, Mclellan A, Birch R, Zuberi SM. A novel inherited mutation in the voltage sensor region of SCN1A is associated with Panayiotopoulos syndrome in siblings and generalized epilepsy with febrile seizures plus. *J Child Neurol* 2009;24(4):503–508.

20. Caraballo RH, Astorino F, Cersosimo R, Soprano AM, Fejerman N. Atypical evolution in childhood epilepsy with occipital paroxysms (Panayiotopoulos type). *Epileptic Disorders* 2001;3:157–162.

21. Glauser T, et al. ILAE treatment guidelines: evidence-based analysis of antiepileptic drug efficacy and effectiveness as initial monotherapy for epileptic seizures and syndromes. *Epilepsia* 2006;47(7):1094–1120.

22. Aebi A, et al. Levetiracetam efficacy in epileptic syndromes with continuous spikes and waves during slow sleep: experience in 12 cases. *Epilepsia* 2005;46(12):1937–1942.

23. Caraballo R, Cersósimo R, de los Santos C. Levetiracetam-induced seizure aggravation and continuous spikes-waves during slow-sleep in children with refractory epilepsies. *Epileptic Disord* 2010;12(2):146–150.

24. Chahine LM, Mikati MA. Benign pediatric localization-related epilepsies. Syndromes in childhood. *Epileptic Disord* 2006;8:243–258.

25. Gastaut H, Roger J, Bureau M. Benign epilepsy of childhood with occipital paroxysms. Up-date. In: Roger J, Bureau M, Dravet C, Dreifuss FE, Perret A, Wolf P (eds), *Epileptic Syndromes in Infancy, Childhood and Adolescence.* London: John Libbey & Company Ltd, 1992; pp. 201–217.

26. Caraballo R, Cersósimo R, Fejerman R. Childhood occipital epilepsy of Gastaut: study of 33 patients. *Epilepsia* 2008a; 49(2):288–297.

27. Grosso S, et al. Late-onset childhood occipital epilepsy (Gastaut type) a family study. *Eur J Paediatr Neurol* 2008; 12(5):421–426.

28. Taylor I, Berkovic S, Kivity S, Scheffer I. Benign occipital epilepsies of childhood: clinical features and genetics. *Brain* 2008;131:2287–2294.

29. Caraballo R, et al. Childhood absence epilepsy and electroencephalographic focal abnormalities with or without clinical manifestations. *Seizures* 2008b;17:617–624.

30. Fejerman N, Caraballo R, Tenembaum SN. Atypical evolutions of benign localization-related epilepsies in children: are they predictable? *Epilepsia* 2000;41(4):380–390.

31. Caraballo RH, Cersosimo RO, Fejerman N. Late-onset, "Gastaut type", childhood occipital epilepsy: an unusual evolution. *Epileptic Disord* 2005;7:341–346.

CHAPTER 27

Autosomal Dominant Nocturnal Frontal Lobe Epilepsy

Christopher Derry and Ingrid E. Scheffer

▶ INTRODUCTION

Autosomal dominant nocturnal frontal lobe epilepsy (ADNFLE) is a familial focal epilepsy syndrome characterized by frontal lobe seizures occurring predominantly during light sleep. Although not a common condition, it is increasingly recognized, with over 100 families reported.[1] It was first described in 1994 in families from Australia, Canada, and the United Kingdom,[2] and subsequently became the first human epilepsy for which an underlying genetic defect was identified. The first mutation to be discovered was in the *CHRNA4* gene encoding the α4 subunit of the nicotinic acetylcholine receptor (nAChR),[3] a ligand-gated ion channel. The subsequent discovery of further nAChR subunit gene mutations in ADNFLE,[4–6] along with ion channel gene mutations in various other familial epilepsy syndromes, led to the concept of channelopathies as the fundamental basis to many epilepsy syndromes.[7]

CLINICAL, ELECTROGRAPHIC, AND IMAGING FINDINGS IN ADNFLE

Clinical Features

Seizure onset is usually in childhood, typically between 8 and 11 years of age, although onset ranges from 1 to 52 years.[8,9] Seizures tend to occur in clusters and arise almost exclusively from sleep, with children usually having 6–8 seizures per night occurring over a few hours.[8] Seizures most commonly occur as the individual is falling off to sleep, or in the morning toward the end of the normal sleep period. Less commonly seizures occur sporadically throughout the night. Around 25% of patients also have occasional daytime seizures during periods of poor control.[8,9]

Semiology is consistent with frontal lobe seizures, with rare secondarily generalized tonic–clonic seizures in some individuals. Although seizure semiology can vary markedly between patients with ADNFLE, it is usually highly stereotyped within a given individual. Subjects are often woken by a nonspecific aura but more frequent auras include a shiver, a feeling of "breath being stuck in the throat," or sensory phenomena in the limbs.[8] Vocalization, which may be a grunt, moan, or a single word, is very common at onset, and may continue throughout the event.[8] Motor features are usually prominent, and may take a variety of forms such as frenetic bipedal automatisms, rhythmic axial movements, and asymmetric tonic posturing. Tonic posturing may be severe such that some individuals have bent their bed-head when holding on to it during a seizure. Other individuals have seizures that appear like a generalized tonic–clonic seizure but awareness is preserved. The appearance of the seizure may be bizarre, and misdiagnosis is not uncommon.[8,9] Consciousness is often preserved through the seizures, or may vary in different attacks in an individual, and is usually associated with a sense of fear or panic during the seizure. Not surprisingly, frequent attacks may cause a child to become scared of falling asleep. Seizures are brief, typically less than 1 minute in duration, and are highly stereotyped. They tend to occur in clusters of, on average, around eight seizures per night, although up to 70 events per night have been recorded in some individuals.[8] Although nocturnal frontal lobe seizures may manifest in a wide variety of ictal behaviors, in general, they can be subdivided into three broad categories for descriptive purposes based on duration.[10] *Paroxysmal arousals* are brief, stereotyped arousals, usually lasting 20 seconds or less; *paroxysmal nocturnal dystonia* describes events lasting up to 2 minutes with prominent dystonic components and often other frontal lobe features; and *epileptic nocturnal wanderings*, where the subject leaves the bed and may walk or run around, often in an agitated fashion, performing semipurposeful behaviors, last longer. Most individuals display more than one of these patterns, including subtle, brief attacks that are simply the beginning of longer seizures if scrutinized carefully on video-EEG monitoring. Epileptic nocturnal wanderings are relatively uncommon.[10]

ADNFLE is usually considered to be a relatively mild disorder. However, there is significant variability both within and between families, in terms of both the severity of epilepsy,[9] the semiology of the seizures[11] and the associated comorbidity. Although in some cases, seizures may be frequent and difficult to treat in childhood and adolescence, in general, they resolve or improve substantially as the individual reaches adult life.[8,9] However, more recently, families have been reported with a more severe ADNFLE phenotype,[12] with frequent refractory seizures associated with cognitive impairment and psychiatric symptoms, and in some cases with cognitive decline. Moreover, recent detailed neuropsychological studies have suggested that subtle cognitive deficits are present in many other, apparently intellectually normal, individuals with ADNFLE. Impaired cognitive flexibility appears to be the core deficit,[13] but more widespread impairments in memory and general intellectual function may also be present.[14]

Ictal and Interictal EEG

Interictal EEG. The interictal EEG is usually normal in wakefulness; during sleep, interictal epileptiform abnormalities may be seen in up to 50% of cases, but even when present, are often sparse.[8,9] Nonspecific abnormalities such as frontal theta and delta slowing may occur in some patients.

Ictal EEG. Seizures typically arise from stage 2 NREM sleep, but may also occur in stage 3 or 4. The ictal EEG is often difficult to interpret, frequently being obscured by muscle and motion artifact. When ictal electrographic patterns are discernable they are usually poorly localized, although typically show a frontal predominance. Ictal patterns may comprise rhythmic sharp waves or repetitive 8–11 Hz spikes, but frank recruiting rhythms are rarely seen;[11] more often, nonspecific patterns such as diffuse flattening or rhythmic frontal theta or delta rhythms are recorded.[8–11] In about 25% of cases, both interictal and ictal EEG are normal.[9] Therefore, EEG alone may be of limited diagnostic value; inpatient video-EEG monitoring, with the ability to analyze the stereotypy of seizure semiology, may be required in cases of diagnostic uncertainty. video-EEG monitoring may lead to the identification of attacks of variable duration such as paroxysmal arousals and seizures of longer duration occurring in one individual. The briefest awakenings may be dismissed as simply arousals until they are directly compared with the clear-cut seizures and seen to be a fragment of the characteristic semiology.

Neuroimaging

Computerized tomography and magnetic resonance imaging (MRI) studies are normal in ADNFLE.[8,9] Interictal abnormalities of[18] fludeoxyglucose (FDG) positron emission tomography (PET) have been reported showing frontal hypometabolism without a characteristic pattern.[11] PET studies in individuals with ADNFLE using a specific $\alpha 4\beta 2$ PET ligand ([^{18}F]-F-A-85380) showed increased binding in brainstem and epithalamus, but reduced binding in mesial frontal regions, when compared to controls.[15] Ictal single photon emission computerised tomography (SPECT) studies may show frontal hyperperfusion relative to the interictal state (Fig. 27–1).

DIFFERENTIAL DIAGNOSIS

The diagnosis of ADNFLE may be difficult for two reasons. Firstly, making a correct diagnosis of nocturnal frontal lobe epilepsy (NFLE) in an individual is not always straightforward; and secondly, the familial nature of the condition may not be obvious.

By far the biggest practical problem in clinical practice is the distinction of NFLE from NREM arousal parasomnias such as night terrors and somnambulism that may occur in children and adults. However, a careful history, will usually be sufficient to distinguish these disorders. The most important historical features indicating NFLE as opposed to benign parasomnias are: the timing of events (in NFLE this is often within 30 minutes of sleep onset, whereas parasomnias typically occur after 1–2 hours of sleep); the number of events per night (in NFLE, there are often multiple events in a single night, whereas parasomnias rarely occur more than once or, at most, twice per night); the duration of events, which may be brief or prolonged in parasomnias, but in NFLE are almost invariably brief (usually less than 1 minute); and the presence of an aura (very common in at least a proportion of seizures in individuals with NFLE, but almost never a feature of parasomnias). Extensive wandering is rare in NFLE, although may occasionally occur and is nondirected, but is common in parasomnias and often partially directed (such as voiding in a drawer instead of the toilet). Conversely, lucid recall for events is common in at least a proportion of seizures in NFLE, but is very uncommon in parasomnias (although some vague recollection may be reported). If these features are explicitly discussed with the patient and witness when taking the history, a correct diagnosis will be reached in most cases, often during the initial clinical consultation.

The frontal lobe epilepsy and parasomnias (FLEP) scale, a simple validated clinical scale that addresses these aspects of the history, may be used to assist the clinician in arriving at the correct diagnosis (Table 27–1).[16] In cases where diagnostic uncertainty remains despite a rigorous history, recording of events using video-EEG monitoring is usually required; however, this is not always achievable if attacks are relatively infrequent. Other sleep disorders that can sometimes cause potential confusion with NFLE and should be considered in the child with nocturnal attacks include rhythmic movement disorder of sleep, sleep-related breathing disorders, and psychogenic nonepileptic attacks.

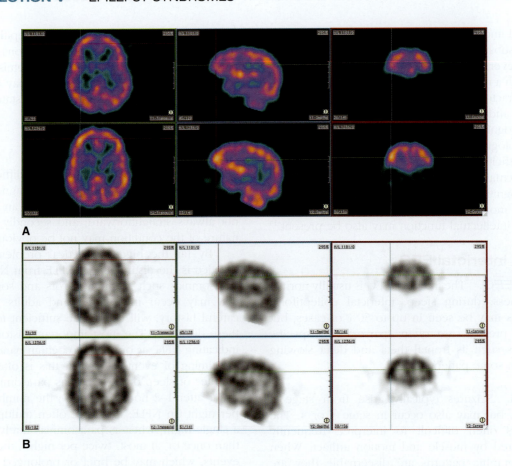

Figure 27–1. Interictal (**A**) and ictal (**B**) technetium-99m-HMPAO SPECT scans of a 4-year-old girl with ADNFLE (the ictal injection was administered 18 seconds into a seizure of 28 seconds duration). The ictal study shows right frontal hyperperfusion relative to the interictal study (left panel axial images, middle parasagittal, right coronal).

Even after NFLE has been correctly diagnosed in an individual, the familial nature of ADNFLE may be elusive, and a meticulous family history is necessary if the condition is to be recognized. This is due, at least in part, to the unusual seizure semiology and characteristic intrafamilial variability in seizure severity and frequency in ADNFLE. Mildly affected family members may have never sought medical attention, and even in more severe cases, misdiagnosis is common due to the unusual seizure semiology.[2] The clinician should also, therefore, ask about a family history of nocturnal events and sleep, parasomnias or pseudoseizures (particularly from sleep). In an individual with known NFLE, such a family history should raise the suspicion of ADNFLE.

CLINICAL GENETICS

ADNFLE is inherited in classic Mendelian autosomal dominant fashion with incomplete (70%–80%) penetrance,[3,4,8,9,17] and displays striking phenotypic heterogeneity. As discussed earlier, individuals with the same underlying genetic mutation, even within the same family, demonstrate significant phenotypic variability both in terms of disease severity and in seizure semiology. In addition, there is also clear genetic heterogeneity; the spectrum of features seen in families with ADNFLE appears to be largely indistinguishable in families with mutations of the α4 and β2 nAChR subunit genes,[18] and individual mutations are not, in general, associated with any distinctive clinical features. However, a possible exception is the ser252leu mutation of the α4 subunit gene that has been reported in three families and may be associated with increased rates of mental retardation and refractoriness to antiepileptic medication.[19]

MOLECULAR GENETICS

To date, all mutations identified in ADNFLE have been in genes coding for subunits of the nAChR (Table 27–2). Four mutations have been identified in the gene coding for the nAChR α4 subunit (*CHRNA4*),[3,17,20,21] and three mutations have been identified in *CHRNB2*, the gene coding for the nAChR β2 subunit.[4,6,22] These mutations have subsequently

▶ **TABLE 27-1.** THE FRONTAL LOBE EPILEPSY AND PARASOMNIAS SCALE

Clinical Feature		Score
Age at onset		
At what age did the patients have their first clinical event?	<55 yr	0
	>55 yr	−1
Duration		
What is the duration of a typical event?	<2 min	+1
	2–10 min	0
	>10 min	−2
Clustering		
What is the typical number of events to occur in a single night?	1 or 2	0
	3–5	+1
	>5	+2
Timing		
At what time of night do the events most commonly occur?	Within 30 min of sleep onset	+1
	Other times (including if no clear pattern identified)	0
Symptoms		
Are the events associated with a definite aura?	Yes	+2
	No	0
Does the patient ever wander outside the bedroom during the events?	Yes	−2
	No (or certain)	0
Does the patient perform complex, directed behaviors (e.g., picking up objects, dressing) during events?	Yes	−2
	No (or uncertain)	0
Is there a clear history of prominent dystonic posturing, tonic limb extension, or cramping during events?	Yes	+1
	No (or uncertain)	0
Stereotypy		
Are the events highly stereotyped or variable in nature?	Highly stereotyped	+1
	Some variability/uncertain	0
	Highly variable	−1
Recall		
Does the patient recall the events?	Yes, lucid recall	+1
	No or vague recollection only	0
Vocalization		
Does the patient speak during the events and, if so, is there subsequent recollection of this speech?	No	0
	Yes, sounds only or single words	0
	Yes, coherent speech with incomplete or no recall	−2
	Yes, coherent speech with recall	+2
Total score		

A score of 0 or less indicates the patient is very likely to have parasomnias, a diagnosis of greater than +3 indicates the patient is very likely to have epilepsy, and a diagnosis of +1 to +3 indicates that epilepsy is likely but that the diagnosis is uncertain.
Source: Adapted from Derry CP, Davey M, Johns M, Kron K, Glencross D, Marini C, Scheffer IE, et al (2006). Distinguishing sleep disorders from seizures: diagnosing bumps in the night. *Archives of neurology,* 63(5), 705–709. doi:10.1001/archneur.63.5.705.

been identified in other families with ADNFLE from various ethnic backgrounds, including European, Middle Eastern, Korean, and Japanese.[8,19,23]

As a result of these findings, ADNFLE is generally considered a disorder of the neuronal nicotinic nAChR, a ligand-gated ion channel that is distributed widely throughout the central nervous system. This receptor has a heteropentameric structure, comprising various combinations of α and β subunits; the α4β2 subtype (two α subunits and three β) is the predominant form expressed in the human brain. Its function is not fully understood, although it may

be important in the modulation of neurotransmitter release in a number of systems, and appears to play a role in the regulation of gene expression during development.[24]

Until recently, the α4β2 nAChR subtype was thought to be the only receptor involved in ADNFLE. However, the recent discovery of α2 subunit involvement in one family[5] suggests that other nAChR subunits may be important in some cases. To complicate the situation further, an association was reported between polymorphisms in the promoter region of the corticotrophin releasing hormone (CRH) and ADNFLE in

▶ **TABLE 27–2.** SUMMARY OF THE IDENTIFIED GENETIC MUTATIONS IN ADNFLE. NOTE THAT THE POLYMORPHISMS REPORTED IN THE CRH GENE PROMOTER REGION (*) HAVE NOT BEEN CONFIRMED AS PATHOGENIC AND REPLICATION OF THIS FINDING IS AWAITED

Gene	Gene Product	Mutation/Polymorphism	Key References
CHRNA2	α2 subunit of nAChR	CHRNA4 Ser248Phe	3, 18, 33, 34
		CHRNA4 Ser252Leu	19, 21, 35, 36
		CHRNA4 776insGCT	17
		CHRNA4 Thr265Iso	20
CHRNB2	β2 subunit of the nAChR receptor	CHRNB2 V287L	4
		CHRNB2 Val287Met	6
		CHRNB2 I312M	22
CHRNA2	α2 subunit of the nAChR receptor	CHRNA2 I279N	5
CRH	Corticotrophin releasing hormone	CRH 1470C-A*	37
		CRH 1166G-C*	

some families.[37] Although this finding has not yet been replicated, it raises the possibility that alternative, non-nAChR–mediated, mechanisms may be involved in some instances.

In fact, despite the considerable evidence for involvement of the nAChR in ADNFLE, only a minority of families (probably less than 10% overall) is accounted for by recognized nAChR mutations.[25] Screening studies in sporadic NFLE and ADNFLE patients have had a very low positive rate for nAChR mutations.[25,26] The molecular basis of the remaining cases remains unclear and is a focus of ongoing research.

PROGNOSIS

ADNFLE is usually a relatively benign epilepsy syndrome, and the prognosis is usually favorable. Most affected individuals have mild epilepsy, being either easily controlled on antiepileptic drugs, or in some cases requiring no medical treatment. Although some cases may be refractory in childhood, seizure control tends to improve considerably in adulthood. Seizures resolve in the majority of patients by adult life; however, some adults report subtle remnants of their earlier seizures occurring into their sixties.[8] In families, a few individuals may have highly refractory seizures that are not controlled despite multiple antiepileptic drugs.[8] Comorbidities have been reported relatively infrequently, and most individuals are said to be of normal intellect although it is increasingly recognized that many have subtle neuropsycholgical deficits on detailed assessment.[13,14]

However, as discussed earlier, recent reports indicate that ADNFLE may sometimes have a more pernicious presentation. Some individuals have been reported in whom epilepsy is severe and refractory throughout their lives, with periods of very frequent seizure activity and frank status epilepticus. In addition, significant rates of psychiatric and cognitive morbidity have been

reported in several families, suggesting that ADNFLE may confer a predisposition to such conditions.[19,27–29] Early diagnosis and optimal treatment of ADNFLE is likely to be important in minimizing the development of such sequelae.

TREATMENT

ADNFLE is not a common disorder, and data to guide its effective treatment are limited. However, anecdotally, seizures in ADNFLE tend to respond well to treatment with antiepileptic drugs in the majority of patients. A number of authors have reported particular success with carbamazepine,[8,9] and indeed there is laboratory evidence to indicate that the mutant α4β2 nAChR is particularly sensitive to this drug.[30] Acetazolamide has also been reported to be helpful in resistant cases.[31] In a single patient with a known α4 nAChR receptor subunit mutation, nicotine (administered via patch) was found to be an effective treatment.[32]

Surgical treatment has no recognized place in the treatment of ADNFLE. In most cases, the condition is easily controlled with medical therapy, and the genetic basis of the disorder, combined with normal MRI imaging and the absence of clearly localizing features on ictal or interictal EEG makes surgery not a feasible option in the small number of drug-resistant individuals. If sufficient data existed to suggest a surgically amenable epileptogenic zone, it is not known if this would be effective as seizures may then arise from another region as all cells contain the genetic defect.

GENETIC COUNSELING

Individuals with ADNFLE should be offered genetic counseling as they have a 50% risk of passing on the genetic mutation that has a 70% penetrance for clinical seizures. They should be counseled about the variable nature of the nocturnal attacks to facilitate earlier diagnosis and treatment. They should also be monitored for potential cognitive and psychiatric morbidity that occurs in some families. Prenatal testing could be offered where a known genetic mutation exists with appropriate planning.

REFERENCES

1. Combi RL, et al. Autosomal dominant nocturnal frontal lobe epilepsy—a critical overview. *J Neurol* 2004;251(8):923–934.
2. Scheffer IE, et al. Autosomal dominant frontal epilepsy misdiagnosed as sleep disorder. *Lancet* 1994;343(8896):515–517.
3. Steinlein OK, et al. A missense mutation in the neuronal nicotinic acetylcholine receptor alpha 4 subunit is associated with autosomal dominant nocturnal frontal lobe epilepsy. *Nat Genet* 1995;11(2):201–203.
4. De Fusco M, et al. The nicotinic receptor beta 2 subunit is mutant in nocturnal frontal lobe epilepsy. *Nat Genet* 2000;26(3):275–276.
5. Aridon P, Marini C, DiResta C, Brilli E, De Fusco M, Politi F, Parrini E, Manfredi I, Pisano T, Pruna D, Curia G, Cianchetti C, Pasqualetti M, Becchetti A, Guerrini R, Casari G. Increased sensitivity of the neuronal nicotinic receptor a2 subunit causes familial epilepsy with nocturnal wandering and ictal fear. *Am J Hum Genet* 2006;79:342–350.
6. Phillips HA, et al. CHRNB2 is the second acetylcholine receptor subunit associated with autosomal dominant nocturnal frontal lobe epilepsy. *Am J Hum Genet* 2001;68(1):225–231.
7. Helbig I, Scheffer IE, Mulley JC, Berkovic SF. Navigating channels and beyond: unravelling the genetics of the epilepsies. *Lancet Neurol* 2008;7(3):231–245.
8. Scheffer IE, et al. Autosomal dominant nocturnal frontal lobe epilepsy. A distinctive clinical disorder. *Brain* 1995;118(Pt 1):61–73.
9. Oldani A, et al. Autosomal dominant nocturnal frontal lobe epilepsy. A video-polysomnographic and genetic appraisal of 40 patients and delineation of the epileptic syndrome. *Brain* 1998;121(Pt 2):205–223.
10. Provini F, et al. Nocturnal frontal lobe epilepsy. A clinical and polygraphic overview of 100 consecutive cases. *Brain* 1999;122(Pt 6):1017–1031.
11. Hayman M, et al. Autosomal dominant nocturnal frontal lobe epilepsy: demonstration of focal frontal onset and intrafamilial variation. *Neurology* 1997;49(4):969–975.
12. Derry C, et al. Severe autosomal dominant nocturnal frontal lobe epilepsy associated with psychiatric disorders and intellectual disability. *Epilepsia* 2008;49:2125.
13. Wood A, et al. Neuropsychological function in patients with a single gene mutation associated with autosomal dominant nocturnal frontal lobe epilepsy. *Epilepsy Behav* 2010;17(4):531–535.
14. Picard F, et al. Neuropsychological disturbances in frontal lobe epilepsy due to mutated nicotinic receptors. *Epilepsy Behav* 2009;14(2):354–359.
15. Picard F, et al. Alteration of the in vivo nicotinic receptor density in ADNFLE patients: a PET study. *Brain* 2006;129(Pt 8):2047–2060.
16. Derry CP, et al. Distinguishing sleep disorders from seizures: diagnosing bumps in the night. *Arch Neurol* 2006;63(5):705–709.
17. Steinlein OK, et al. An insertion mutation of the CHRNA4 gene in a family with autosomal dominant nocturnal frontal lobe epilepsy. *Hum Mol Genet* 1997;6(6):943–947.
18. McLellan A, et al. Phenotypic comparison of two Scottish families with mutations in different genes causing autosomal dominant nocturnal frontal lobe epilepsy. *Epilepsia* 2003;44(4):613–617.
19. Cho YW, et al. A Korean kindred with autosomal dominant nocturnal frontal lobe epilepsy and mental retardation. *Arch Neurol* 2003;60(11):1625–1632.
20. Leniger T, et al. A new Chrna4 mutation with low penetrance in nocturnal frontal lobe epilepsy. *Epilepsia* 2003;44(7):981–985.
21. Hirose S, et al. A novel mutation of CHRNA4 responsible for autosomal dominant nocturnal frontal lobe epilepsy. *Neurology* 1999;53(8):1749–1753.
22. Bertrand D, et al. The CHRNB2 mutation I312M is associated with epilepsy and distinct memory deficits. *Neurobiol Dis* 2005;20(3):799–804.
23. Ito M, et al. Electroclinical picture of autosomal dominant nocturnal frontal lobe epilepsy in a Japanese family. *Epilepsia* 2000;41(1):52–58.
24. Role LW, Berg DK. Nicotinic receptors in the development and modulation of CNS synapses. *Neuron* 1996;16(6):1077–1085.
25. Combi R, et al. Evidence for a fourth locus for autosomal dominant nocturnal frontal lobe epilepsy. *Brain Res Bull* 2004;63(5):353–359.
26. Gu W, Bertrand D, Steinlein OK. A major role of the nicotinic acetylcholine receptor gene CHRNA2 in autosomal dominant nocturnal frontal lobe epilepsy (ADNFLE) is unlikely. *Neurosci lett* 2007;422(1):74–76.
27. Magnusson A, et al. Schizophrenia, psychotic illness and other psychiatric symptoms in families with autosomal dominant nocturnal frontal lobe epilepsy caused by different mutations. *Psychiatr Genet* 2003;13(2):91–95.
28. Khatami R, et al. A family with autosomal dominant nocturnal frontal lobe epilepsy and mental retardation. *J Neurol* 1998;245(12):809–810.
29. Derry CP, Heron SE, Phillips F, Howell S, MacMahon J, Phillips HA, Duncan JS, Mulley JS, Berkovic SF, Scheffer IE. Severe autosomal dominant nocturnal frontal lobe epilepsy associated with psychiatric disorders and intellectual disability. *Epilepsia* 2008;49(12):2125–2129.
30. Picard F, et al. Mutated nicotinic receptors responsible for autosomal dominant nocturnal frontal lobe epilepsy are more sensitive to carbamazepine. *Epilepsia* 1999;40(9): 1198–1209.
31. Varadkar S, Duncan JS, Cross JH. Acetazolamide and autosomal dominant nocturnal frontal lobe epilepsy. *Epilepsia* 2003;44(7):986–987.
32. Willoughby JO, Pope KJ, Eaton V. Nicotine as an antiepileptic agent in ADNFLE: an N-of-one study. *Epilepsia* 2003;44(9):1238–1240.
33. Steinlein OK, et al. Independent occurrence of the CHRNA4 Ser248Phe mutation in a Norwegian family with nocturnal frontal lobe epilepsy. *Epilepsia* 2000;41(5):529–535.

34. Saenz A, et al. Autosomal dominant nocturnal frontal lobe epilepsy in a Spanish family with a Ser252Phe mutation in the CHRNA4 gene. *Arch Neurol* 1999;56(8):1004–1009.

35. Phillips HA, et al. A de novo mutation in sporadic nocturnal frontal lobe epilepsy. *Ann Neurol* 2000;48(2):264–267.

36. Rozycka A, et al. Evidence for S284L mutation of the CHRNA4 in a white family with autosomal dominant nocturnal frontal lobe epilepsy. *Epilepsia* 2003;44(8):1113–1117.

37. Combi R, et al. Frontal lobe epilepsy and mutations of the corticotropin-releasing hormone gene. *Ann Neurol* 2005;58(6):899–904.

38. Berkovic SF, et al. Familial partial epilepsy with variable foci: clinical features and linkage to chromosome 22q12. *Epilepsia* 2004;45(9):1054–1060.

CHAPTER 28

Infantile Spasms and West Syndrome

Cristina Yip Go and O. Carter Snead, III

▶ OVERVIEW

In 1841, Dr. William J. West penned a letter to Lancet in which he described an unusual condition in his 4-month-old son, James, that was characterized by "… slight bobbings of the head forward"…which "… increased in frequency, and at length became so powerful, as to cause a compete heaving of the head forward toward his knees, and then immediately relaxing in an upright position. … these bowings and relaxings would be repeated alternately at intervals of a few seconds, and repeated from ten to twenty or more times at each attack, which attack would not continue more than two or three minutes; he sometimes has two, three, or more attacks in the day …." Dr. West went on to describe a reduction in a developmental trajectory in his child that was normal prior to the onset of these events: he states that since the onset of the spells his son "… neither possesses the intellectual vivacity, or the power of moving his limbs, of a child of his age." This remarkable letter, now over 160 years old, remains the most eloquent clinical description of what we now know as infantile spasms. It describes the relentless nature of the condition, the early age of onset, the classical clinical presentation, and the developmental regression associated with infantile spasms.[1]

In 1952, Gibbs and Gibbs[2] described the classical interictal electroencephalographic (EEG) pattern associated with infantile spasms, called hypsarrhythmia. This EEG is characterized by a chaotic and disorganized background of high-voltage, asynchronous spike and slow-wave activity. Although hypsarrhythmia is certainly characteristic of infantile spasms, it should be remembered that the EEG findings in infantile spasms are dynamic and hypsarrhythmia is but a point on a continuum of epileptiform changes observed on the EEG in this disorder. Therefore, the absence of hypsarrhythmia in the presence of clinical evidence of infantile spasms and other types of epileptiform abnormalities on the EEG does not in any way exclude the diagnosis of infantile spasms.

The term West Syndrome refers to an age-related triad of epileptic spasms, developmental regression, and hypsarrhythmia on EEG. Although this triad may be used synonymously with infantile spasms, the latter should refer strictly to the massive myoclonus because infantile spasms may occur in the absence of either hypsarrhythmia or mental retardation. The incidence of infantile spasm is 1 per 2000–4000 live births[3,4] and the prevalence rate is 0.15–0.2 per 1000 children of age 10 years or younger.[5] It is slightly more common in males, accounting for about 60% of cases, and a family history exists in 3%–6%.

▶ CLINICAL FEATURES

CLINICAL MANIFESTATIONS

The epileptic syndrome of infantile spasms begins in infancy, with initial onset mostly between 3 and 7 months of life in more than 50% of cases. Over 90% of cases begin before 12 months of life.[6]

The clinical spasms are brief and sudden contractions of the axial musculature, which may occur in clusters several times a day. Although there is no predilection for day or night, they appear to be temporally related to sleep. They tend to occur upon awakening or as the infant falls asleep. Spasms are occasionally triggered by loud noises usually associated with arousal from sleep but are not exacerbated by photic stimulation. They are clinically distinct from myoclonic and tonic seizures with an initial contraction phase followed by a more sustained tonic phase.[7] The spasms can be divided into flexor, extensor, or mixed depending on the muscle groups involved. Most infants have more than one type, and the type observed may be influenced by the body position at the time the spasm occurs. They can be symmetric or asymmetric. Mixed spasms are most common, followed by flexor spasms, with extensor type being the least common.[6]

Flexor spasm is the most characteristic of West syndrome. The infant appears to be in a self-hugging posture with sudden adduction or abduction of the arms. When abdominal muscles are involved, the infant may bend at the waist, giving rise to the term, "jackknife" seizure. The combination of jackknife seizure plus adduction of the arms with or without neck flexor muscle involvement is called "salaam" seizures.

Extensor spasms are characterized by abrupt extension of the neck, trunk, and legs with extension and abduction of the arms, simulating a Moro reflex. The mixed flexor-extensor spasms are a combination of leg extension with flexion of neck, trunk, and arms. The spasms may manifest as head nods when only the neck flexor muscles are involved. In children who are walking, drop attacks may be the initial manifestation. The type of spasms does not seem to be affected by etiology nor the prognosis; however, the symmetry of spasms is important because the presence of asymmetry may indicate focal cortical brain pathology.[7]

Developmental regression is an important, but not invariable component of infantile spasms. However, the long-term prognosis for unselected cases of infantile spasms is generally poor with well over 50% of children having significant cognitive impairment after infantile spasms. In one-third of cases, development is normal before onset.[8] Previously normal infants may have developmental regression with the onset of infantile spasm. Axial hypotonia and loss of hand grasp are the frequently lost skill. Guzzetta et al noted that the development of visual inattention expressed as loss of eye contact has a negative prognostic significance.[9]

ETIOLOGY

Infantile spasms may be classified into three main groups— symptomatic, idiopathic, and cryptogenic. Symptomatic cases are those where there is structural brain abnormality or metabolic cause in a child with preexisting neurologic abnormality. The term cryptogenic infantile spasms is used when there are no apparent causes identified although a cause is suspected, usually because the child is developmentally delayed or has some other neurological impairment before the onset of the spasms. Idiopathic is used to describe children with no identifiable cause and who have a normal neurological examination and normal development prior to the onset of infantile spasms.

Cryptogenic cases account for 9%–15% of infantile spasms cases.[10] The number of symptomatic cases has increased over the years due to advancement in neuroimaging techniques such as magnetic resonance imaging (MRI) and positron emission tomography (PET) that facilitate better detection of subtle brain abnormalities causing infantile spasms.

The symptomatic cases can be further classified into three etiologic subgroups depending on the timing of presumed causes: prenatal, perinatal, and postnatal.[11]

Tuberous sclerosis (TS) is a major cause of infantile spasms, with up to 50% of all patients with TS presenting with infantile spasms which peak between 4 and 6 months of age.[12] The number of diseases that can cause infantile spasms is enormous but the major categories include cortical dysgenesis, chromosomal aberrations and genetic syndromes, infections, certain metabolic conditions and vitamin deficiency, vascular insult, and tumors and trauma (Table 28–1).

▶ **TABLE 28–1. DISORDERS ASSOCIATED WITH SYMPTOMATIC INFANTILE SPASMS**

Etiology	Examples
Cortical dysgenesis	Cortical dysplasia
	Laminar heterotropia
	Lissencephaly
	Hemimegalencephaly
	Septal dysplasia
	Schizencephaly
	Pachygyria
	Porencephaly
	Microgyria
	Agenesis of corpus callosum
Chromosomal aberrations and genetic syndromes	Tuberous sclerosis
	Incontinentia pigmenti
	Neurofibromatosis
	Sturge Weber syndrome
	Aicardi's syndrome
	Down's syndrome
Infections	CMV
	Toxoplasma
	Herpes encephalitis
	Bacterial meningitis
	Brain abscess
Metabolic	Inborn errors of metabolism: phenylketonuria, amino acid and organic acidopathies, nonketotic hyperglycinemia
	Pyridoxine deficiency/dependency
	Mitochondrial disorders
	Neonatal hypoglycemia
Vascular	Hypoxic-ischemic insult
	Hemorrhagic insult
Tumors	Ependymomas
	Gliomas
	Gangliogliomas
	Choroids plexus papillomas
Trauma	

▶ DIAGNOSTIC WORKUP

A comprehensive evaluation of children with infantile spasms includes a complete history and physical examination including Wood's lamp evaluation as well as an initial EEG. Once a diagnosis of infantile spasms is made, an extensive search for the etiology such as structural brain abnormalities with neuroimaging studies, metabolic and chromosomal abnormalities should be performed.

EEG

The characteristic interictal EEG finding of infantile spasms is the hypsarrhythmia pattern described by Gibbs and Gibbs,[2] which consists of a disorganized and asynchronous background pattern of high-amplitude

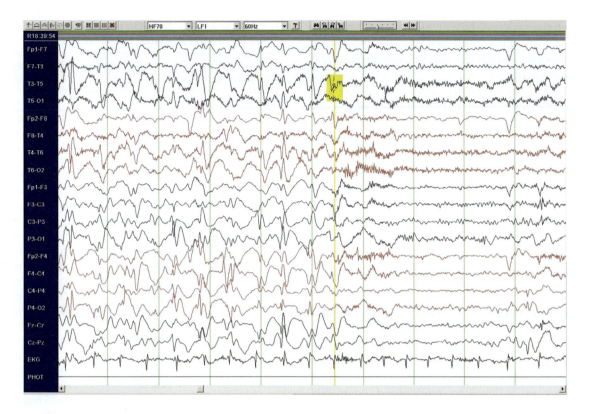

Figure 28–1. EEG showing hypsarrhythmia pattern with electrodecremental fast activity in a 9-month-old child with infantile spasms.

spikes and slow waves (Fig. 28–1). It may be present during wakefulness and sleep. However, this pattern is seen most often during early infancy in approximately 66% of cases. The chaotic pattern becomes more organized by early childhood, and may evolve into the generalized sharp and slow-wave pattern seen in Lennox–Gastaut syndrome.

Kellaway et al[6] described several ictal EEG patterns associated with infantile spasms. The electrodecremental response, described as high-voltage sharp- or slow-wave discharges followed by generalized voltage attenuation lasting more than 1 second, is the most common, occurring in more than 70% of recorded spasms. Other types include various combinations of generalized sharp- and slow-wave discharges and electrodecremental fast activity (Fig. 28–1).

Focal EEG abnormalities can be seen in a subset of patients with infantile spasms.[13,14] The combination of asymmetric spasms and focal or asymmetric hypsarrhythmia pattern with focal ictal discharges strongly suggest the presence of focal brain lesion.

NEUROIMAGING STUDIES

Although computerized tomography (CT) scans are readily available and can detect some underlying focal or diffuse brain pathology, MRI is much more sensitive in picking up smaller lesions including neuronal migrational anomalies, abnormal myelination, and demarcation of the gray and white mater.[15] However, it should be remembered that MRI in a child less than 2 years of age, which includes the vast majority of patients with new onset spasms, could still miss cortical migrational abnormalities because of immaturity of white matter.

The value of interictal PET scans in revealing focal areas of hypometabolism, which may correlate with cortical dysplasia in some cases where MRI is normal, was first reported by Chugani et al[16] and subsequently validated by others.[17]

LABORATORY TESTS

Blood and urine tests can be done to search for metabolic, genetic, and infectious etiologies that cause symptomatic infantile spasms. They also serve as baseline studies before initiation of treatment.

Blood tests should include but not be limited to: complete blood count (CBC) and differential count, electrolytes (sodium, potassium, chloride, bicarbonate, calcium, magnesium, phosphate), pH, lactate, blood urea nitrogen (BUN), creatinine, glucose, creatine phosphokinase (CPK), aspartate aminotransferase (AST), alanine transaminase (ALT), total bilirubin, alkaline phosphatase, thyroid function, serum amino acid screen, cytomegalovirus (CMV) and toxoplasma IgG and IgM, and/or polymerase chain reaction (PCR) studies. Chromosomal studies can also be done especially if there is a family history.

Urine tests should include urinalysis, amino acid screen, organic acid screen, CMV culture, or PCR. Electrocardiogram and chest X-ray should be performed especially if cardiac examination is abnormal. Ophthalmology, cardiology, and genetics consultations can also be requested as needed.

▶ MANAGEMENT

MEDICAL

Hormonal Therapy

Adrenocorticotrophic hormone and prednisone. In 1958, Sorel and Dusaucy-Bauloye[18] demonstrated the efficacy of adrenocorticotrophic hormone (ACTH) in treating infantile spasms. Oral corticosteroids like prednisone have also been found to be effective by Hrachovy et al.[19,20] Two randomized controlled studies[20,21] showed the superiority of ACTH to oral prednisone. The dose and duration of treatment with ACTH vary among different institutions and among different countries.[22–24] Snead et al[25] showed that high-dose ACTH resulted in up to 93% seizure control and found an all-or-none treatment response to ACTH similar to that reported by Hrachovy et al.[20] The United Kingdom Infantile Spasms Study (UKISS) comparing vigabatrin with either high-dose ACTH or oral prednisolone[35] showed similar efficacy of the two hormonal therapies with similar side-effect profiles.

The side effects associated with hormonal therapy, which occurs in about 37% of cases, include hypertension, irritability, susceptibility to infections, increased body weight, hypotonia, drowsiness, electrolyte disturbance, and reversible cerebral atrophy. Because of the relatively high incidence of side effects, treatment with ACTH or oral steroids should only be used for short periods of time, usually ranging from 2 to 6 weeks depending on the treatment schedule. A suggested protocol using synacthen (cosyntropin or tetracosactide) is included based on the study done by Snead et al[25] with 0.25 mg of synacthen equivalent to 25 units of corticotrophin (Table 28–2).

Vigabatrin

Vigabatrin [gamma vinyl, gamma-aminobutyric acid (GABA)] is a specific, irreversible inhibitor of GABA-transaminase that is available in Canada, Europe, and in 2009, also became available in the USA. It has been shown to be effective and safe in the treatment of

▶ **TABLE 28–2. SUGGESTED SCHEDULE FOR ACTH IN INFANTILE SPASMS**[a]

Week Number	Date of Injection	Dose Given Intramuscularly
Week 1	Day 1	1.9 mg/m^2
	Day 3	1.9 mg/m^2
	Day 5	1.9 mg/m^2
	Day 7	1.9 mg/m^2
Week 2	Day 9	0.94 mg/m^2
	Day 11	0.94 mg/m^2
	Day 13	0.94 mg/m^2
Evaluate after 2 weeks. Responders will finish protocol on the following taper schedule		
Week 3	Day 15	0.94 mg/m^2
	Day 17	0.94 mg/m^2
	Day 19	0.94 mg/m^2
	Day 21	0.94 mg/m^2
Week 4	Day 23	0.94 mg/m^2
	Day 25	0.94 mg/m^2
	Day 27	0.94 mg/m^2
Week 5	Day 29	0.75 mg/m^2
	Day 31	0.75 mg/m^2
	Day 33	0.75 mg/m^2
	Day 35	0.75 mg/m^2
Week 6	Day 37	0.75 mg/m^2
	Day 39	0.75 mg/m^2
	Day 41	0.75 mg/m^2
Week 7	Day 43	0.63 mg/m^2
	Day 45	0.63 mg/m^2
	Day 47	0.63 mg/m^2
	Day 49	0.63 mg/m^2
Week 8	Day 51	0.5 mg/m^2
	Day 53	0.5 mg/m^2
	Day 55	0.5 mg/m^2
Week 9	Day 57	0.38 mg/m^2
	Day 59	0.38 mg/m^2
	Day 61	0.38 mg/m^2
Week 10	Day 63	0.25 mg/m^2
	Day 65	0.25 mg/m^2
	Day 67	0.25 mg/m^2
	Day 69	0.25 mg/m^2
Week 11	Day 71	0.13 mg/m^2
	Day 73	0.13 mg/m^2
	Day 75	0.13 mg/m^2
	Day 77	0.13 mg/m^2
Week 12	Day 79	0.06 mg/m^2
	Day 81	0.06 mg/m^2
	Day 83	0.06 mg/m^2. Then stop ACTH.

[a]This protocol was developed and used at the Hospital for Sick Children, Toronto, Ontario.

infantile spasms especially in cases due to tuberous sclerosis.[26–28] Cessation of spasms with vigabatrin is seen in 48%–68% of infants,[26,29] with the best responders seen in patients with tuberous sclerosis and cerebral

▶ **TABLE 28–3.** VIGABATRIN REGIMEN*a*

Day 1	50 mg/kg per day PO divided BID
Day 2	100 mg/kg per day PO divided BID
Day 3	125 mg/kg per day PO divided BID
Day 4	150 mg/kg per day PO divided BID and maintain same dose for 6 months

The patient is reviewed after 2 weeks for response of treatment. If clinical spasms resolved and EEG showed resolution of hypsarrhythmia, continue high-dose vigabatrin for a minimum of 6 months.
Arrange for baseline electroretinogram (ERG) before initiating treatment and follow up ERG every 3 months while patient is on vigabatrin therapy.
*a*This protocol is used at the Hospital for Sick Children, Toronto, Ontario.
Note: BID, twice a day.

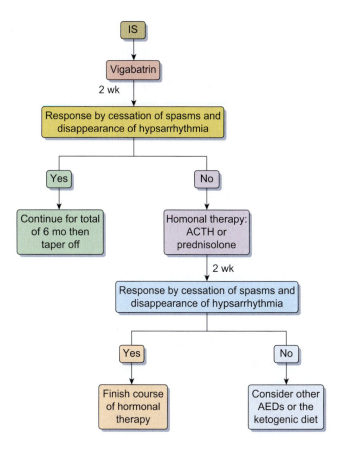

Figure 28–2. Treatment algorithm for newly diagnosed infantile spasms. This algorithm is used at the Hospital for Sick Children Toronto, Ontario, Canada.

malformations. Vigevano et al[29] noted that a therapeutic response can be detected within 1–2 weeks of treatment. The dose is 150 mg/kg per day divided twice a day (Table 28–3).

A major concern with vigabatrin treatment is the constriction of visual fields due to retinal toxicity documented in several studies.[30–32] Baseline visual field testing should be performed before initiation of vigabatrin therapy and should be performed regularly during treatment. Other side effects associated with vigabatrin include drowsiness, hypotonia, and irritability, which occur in 13% of cases.

ACTH Versus Vigabatrin

The practice parameter for the medical treatment of infantile spasms released by the American Academy of Neurology (AAN) and the Child Neurology Society in 2004 and subsequently endorsed by the American Epilepsy Society, reported that ACTH is probably effective for the short-term treatment of infantile spasms but there is insufficient evidence to recommend the optimum dosage and duration of treatment. There is insufficient evidence to determine whether oral corticosteroids are effective. Vigabatrin is possibly effective for the short-term treatment of infantile spasm and is possibly also effective for children with tuberous sclerosis. Concerns about retinal toxicity suggest that serial ophthalmologic screening is required in patients on vigabatrin; however, the data are insufficient to make recommendations regarding the frequency or type of screening. The practice parameter concluded that ACTH is probably an effective agent in the short-term treatment of infantile spasms and that vigabatrin is possibly effective.[33] A number of studies have compared the efficacy and tolerability of hormonal therapy to vigabatrin.[29,34,35] Cessation of spasms was more likely (up to 74%) in patients assigned to hormonal treatments when compared to those taking vigabatrin (48%–54%). Disappearance of EEG abnormalities also occurred sooner in patients on hormonal therapy. However, long-term follow-up did

not show significant difference in prognosis between the ACTH and vigabatrin groups. Because of the efficacy, safety, and tolerability of vigabatrin, many authors have concluded that vigabatrin[26–29] may be considered a first choice in the initial treatment for infantile spasms regardless of the cause. Thus, in Canada, our practice is to initiate treatment with vigabatrin with all the caveats detailed previously, via the protocol outlined in Figure 28–2 for 2 weeks. If there are not both complete cessation of spasms and marked improvement of the EEG at the end of that time, ACTH is then started using the protocol outlined in Table 28–3.

OTHER MEDICAL TREATMENT OF INFANTILE SPASMS

The AAN infantile spasms practice parameter published in 2004[33] concluded that there is insufficient evidence to recommend any treatment of infantile spasms other than ACTH or vigabatrin. However, a number of studies employing other medical treatment modalities in the treatment of infantile spasms are being published and are reviewed later.

Zonisamide

Zonisamide is an anticonvulsant drug chemically classified as a sulfonamide. It was approved for use in the US in 2000 as adjunctive treatment of partial seizures. Although zonisamide's exact mechanism is unknown, its action on calcium and sodium channels as well as some carbonic anhydrase inhibiting activity may be contributory to its antiseizure activity. Several Japanese studies[36–38] suggest that zonisamide may be useful in the treatment of infantile spasms. A more recent study performed on 23 patients with infantile spasms by Lotze and Wilfong[39] demonstrated a 26% cessation of spasms and clearing of hypsarrhythmia with the mean latency time from onset to complete spasm control of 19 days. The dose ranged from 8 to 32 mg/kg per day. The main side effect is anorexia and somnolence. It should be avoided in patients with history of allergic reactions to sulfonamides.

Topiramate

Topiramate is a sulfamate-substituted monosaccharide with a broad range of antiseizure activities. Glauser et al[40] showed in a pilot study the efficacy of topiramate in children with refractory infantile spasms. Forty-five percent of children became spasm free and the response was sustained with long-term use.[41] Side effects include anorexia and weight loss, somnolence, and psychomotor slowing. Nephrolithiasis may also be seen especially with long-term use. It is an effective and well-tolerated medication that may be considered in children with infantile spasms refractory to other treatment.

Valproic Acid

Valproic acid has been used in the treatment of infantile spasms with several studies reporting cessation of spasms in 40%–73% of cases[42–44] and resolution of hypsarrhythmia in 91% at 6 months.[42,43] Relapse rate is 23%. The dose ranged from 25 to 100 mg/kg per day. The greatest concern with the use of valproic acid in children under the age of 2 is the risk for severe and fatal hepatotoxicity and metabolic disturbances[45–47] due to the accumulation of toxic valproic acid metabolites, particularly 4-en-valproic acid.

Nitrazepam

Nitrazepam is a benzodiazepine that has been shown in several studies to be useful in the treatment of infantile spasms.[48–50] With a dose ranging from 0.5 to 3.5 mg/kg per day, cessation of spasms was reported in 30%–54% with resolution of hypsarrhythmia in 46% and a relapse rate of about 15%. Side effects include sedation but may induce paradoxical hyperactivity and irritability.

Pyridoxine (Vitamin B6)

High-dose pyridoxine of 100–400 mg/kg per day has been used in the treatment of infantile spasms.[51–53] Response rate ranged from 13% to 29%.

Ketogenic Diet

The Ketogenic diet has been used for more than 80 years in patients with refractory epilepsies. This high-fat, adequate-protein, and low-carbohydrate diet was reported to be effective (more than 90% seizure reduction) in 39%–46% of children with infantile spasms.[54,55] It can be considered in children with infantile spasms who have failed hormonal and anticonvulsant therapy. The side effects associated with being on the ketogenic diet include hyperlipidemia, constipation, increased risk of nephrolithiasis, and potential dehydration.

SURGERY

In children with infantile spasms who present with asymmetric spasms, focal neurologic abnormalities on examination, EEG with focal or lateralizing features and radiologic evidence of structural abnormality, epilepsy surgery should be considered[16,17,56,57] even if they have responded to medical therapy. Jonas et al[58] noted that better postsurgery seizure and neurodevelopmental outcomes are seen in patients with infantile spasms that responded to medical therapy with resolution of hypsarrhythmia prior to surgery.

► PROGNOSIS

More than 150 years after this condition was described by West, infantile spasms continues to be a challenge to neurologists, with the best form of therapy still being debated upon. The prognosis of West syndrome in terms of neurodevelopmental progress and the development of other types of seizures remain poor despite treatment. Although the clinical spasms and EEG hypsarrhythmia pattern tend to disappear spontaneously by 3–4 years of age, up to 60% of these children will go on to develop other types of seizures.[11,59,60] There are conflicting results on whether better initial control of spasms or the time to initiate treatment affect the long-term outcome of children with infantile spasms. The AAN practice parameter concluded that there is insufficient evidence to conclude that successful treatment of infantile spasms improves the long-term prognosis. However, the UKISS reported that better initial control of spasms by hormonal treatment in cryptogenic or idiopathic cases of infantile spasms may lead to improved developmental outcome.[61] This is also reported in another study done by Kivity et al[62] which suggested that long-term prognosis of cryptogenic infantile spasms is good to excellent provided that the treatment is started within 1 month after the onset of spasms. Other studies[19,59] noted that delay in initiation of treatment from the onset of spasms had no influence on long-term outcomes. However, most studies reported similarly that neurodevelopment prognosis is better in idiopathic or cryptogenic cases, with up to 40% regaining normal development at long-term follow-up.[11,59,61–63]

▶ PATHOPHYSIOLOGY

Although a number of hypotheses have been put forward to explain the mechanisms that underpin infantile spasms,[64] virtually nothing is really known about the pathogenesis of this age-dependent phenomenon. There is circumstantial evidence that implicates brainstem involvement in this disorder,[65] but until an animal model of infantile spasms is developed,[66] it is unlikely that a precise mechanism will be elucidated. In fact, there may well be more than one mechanism at play in the pathogenesis of infantile spasms. Similarly, unraveling of the mechanism by which ACTH and vigabatrin exert their unique therapeutic effects in this disorder also await the development of an animal model of infantile spasms.[66]

REFERENCES

1. West W. On a peculiar form of infantile convulsions. *Lancet* 1841;1:724–725.
2. Gibbs FA, Gibbs EL. *Atlas of Electroencephalography Vol 2: Epilepsy.* Cambridge, MA. Addison-Wesley, 1952.
3. Hurst DL. Epidemiology. In: Dulac O, Bernardina BD, Chugani HT (eds), *Infantile Spasms and West Syndrome.* London: WB Saunders, 1994.
4. Sidenvall R, Eeg-Olofsson O. Epidemiology of infantile spasms in sweden. *Epilepsia* 1995;36:572–574.
5. Cowan LD, Bodensteiner JB. Prevalence of epilepsies in children and adolescents. *Epilepsia* 1989;30:94–106.
6. Kellaway P, et al. Precise characterization and quantification of infantile spasms. *Ann Neurol* 1979;6:214–218.
7. Fusco L, Vigevano F. Ictal clinical electrographic findings of spasms in West syndrome. *Epilepsia* 1993;34:671–678.
8. Kurokawa T, et al. West syndrome and Lennox–Gastaut syndrome: a survey of natural history. *Pediatrics* 1980;65:81–88.
9. Guzzetta F, et al. Development of visual attention in West syndrome. *Epilepsia* 2002;43(7):754–763.
10. Matsumoto A, et al. Long-term prognosis after infantile spasms: a statistical study of prognostic factors in 200 cases. *Dev Med Child Neurol* 1981;23(1):51–65.
11. Hamano SI, et al. long-term follow up study of west syndrome: differences of outcome among symptomatic etiologies. *J Pediatr* 2003;143:231–235.
12. Riikonen R, Simell O. Tuberous sclerosis and infantile spasms. *Dev Med Child Neurol* 1990;32:203–209.
13. Donat JF, Wright FS. Unusual variants of infantile spasms. *J Child Neurol* 1996;6:313–318.
14. Donat JF, Lo WD. Asymmetric hypsarrhythmia and infantile spasms in west syndromes. *J Child Neurol* 1994;9:290–296.
15. van Bogaert P, et al. Value of magnetic resonance imaging in West syndrome of unknown etiology. *Epilepsia* 1993:34(4):701–706.
16. Chugani HT, et al. Infantile spasms: I. PET identifies focal cortical dysgenesis in cryptogenic cases for surgical treatment. *Ann Neurol* 1990;27:406–413.
17. Kramer U, Sue WC, Mikati MA. Focal features in West syndrome indicating candidacy for surgery. *Pediatr Neurol* 1997;16:213–217.
18. Sorel L, Dusaucy-Bauloye A. A propos de cas d'hypsarrhythmia de Gibbs: son traitment spectaculaire par l'ACTH. *Acta Neurol Belg* 1958;58:130–141.
19. Hrachovy RA, et al. A controlled study of prednisone therapy in infantile spasms. *Epilepsia* 1979;20:403–477.
20. Hrachovy RA, et al. Double-blind study of ACTH vs prednisone therapy in infantile spasms. *J Pediatr* 1983;103:641–645.
21. Baram TZ, et al. High-dose corticotropin (ACTH) versus prednisone for infantile spasms: a prospective, randomized, blinded study. *Pediatrics* 1996;97:375–379.
22. Bobele GB, Bodensteiner JB. The treatment of infantile spasms by child neurologists. *J Child Neurol* 1994;9:432–435.
23. Appleton RE. The treatment of infantile spasms by paediatric neurologists in the UK and Ireland. *Dev Med Child Neurol* 1996;38:278–279.
24. Ito M, Seki T, Takuma Y. Current therapy for West syndrome in japan. *J Child Neurol* 2000;15:424–428.
25. Snead OC 3rd, et al. Treatment of infantile spasms with high-dose ACTH: efficacy and plasma levels of ACTH and cortisol. *Neurol* 1989;39:1027–1031.
26. Aicardi J, et al. Vigabatrin as initial therapy for infantile spasms: a European retrospective study. *Epilepsia* 1996:37(7):638–642.
27. Chiron C, et al. Randomized trial comparing vigabatrin and hydrocortisone in infantile spasms due to tuberous sclerosis. *Epilepsy Res* 1997;26(2):389–395.
28. Elterman RD, et al. Randomized trial of vigabatrin in patients with infantile spasms. *Neurol* 2001;57:1416–1421.
29. Vigevano F, Cilio MR. Vigabatrin versus ACTH as first-line treatment for infantile spasms: a randomized, prospective study. *Epilepsia* 1997;38(12):1270–1274.
30. Eke T, Talbot JF, Lawden MC. Severe persistent visual field constriction associated with vigabatrin. *BMJ* 1997;314:180–181.
31. Wild JM, et al. Characteristics of a unique visual field defect attributed vigabatrin. *Epilepsia* 1999;40:1784–1794.
32. Gross-Tsur V, et al. Visual impairment in children with epilepsy treated with vigabatrin. *Ann Neurol* 2000;48:60–64.
33. Mackay MT, et al. Practice parameter: medical treatment of infantile spasms. Report of the american academy of neurology and the child neurology society. *Neurol* 2004;62:1668–1681.
34. Lux AL, et al. The United Kingdom infantile spasms study comparing vigabatrin with prednisolone or tetracosactide at 14 days: a multicentre, randomized controlled trial. *Lancet* 2004;364:1773–1778.

35. Cosette P, Riviello JJ, Carmant L. Brief communications: ACTH versus vigabatrin therapy in infantile spasms: a retrospective study. *Neurol* 1999;52:1691.

36. Suzuki Y, et al. Zonisamide monotherapy in newly diagnosed infantile spasms (2nd Report) [Japanese]. *No To Hattatsu* 2000;32:S204. Abstract.

37. Suzuki Y. Zonisamide in West syndrome. *Brain Dev* 2001;23:658–661.

38. Suzuki Y, et al. Long term response to zonisamide in patients with west syndrome. *Neurol* 2002;58:1556–1559.

39. Lotze TE, Wilfong AA. Zonisamide treatment for symptomatic infantile spasms. *Neurol* 2004;62:296–298.

40. Glauser TA, Clark PO, Strawsburg R. A pilot study of topiramate in the treatment of infantile spasms. *Epilepsia* 1998;39:1324–1328.

41. Glauser TA, Clark PO, McGee K. Long-term response to topiramate in patients with West syndrome. *Epilepsia* 2000;41(S1):S91–S94.

42. Bachman DS. Use of valproic acid in treatment of infantile spasms. *Arch Neurol* 1982;39:49–52.

43. Siemes H, et al. Therapy of infantile spasms with valproate: results of a prospective study. *Epilepsia* 1988;29:553–560.

44. Fisher E, et al. Valproate metabolites in serum and urine during antiepileptic therapy in children with infantile spasms: abnormal metabolite pattern associated with reversibly hepatotoxicity. *Epilepsia* 1992;33:165–171.

45. Bryant AE, Dreifuss FE. Valproic acid hepatic fatalities. III. U.S. experience since 1986. *Neurol* 1996;46:465–469.

46. Murphy JV, Groover RV, Hodge C. Hepatotoxic effects in a child receiving valproate and carnitine. *J Pediatr* 1993;123:318–320.

47. Buck M. Valproic acid in the treatment of pediatric seizures. *Pediatr Pharm* 1997;3(3):1–4.

48. Volzke E, Doose H, Stephan E. The treatment of infantile spasms and hypsarrhythmia with mogadon. *Epilepsia* 1967;8:64–70.

49. Chamberlain MC. Nitrazepam for refractory infantile spasms and the Lennox–Gastaut syndrome. *J Child Neurol* 1996;11:31–34.

50. Dreifuss F, et al. Infantile spasms. Comparative trial of nitrazepam and corticotropin. *Arch Neurol* 1986;43:1107–1110.

51. Ohtsuka Y, et al. Pyridoxal phosphate in the treatment of the west syndrome. In: Akimoto H, Kazamatsuri H, Seino M, Ward AA Jr (eds), *Advances in Epileptology. XIIIth Epilepsy International Symposium.* New York: Raven Press, 1982, pp. 311–313.

52. Ohtsuka Y, et al. Treatment of the West syndrome with high dose pyridoxal phosphate. *Brain Dev* 1987;9:418–421.

53. Pietz J, et al. Treatment of infantile spasms with high-dosage vitamin B6. *Epilepsia* 1993;34:757–763.

54. Freeman JM, et al. The efficacy of the ketogenic diet – 1998: a prospective evaluation of intervention in 150 children. *Pediatr* 1998;102:1358–1363.

55. Kossoff EH, et al. Efficacy of the ketogenic diet for infantile spasms. *Pediatr* 2002;109:780–783.

56. Churgani HT, et al. Surgery for intractable infantile spasms: neuroimaging perspectives. *Epilepsia* 1993;34(4):764–771.

57. Holmes G. Surgery for intractable seizures in infancy and early childhood. *Neurol* 1993;43:S33–S42.

58. Jonas R, et al. Surgery for symptomatic infant-onset epileptic encephalopathy with or without infantile spasms. *Neurol* 2005;64:746–750.

59. Glaze DG, et al. Prospective study of outcome of infants with infantile spasms treated during controlled studies of ACTH and prednisone. *J Pediatr* 1988;112:389–396.

60. Camfield P, et al. Infantile spasms in remission may re-emerge as intractable epileptic spasms. *Epilepsia* 2003;44:1592–1595.

61. Lux AL, et al. The United Kingdom infantile spasms study (UKISS) comparing hormone treatment with vigabatrin on developmental and epilepsy outcomes to age 14 months: a multicentre randomized trial. *Lancet Neurol* 2005;4:712–717.

62. Kivity S, et al. Long-term cognitive outcomes of a cohort of children with cryptogenic infantile spasms treated with high-dose adrenocorticotropic hormone. *Epilepsia* 2004;45:255–262.

63. Riikonen R. A long term follow up study of 214 children with the syndrome of infantile spasms. *NeuroPediatr* 1982;13:14–23.

64. Rho JM. Basic science behind the catastrophic epilepsies. *Epilepsia* 2004;45(Suppl 5):5–11.

65. Frost JD, Hrachovy RA. *Infantile Spasms, Diagnosis, Management, and Prognosis.* Boston: Kluwer Academic Publishers, 2003.

66. Stafstrom CE, Moshe SL, Swann JW, Nehlig A, Jacobs MP, Schwartzkroin PA. Models of pediatric epilepsies: strategies and opportunities. *Epilepsia* 2006;47:1407–1414.

CHAPTER 29

Lennox–Gastaut and Related Syndromes

Diego A. Morita and Tracy A. Glauser

▶ DEFINITION

The clinical features of the Lennox–Gastaut syndrome (LGS) have been recognized for more than 200 years. The current definition of LGS by the International League Against Epilepsy (ILAE) classification is: "LGS manifests itself in children aged 1–8 years, but appears mainly in preschool-age children. The most common seizure types are tonic-axial, atonic, and absence seizures, but other types such as myoclonic, generalized tonic–clonic seizures (GTCS), or partial seizures are frequently associated with this syndrome. Seizure frequency is high, and status epilepticus is frequent (stuporous states with myoclonias, tonic, and atonic seizures). The electroencephalography (EEG) usually has abnormal background activity, slow spike-waves less than 3 Hz and, often, multifocal abnormalities. During sleep, bursts of fast rhythms (10 Hz) appear. In general, there is mental retardation. Seizures are difficult to control, and the development is unfavorable. In 60% of cases, the syndrome occurs in children suffering from a previous encephalopathy, but is primary in other cases."

A triad of basic elements for diagnosing LGS is typically based on this definition, and tailored by clinical experience and research:

- Multiple types of seizures including tonic seizures, atypical absences, and atonic seizures
- An EEG pattern consisting of interictal diffuse slow spike and wave discharges occurring at a 1.5–2 Hz frequency
- Global cognitive dysfunction.

This is no consensus about the minimal necessary and sufficient criteria to diagnose LGS. Some investigators do not consider cognitive dysfunction indispensable for diagnosis, especially at onset, if the seizures and EEG pattern are typical. Others use stricter EEG criteria requiring that the diagnostic EEG pattern include bursts of generalized fast spikes (10 Hz) during nonrapid eye movement (NREM) sleep.

▶ EPIDEMIOLOGY

LGS accounts for 1%–4% of all cases of childhood epilepsy, but 10% of cases that start in the first 5 years of life. The annual incidence of LGS in childhood is 2 per 100,000 children while its prevalence ranges from 0.1 to 0.28 per 1000 in Europe and the United States. Males are affected more often than females but this gender difference is not statistically significant. There are no racial differences in the occurrence of LGS. The mean age at epilepsy onset is 26–28 months (range 1 day-14 years).

Patients are considered to have idiopathic LGS if there is normal psychomotor development before the onset of symptoms, if there are no underlying disorders or definite presumptive causes, and if there are no neurologic or neuroradiologic abnormalities. In contrast, patients have symptomatic LGS if there is an identifiable cause for the syndrome. Population-based studies reveal that 22%–30% of patients have idiopathic LGS, while 70%–78% have symptomatic LGS.

Pathologies responsible for LGS include encephalitis/meningitis, tuberous sclerosis, brain malformations (e.g., cortical dysplasias), birth injury, hypoxic–ischemic injury, frontal lobe lesions, and trauma. Infantile spasms precede the development of LGS in 9%–41% of cases. Some investigators consider cryptogenic cases in which there is no identified cause or when a cause is suspected and the epilepsy is presumed to be symptomatic as a distinct etiological category.

▶ CLINICAL MANIFESTATIONS

Cognitive dysfunction, psychiatric symptoms, and multiple seizures types are common clinical manifestations. Factors associated with cognitive dysfunction are symptomatic LGS, a previous history of West syndrome, onset of symptoms before 12–24 months of age, and higher seizure frequency. A significant correlation exists between age of onset of seizures and mental deterioration, with a favorable cognitive outcome more likely to occur in patients with a later age of LGS onset. Psychiatric symptoms in young children consist of mood instability and personality disturbances, while slowing or arrest of psychomotor development and educational progress characterize the neuropsychological symptoms. Character problems predominate in older children, and acute psychotic episodes or chronic forms of psychosis with aggressiveness, irritability, or social isolation may occur.

Several types of seizures occur in LGS including tonic, atonic, myoclonic, and atypical absences, often associated with other less common types.

TONIC SEIZURES

Tonic seizures are said to be the most characteristic type of seizure occurring in 17%–95% of children with LGS. Tonic seizures are more frequent during NREM sleep and researchers who have systematically obtained sleep tracings report a higher prevalence. Tonic seizures may be subdivided into[1] axial tonic characterized by involvement of the head and trunk with head and neck flexion contraction of masticatory muscles and eventual vocalizations[2] axorhizomelic tonic characterized by tonic involvement of the proximal upper limbs with elevation of the shoulders and abduction of the arms and[3] global tonic characterized by contraction of the distal extremities, sometimes leading to a sudden fall or mimicking infantile spasms.

ATYPICAL ABSENCES

The reported frequency of atypical absence seizures ranges from 17% to 100%. The frequency of seizure types in most studies is based on parental seizure counts and chart reviews or is unspecified. This retrospective methodology is prone to subjective bias as, for example, a parent's limited ability to recognize and identify atypical absences correctly. Furthermore, atypical absences are often difficult to diagnose due to their subtle onset and incomplete loss of consciousness permitting continuation of ongoing activities.

ATONIC SEIZURES, MASSIVE MYOCLONIC SEIZURES, AND MYOCLONIC-ATONIC SEIZURES

Atonic seizures, massive myoclonic seizures, and myoclonic-atonic seizures are all typical of patients with LGS but may be difficult to differentiate by clinical observation alone. Their reported frequency ranges from 10% to 56%. All can result in sudden and precipitous falls associated with craniofacial injury ("drop attacks" and "Sturzanfalle"). Movement may be limited to the head only characterized by the head falling on the chest ("head drop," "head nod," and "nictatio capitis"). Notably, pure atonic seizures are the exception rather than the rule as most atonic seizures have been shown to have a tonic or myoclonic component.

OTHER SEIZURE TYPES

GTCS are reported to occur in 15% of patients with LGS while complex partial seizures occur in 5%. Status epilepticus associated with several different seizure types (absence status epilepticus, tonic status epilepticus, nonconvulsive status epilepticus) is not uncommon and often displays prolonged duration and resistance to treatment.

▶ EEG FEATURES

INTERICTAL MANIFESTATIONS

The interictal EEG is characterized by a slow background that may be constant suggesting an underlying encephalopathy or more variable in presentation. The hallmark of the waking interictal EEG in LGS is the occurrence of generalized slow spike-wave discharges. This pattern consist of bursts of irregular bilateral spikes or sharp waves followed by a sinusoidal 35–400 milliseconds slow waves of high-amplitude ranging from 200 to 800 µV that can be symmetrical or asymmetrical. The amplitude is often higher in the anterior region and in the frontal or frontocentral areas but may predominate in the posterior head regions. The frequency of the slow spike-wave activity is typically between 1.5 and 2.5 Hz.

Slow spike-waves are usually not activated by photic stimulation. Hyperventilation rarely induces slow spike-waves, although cognitive delay may prevent adequate cooperation. During NREM sleep, discharges are more generalized, occur more frequently, and consist of polyspikes and slow waves. There is a decrease in spike-wave activity in REM sleep and a reduction in the total duration of REM sleep during periods of frequent seizures.

ICTAL MANIFESTATIONS

Several seizure types occur in LGS including tonic, atonic, myoclonic, and atypical absences, often in association with less common types. The tonic seizure EEG is characterized by a diffuse rapid (10–13 Hz), low-amplitude activity, mainly in the anterior and vertex areas (recruiting rhythm) that progressively decreases in frequency and increases in amplitude. The atypical absence seizure EEG is characterized by diffuse slow (2–2.5 Hz) and irregular spike-waves that may be difficult to differentiate from interictal bursts. The EEG in atonic seizures, massive myoclonic seizures, and myoclonic-atonic seizures is characterized by slow spike-waves, polyspike and waves, or rapid diffuse rhythms.[22,26] Simultaneous video-EEG recording and polygraphy is often required for precise diagnosis. In 95% of affected patients, all three types of seizures occur in the same patient.

▶ PATHOPHYSIOLOGY

The pathophysiology of LGS is not well known as there are no animal models. Several possible pathophysiologies have been proposed including developmental, immunologic, and metabolic.

▶ DIAGNOSTIC EVALUATION

Neuroimaging is an important part of the search for an underlying etiology in patients with LGS. Magnetic resonance imaging (MRI) is the preferred neuroimaging modality and computerized tomography (CT) scanning is indicated only in highly selected situations (e.g., evaluation of suspected intracranial injury and/or hematoma in a patient with head trauma resulting from an atonic and/or tonic seizure). No current indications exist for routine positron emission tomography (PET) or single-proton emission computed tomography (SPECT) scanning in patients with LGS unless a localized primary epileptogenic zone is suspected as a source for secondary bilateral synchrony. In this situation, patients with LGS may become potential epilepsy surgery candidates and further work-up is fully justified.

The EEG evaluation of patients with suspected LGS is critical, since a correct diagnosis depends on the presence of specific electrographic findings. Recording of a prolonged EEG is desirable as a routine 30-minute tracing may not capture both awake and asleep electrographic activity and thus may miss crucial findings. It is important to capture and classify each of the patient's multiple seizure types. Video-EEG telemetry should be strongly considered as it may also help to educate parents on which patient "events" are seizures and which are nonepileptic behaviors.

▶ TREATMENT

OVERVIEW

The goals of LGS treatment are the same as for all epilepsy patients: improving quality of life with the fewest seizures (hopefully none), the fewest treatment side effects, and the least number of medications. As LGS may be treatment resistant, achieving all of these goals is often challenging. Medication resistance typically leads to the use of polytherapy, more drug-drug interactions, increased side effects, and a reduced quality of life. Potential treatment modalities in LGS include pharmacologic, dietary, and surgical therapies. Traditionally, pharmacologic treatment is the first approach.

PHARMACOLOGIC TREATMENT

Expert Consensus

For decades, the paucity of pediatric epilepsy evidence-based data and clinical guidance resulted in clinicians relying frequently on clinical judgment. A survey sent to 41 American pediatric epileptologists revealed that valproate (VPA) was the initial treatment of choice followed by topiramate (TPM) as the next option and lamotrigine (LTG) as another first line choice. A similar survey sent to 57 European physicians specializing in pediatric epilepsy concurred that VPA was the agent of first choice. If there was no response to VPA, the next choice was LTG with TPM being another first line selection. Significantly no randomized controlled studies with VPA have been undertaken in patients with LGS. Covanis and collaborators reported their findings on the open-label use of VPA in 336 patients, of which 38 had "myoclonic-astatic epilepsy." VPA reduced the number of seizures, primarily drop attacks but also atypical absences and myoclonic seizures, with seven becoming seizure free.

Randomized Controlled Trial Evidence

The gold standard for evaluation of the safety and efficacy of an anticonvulsant medication is the randomized, double-blind, placebo-controlled clinical trial. During the past two decades, seven drugs have undergone this rigorous testing to determine safety and efficacy in patients with LGS: cinromide, intravenous immunoglobulin (IVIG), felbamate (FBM), LTG, TPM, rufinamide (RFM), and clobazam (CLB). The latter five antiepileptic drugs (AEDs) successfully demonstrated efficacy against seizures in patients with LGS, whereas the first two did not.

Felbamate

FBM was found to be effective and well tolerated in patients with LGS in a randomized, double-blind, placebo-controlled adjunctive therapy trial[34] involving 73 patients aged 4–36 years. The target FBM dose in the double-blind portion was 45 mg/kg per day (maximum 3600 mg/day). The total seizure frequency decreased by 19% in the FBM group compared with a 4% increase in seizures in the placebo group ($p < 0.002$). Patients treated with FBM had a 34% reduction in atonic seizures, whereas patients receiving placebo experienced a 9% reduction ($p < 0.01$). The responder rate (percentage of patients experiencing at least a 50% reduction) for atonic seizures was 57% for the FBM group compared to 9% in the placebo group ($p < 0.001$). Likewise, the percentage of patients experiencing at least a 50% reduction in total seizure frequency was 50% for the FBM group compared to 11% in the placebo group ($p < 0.001$). Global evaluation scores were significantly better in the FBM-treated arm. Most side-effects were of mild or moderate severity. The types and frequency of side effects were similar in the two treatment groups. Long-term efficacy was confirmed in a 12-month follow-up of patients who completed the controlled part of the study.[35]

Unfortunately, treatment with FBM is hampered by the risk for idiosyncratic reactions including aplastic anemia and hepatotoxicity.[36,37] The most common severe FBM-associated idiosyncratic reaction is aplastic anemia, with an incidence of approximately 127 cases per 100,000 treated with FBM (approximately 1 in 4000–8000 FBM-treated patients). This compares unfavorably with an incidence of 2–6 per 100,000 people in the general population.[36,38–40] Other reports estimate the risk of aplastic anemia in patients receiving FBM to be 1:3000, with a death rate of 1 in 10,000 FBM-treated patients.[39,41] In perspective, this estimated risk is approximately 20 times greater than that for carbamazepine-associated aplastic anemia.[36] Factors that increase the risk of FBM-associated aplastic anemia include: Caucasian ethnicity, adult usage, female sex, history of autoimmune disorder, positive antinuclear antibody titer, history of prior AED toxicity or allergy, prior cytopenia, and treatment with FBM for less than 1 year.[36,37,42]

The second most common severe FBM-associated idiosyncratic reaction is hepatotoxicity, which was reported in 18 patients receiving FBM, with an estimated incidence of 64–164 per 100,000 (approximately 1 in 18,500–25,000 FBM-treated patients).[36] This suggests a similar frequency of FBM-associated hepatotoxicity and VPA-associated hepatotoxicity.[36] Based on the reported five FBM-related liver failure fatalities, which occurred in approximately 130,000–170,000 exposed persons, the estimated incidence lies between 1 per 26,000–34,000 exposures. In perspective, the risk of hepatic-related fatalities in the population taking VPA is between 1 in 10,000–49,000; the highest risk is 1 in 500 in patients younger than 2 years of age.[37] Although there is no evidence that routine laboratory monitoring of blood counts and liver function during FBM therapy anticipates these severe idiosyncratic reactions,[36] it is suggested that careful clinical monitoring and routine laboratory testing is performed, and the drug is discontinued if no significant clinical benefit is observed after 3–6 months of therapy.

Lamotrigine

LTG was found to be safe and effective in patients with LGS in a randomized, double-blind, placebo-controlled, adjunctive therapy trial.[43] A total of 169 patients were enrolled and randomized, 79 to LTG and 90 to placebo adjunctive therapy. Patients treated with LTG experienced a greater median percent reduction from baseline in weekly seizure counts (for drop attacks, tonic–clonic seizures, and all major seizures—defined as drop attacks plus tonic clonic seizures) compared with patients on the placebo treatment arm. The percentage of patients experiencing at least a 50% reduction in seizures for major seizures (drop attacks and tonic–clonic seizures) was greater in the LTG group (33%) than in the placebo

group (16%, $p < 0.01$). Significantly, more LTG-treated patients had a reduction of at least 50% in drop attacks, 37%, compared with 22% of the patients receiving placebo ($p < 0.04$). Likewise, for tonic–clonic seizures, 43% of the patients treated with LTG responded, compared with 20% of placebo-treated patients ($p < 0.007$).[43]

Unfortunately, LTG is associated with severe idiosyncratic reactions, predominantly involving the skin. The most common is a rash affecting 10%–12% of LTG patients.[44–46] Although it usually resolves following LTG withdrawal, this dermatologic reaction can progress to erythema multiforme, Stevens-Johnson syndrome, or toxic epidermal necrolysis.[39,44,47] Stevens-Johnson syndrome and toxic epidermal necrolysis are severe related mucocutaneous disorders with mortality rates of 5% and 30%, respectively.[44] Based on data from clinical trials and postmarketing reports, the risk of a potentially life-threatening rash in adults is 0.3% and higher in children 16 years old and younger (up to approximately 1%).[47]

Risk factors for LTG-associated severe dermatologic reactions include younger age (children more than adults), concomitant VPA use, a rapid rate of LTG titration, and a high LTG starting dose.[39,47,48] Clinicians should pay careful attention to initial LTG starting dose, titration rate, and comedications. The prompt evaluation of any rash is recommended.

Despite the risk of idiosyncratic reactions, LTG is a very valuable medication for patients with LGS and should be considered for use as soon as the diagnosis of LGS is made.

Topiramate

TPM was found to be well tolerated and effective as adjunctive therapy for patients with LGS in a multicenter, double-blind, placebo-controlled trial.[49] A total of 98 patients with LGS, ages 1–30 years, were randomized to receive either TPM adjunctive therapy ($n = 46$, target dose of 6 mg/kg per day) or placebo adjunctive therapy ($n = 50$). The median percent change from baseline in average monthly seizure rate for drop attacks was a 14.8% reduction for the TPM group, while there was an increase of 5.1% in the placebo group ($p < 0.041$). The responder rate for major seizures (drop attacks and tonic–clonic seizures) was greater in the TPM group (15/46, 33%) than in the placebo group (4/50, or 8%; $p < 0.002$). Although the responder rate for drop attacks in the TPM group was higher than in the placebo group (28% vs. 14%), this finding did not reach statistical significance.[49] Using parental global evaluations, TPM-treated patients demonstrated greater improvement in seizure severity than did placebo-treated patients ($p < 0.037$).

Long-term efficacy was demonstrated in the open-label extension portion of the previously mentioned trial, in which 97 patients were followed and had their TPM dose adjusted as clinically indicated.[50] The mean TPM dose in patients who completed 6 months of therapy was 10 mg/kg per day. For patients who completed 6 months of TPM therapy, drop attacks were reduced at least 50% in 55% of patients. In addition, 15% of patients were free of drop attacks for at least 6 months at the last visit. The median percent reduction in drop attacks was 56% and the median percent reduction in overall seizure frequency was 44%. Forty-five percent of the patients had at least a 50% reduction in all seizure types, and 2% were seizure-free for the previous 6 months. The most common adverse events were somnolence, injury, and anorexia. Behavioral problems during the last 6 months of TPM long-term therapy were reported in only 5% of the patients. During long-term therapy, TPM is effective and well tolerated in controlling drop attacks and seizures associated with LGS.[50]

Rufinamide

The efficacy and tolerability of RFM adjunctive therapy for patients with LGS was studied in a multicenter, double-blind, placebo-controlled, randomized, parallel-group study.[51,52] Patients enrolled were between 4 and 30 years of age, had 90 seizures in the month prior to the 28-day baseline phase, and were taking one to three concomitant AEDs. The treatment phase consisted of 14 days of titration and 70 days of maintenance, with a target RFM dose of 45 mg/kg per day. Overall, 138 patients with a mean age of 14.1 years (range 4–37 years), were randomized to either RFM ($n = 74$) or placebo ($n = 64$). The median dose in both groups was 1800 mg/day (42–45 mg/kg per day).[51,52]

The median percent reduction in total seizure frequency per 28 days relative to baseline was significantly higher in the RFM group compared to the placebo group (32.7% vs. 11.7%, $p = 0.0015$). In the RFM group, the median percent reduction in tonic–atonic seizure frequency per 28 days relative to the baseline phase was significantly higher compared with the placebo group (42.5% vs. 1.4%, $p < 0.0001$). The tonic–atonic seizure responder rate was also significantly higher in the RFM group compared with the placebo group (42.5% vs. 16.7%, $p = 0.0020$).[51,52]

The most common adverse events experienced included somnolence, vomiting, pyrexia, and diarrhea. A lower percentage of patients in the RFM group (17.6%) experienced cognitive/psychiatric adverse events of interest, such as psychomotor hyperactivity and lethargy, compared with the placebo group (23.4%). RFM was efficacious and well tolerated as an adjunctive therapy for the treatment of resistant seizures in patients with LGS.[51,52]

Clobazam

A randomized, double-blind, placebo-controlled, parallel-group, multicenter study of CLB as adjunctive therapy in patients with LGS was reported in 2011.[53] Patients were eligible to participate if they had onset of LGS before age 11 years, one or more type of generalized seizure, including drop seizures, for 6 or more months and a previous EEG reporting generalized, slow spike and wave discharges. A total of 238 patients with LGS (ages 2–54 years) were randomized to placebo or CLB 0.25 mg, 0.5 mg, or 1 mg/kg per day. The study included a 4-week baseline, followed by a 3-week titration and a 12-week maintenance period.

The mean percentage reduction in average weekly rate of drop seizures from baseline to maintenance period was 41.2% ($p = 0.012$) for the 0.25 mg/kg per day group, 49.4% ($p = 0.0015$) for the 0.5 mg/kg per day group and 68.3% ($p < 0.0001$) for the 1 mg/kg per day group, compared to 12.1% for placebo, showing a linear trend ($p < 0.0001$) of increasing efficacy with increasing doses. In addition, the mean percentage reduction in average weekly rate of total (drop and nondrop) seizures was 9.3% for placebo, compared to 34.8% ($p = 0.0414$), 45.3% ($p = 0.0044$), and 65.3% ($p = < 0.0001$) for the CLB 0.25, 0.5, and 1 mg/kg per day groups, respectively. Likewise, responder rates (≥50% seizure reduction in drop seizures from baseline to maintenance) increased with increasing CLB doses. The percentage of responders was 31.6% for placebo, vs. 43.4%, 58%, and 77.6% for the low-, medium-, and high-dose CLB groups.

The most frequent adverse events reported for CLB were somnolence (21.8% for all CLB groups vs. 11.9% for placebo), pyrexia (12.8% vs. 3.4%), upper respiratory infections (12.3% vs. 10.2%), and lethargy (10.1% vs. 5.1%).

Open-Label Uncontrolled Trial Evidence

Based on open-label uncontrolled trials other potential useful AEDs include (in alphabetical order): adrenocorticotropic hormone (ACTH),[54,55] corticosteroids,[22,56,57] IVIG,[58,59] levetiracetam,[60] vigabatrin,[61] and zonisamide (ZNS).[62]

Both ACTH and corticosteroid therapy are proposed to be effective against the seizures associated with LGS. Roger proposes that prolonged corticosteroid therapy initiated at the onset of cryptogenic LGS can yield "excellent" results.[22] Despite this effectiveness, there are multiple potentially significant side effects associated with therapy, and relapse frequently occurs when the drugs are withdrawn.[25,54–57,63]

The efficacy of adjunctive high-dose IVIG in patients with LGS has been investigated in several open-label trials.[58] The results of these trials were very encouraging, with 30%–92% of LGS patients on IVIG experiencing at least a 50% seizure reduction during treatment.[58] Dosing schedules varied between studies. Despite encouraging earlier results, later well-controlled trials failed to confirm the effectiveness of IVIG against seizures associated with LGS.[64,65]

A small retrospective study of six patients showed a reduction in tonic–clonic, atonic, atypical absence, and myoclonic seizures when levetiracetam was added as adjunctive therapy.[60]

Six studies involving 78 patients treated with vigabatrin showed that 15% of these patients became completely seizure-free and 44% of the patients had at least 50% reduction in their seizure frequency.[61,66–70] The best results were noted in an open-label, dose-ranging, adjunctive therapy study of vigabatrin in 20 children with LGS in which monotherapy with valproic acid did not control their seizures. Seventeen children (85%) experienced at least 50% reduction in their seizure frequency, and eight children (40%) were seizure-free at doses ranging from 1 to 3 g/day at study end.[61] The authors concluded that vigabatrin and valproic acid duo therapy was effective and well tolerated in children with LGS.[61]

The most common adverse effects of vigabatrin are generally central nervous system related and include hyperactivity, agitation, weight gain, drowsiness, insomnia, facial edema, ataxia, stupor, and somnolence.[39,68,71,72] Not only can vigabatrin exacerbate myoclonic seizures and even absence seizures in some patients, but can also cause visual field constriction in children.[67,68,71,73,74] The aforementioned side effects significantly limit consideration of vigabatrin as long-term therapy for patients with LGS.[39]

The effectiveness of ZNS in LGS has been investigated in three small studies in Japan. Although Sakamoto reported that ZNS was "effective" in 39% of patients with LGS, the definition of effectiveness was not clear.[62] In another study, Yamatogi reported that 50% of 20 Lennox–Gastaut patients treated with ZNS had at least 50% reduction in seizure frequency.[75] Iinuma found that 26% (10 of 39) of patients with LGS treated with ZNS responded with a 50% or greater reduction in seizure frequency.[76]

DIETARY TREATMENT

In a recent study, Freeman, Vining, and collaborators reported their findings of a blinded, crossover, placebo-controlled trial.[77] Twenty children with LGS were fasted for 36 hours, and introduced to the ketogenic diet. Glucose or saccharine were randomly used in a blinded fashion to negate or sustain the effect of the diet. In a preliminary study, these investigators were able to negate urinary ketosis in patients on the ketogenic diet

by giving a drink containing glucose, creating therefore a placebo arm.[85] In the most recent study, although there was a reduction in parent-reported clinical events between the glucose and saccharine arms, the difference did not reach statistical significance. Likewise, there was no statistical difference in EEG-identified events between the two arms. Unexpectedly, the patients in the glucose arm still showed trace to moderate ketones, creating in fact an active control arm rather than a placebo arm.

SURGICAL TREATMENT

There are no double-blind trials examining the efficacy of surgical intervention in patients with LGS. However, open-label uncontrolled studies have reported surgical procedures to be beneficial for patients with LGS, including corpus callosotomy, focal resection (rarely), and electrical stimulation, in particular, vagus nerve stimulation (VNS) and the electrical stimulation of the centromedian thalamic nuclei.[78,79]

Corpus callosotomy is effective in reducing drop attacks but typically does not appear to be helpful for other seizure types.[25,80,81] A study from Taiwan reported that anterior corpus callosotomy was effective for "all kinds of medically intractable seizures, especially generalized" in a cohort of 74 patients (80% had LGS).[82] In general, callosotomy is considered palliative rather than curative, and although it can occur, seizure freedom is rare.[82,83]

In the largest cohort of LGS patients treated with VNS, Frost reported the effectiveness, tolerability, and safety of VNS therapy in 50 patients (median age 13 years) with LGS. At 6 months after VNS implantation, a median reduction of 58% in seizure frequency was seen. Quality of life was improved in some patients and the most common adverse effects were voice change and coughing during stimulation.[84]

In rare cases, resection of a localized lesion (e.g., vascular lesion or tumor) was reported to improve seizure control in patients with LGS.[25,85]

TREATMENT ALGORITHM

From a practical viewpoint, by the time a clinician makes a diagnosis of LGS, the patient has usually been diagnosed with generalized epilepsy and started treatment with a broad spectrum AED (e.g., valproic acid, levetiracetam, TPM, or LTG) (Fig. 29–1). Once a diagnosis of LGS has been established, it is important to remove AEDs that do not have strong clinical trial evidence of efficacy (unless the patient appears to be significantly benefiting from them) and discuss with the patient's family the variety of AEDs with clinical trial evidence for effectiveness against seizures associated with LGS.

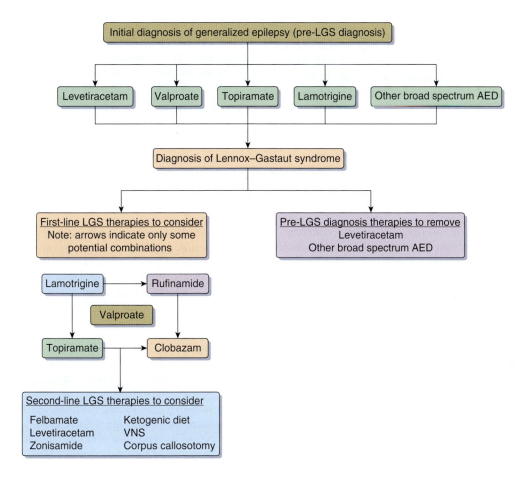

Figure 29–1. Diagnosis and treatment algorithm.

There is no clear difference in efficacy among the five AEDs (FBM, LTG, TPM, RFM, and CLB) with randomized controlled trial data in LGS. However many clinicians continue to have concerns about the potential for idiosyncratic reactions with FBM; as such it is not usually considered a first line AED for LGS. It is reasonable to consider the remaining four AEDs (along with valproic acid) as first line medications for LGS.

These four AEDs (along with valproic acid) are often used either as monotherapy or more commonly as polytherapy (Fig. 29–1). Many clinicians will select "a foundation" AED upon which to implement a series of polytherapy trials. This foundation AED is the medication to which the patient exhibits the best combination of seizure control and tolerability.

It is important to have families maintain seizure diaries that list each seizure type separately. These diaries provide the objective data needed to determine whether the addition of a new AED to the foundation AED has made a substantial (>50% reduction) difference in one or more seizure types. Coupling these seizure diaries with some objective measure of quality of life or seizure severity can be useful in the overall assessment of a particular AED or AED combination.

If the aforementioned therapies are unsuccessful either individually or in combination, then second line therapies such as FBM, ketogenic diet, VNS, corpus callosotomy, levetiracetam, and ZNS should be considered.

▶ PROGNOSIS

The long-term prognosis is variable but overall is unfavorable. Several studies have prospectively followed cohorts of children with LGS and demonstrated persistence of typical characteristics over time in many of these children. Long-term follow-up reveals that few become seizure-free (20, 123). Poorer prognosis is associated with symptomatic LGS, particularly with a prior history of West syndrome, early seizure onset, higher seizure frequency, and a persistently slow EEG background. In one report, tonic seizures became more difficult to control over time and persisted (97.8% of the patients) while myoclonic and atypical absences appeared easier to control, persisting in 22.5–39.3% of patients, respectively. The characteristic diffuse slow spike-wave pattern of LGS gradually disappears with age and is replaced by focal epileptic discharges often at multiple independent spikes. This may reflect that subcortical epileptic discharges are suppressed while focal cortical discharges gain preponderance with brain maturation. Mortality is reported to range from 3% (mean follow-up of 8.5 years) to 7% (mean follow-up of 9.7 years).

REFERENCES

1. Proposal for revised classification of epilepsies and epileptic syndromes. Commission on classification and terminology of the international league against epilepsy. *Epilepsia* 1989;30(4):389–399.
2. Gastaut H. The Lennox–Gastaut syndrome: comments on the syndrome's terminology and nosological position amongst the secondary generalized epilepsies of childhood. *Electroencephalogr Clin Neurophysiol Suppl* 1982;35:71–84.
3. Beaumanoir A, Blume Warren. In: Roger J, Bureau M, Dravet C, Genton, P; Tassinari, C; Wolf, P (eds), *The Lennox–Gastaut Syndrome*. Montrouge: John Libbey Eurotext, 2005.
4. Farrell K. Classifying epileptic syndromes: problems and a neurobiologic solution. *Neurology* 1993;43(11 Suppl 5):S8–S11.
5. Aicardi J. Epileptic syndromes in childhood. *Epilepsia* 1988;29(Suppl 3):S1–S15.
6. Livingston JH. The Lennox–Gastaut syndrome. *Dev Med Child Neurol* 1988;30(4):536–540.
7. Dulac O, N'Guyen T. The Lennox–Gastaut syndrome. *Epilepsia* 1993;34(Suppl 7):S7–S17.
8. Ohtahara S. Lennox–Gastaut syndrome. Considerations in its concept and categorization. *Jpn J Psychiatry Neurol* 1988;42(3):535–542.
9. Oguni H, Hayashi K, Osawa M. Long-term prognosis of Lennox–Gastaut syndrome. *Epilepsia* 1996;37(Suppl 3):44–47.
10. Trevathan E, Murphy CC, Yeargin-Allsopp M. Prevalence and descriptive epidemiology of Lennox–Gastaut syndrome among Atlanta children. *Epilepsia* 1997;38(12):1283–1288.
11. Yaqub BA. Electroclinical seizures in Lennox–Gastaut syndrome. *Epilepsia* 1993;34(1):120–127.
12. Hauser WA. The prevalence and incidence of convulsive disorders in children. *Epilepsia* 1994;35:(Suppl 2):S1–S6.
13. Kramer U, Nevo Y, Neufeld MY, Fatal A, Leitner Y, Harel S. Epidemiology of epilepsy in childhood: a cohort of 440 consecutive patients. *Pediatr Neurol* 1998;18(1):46–50.
14. Prats JM, Garaizar C. [Etiology of epilepsy in adolescents]. *Rev Neurol* 1999;28(1):32–35.
15. Beilmann A, Talvik T. Is the international league against epilepsy classification of epileptic syndromes applicable to children in Estonia? [In process citation]. *Europ J Paediatr Neurol* 1999;3(6):265–272.
16. Cavazzuti GB. Epidemiology of different types of epilepsy in school age children of Modena, Italy. *Epilepsia* 1980; 21(1):57–62.
17. Steffenburg U, Hedstrom A, Lindroth A, Wiklund LM, Hagberg G, Kyllerman M. Intractable epilepsy in a population-based series of mentally retarded children. *Epilepsia* 1998;39(7):767–775.
18. Heiskala H. Community-based study of Lennox–Gastaut syndrome. *Epilepsia* 1997;38(5):526–531.
19. Rantala H, Putkonen T. Occurrence, outcome, and prognostic factors of infantile spasms and Lennox–Gastaut syndrome. *Epilepsia* 1999;40(3):286–289.
20. Beilmann A, Napa A, Soot A, Talvik I, Talvik T. Prevalence of childhood epilepsy in Estonia. *Epilepsia* 1999;40(7):1011–1019.
21. Beaumanoir A. The Lennox–Gastaut syndrome: a personal study. *Electroencephalogr Clin Neurophysiol Suppl* 1982; 35:85–99.
22. Roger J, Dravet C, Bureau M. The Lennox–Gastaut syndrome. *Cleve Clin J Med* 1989;56(Suppl Pt 2):S172–S180.
23. Chevrie JJ, Aicardi J. Childhood epileptic encephalopathy with slow spike-wave. A statistical study of 80 cases. *Epilepsia* 1972;13(2):259–271.
24. Ohtsuka Y, Amano R, Mizukawa M, Ohtahara S. Long-term prognosis of the Lennox–Gastaut syndrome. *Jpn J Psychiatry Neurol* 1990;44(2):257–264.
25. Aicardi J. Epilepsy. In: Procopis PG, Rapin I (eds), *Children*. New York: Raven Press, 1994; 2nd edn.
26. Markand ON. Slow spike-wave activity in EEG and associated clinical features: often called 'Lennox' or 'Lennox–Gastaut' syndrome. *Neurology* 1977;27(8):746–757.
27. Goldsmith IL, Zupanc ML, Buchhalter JR. Long-term seizure outcome in 74 patients with Lennox–Gastaut syndrome: effects of incorporating MRI head imaging in defining the cryptogenic subgroup. *Epilepsia* 2000;41(4):395–399.
28. Bare MA, Glauser TA, Strawsburg RH. Need for electroencephalogram video confirmation of atypical absence seizures in children with Lennox–Gastaut syndrome. *J Child Neurol* 1998;13(10):498–500.
29. Ikeno T, Shigematsu H, Miyakoshi M, Ohba A, Yagi K, Seino M. An analytic study of epileptic falls. *Epilepsia* 1985;26(6):612–621.
30. van Engelen BG, de Waal LP, Weemaes CM, Renier WO. Serologic HLA typing in cryptogenic Lennox–Gastaut syndrome. *Epilepsy Research* 1994;17(1):43–47.
31. Wheless JW, Clarke DF, Carpenter D. Treatment of pediatric epilepsy: expert opinion, 2005. *J Child Neurol* 2005;20(Suppl 1):S1–S56; quiz S9–S60.
32. Wheless JW, Clarke DF, Arzimanoglou A, Carpenter D. Treatment of pediatric epilepsy: European expert opinion, 2007. *Epileptic Disord* 2007;9(4):353–412.
33. Covanis A, Gupta AK, Jeavons PM. Sodium valproate: monotherapy and polytherapy. *Epilepsia* 1982;23(6):693–720.
34. Ritter FJ. Efficacy of felbamate in childhood epileptic encephalopathy (Lennox–Gastaut syndrome). *N Engl J Med* 1993;328(Jan. 7):29–33.
35. Jensen PK. Felbamate in the treatment of Lennox–Gastaut syndrome. *Epilepsia* 1994;35:(Suppl 5):S54–S57.
36. Pellock JM. Felbamate. *Epilepsia* 1999;40(Suppl 5):S57–S62.
37. Pellock JM, Faught E, Leppik IE, Shinnar S, Zupanc ML. Felbamate: consensus of current clinical experience. *Epilepsy Res* 2006;71(2–3):89–101.
38. Patton W, Duffull S. Idiosyncratic drug-induced haematological abnormalities. Incidence, pathogenesis, management and avoidance. *Drug Saf* 1994;11(6):445–462.

39. Pellock JM. New antiepileptic drugs in pediatric epilepsy syndromes. *Pediatrics* 1999;104(5 Part 1):1106–1116.

40. Kaufman DW, Kelly JP, Anderson T, Harmon DC, Shapiro S. Evaluation of case reports of aplastic anemia among patients treated with felbamate. *Epilepsia* 1997; 38(12):1265–1269.

41. Bourgeois BF. Felbamate [published erratum appears in *Semin Pediatr Neurol* 1998;5(1):76]. *Semin Pediatr Neurol* 1997;4(1):3–8.

42. Pellock JM, Brodie MJ. Felbamate: 1997 update. *Epilepsia* 1997;38(12):1261–1264.

43. Motte J, Trevathan E, Arvidsson JF, Barrera MN, Mullens EL, Manasco P. Lamotrigine for generalized seizures associated with the Lennox–Gastaut syndrome. *N Engl J Med* 1997;337(25):1807–1812.

44. Pellock JM. Overview of lamotrigine and the new antiepileptic drugs: the challenge. *J Child Neurol* 1997; 12(Suppl 1):S48–S52.

45. Schlienger RG, Shapiro LE, Shear NH. Lamotrigine-induced severe cutaneous adverse reactions. *Epilepsia* 1998;39(Suppl 7):S22–S26.

46. Pellock JM, Watemberg N. New antiepileptic drugs in children: present and future. *Semin Pediatr Neurol* 1997; 4(1):9–18.

47. Matsuo F. Lamotrigine. *Epilepsia* 1999;40(Suppl 5):S30–S36.

48. Pellock J. Overview of lamotrigine and the new antiepileptic drugs: the challenge. *J Child Neurol* 1997;12:S48–S52.

49. Sachdeo RC, Glauser TA, Ritter F, Reife R, Lim P, Pledger G. A double-blind, randomized trial of topiramate in Lennox–Gastaut syndrome. *Neurology* 1999;52(9):1882–1887.

50. Glauser TA, Levisohn PM, Ritter F, Sachdeo RC. Topiramate in Lennox–Gastaut syndrome: open-label treatment of patients completing a randomized controlled trial. Topiramate YL Study Group. *Epilepsia* 2000;41(Suppl 1): S86–S90.

51. Glauser T, Kluger G, Krauss GL, Perdomo C, Arroyo S. Short term and long-term efficacy and safety of rufinamide as adjunctive therapy in patients with inadequately controlled Lennox Gastaut syndrome. *Neurology* 2006;Z66(Suppl 2):36.

52. Glauser T, Kluger G, Sachdeo RC, Krauss GL, Perdomo C, Arroyo S. Efficacy and safety of rufinamide adjunctive therapy in patients with Lennox–Gastaut syndrome (LGS): a multicenter, randomized, double-blind, placebo-controlled, parallel trial. *Neurology* 2005;64:1826.

53. Ng YT, Conry JA, Drummond R, Stolle J, Weinberg MA. Randomized, phase III study results of clobazam in Lennox–Gastaut syndrome. *Neurology* 2011;77(15):1473–1481.

54. Brett E. The Lennox–Gastaut syndrome: therapeutic aspects. In: Niedermeyer E, Degen R (eds), *The Lennox–Gastaut Syndrome*. New York: Alan Liss, 1988, pp. 317–339.

55. Yamatogi Y, et al. Treatment of the Lennox syndrome with ACTH: a clinical and electroencephalographic study. *Brain Dev* 1979;1:267–276.

56. Snead O, Benton J, Myers C. ACTH and prednisone in childhood seizure disorders. *Neurology* 1983;33:966–970.

57. Wheless JW, Constantinou JEC. Lennox–Gastaut syndrome. *Pediatr Neurol* 1997;17(3):203–211.

58. Duse M, Notarangelo LD, Tiberti S, Menegati E, Plebani A, Ugazio AG. Intravenous immune globulin in the treatment of intractable childhood epilepsy. *Clin Exp Immunol* 1996; 104(Suppl 1):71–76.

59. van Engelen BG, Renier WO, Weemaes CM, Strengers PF, Bernsen PJ, Notermans SL. High-dose intravenous immunoglobulin treatment in cryptogenic West and Lennox–Gastaut syndrome; an add-on study. *Eur J Pediatr* 1994;153(10):762–769.

60. De Los Reyes EC, Sharp GB, Williams JP, Hale SE. Levetiracetam in the treatment of Lennox–Gastaut syndrome. *Pediatr Neurol* 2004;30(4):254–256.

61. Feucht M, Brantner-Inthaler S. Gamma-vinyl-GABA (vigabatrin) in the therapy of Lennox–Gastaut syndrome: an open study. *Epilepsia* 1994;35(5):993–998.

62. Sakamoto K, et al. Effects of zonisamide on children with epilepsy. *Curr Ther Res* 1988;43(3):378–383.

63. Bourgeois BFD. Antiepileptic drugs in pediatric practice. *Epilepsia* 1995;36(2):S34–S45.

64. Illum N, et al. Intravenous immunoglobulin: a single-blind trial in children with Lennox–Gastaut syndrome. *Neuropediatrics* 1990;21(2):87–90.

65. van Rijckevorsel-Harmant K, Delire M, Schmitz-Moorman W, Wieser HG. Treatment of refractory epilepsy with intravenous immunoglobulins. Results of the first double-blind/dose finding clinical study. *Int J Clin Lab Res* 1994; 24(3):162–166.

66. Livingston J, Beaumont D, Arzimanoglou A. Vigabatrin in the treatment of epilepsy in children. *Br J Clin Pharmacol* 1989;27:109S–112S.

67. Gibbs J, Appleton R, Rosenbloom L. Vigabatrin in intractable childhood epilepsy: a restrospective study. *Pediatr Neurol* 1992;8:338–340.

68. Luna D, Dulac O, Pajot N. Vigabatrin in the treatment of childhood epilepsies. A single-blind placebo-controlled study. *Epilepsia* 1989;30:430–437.

69. Fois A, Buoni S, Bartolo RD. Vigabatrin treatment in children. *Childs Nerv Syst* 1994;10:244–248.

70. Maldonado C, Castello J, Fuentes E. Vigabatrin in the management of Lennox–Gastaut syndrome. *Epilepsia* 1995; 36:S102.

71. Dulac O, et al. Vigabatrin in childhood epilepsy. *J Child Neurol* 1991;(Suppl 2):S30–S37.

72. Shields WD, Sankar R. Vigabatrin. *Semin Pediatr Neurol* 1997;4(1):43–50.

73. Appleton RE. Vigabatrin in the management of generalized seizures in children. *Seizure* 1995;4(1):45–48.

74. Sankar R, Wasterlain CG. Is the devil we know the lesser of two evils? Vigabatrin and visual fields. *Neurology* 1999;52(8):1537–1538.

75. Yamatogi Y, Ohtahara S. Current topics of treatment. In: Ohtahara S, Roger J (eds), *Proceedings of the International Symposium, New Trends in Pediatric Epileptology*. Okayama: 1991, pp. 136–148.

76. Iinuma K, Haginoya K. Clinical efficacy of zonisamide in childhood epilepsy after long-term treatment: a postmarketing, multi-institutional survey. *Seizure* 2004; 13(Suppl 1):S34–S39; discussion S40.

77. Freeman JM, Vining EP, Kossoff EH, Pyzik PL, Ye X, Goodman SN. A blinded, crossover study of the efficacy of the ketogenic diet. *Epilepsia* 2009;50(2):322–325.

78. Arzimanoglou A, Guerrini R, Aicardi J. *Aicardi's Epilepsy In Children*. Philadelphia: Lippincott Wilkins & Williams, 2004; 3rd ed.

79. Velasco AL, et al. Neuromodulation of the centromedian thalamic nuclei in the treatment of generalized seizures and the improvement of the quality of life in patients with Lennox–Gastaut syndrome. *Epilepsia* 2006;47(7):1203–1212.

80. Wheless J. Evaluation of children for epilepsy surgery. *Pediatr Ann* 1991;20:41–49.

81. Baumgartner J, Clifton G, Wheless J. Corpus callostomy. *Tech Neurosurg* 1995;1:45–51.

82. Kwan SY, et al. Seizure outcome after corpus callosotomy: the Taiwan experience. *Childs Nerv Syst* 2000;16(2):87–92.

83. Farrell KTI W. *Encephalopathic Generalized Epilepsy and Lennox–Gastaut Syndrome*. Wyllie E (ed). Philadelphia: Lippincott Wilkins & Williams, 2006.

84. Frost M, et al. Vagus nerve stimulation in children with refractory seizures associated with Lennox–Gastaut syndrome. *Epilepsia* 2001;42(9):1148–1152.

85. Angelini L, Broggi G, Riva D, Lazzaro Solero C. A case of Lennox–Gastaut syndrome successfully treated by removal of a parietotemporal astrocytoma. *Epilepsia* 1979; 20(6):665–669.

86. Roger J, et al. [Lennox–Gastaut syndrome in the adult]. *Rev Neurol* 1987;143(5):401–405.

87. Ohtahara S, Ohtsuka Y, Kobayashi K. Lennox–Gastaut syndrome: a new vista. *Psychiatry Clin Neurosci* 1995; 49(3):S179–S183.

88. Yagi K. Evolution of Lennox–Gastaut syndrome: a long-term longitudinal study. *Epilepsia* 1996;37(Suppl 3):48–51.

89. Ohtsuka Y, Ohmori I, Oka E. Long-term follow-up of childhood epilepsy associated with tuberous sclerosis. *Epilepsia* 1998;39(11):1158–1163.

CHAPTER 30

Acquired Epileptic Aphasia (Landau–Kleffner Syndrome)

Edouard Hirsch

► CLINICAL PRESENTATION AND DIAGNOSIS

Acquired epileptic aphasia[1] is an epileptic syndrome described in the International Classification of Epilepsies by the eponym Landau–Kleffner syndrome (LKS). Typical LKS[2,3] is part of the epileptic encephalopathy of late childhood defined by[1]: age of onset ranging from 3 to 10 years in children with previously normal language development;[2] insidious or abrupt acquired aphasia with verbal auditory agnosia; behavior disturbances (attention deficit and hyperactivity);[3] seizures that may be nocturnal, focal motor, secondarily generalized, or atypical absences with an awake electroencephalographic (EEG) showing focal or multifocal spikes-and-waves predominantly over the temporal regions (Fig. 30–1);[4] and sleep EEG reveals activation of interictal EEG abnormalities and, during the course of the syndrome in the acute phase, nonrapid eye movement (NREM) subcontinuous or continuous spike-waves during sleep (CSWS) (Fig. 30–1).

Typical LKS is not related to nonconvulsive status epilepticus, which presents as a subacute progressive aphasia in adults,[4] or acquired lesions with seizures such as cysticercosis[5] or astrocytoma.[6] LKS represents a subtype of idiopathic focal epilepsies with acquired cognitive deficits.[7,8] Other subtypes of idiopathic focal epilepsies related to LKS are described by several terms in the literature: acquired opercular syndrome with epilepsy, frontal epilepsy with or without autistic regression, atypical partial benign epilepsy or pseudo-Lennox–Gastaut syndrome, and idiopathic or symptomatic CSWS[8] (Table 30–1)

De Saint-Matin et al[9] suggested a terminology for symptoms of LKS and related epilepsies that included three major categories: "classical focal seizures," "spike-wave-related symptoms," and "paraictal symptoms" (see Fig. 30–2 for definition). The variability in clinical expression probably reflects the implication of different pathophysiological mechanisms, which in turn could explain differences in responses to treatment.

ETIOLOGY AND PATHOPHYSIOLOGY

LKS is included in the focal idiopathic group of epilepsies but its causes remain unknown. Two main hypotheses are proposed. The first favors genetic predisposition as an underlying cause, despite the absence of identified genes in typical LKS patients. Autoantibodies have also been suggested as either a cause or consequence of LKS,[9,10] driven by the improvement in patients treated with immunoglobulin[11] or steroids.[12]

Landau and Kleffner[1] suggested that "persistent convulsive discharges in brain tissue, largely concerned with linguistic communication, result in the functional ablation of these areas for normal linguistic behavior." Epileptic discharges in the sleep recorded EEG also favor this initial suggestion. Although several studies reveal parallel fluctuation of the aphasia and EEG abnormalities,[13] the causal relationship between epileptiform EEG discharges and the language defect remains a matter of debate.[14]

LKS is related to a focal dysfunction in the temporal cortex.[2,3] Although the EEG may show both focal discharges and bilateral generalized abnormalities, neurophysiological and positron emission tomography (PET) findings provide strong evidence in favor of focal cerebral dysfunction involving the temporal cortex.[15–17] To date, no specific anatomic abnormalities have been detected in LKS. However, recently, Takeoka et al[18] performed volumetric magnetic resonance imaging (MRI) analysis of several neocortical regions and subcortical substructures in four children with typical LKS without obvious anatomical abnormalities. They evidenced bilateral volume reduction in the superior temporal areas, specifically the planum temporale and superior temporal gyrus where receptive language is localized. However, it is not clear if cortical volume reduction is a cause or effect of paroxysmal epileptic activity in LKS.

Since 1992, neurophysiological, metabolic, and neuroanatomical studies have led to the view that LKS is an acquired aphasia secondary to an epileptogenic disturbance affecting a cortical area involved in verbal processing. This fits with the early suggestion of a "functional ablation" caused by persistent abnormal epileptic activity in cortical areas subserving language. According to these electrophysiological features, epileptic aphasia would then constitute a subgroup of the CSWS syndrome in which the epileptic discharges arise from the temporal cortex. However, the abnormal neuronal activity (related to the epileptic focus)

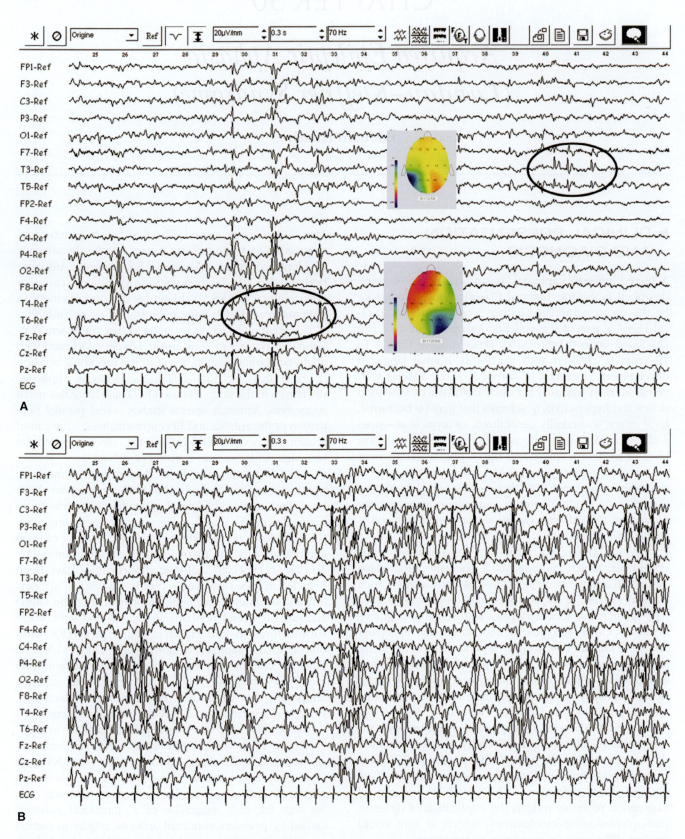

Figure 30–1. Awake (**A**) and sleep (**B**) EEG in 6-year-old girls with auditory agnosia in a typical case of Landau–Kleffner syndrome.

▶**TABLE 30–1. COMPARISON OF DIAGNOSIS AND TREATMENTS OF LANDAU–KLEFFNER SYNDROME WITH RELATED EPILEPTIC SITUATIONS**

	Landau–Kleffner Syndrome	Acquired Opercular Deficit	Frontal Deficit with or without Autistic Regression	Atypical BECST	CSWS
Onset (years)	3–10	2–10	3–10	3–10	3–10
Acquired cognitive symptoms "paraictal"	Auditory agnosia Expressive aphasia Attention deficits	Dysphasia Aphasia Drooling Attention deficits	Behavioral Attention deficits	Attention Short-term memory Deficits	All types
Seizures types	None Focal motor Atypical absences	None Focal motor	None Focal motor Atypical absences	None Focal motor Atypical absences	None Focal motor Atypical absences
Awake EEG	Multifocal, bilateral Posterior temporal	Multifocal Bilateral Central	Multifocal Bilateral Frontal	Multifocal Bilateral Central	Multifocal Bilateral
Sleep EEG	Major activation To CSWS	Major activation To CSWS	Major activation To CSWS	Major activation To CSWS	CSWS By definition
MRI finding	Normal or subtle Abnormalities	Normal or subtle Abnormalities	Normal or subtle Abnormalities	Normal or subtle Abnormalities	Normal or thalamus lesion Polymicrogyria
Treatment First line	Benzodiazepines	Benzodiazepines	Benzodiazepines	Benzodiazepines	Benzodiazepines
Treatment Second line	Steroids	Sulthiam	Ethosuximide	Sulthiam	Ethosuximide
Treatment Third line	Subpial transection	Steroids	Steroids	Ethosuximide	Steroids

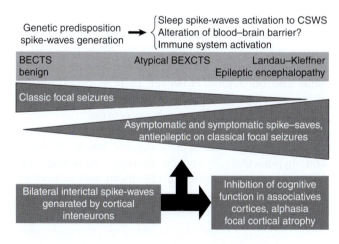

Figure 30–2. Unified hypothesis about Landau–Kleffner syndrome pathophysiology, benign epilepsy with centrotemporal spikes, CSWS. "Classical focal seizures" constitute the electroclinical development and propagation of a focal cortical neuronal discharge. "Spike-and-wave-related symptoms" are brief neurological or neuropsychological phenomena having a relatively strict temporal correlation with individual components of isolated focal or generalized spikes and waves. "Paraictal symptoms" consist of acquired progressive and fluctuating motor or cognitive deficits and are not directly correlated with Todd paralysis.

not only has immediate consequences on the function of the involved cortical area (epileptic functional inhibition), but also induces a permanent dysfunction that might explain, in some cases, the poor long-term verbal outcome.

Taken together, the previously mentioned discussion can be used to formulate a unified speculative hypothesis about LKS pathophysiology (Fig. 30–2). Genetic predisposition induces hyperexcitability and synchronization of gabaergic interneurons in the perisylvian cortices responsible for spike-wave generation. Major spike-wave activation during NREM sleep following thalamocortical uncoupling may lead to an alteration of the blood brain barrier, which might in turn provoke an immune reaction with synthesis of different autoantibodies. This interneuron hyperactivity might have an antiepileptic effect on the classical focal seizures, with an associated inhibition of function in the associative cortices responsible for auditory agnosia. Long-term effects of spike-waves might manifest in focal atrophy in the superior temporal gyri, which may explain the poor verbal outcome in some cases of LKS.

▶ TREATMENT

Classical focal seizures (focal motor seizures), spike-wave-related symptoms (negative myoclonia, CSWS), and

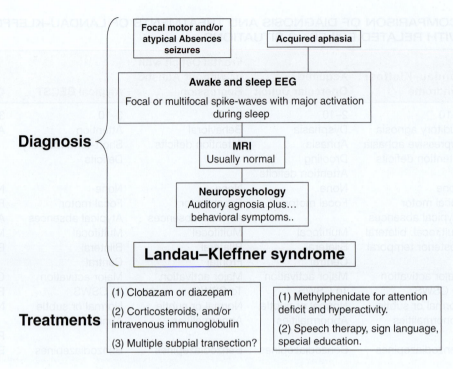

Figure 30–3. Diagnosis and treatment algorithm.

paraictal symptoms (aphasia) probably reflect different pathophysiological mechanisms, which in turn could explain different sensitivities to treatment. For example, carbamazepine is effective for classical focal seizures but could have a paradoxical effect on spike-wave-related and paraictal symptoms.[9] No controlled clinical trials have been undertaken on the therapeutic options for LKS, and only open-label data are available.

Early diagnosis and initiation of prompt medical treatment appear important for improving long-term prognosis[2,11] (Fig. 30–3). In addition, several antiepileptic drugs are reportedly beneficial in treating this syndrome. These include valproic acid, diazepam, ethosuximide, clobazam, and clonazepam.[12] Reports on the efficacy of lamotrigine, sulthiame, felbamate, nicardipine, vigabatrin, levetiracetam, vagus nerve stimulation, and the ketogenic diet are insufficient and more data is needed. Carbamazepine and possibly phenobarbital and phenytoin may exacerbate the syndrome.[12]

As initial therapy, monotherapy with clobazam or diazepam is often empirically chosen (Marescaux et al, 1990, Mikati and Shamseddine, 2005). Subsequently, other antiepileptic drugs, corticosteroids, or intravenous immunoglobulin (IVIG) therapy are often used. Corticosteroid therapy should probably not be delayed more than 1–4 months after the initial diagnosis.[11,12] Various corticosteroid regimens including oral prednisone and, recently, high doses of intravenous pulsed corticosteroids, (as well as corticotropin or adrenocorticotropic hormone) are reportedly effective in LKS. Of these, oral

corticosteroids are used more often and maintained for longer periods to prevent relapses. Immunoglobulins have only been administered in a few patients but have been associated with a transitory dramatic response.[11,19]

Surgical treatment utilizing multiple subpial transection, is reserved for patients who have not responded to multiple medical therapies. It has been followed in selected cases by a marked improvement in language skills and behavior.[16] However, there is no consensus about which patients are candidates for this treatment and its effectiveness has not been proven.[20]

Behavioral symptoms may improve with methylphenidate treatment, specifically for attention deficit and hyperactivity.[12] Speech therapy, including sign language, and a number of classroom and behavioral interventions are also helpful in managing LKS, and should be used in all patients.[21]

REFERENCES

1. Landau WM, Kleffner FR. Syndrome of acquired aphasia with convulsive disorder in children. *Neurology* 1957;7:523–530.
2. Smith MC, Hoeppner TJ. Epileptic encephalopathy of late childhood: Landau–Kleffner syndrome and the syndrome of continuous spikes and waves during slow-wave sleep. *J Clin Neurophysiol* 2003;20:462–472.
3. Hirsch E, et al. Landau–Kleffner syndrome is not an eponymic badge of ignorance. *Epilepsy Res* 2006;70:(Suppl 1):S239–S247.

4. Chung PW, et al. Nonconvulsive status epilepticus presenting as a subacute progressive aphasia. *Seizure* 2002; 11:449–454.

5. Otero E, et al. Acquired epileptic aphasia (the Landau–Kleffner syndrome) due to neurocysticercosis. *Epilepsia* 1989;30:569–572.

6. Solomon GE, et al. Intracranial EEG monitoring in Landau–Kleffner syndrome associated with left temporal lobe astrocytoma. *Epilepsia* 1993;34:557–560.

7. Hirsch E, et al. The eponym "Landau–Kleffner Syndrome" should not be restricted to childhood acquired aphasia with epilepsy. In: Beaumanoir A, Deonna T, Mira L, Tassinari CA (eds), *Continuous Spikes and Waves During Slow Sleep*. London: John Libbey and Company Ltd, 1995; pp. 57–62.

8. Tassinari CA, et al. Encephalopathy with electrical status epilepticus during slow sleep or ESES syndrome including the acquired aphasia. *Clin Neurophysiol* 2000;111:(Suppl 2):S94–S10.

9. Saint-Martin AD, et al. Semiology of typical and atypical Rolandic epilepsy: a video-EEG analysis. *Epileptic Disord* 2001;3:173–182.

10. Connolly AM, et al. Serum autoantibodies to brain in Landau–Kleffner variant, autism, and other neurologic disorders. *J Pediatr* 1999;34:607–613.

11. Mikati MA, Shamseddine AN. Management of Landau–Kleffner syndrome. *Paediatr Drugs* 2005;7(6):377–389.

12. Marescaux C, et al. Landau–Kleffner syndrome: a pharmacologic study of five cases. *Epilepsia* 1990;31:768–777.

13. Beaumanoir A. The Landau–Kleffner syndrome. In: Roger J, Bureau M, Dravet C, Dreifuss FE, Perret A, Wolf P (eds), *Epileptic Syndromes in Infancy, Childhood and Adolescence*. London: John Libbey and Company Ltd, 1992; 2nd edn.

14. Pearl PL, Carrazana EJ, Holmes GL. The Landau–Kleffner syndrome. *Epilepsy Curr* 2001;1:39–45.

15. Maquet P, et al. Regional cerebral glucose metabolism in children with deterioration of one or more cognitive functions and continuous spike-and-wave discharges during sleep. *Brain* 1995;118:1492–1520.

16. Morrell F, et al. Landau–Kleffner syndrome. Treatment with subpial intracortical transection. *Brain* 1995;118:1529–1546.

17. Paetau R. Sound triggers spikes in Landau–Kleffner syndrome. *J Clin Neurophysiology* 1994;11:231–241.

18. Takeoka M, et al. Bilateral volume reduction of the superior temporal areas in Landau–Kleffner syndrome. *Neurology* 2004;63:1289–1292.

19. Lagae LG, et al. Successful use of intravenous immunoglobulins in Landau–Kleffner syndrome. *Pediatr Neurol* 1998;18:165–168.

20. Irwin K, et al. Multiple subpial transection in Landau–Kleffner syndrome. *Dev Med Child Neurol* 2001;43:248–252.

21. Perez ER, Davidoff V. Sign language in childhood epileptic aphasia (Landau–Kleffner syndrome). *Dev Med Child Neurol* 2001;43:739–744.

CHAPTER 31

Reflex Epilepsy

Yushi Inoue

▶ INTRODUCTION

Epilepsies characterized by seizures with a specific mode of precipitation occur in 4%–7% of patients with epilepsy.[1] More general factors such as stress, sleep deprivation, and fatigue may contribute to the exacerbation of seizures in up to 62% of patients.[2] Precipitants may be divided into simple and complex: simple precipitants include elementary sensory stimuli such as flickering light, color, patterns, somatosensory, proprioceptive, or startle, whereas complex precipitation implies relatively elaborate stimuli such as music and other complex auditory materials, eating, language, thinking, praxis, and experience/emotion.

These precipitants apparently relate to specific local or regional cortical function, and some precipitants activate symptomatic and focal epileptogenesis, whereas others activate idiopathic and generalized epileptogenesis. This chapter deals with reflex epilepsy or seizures in patients with idiopathic generalized epilepsy (IGE).

▶ SIMPLE PRECIPITATION

Somatosensory or proprioceptive stimuli usually induce focal seizures in patients with epilepsies of symptomatic or probable symptomatic origin, although there are some reports in patients with idiopathic epilepsy. Tapping may induce extreme spikes in children with benign Rolandic epilepsy,[3] hot water precipitates focal seizures in familial cases,[4] and specific auditory triggers (some also with complex linguistic modality) may operate in patients with lateral temporal lobe epilepsy with the *LGI1* gene mutation.[5]

The common form of startle epilepsy occurs in patients with symptomatic etiology. However, Ricci et al[6] and subsequent authors described several infants with myoclonic jerks provoked by startle stimuli and later by noise or contact. Seizure occurred before the age of 2 years, and seizure remission was rapid. The electroencephalographic (EEG) shows brief generalized polyspikes- or spike-wave complexes with the myoclonic jerks. This idiopathic type was designated as reflex myoclonic startle epilepsy in infancy and may be included in the syndrome of benign myoclonic epilepsy in infancy.[7]

Seizure induction by other sensations such as smell usually occurs in patients with a symptomatic etiology.

VISUALLY INDUCED SEIZURES

Visual sensitivity is the most common simple precipitant in patients with idiopathic generalized epileptogenesis and includes both flicker sensitivity and pattern sensitivity.[8] A prevalence of photosensitivity, an abnormal response of the EEG to light stimulation consisting of a photoparoxysmal response (PPR), is estimated in the range of 0.3%–3%, although many studies are limited by subject-selection bias.[9] Photosensitivity is higher in the young and female population. About one-third of photosensitive patients have epileptiform EEG abnormalities on viewing stationary striped patterns, and only a minority of patients sensitive to pattern are not sensitive to flicker.

The prevalence of visually induced seizures in the general population is <1 per 10,000, and the incidence 1 per 91,000 in the overall population.[9] The Pokemon incident in Japan (1997) revealed that three of four photosensitive individuals had been unaware of their photosensitivity.

Sunlight, discotheque strobes, television viewing, movie screens, public displays, or videogames are common environmental triggers. Factors such as flicker rate, pattern, luminous intensity, color, size, location, and stimulus duration contribute to seizure precipitation.[10] Intensities of 0.2–1.5 million candlepower are in range to trigger seizures. Frequency (flash rate) in the range of 15–25 Hz is most provocative.[9] Patients with IGE are sensitive to the intermittent light stimulation containing wavelength spectra of approximately 700 nm.[11]

Pattern sensitivity is enhanced by pattern vibration. Some patients are sensitive to eye closure. Abolition of central vision and fixation may also precipitate seizures. Some patients induce attacks with maneuvers producing visual stimulation. Game play may involve not only photo- or pattern stimuli, but also specific nonvisual triggers such as thinking, possibly with decision making, and hand movement, in addition to nonspecific factors such as fatigue by prolonged play and sleep deprivation.[12]

To avoid the risk of triggering seizures, the followings practices are recommended:[13–15] limiting bright flashes at >3Hz; light–dark stationary, oscillating, or reversing patterns should not have more than five stripes, unless they are restricted to <25% of the screen or are <50 cd/m² in brightness. Transition to or from saturated red is also considered to be a risk. People with epilepsy or known photosensitivity are advised to sit >2 m from any screen, to use good ambient lighting to reduce contrast, to avoid looking at rapidly flashing lights or alternating geometric patterns. Closing one eye or looking away from the image is of more benefit than closing both eyes. The effectiveness of nonpharmacologic treatment using sunglasses in controlling PPR was also reported.[16,17]

Binnie[18] reviewed mechanisms of photosensitivity with respect to activation of generalized seizures, and concluded that the visual cortex plays a crucial role in photogenic epileptogenesis and the generalization of discharges is secondary. He suggested that cortical hyperexcitability in generalized epilepsy is not uniform and may differ in degree and extent.

Myoclonus, absences, and generalized tonic–clonic seizures (GTC) are the typical clinical manifestations, but visual symptoms and lateralizing features may occur. Taylor et al[19] noted previously unrecognized focal clinical and EEG occipital features in juvenile myoclonic epilepsy (JME) and suggested an overlap between JME and idiopathic photosensitive occipital lobe epilepsy, a syndrome defined as an idiopathic localization-related epilepsy with seizures of phosphen, blindness, or blurring of vision, often followed by head and eye deviation.[20]

▶ COMPLEX PRECIPITANTS

Complex precipitants involve higher brain function or mental processes, often associated with emotion. These complex triggers include: (1) verbal precipitation such as talking, reading, and writing; (2) nonverbal precipitation such as hearing music, game playing, decision making, drawing, solving mathematics, spatial thinking; and lastly (3) specific emotional precipitants.

Seizures induced by higher brain function may also be due to idiopathic or symptomatic etiologies, and may be focal or generalized. The latency from provocation is generally longer than for simple reflex seizures. The triggers often overlap. There may also be a contribution from nonspecific factors such as sleep deprivation.

In 1954, Bickford et al[21] reported reflex idiopathic epilepsy induced by reading. He described three cases where prolonged reading gave rise to convulsions preceded by an aura of clicking or jaw movement. There were subsequent descriptions of seizures induced by various other cognitive activities such as calculating, writing, game playing, using language, decision making, drawing, and thinking, the majority of which were generalized.

Music or related stimuli, eating and emotion/experience principally induce focal seizures with symptomatic pathology, although Woods et al[22] mentioned an exceptional case of IGE in which absence seizures were frequently induced by talking about emotional personal history. The rarity of experience/emotion induction in IGE may be a unique feature of this type of epilepsy.

LANGUAGE INDUCTION

Lee et al[23] described a case of language-induced epilepsy of cortical origin after probable left middle cerebral artery stroke. In this case, speaking-induced jaw jerking, silent-reading induced jerking of the right face, jaw and neck, reading aloud induced stuttering, and writing induced dysgraphia. In contrast to this apparently focal form of epilepsy, Geschwind and Sherwin[24] reported a case where seizures were triggered by three modalities of language, that is, reading, writing, and speaking, and the ictal EEG showed bilaterally symmetrical spike and polyspike-wave complexes. The authors assumed that the electrical focus resided in some portion of the so-called centrencephalic system. They used the term "language-induced epilepsy" and drew attention to a close link to cases designated as primary reading or writing-induced epilepsy described later.

Primary reading epilepsy (PRE) is a well-known idiopathic syndrome.[25] Mean age of seizure onset is 17–18 years. Reading induces localized, rarely bilateral perioral reflex myoclonus (PORM) and may manifest as stuttering irrespective of the content of the reading. Reading aloud is more provocative than silent reading. Talking, writing, and reading of musical scores can also precipitate seizures. Transformation of linguistic material into speech may be affected.

The EEG is normal in 80% of cases, but reading activates sharp waves or single, rarely repetitive spike-wave (SW) complexes unilaterally or bilaterally, often in the parieto-temporal region. There may be unilateral facial myoclonias with bilateral EEG discharges, and bilateral myoclonias with unilateral discharges. These findings are not typical of focal epilepsy, but show similarities to generalized epilepsy.

Mayer et al[26] examined the nature of the specific precipitant in JME by sending a questionnaire to 86 patients. They found that PORM was induced by talking and reading in half of the responders. Speaking and reading activated EEG paroxysmal discharges in 36% of cases. The PORM seen in JME was indistinguishable from that seen in PRE. The seizures in JME may also manifest as myoclonic movement or sensation of orolaryngeal muscles. Therefore, these findings suggest a close relationship between PRE and JME.

PRAXIS OR THINKING INDUCTION

Chuang et al[27] investigated cases of seizures induced by games or game-related materials, and noted two subtypes. The first was attributed to focal or diffuse pathologic changes of cortex with advancing age at seizure onset. A second subtype had both game-induced and spontaneous seizures: absence, myoclonus, or GTC. Seizure onset was during adolescence and seizures were usually responsive to antiepileptic drugs. This latter group has often been reported as epilepsy with praxis-induced or thinking-induced seizures as part of the IGE.

In praxis-induced seizures, both the seizures and discharges are precipitated by thinking about a task in a sequential fashion, making decisions, and making responses with a part of the body under stressful circumstances. The most effective precipitants often involve spatial processing and ideation or execution of praxis. Transcoding processes of thinking into voluntary or intentional acts appear to be affected. Praxis is not necessarily accompanied by actual movement, but includes ideation of motor activity.[28] Cases where precipitation does not include real movement are referred as thinking-induced epilepsy, and the relation between this kind of thought and praxis is not entirely understood.[29] The induced seizures are myoclonus, absence, and GTC.

Matsuoka et al[30] studied 480 patients with EEG during neuropsychological tasks including reading, speaking, writing, written and arithmetic calculation, and spatial construction, and found 38 patients in whom paroxysmal EEG features or seizures were triggered by various praxis activities; 36 patients had IGE. Effective triggers included writing, spatial construction, and calculation.

Guaranha et al[31] performed a similar comprehensive neuropsychological activation study in 76 JME patients and found some form of provocative effect in 38.2%. Action-programming tasks (reading aloud, speaking, writing, written calculation, drawing, and spatial construction) were more effective than thinking (reading silently and mental calculation) in provoking epileptiform discharges (23.7% vs. 11%). They also found inhibitory effects using these tasks in 90.3%, which supports the possibility of nonpharmacologic therapeutic interventions in JME.

Therefore, precipitants in praxis sensitivity include higher cortical activity involving spatiomanual pathways. The seizures induced by praxis are typical of the juvenile idiopathic generalized epilepsies, and unprovoked seizures are common.

There are, as already stated, many similarities between PRE and epilepsy with praxis-sensitive seizures. Both have juvenile onset, are idiopathic with a benign course, and show a good response to similar drugs (especially valproate). Both involve higher cortical and motor performances together, and ictal motor symptoms arise in the motor segment where the precipitating activity takes place.[25]

▶ IDIOPATHIC REFLEX EPILEPSIES

An epileptic seizure can be induced by brain activity that either reduces seizure threshold or activates seizure initiation, or both. Such brain activity may be general or specific. A more general or nonspecific brain activity is usually not regarded as a seizure precipitant, but specific activities relating to seizure induction have attracted attention. Each specific activity usually corresponds to a regional network in the brain, so that the induced seizure may be expected to be of focal or regional nature. Musicogenic epilepsy represents a typical example of a specific precipitation with induced focal seizures arising from a local epileptogenic zone: a temporal lobe seizure is induced by hearing certain music, often accompanied with emotion.

However, there are cases where a specific precipitant induces generalized seizure expression, such as visually induced seizure with generalized spike-waves in the EEG, talking-induced PORM or praxis-induced myoclonus in patients with JME.

These observations may offer clues to our understanding of the epileptogenic mechanisms of generalized epilepsy. The so-called diffuse hyperexcitability of generalized epilepsy may in fact not be uniform and may differ in both degree and extent, activating "generalized" or bilateral epileptogenic mechanisms in response to a stimulus to a localized region or network. Ferlazzo et al[32] suggested that when a hyperexcitable area receives appropriate afferent volleys and a critical mass of cortex is activated, epileptic activity is produced that ultimately involves the cortico-reticular or cortico-cortical pathways, with the final result of a generalized or bilateral epileptic event.

These observations also shed insight into the understanding of idiopathic epilepsy. The vast majority of cases with visual sensitivity, reading, language, and praxis/thinking precipitation belong to idiopathic epilepsy (Fig. 31–1). Idiopathic epilepsy may thus have

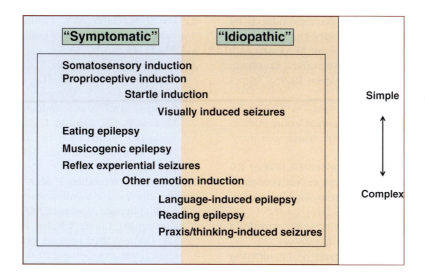

Figure 31–1. Schematic representation of the various seizure precipitants in relation to idiopathic or symptomatic etiology.

an increased hereditary regional vulnerability, at least in certain parts or networks in the brain[33] (Fig. 31–2). This regional characteristic appears to be closely connected with or accessible to generalized mechanisms or networks, as observed in the similarities between PRE or idiopathic photosensitive occipital lobe epilepsy and JME. A complex interplay of genetic and maturational factors may underlie this regionalization and generalization in idiopathic susceptibility, with age-dependent expressions.

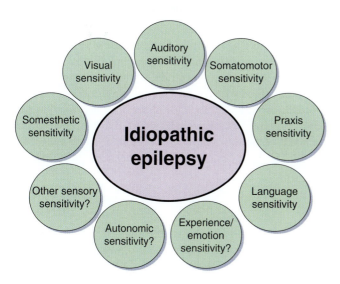

Figure 31–2. Spectrum of reflex induction observed in patients with idiopathic epilepsy.

REFERENCES

1. Panayioyopoulos CP. Epilepsies characterized by seizures with specific modes of precipitation (reflex epilepsies). In: Wallace S (ed), *Epilepsy in Children*. London: Chapman & Hill, 1996, pp. 355–375.
2. Frucht MM, Quigg M, Schwaner C, Fountain NB. Distribution of seizure precipitants among epilepsy syndromes. *Epilepsia* 2000;41:1534–1539.
3. Manganotti P, Miniussi C, Santorum E, Tinazzi M, Bonato C, Marzi CA, Fiaschi A, Dalla Bernardina B, Zanette G. Influence of somatosensory input on paroxysmal activity in benign rolandic epilepsy with 'extreme somatosensory evoked potentials'. *Brain* 1998;121:647–658.
4. Satishchandra P, Ullal GR, Shankar SK. Trigger mechanisms in hot-water epilepsy. In: Wolf P, Inoue Y, Zifkin B (eds), *Reflex Epilepsies*. Montrouge: John Libbey Eurotext, 2004, pp. 105–114.
5. Michelucci R, Pasini E, Nobile C. Lateral temporal lobe epilepsies: clinical and genetic features. *Epilepsia* 2009;50 (Suppl 5):52–54.
6. Ricci S, Cusmai R, Fusco L, Vigevano F. Reflex myoclonic epilepsy in infancy: a new age-dependent idiopathic epileptic syndrome related to startle reaction. *Epilepsia* 1995;36:342–348.
7. Dravet C, Bureau M. Benign myoclonic epilepsy in infancy. In: Roger J, Bureau M, Dravet C, Genton P, Tassinari CA, Wolf P (eds), *Epileptic Syndromes in Infancy, Childhood and Adolescence*. Montrouge: John Libbey, 2005; 4th edn: pp. 77–88.
8. Covanis A. Photosensitivity in idiopathic generalized epilepsies. *Epilepsia* 2005;46(Suppl 9):67–72.
9. Fisher RS, Harding G, Erba G, Barkley GL, Wilkins A; Epilepsy Foundation of America Working Group. Photic- and pattern-induced seizures: a review for the Epilepsy Foundation of America Working Group. *Epilepsia* 2005;46:1426–1441.

10. Zifkin BG, Inoue Y. Visual reflex seizures induced by complex stimuli. *Epilepsia* 2004;45(Suppl 1):27–29.

11. Takahashi Y, Fujiwara T, Yagi K, Seino M. Wavelength dependence of photoparoxysmal responses in photosensitive patients with epilepsy. *Epilepsia* 1999;40 (suppl 4):23–27.

12. Millett CJ, Fish DR, Thompson PJ, Johnson A. Seizures during video-game play and other common leisure pursuits in known epilepsy patients without visual sensitivity. *Epilepsia* 1999;40(Suppl 4):70–74.

13. Harding G, Wilkins AJ, Erba G, Barkley GL, Fisher RS. Photic- and pattern-induced seizures: expert consensus of the Epilepsy Foundation of America Working Group. *Epilepsia* 2005;46:1423–1425.

14. Binnie CD, et al. Video games and epileptic seizures: a consensus statement. *Seizure* 1994;3:245–246.

15. Takahashi Y, Fujiwara T. Effectiveness of broadcasting guidelines for photosensitive seizure prevention. *Neurology* 2004;62:990–993.

16. Capovilla G, et al. Suppressive efficacy by a commercially available blue lens on PPR in 610 photosensitive epilepsy patients. *Epilepsia* 2006;47:529–533.

17. Parra L, Lopes da Silva FH, Stroink H, Kalitzin S. Is colour modulation an independent factor in human visual photosensitivity? *Brain* 2007;130:1679–1689.

18. Binnie CD. Evidence of reflex epilepsy on functional systems in the brain and "generalised" epilepsy. In: Wolf P, Inoue Y, Zifkin B (eds), *Reflex Epilepsies*. Montrouge: John Libbey Eurotext, 2004, pp. 7–14.

19. Taylor I, Marini C, Johnson MR, Turner S, Berkovic SF, Scheffer IE. Juvenile myoclonic epilepsy and idiopathic photosensitive occipital lobe epilepsy: is there overlap? *Brain* 2004;127:1878–1886.

20. Guerrini R, et al. Idiopathic photosensitive occipital lobe epilepsy. *Epilepsia* 1995;36:883–891.

21. Bickford RG, Whelan JL, Klass DW, Corbin KB. Reading epilepsy: clinical and electroencephalographic studies of a new syndrome. *Trans Amer Neurol Assoc* 1956;81:100–102.

22. Woods RJ, Gruenthal M. Cognition-induced epilepsy associated with specific emotional precipitants. *Epilepsy Behav* 2006;9:360–362.

23. Lee SI, Sutherling WW, Persing JA, Butler AB. Language-induced seizure: a case of cortical origin. *Arch Neurol* 1980; 37:433–436.

24. Geschwind N, Sherwin I. Language-induced epilepsy. *Arch Neurol* 1967;16:25–31.

25. Wolf P, Inoue Y. Complex reflex epilepsies: reading epilepsy and praxis induction. In: Roger J, Bureau M, Dravet Ch, Genton P, Tassinari CA, Wolf P (eds), *Epileptic Syndromes in Infancy, Childhood and Adolescence*. Montrouge: John Libbey, 2005; 4th edn: pp. 347–358.

26. Mayer TA, Schroeder F, May TW, Wolf P. Perioral reflex myoclonias: a controlled study in patients with JME and focal epilepsies. *Epilepsia* 2006;47:1059–1067.

27. Chuang YC, Chang WN, Lin TK, Lu CH, Chen SD, Huang CR. Game-related seizures presenting with two types of clinical features. *Seizure* 2006;15:98–105.

28. Inoue Y, Seino M, Tanaka M, Kubota H, Yamakaku K, Yagi K. Epilepsy with praxis-induced seizures. In: Wolf P (ed), *Epileptic Seizures and Syndromes*. London: John Libbey, 1994, pp. 81–91.

29. Inoue Y, Zifkin B. Praxis induction and thinking induction: one or two mechanisms? A controversy. In: Wolf P, Inoue Y, Zifkin B (eds), *Reflex Epilepsies*. Paris: John Libbey Eurotext, 2004, pp. 41–55.

30. Matsuoka H, et al. Neuropsychological EEG activation in patients with epilepsy. *Brain* 2000;123:318–330.

31. Guaranha MS, da Silva Sousa P, de Araujo-Filho GM, Lin, K., Guilhoto, L.M., Caboclo, L.O., Yacubian, E.M. Provocative and inhibitory effects of a video-EEG neuropsychologic protocol in juvenile myoclonic epilepsy. *Epilepsia* 2009;50:2446–2455.

32. Ferlazzo E, Zifkin BG, Andermann E, Andermann F. Cortical triggers in generalized reflex seizures and epilepsies. *Brain* 2005;128:700–710.

33. Wolf P, Berkovic S, Genton P, Binnie C, Anderson VE, Draguhn A. Regional manifestations of idiopathic epilepsy. In: Wolf P (ed), *Epileptic Seizures and Syndromes*. London: John Libbey, 1994, pp. 265–281.

SECTION VI
Epilepsy and Neurological Disorders

CHAPTER 32

Tuberous Sclerosis Complex

Susan Koh and Michael Duchowny

► CLINICAL OVERVIEW

Tuberous sclerosis complex (TSC) is an inherited neurocutaneous disease of cell differentiation and proliferation affecting multiple organs with hamartomas or abnormal neuronal migration. It was first described by Bourneville in 1880, and the incidence of tuberous sclerosis in the population is reported to be 1/6000 to 1/10,000.[1,2] Cortical tubers and subependymal nodules (SEN) are the hallmark pathological findings in children. TSC is caused by aberrant neuronal migration and differentiation. Radial glial fibers guide migration of neurons during development from the 3rd to 5th month of gestation, and if there is a disruption in one tract, hamartomas may develop. This process of abnormal differentiation also explains the occurrence of hamartomas outside the CNS.[3]

Tubers and other migrational defects typically arise in the cerebrum rather than the cerebellum or brainstem, although subcortical involvement occurs rarely. It is unknown whether seizures originate from dysplastic neurons or neurons in surrounding cortex. Tubers form during gestation, and all brain tubers do not change in number or location during postnatal life. Pathological examination of cortical tubers reveals sclerotic white patches within the gyri and few neurons. Most neurons are large and bizarrely shaped with 2–3 nuclei located peripherally and prominent nucleoli. Fibrillary astrocytic proliferation and large glial cells are also present.[4]

Magnetic resonance imaging (MRI) scans are better in defining tubers than computerized tomography

(CT) scans. Tubers occur at the cortical gray white interface and are most frequent in the parietal and frontal lobes. Calcification is less common in tubers than in subependymal nodules (SEN). Myelination helps distinguish tubers from white matter and, tubers therefore become more evident in older children. T2 weighted imaging and fluid attenuation inversion recovery imaging (FLAIR) is more accurate for viewing tubers compared to T1 imaging.[5] In children, tubers are hypointense on T1 weighted imaging and hyperintense on T2 weighted imaging and FLAIR. FLAIR also provides better resolution of small subcortical tubers but is not useful for SEN due to CSF flow artifact caused by the inflow of noninverted CSF especially at the foramen of Monroe. White matter radial lines occur in 20–30% of patients and consist of hyperintense linear lesions perpendicular to cortex that extend to the periventricular white matter on T2 weighted imaging.[5]

SEN do not cause seizures and are located in the anterior lateral ventricles. They are hamartomas composed of round or oval cells with whorls of fibrillary glial tissue and deposition of amyloid or calcification within the nodule and usually lie around the foramen of Monroe adjacent to the ventricle.[6] SENs are less than 1 cm and rarely enhance. On MRI, SENs are better seen on T1 weighted images as the lesions are isointense to white matter and hyperintense to gray matter. SENs calcify with age and are well visualized on CT scans in adults.[5,7]

SEN may enlarge over time and may transform into a subependymal giant cell astrocytoma (SEGA).

SEGAs are benign tumors occurring in 10% of patients with TSC.[8] SEGAs typically occur at the Foramen of Monroe. They may obstruct the ventricle in older patients and lead to increased intracranial pressure. There is minimal correlation between the lesion's histology and clinical aggressiveness and it is not known why growth takes place. SEGAs are pathologically similar to SEN; however, on neuroimaging, SEGAs are larger, usually greater than 10 mm in diameter[8] and enhance with contrast. MRI is the procedure of choice for their diagnosis and follow-up as serial scans do not produce radiation exposure.

▶ GENETICS

TSC is inherited through autosomal dominance with variable penetrance. Therefore, many parents may carry the gene but do not show symptoms due to high phenotypic variability.[9] It is important to perform a Wood's lamp examination, ophthalmologic exam, renal ultrasound or even a CT or MRI scan on parents for purposes of genetic counseling; when a parent carries the gene, the risk of conceiving another affected child is 50% compared to having a child with a spontaneous mutation where subsequent risk is 1:10,000, the same as the general population. In addition, there is a high sporadic mutation rate of 60%.[10–12]

There are presently two confirmed genetic TSC loci on chromosome 9 (TSC 1 on 9p34.3) and chromosome 16 (TSC 2 on 16p13.3).[13,14] Most patients with a family history for TSC have the TSC 1 mutation[15] that produces hamartin and is associated with less severe symptoms. A smaller proportion carries the TSC 2 mutation that produces tuberin. Both genes are tumor suppressor genes and negative growth regulators.[13] The interaction between the 2 proteins, the tuberin–hamartin complex, is important in controlling cell growth.[16] Genetic blood markers are available to screen for potential TS patients although there is a high false negative rate of 15%.[17]

▶ CLINICAL MANIFESTATIONS

The clinical manifestations of TSC are varied and affect multiple organ systems. The most common symptoms consist of cutaneous findings (96%), seizures (84%), mental retardation (45%), and autism (50%).[18] In later life, renal manifestations and SEGAs produce the greatest morbidity and mortality. In terms of dermatological symptoms, ash leaf spots or hypopigmented macules are often present at birth or early infancy and best viewed with Wood's lamp. This lesion is nonspecific as it occurs in asymptomatic individuals; thus only 3 or more findings are considered significant. Shagreen patches may also appear at birth on the trunk or buttocks. They are typically flesh colored and have a raised surface similar to an orange peel. Other dermatological lesions such as ungual fibromas in the nail beds and facial angiofibromas in the malar distribution become more prevalent in adolescence.

Cardiac rhabdomyomas usually present at birth and diminish in size with age. Arrhythmias are rare. Echocardiograms can exclude this diagnosis; Ophthalmologic lesions such as retinal hamartomas or mulberry lesions rarely impair vision and remain static. Renal angiomyolipomas, cysts, and carcinomas may worsen with age; polycystic kidneys have been reported in children.[19] Angiomyolipomas may rupture with maturity and ultrasound surveillance is indicated for lesions larger than 4 cm. Renal cysts may cause hypertension and renal insufficiency.[20] Pulmonary lesions occur rarely in women with TSC and may produce spontaneous pneumothoraces.[21]

Neurological manifestations occur in 85% of patients with TSC and are the predominant cause of morbidity in children. These include behavioral issues (attention deficit, psychosis) seizures, autism, mental retardation, sleep abnormalities, hydrocephalus, or visual disturbances from SEGA-induced third ventricular obstruction. SEGAs are usually removed surgically; an ongoing trial is assessing the efficacy of rapamycin to shrink tumor growth.

Epilepsy is the most common presenting feature in TSC (while more common, skin lesions are rarely the presenting lesion) and occurs in 80–90% of patients; onset is usually before age 2 years.[22] Epilepsy in TSC is often intractable and only 14% of patients achieve spontaneous remission.[23] However, many trials were performed prior to the use of newer anticonvulsants.[24]

Seizures may occur in the neonatal period.[25] While all seizure types may occur in TSC, the most common presentation is infantile spasms (IS) that occurs in 1/3 of TSC patients. TSC accounts for 25% of all patients presenting with IS.[26] Most TSC children with IS eventually develop Lennox–Gastaut or complex partial seizures (CPS).[26,27]

A high proportion of patients with TSC present with IS in the first year of life while older children more commonly present with partial epilepsy.[28] Seizure onset after 12 months is typically associated with partial seizures as the sole type.[29] In addition, TSC patients with partial seizures typically evidence better development than TSC patients with IS. Fukshima (2001) found that 64% of partial seizures are controlled with medications.[27] Partial seizures can coexist or predate the occurrence of IS suggesting that IS may result from rapid secondary generalization. Rapid secondary bilateral synchrony mimics primary generalized seizures if there is rapid spread of seizures propagating from a frontal tuber through the anterior commissure.[30,31]

It has been suggested that high tuber counts, especially in the frontal lobes, increase the likelihood of intractable seizures and mental retardation (MR). However, this observation is controversial as normal IQs are documented in women with high tuber counts on MRI. 5–10 tubers correlated to an increased likelihood of MR although there is no minimum tuber count associated with MR or increased seizures.[32] In addition, there is no correlation between the number of tubers on FLAIR imaging and IQ.

Newer imaging studies may show more tubers than the neuroimaging techniques in past which might also negate this finding. A study by Wong & Khong[33] looked at MRI scans and found that neither tuber count nor location had any influence over MR, autism, epilepsy, IS or age of seizure onset less than 1 year. Only the presence of cortical tubers in parietal and occipital region correlated with IS. Another study by Doherty found that autism occurred more commonly in patients with occipital lobe tubers, and that an increased tuber count was associated with IS and TSC2 mutations.[34] However, seizure control and MR were not associated with tuber count.

In addition, there is a correlation with tubers and cortical dysplasias. For example, there is a series of patients who had a solitary lesion removed during surgery and pathology findings of tuberous sclerosis were found rather than cortical dysplasia. In these patients, there are no skin stigmata for TSC.[35] Another study reported changes in MR imaging with time in a child with TSC and hemimegalencephaly.[36] TSC forms a histopathological spectrum with cortical dysplasias, which makes this close association possible. One study revealed hippocampal abnormalities on MRI in a series of tuberous sclerosis patients.[37]

Mental retardation occurs in 60% of patients with TSC[38–40] and is often associated with seizures, especially ones that begin before age 2 years. Chou[41] demonstrated that MR was associated with poor seizure control, especially for generalized tonic clonic seizures. However, 1/3 of patients with seizures show normal cognition. Winterkorn et al[42] found that 57% of TSC patients had normal IQ/DQ scores and that MR was associated with intractable seizures and the presence of the TSC2 mutation.

Goh[43] reviewed 50 patients with TSC and IS and found that 64% of patients had IQs less than 70. There was an association with increased duration of IS, prolonged time from treatment initiation until the cessation of IS, and poor control of seizures after IS. Fukushima[27] documented 50 patients with TSC who presented with IS and were monitored for 10 years; Patients who developed other seizure types, especially generalized seizures, tended to have lower IQ scores. Dyspraxia, speech delay, visuospatial disturbances, dyscalculia or memory problems may also occur[43] especially in patients with high tuber counts.[44]

Aggression and psychosis occur in 13% of patients with no history of IS.[45,46] 25–50% of patients with TSC manifest autism[47] but it is unclear whether autism in TSC is the direct result of mutation in the TSC gene or a secondary effect of factors such as the associated structural brain abnormalities or epileptic encephalopathy.[48]

► **TABLE 32–1.** DEFINITE TSC: EITHER TWO MAJOR FEATURES OR ONE MAJOR FEATURE PLUS TWO MINOR FEATURES. PROBABLE TSC: ONE MAJOR PLUS ONE MINOR FEATURE. SUSPECTED TSC: EITHER ONE MAJOR FEATURE OR TWO OR MORE MINOR FEATURES

Major Features
- Multiple nontraumatic ungual or periungual fibromas
- Hypomelanotic macules (more than 3)
- Shagreen patch (connective tissue nevus)
- Cortical tuber
- Subependymal nodule or giant cell astrocytoma
- Multiple retinal nodular hamartomas
- Facial angiofibromas or forehead plaque
- Cardiac rhadomyomas, single or multiple
- Lymphangiomyomatosis
- Renal angiomyolipomas

Minor Features
- Multiple, randomly distributed pits in dental enamel
- Hamartomatous rectal polyps
- Bone cysts
- Cerebral white matter radial migration lines
- Gingival fibromas
- Nonrenal hamartomas
- Retinal achromic patch
- Confetti skin lesions
- Multiple renal cysts

Autism may result from tubers in anterior or posterior brain areas,[40] the temporal lobes or cerebellum.[49] Alternatively, autism may result from an interaction of seizures, tuber location, cognitive impairment, or linkage between the TSC and an autism susceptibility genes.[50]

► DIAGNOSTIC CRITERIA

The diagnosis of TSC is based on clinical criteria established through a consensus conference (see Table 32–1).[51] Increased weight was given to histologically confirmed lesions rather than to nonspecific findings. In addition, many of the findings, especially dermatological, may be apparent only at certain developmental stages. Patients may need to be reexamined to see if criteria are met. When both lymphagniomyomatosis and renal angiomyolipomas are present, other features of tuberous sclerosis must be present before entertaining a definitive diagnosis (Table 32–1).

► OPTIMAL TREATMENT REGIMEN

There is no one treatment that is specific for all patients with tuberous sclerosis, and treatment is purely symptomatic. Epilepsy is treated medically according to seizure type However, TSC patients are more prone to intractable epilepsy. The demonstration of multiple drug resistance protein-1 in cortical tubers which suggests a possible cellular mechanism for pharmacoresistance in TSC.[52]

Vigabatrin is often the first-line drug for treating IS in TSC patients as ACTH is associated with a higher relapse rate[53] and the need for extended administration. Approximately 95% of TSC patients with infantile spasms become seizure-free with vigabatrin.[26,54] Jambaque[55] found that most patients given vigabatrin remained spasm-free or had rare partial seizures. With successful treatment, DQ scores were higher after vigabatrin-induced cessation of IS and autistic behavior improved. Vigabatrin is usually effective after fewer than 10 days of treatment at a dose of 100 mg/kg per day.[26] Another study comparing low and high dose vigabatrin found that response time was shorter with high dose compared to low dose vigabatrin in TSC patients.[56]

Retinal toxicity and visual field deficits are reported with vigabatrin; one study found that 50% of patients develop partial blindness that is progressive and irreversible.[26] However, blindness is associated with prolonged administration that is rarely necessary in IS. Frequent eye examinations and electroretinograms have been advocated but are difficult to assess in small children. There is no consensus as to how often to perform the examination or what type of screening should be used.[57] It has been suggested that vigabatrin be withdrawn after a spasm-free interval greater than one year.[58]

Epilepsy surgery is a potential option for TSC children with intractable partial epilepsy who fail more than 2 anticonvulsants. The seizure focus is localized to one epileptogenic tuber utilizing MRI, video telemetry, and functional neuroimaging (PET, SPECT). Multiple studies document that localizing and removing the epileptogenic tubers results in seizure freedom.[58–64] TSC patients who are not surgical candidates may benefit from the ketogenic diet[65] and vagal nerve stimulation.[66,67] However both treatment modalities are less effective than resective surgery.[65]

Additional evaluations required in TSC patients include an echocardiogram for rhabomyomas, renal ultrasound to rule out renal cysts or angiomyolipomas, ophthalmologic examination to rule out retinal hamartomas, and genetic screening of the parents. MRI and renal ultrasound should be repeated every 1–3 years to screen for a growing angiomyolipoma or SEGA.

▶ MANAGEMENT ALGORITHM (FIG. 32–1)

In patients with a new onset seizure suspected of TSC, history and physical examination are paramount to diagnosis. The skin exam is particularly important. Ash leaf spots, shagreen patches and sebaceous adenoma are characteristic features of TSC. A family history of neurological disorder may suggest a genetic predisposition. MRI of the brain is indicated to look for cortical tubers or SEN. An electroencephalogram (EEG) can help determine whether seizures are partial or IS and assist in the choice of anticonvulsants. Further testing including ophthalmological examination, echocardiogram and renal ultrasound finding are needed to search for systemic findings that support the diagnosis of TSC. Genetic screening of families is also indicated. Finally, Wood's lamp examination, MRI/CT or renal ultrasound of the parents aids genetic counseling.

Once the diagnosis of TSC is established in a child with new onset seizures, the choice of anticonvulsant therapy is based on the EEG and seizure type. Vigabatrin is suggested as first line drug treatment of IS due to its demonstrated efficacy in TSC patients. ACTH may be substituted if the patient fails vigabatrin. Topiramate, zonisamide, pyridoxine, and benzodiazepines are further options. Valproic acid is rarely used due to potential liver toxicity in children less than 2 years old. Carbamazepine, oxcarbazepine, lamotrigine are options for CPS in children; neonates may respond to phenobarbital. If these medications fail, zonisamide, topiramate, levetiracetam, can be used. There has been a case report concerning the possible use of rapamycin for seizure control.[68] Epilepsy surgical work-up is warranted for patients who have failed several medications.

The epilepsy surgery evaluation of patients with TSC is similar to the evaluation of patients with refractory partial seizures. MR imaging, video EEG and functional neuroimaging such as PET or SPECT assist in seizure localization. Nonconcordant MRI, EEG, and PET/SPECT findings may lower seizure freedom rates.[63] The epileptogenic tuber is often the largest and most calcified, and frequently located in the frontocentral region. Due to lack of calcification in infants less than 18 months, CT is preferable in neonates. However, the MRI evaluation can be normal in 5% of older TSC patients. MRI is often useful in older children lacking CT abnormalities and is diagnostically superior for cortical tubers. CT is also useful as a screening tool in adults as calcification is common.

Many TSC patients, show multifocal interictal spiking and require 3–4 typical seizures to demonstrate a consistent epileptogenic focus Jansen et al[69] found that 90% of TSC patients showed at least one region of consistent interictal epileptiform activity but these patients tended to be older, had partial epilepsy and were not retarded.

Functional neuroimaging may pinpoint the epileptogenic tuber. Tamaki et al[70] studied 19 patients with interictal SPECT and found that 2/3 had an area of hypoperfusion that corresponded with an MRI lesion. Interictal SPECT is less sensitive than ictal SPECT. Koh et al[71] reviewed the ictal SPECT scans of 13 patients with TSC. In 9 patients with localized EEG findings,

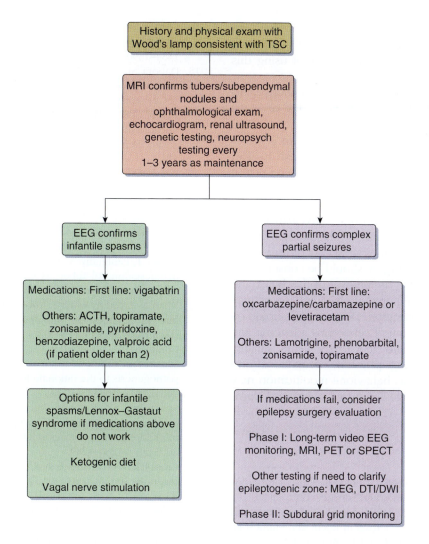

Figure 32–1. Presentation of patient with new onset seizures and possible TSC.

4 had hyperperfused regions on SPECT, which were associated with fast rhythmical alpha patterns and rhythmical epileptiform discharges

PET scan results correlate well with EEG findings.[72,73] AMT-PET may be more sensitive than a FDG-PET for TSC and has a greater correlation with the area of epileptogenesis[74] and frequent interictal abnormalities[75] Both PET and SPECT reveal epileptogenic regions surrounding tubers. Subtraction ictal SPECT coregistered to MRI (SISCOM) may bring out subtle abnormalities than just ictal SPECT alone[76] but has not been tested in TSC patients. PET–MRI fusion may also demonstrate subtle regions of surrounding cortical dysplasia.[77]

Magnetoencephalogram (MEG) provides another noninvasive technique to identify the epileptogenic tuber. In a recent study by Wu et al,[78] MEG was judged to be helpful in the presurgical planning for TSC patients. A study of EEG and MEG in 19 patients

with TSC and epilepsy revealed that MEG sources were closer to epileptogenic tubers than EEG sources.[79]

Diffusion weighted imaging (DWI) and diffusion tensor imaging (DTI) studies reveal that the epileptogenic tuber in TSC exhibits low anistrophic diffusion (FA) and a high ADC ratio (diffusivity ratio). Karadag et al[80] found 7 children with TSC where the ADC was higher in cortical tubers than in controls and lower FA ratio. Another study of 4 patients who underwent DWI[81] calculated diffusion coefficient maps for the epileptogenic and nonepileptogenic tuber. A higher diffusion coefficient for the epileptogenic tuber distinguished this tuber from others.

Subdural grids may ultimately need to be placed to confirm the epileptogenic tuber.[59] Multistage procedures involving grid placement in both cerebral hemispheres have also been performed. In a multistaged procedure, the epileptogenic zone is first removed;

grids then record a second seizure focus that can be excised at a later time. Two studies have shown effectiveness and improved seizure control using this method.[60,61]

Patients who are not candidates for epilepsy surgery may be eligible for the ketogenic diet or vagal nerve stimulation. Kossoff found that 92% of 12 TSC patients had a greater than 50% reduction in seizures with dietary therapy[65] Parain et al[66] studied 10 TSC patients with VNS; 9 achieved at least a 50% reduction in seizures.

TSC patients who do not have seizures or have controlled seizures require periodic surveillance with brain MRI, renal ultrasound, and ophthalmologic examinations every 1–3 years to rule out SEGAs or renal cysts and hamartomas. Neurosurgery should be consulted for clinically significant SEGA as removal of the SEGA and VP shunting may be required. Behavioral issues may require psychiatric intervention. Dermatology should be consulted for laser therapy of sebaceous adenoma and ungual fibromas, especially in teenage years. Finally, neuropsychological testing, physical, occupational and speech therapy as well as behavioral modification may be required at an early age if signs of autism and learning disability appear.

REFERENCES

1. Osborne JP, Fyer A, Webb D. Epidemiology of tuberous sclerosis. *Ann NY Acad Sci* 1991;615:125–127.
2. Wiederholt WC, Gomez MR, Kurland LT. Incidence and prevalence of tuberous sclerosis in Rochester, Minnesota, 1950 through 1982. *Neurology* 1985;35:600–603.
3. Christophe C, et al. MRI spectrum of cortical malformation in tuberous sclerosis complex. *Brain Dev* 2000;22:487–493.
4. Mizuguchi M, Takashima S. Neuropathology of tuberous sclerosis. *Brain Dev* 2001;23(7):508–515.
5. Inoue Y, et al. CT and MR imaging of cerebral tuberous sclerosis. *Brain Dev* 1998;20:209–221.
6. Di Mario FJ. Brain abnormalities in tuberous sclerosis complex. *J Child Neurol* 2004;19:650–657.
7. Baron Y, Barkovich AJ. MR imaging of tuberous sclerosis in neonates and young infants. *AJNR Am J Neuroradiol* 1999;20:907–916.
8. Goh S, Butler W, Thiele EA. Subependymal giant cell tumors in tuberous sclerosis complex. *Neurology* 2004; 63:1457–1461.
9. McClintock WM. Neurological manifestations of tuberous sclerosis complex. *Curr Neurol Neursoci Rep* 2002;2(2): 158–163.
10. Cassidy SB. Tuberous sclerosis in children: diagnosis and course. *Comp Ther* 1984;10:43–51.
11. Fleury P, et al. Tuberous sclerosis: the incidence of sporadic cases versus familial cases. *Brain Dev* 1980;2:107–117.
12. Sampson JR, et al. Genetic aspects of tuberous sclerosis in the west of Scotland. *J Med Genet* 1989;26:28–31.
13. Narayanan V. Tuberous sclerosis complex: genetics to pathogenesis. *Pediatr Neurol* 2003;29(5):404–409.
14. Crino PB, Henske EP. New developments in the neurobiology of the tuberous sclerosis complex. *Neurology* 1999;53(7): 1384–1390.
15. Dabora SL, et al. Mutational analysis in a cohort of 224 tuberous sclerosis patients indicates increased severity of TSC2 compared with TSC1, disease in multiple organs. *Am J Hum Gent* 2001;68:64–80.
16. Cheadle JP, Reeve MP, Sampson JR. Molecular genetic advances in tuberous sclerosis. *Hum Genet* 2000;107:97–114.
17. Roach ES, Sparagana SP. Diagnosis of tuberous sclerosis complex. *J Child Neurol* 2004;19(9):643–649.
18. Gomez MR (ed). Neurologic and psychiatric features. In: *Tuberous Sclerosis*. New York: Raven Press, 1979; pp. 21–36.
19. Ewalt DH, et al. Renal lesion growth in children with tuberous sclerosis *J Urol* 1998;160:141–145.
20. Rosser T, Panigrahy A, McClintock W. The diverse clinical manifestations of tuberous sclerosis complex: a review. *Semin Pedtr Neurol* 2006;13:27–36.
21. Khan N, Javed A, Wazir S, Yousaf M. Tuberous sclerosis—rare presentation as pneumothorax. *J Ayub Med Coll Abottabad* 2003;15(4):60–62.
22. Curatolo P, Bombardieri R, Verdecchia M, Seri S. Intractable seizures in tuberous sclerosis complex: from molecular pathogenesis to the rationale for treatment. *J Child Neurol* 2005;20(4):318–325.
23. Sparagana SP, Delgado MR, Batchelor LL, Roach ES. Seizure remission and antiepileptic drug discontinuation in children with tuberous sclerosis complex. *Arch Neurol* 2003;60(9):1286–1289.
24. Cross JH. Neurocutaneous syndrome and epilepsy—issues in diagnosis and management. *Epilepsia* 2005;46(Supp 10):17–23.
25. Miller SP, et al. Tuberous sclerosis complex and neonatal seizures. *J Child Neurol* 1998;13:619–623.
26. Curatolo P, Verdecchia M, Bombardieri R. Vigabatrin for tuberous sclerosis complex. *Brain Dev* 2001;23:649–653.
27. Fukushima K, Inoue Y, Fujiwara T, Yagi K. Long-term follow-up study of West syndrome associated with tuberous sclerosis. *Brain Dev* 2001;23:698–704.
28. Curatolo P. Epilepsy in tuberous sclerosis. In: Otahara S, Roger J (eds), *New Trends in Pediatric Epileptology*. Osaka, Japan: Danippon Phamaceutical, 1991; pp. 86–93.
29. Roger J, et al. L'epilepsie dans la sclerose tubereuse de Bournville. *Boll Lega Ital Epil* 1984;43:33–38.
30. Cusmai R, et al. Topographic comparative study of magnetic resonance imaging and electroencephalography in 34 children with tuberous sclerosis. *Epilepsia* 1990;31:747–775.
31. Gibbs EL, Gillen HW, Gibbs FA. Disappearance and migration of epileptic foci in childhood. *AMA Am J Dis Child* 1954;88:596–603.
32. Shepherd CW, Houser OW, Gomez MR. MR findings in tuberous sclerosis complex and correlation with seizure development and mental impairment. *AJNR Am J Neuroradiol* 1995;16(1):149–155.
33. Wong V, Khong PL. Tuberous sclerosis complex: correlation of magnetic resonance imaging (MRI) findings with comorbidities. *J Child Neurol* 2006;21(2):99–105.
34. Doherty C, Goh S, Young Poussaint T, Erdag N, Thiele EA. Prognostic significance of tuber count and

location in tuberous sclerosis complex. *J Child Neurol* 2005;20(10):837–841.

35. Hirfanoglu T, Gupta A. Tuberous sclerosis complex with a single brain lesion on MRI mimicking focal cortical dysplasia. *Pediatr Neurol* 2010;42(5):343–347.

36. Balaji R, Kesavadas C, Ramachandran K, Nayak SD, Priyakumari T. Longitudinal CT and MR appearances of hemimegalencepahly in a patient with tuberous sclerosis. *Childs Nerv Syst* 2008;24(3):397–401.

37. Gama HP, da Rocha AJ, Valerio RM, da Silva CJ, Garcia LA. Hippocampal abnormalities in an MR imaging series of patients with tuberous sclerosis. *AJNR Am J Neuroradiol* 2010;31(6):1059–1062.

38. Gomez MR (ed). Criteria for diagnosis. In: *Tuberous Sclerosis.* New York: Raven Press, 1979; pp. 9–20.

39. Webb DW, Fryer AE, Osborne JP. On the incidence of fits and mental retardation in tuberous sclerosis. *J Med Genet* 1991;28:395–397.

40. Jambaque I, et al. Neuropsychological aspects of tuberous sclerosis in relation to epilepsy and MRI findings. *Dev Med Child Neurol* 1991;33:698–705.

41. Chou PC, Chang YJ. Prognostic factors for mental retardation in patients with tuberous sclerosis complex. *Acta Neurol Taiwan* 2004;13(1):10–13.

42. Winterkorn EB, Pulsifer MB, Thiele EA. Cognitive prognosis of patients with tuberous sclerosis complex. *Neurology* 2007;68(1):62–64.

43. Goh S, Kwiatkowki DJ, Dorer DJ, Thiele EA. Infantile spasms and intellectual outcomes in children with tuberous sclerosis complex. *Neurology* 2005;65(2):235–238.

44. Kotagal P, Lachwani DK. Epilepsy in the setting of neurocutaneous syndromes. In: Wyllie E (ed), *The Treatment of Epilepsy, Principles and Practice.* Philadelphia: Lippincott William and Wilkins, 4th edn: pp. 537–545.

45. O Callaghan FJ, et al. The relation of spasms, tubers and intelligence in tuberous sclerosis complex. *Arch Dis Child* 2004;89:530–533.

46. Hunt A, Dennis J. Psychiatric disorder among children with tuberous sclerosis. *Dev Med Child Neurol* 1987;29:190–198.

47. Hunt A. Development, behavior, and seizures in 300 cases of tuberous sclerosis. *J Intellect Disabil Res* 1993;38(Pt 1): 41–51.

48. Wiznitzer M. Autism and tuberous sclerosis. *J Child Neurol* 2004;19(9):675–679.

49. Smalley SL. Autism and tuberous sclerosis. *J Autism Dev Disord* 1998;28:407–414.

50. Zaroff CM, Devinsky O, Miles D, Barr WB. Cognitive and behavioral correlates of tuberous sclerosis complex. *J Child Neurol* 2004;19(11):847–852.

51. Roach ES, Gomez MR, Northrup H. Tuberous sclerosis complex consensus conference: revised clinical diagnostic criteria. *J Child Neurol* 1998;13:624–628.

52. Lazarowski A, Lubienicki F, Camarero S, Pomata H, Bartuluchi M, Sevierver G, Taratuto AL. Multidrug resistance proteins in tuberous sclerosis and refractory epilepsy. *Pediatr Neurol* 2004;30:102–106.

53. Riikonen R, Simell O. Tuberous sclerosis and infantile spasms. *Dev Med Child Neurol* 1990;32:203–209.

54. Aicardi J, et al. Vigabatrin as initial therapy for infantile spasms: a European retrospective study. *Epilepsia* 1996;37: 638–642.

55. Jambaque I, Chiron C, Dumas C, Mumford J, Dulac O. Mental and behavioural outcome of infantile epilepsy treated by vigabatrin in tuberous sclerosis patients. *Epilepsy Res* 2000;38(2–3):151–160.

56. Elterman RD, Shields WD, Mansfield KA, Nakagawa J. US Infantile Spasms Vigabatrin Study Group. Randomized trial of vigabatrin in patients with infantile spasms. *Neurology* 2001;57(8):1416–1421.

57. Mackay MT, Weiss SK, Adams-Webber T, Ashwal S, Stephens D, Ballaban-Gill K, Baram TZ, Duchowny M, Hirtz D, Pellock JM, Shields WD, Shinnar S, Wyllie E, Snead OC 3rd. American Academy of Neurology, Child Neurology Society. Practice parameter: medical treatment of infantile spasms: report of the American Academy of Neurology and the Child Neurology Society. *Neurology* 2004;62(10):1668–1681.

58. Kankirawatana P, Raksadawan N, Balankura K. Vigabatrin therapy in infantile spasms. *J Med Assoc Thai* 2002;85(Suppl 2):S7788–S7783.

59. Koh S, Jayakar P, Dunoyer C, Whiting SE, Resnick TJ, Alvarez LA, Morrison G, Ragheb J, Prats A, Dean P, Gilman J, Duchowny MS. Epilepsy surgery in children with tuberous sclerosis complex: presurgical evaluation and outcome. *Epilepsia* 2000;41(9):1206–1213.

60. Romanelli P, et al. Epilepsy surgery in tuberous sclerosis: multistage procedures with bilateral or multilobar foci. *J Child Neurol* 2002;17:689–692.

61. Romanelli P, Weiner HL, Majjar S, Devinsky O. Bilateral resective epilepsy surgery in a child with tuberous sclerosis: case report. *Neurosurgery* 2001;49(3):732–734.

62. Kagawa K, Chugani DC, Asano E, Juhasz C, Muzik O, Shah A, Shah J, Sood S, Kupsky WJ, Mangner TJ, Chakraborty PK, Chugani HT. Epilepsy surgery outcome in children with tuberous sclerosis complex evaluated with alpha-[11C]methyl-L-trptophan positron emission tomography (PET). *J Child Neurol* 2005;20(5):429–438.

63. Lachhwani DK, Pestana E, Gupta A, Kotagal P, Bingaman W, Wyllie E. Identification of candidates for epilepsy surgery in patients with tuberous sclerosis. *Neurology* 2005; 64(9):1651–1654.

64. Jarrar RG, Buchhalter JR, Raffel C. Long-term outcome of epilepsy surgery in patients with tuberous sclerosis. *Neurology* 2004;62(3):479–481.

65. Kossoff EH, Thiele EA, Pfeifer HH, McGrogan JR, Freeman JM. Tuberous sclerosis complex and the ketogenic diet. *Epilepsia* 2005;46(10):1684–1686.

66. Parain D, Penniello MJ, Berquen P, Delangre T, Billard C, Murphy JV. Vagal nerve stimulation in tuberous sclerosis complex patients. *Pediatr Neurol* 2001;25(3):213–216.

67. Major P, Thiele EA. Vagal nerve stimulation for intractable epilepsy in tuberous sclerosis complex. *Epilepsy Behav* 2008;13(2):357–360.

68. Muncy J, Butler IJ, Koenig MK. Rapamycin reduces seizure frequency in tuberous sclerosis complex. *J Child Neurol* 2009;24(4):477.

69. Janson FE, van Huffelen AC, Bourez-Swart M, van Nieuwenhuizen O. Consistent localization of interictal epileptiform activity on EEGs of patients with tuberous sclerosis complex. *Epilepsia* 2005;46(3):415–419.

70. Tamaki K, Okuno T, Iwasaki Y, Yonekura Y, Konishi J, Mikawa H. Regional cerebral blood flow in relation to

MRI and EEG findings in tuberous sclerosis. *Brain Dev* 1991;13(6):420–424.

71. Koh S, Jayakar P, Resnick T, Alvarez LA, Litt RE, Duchowny M. The localizing value of SPECT in children with tuberous sclerosis complex and refractory partial seizures. *Epileptic Disord* 1999;1(1):41–46.

72. Rintahaka PJ, Chugani HT. Clinical role of positron emission tomography in children with tuberous sclerosis complex. *J Child Neurol* 1997;12(1):42–52.

73. Chugani DC, Chugani HT, Muzik O, Shah JR, Shah AK, Canady A. Mangner TJ, Chakraborty PK. Imaging epileptogenic tubers in children with tuberous sclerosis complex using alpha-[11C]methyl-L-tryptophan positron emission tomography. *Ann Neurol* 1998;44(6):858–866.

74. Asano E, Chugani DC, Muzik O, Shen C, Juhasz C, Janisse J, Ager J, Canady A, Shah JR, Shah AK, Watson C, Chugani HT. Multimodality imaging for improved detection of epileptogenic foci in tuberous sclerosis complex. *Neurology* 2000;54(10):1976–1984.

75. Fedi M, Reutens DC, Andermann F, Okazawa H, Boling W, White C, Dubeau F, Nakai A, Gross DW, Andermann E, Diksic M. Alpha-[11C]-Methyl-L-tryptophan PET identifies the epileptogenic tuber and correlates with interictal spike frequency. *Epilepsy Res* 2003;52(3):203–213.

76. O'Brien TJ, So EL, Cascino GD, Hauser MF, Marsh WR, Meyer FB, Sharbrough FW, Mullan BP. Subtraction SPECT coregistered to MRI in focal malformations of cortical development: localization of the epileptogenic zone in epilepsy surgery candidates. *Epilepsia* 2004;45(4):367–376.

77. Chandra PS, Salamon N, Huang J, Wu JY, Koh S, Vinters HV, Mathern GW. FDG-PET/MRI coregistration and diffusion tensor imaging distinguish epileptogenic tubers and cortex in patients with tuberous sclerosis complex: a preliminary report. *Epilepsia* 2006;47(9):1543–1549.

78. Wu JY, Sutherling WW, Koh S, Salamon N, Jonas R, Yudovin S, Sankar R, Shields WD, Mathern GW. Magnetic source imaging localizes epileptogenic zone in children with tuberous sclerosis complex. *Neurology* 2006;66(8):1270–1272.

79. Jansen FE, Huiskamp G, van Huffelen AC, Bourez-Swart M, Boere E, Gebvbink T, Vincken KL, van Nieurwenhuizen O. Identification of the epileptogenic tuber in patients with tuberous sclerosis: a comparison of high resolution EEG and MEG. *Epilepsia* 2006;47(1):108–114.

80. Karadag D, Mentzel HJ, Gullmar D, Rating T, Lobel U, Brandl U, Reichenbach JR, Kaiser WA. Diffusion tensor imaging in children and adolescents with tuberous sclerosis. *Pediatr Radiol* 2005;35(10):980–983.

81. Jansen FE, Braun KP, van Nieurwenhuizen O, Huiskamp G, Vincken KL, van Huffelen AC, van der Grond J. Diffusion weighted magnetic resonance imaging and identification of the epileptogenic tuber in patients with tuberous sclerosis. *Arch Neurol* 2003;60(11):1580–1584.

CHAPTER 33

Sturge–Weber Syndrome

Alexis Arzimanoglou and Eric Kossoff

► CLINICAL PRESENTATION

Sturge–Weber syndrome (SWS) is a nonfamilial neurocutaneous disorder with a potentially progressive course. The syndrome consists of a nevus flammeus (port-wine stain) involving part of the face, in most of the patients all or part of the area supplied by the trigeminal nerve (V_1 distribution most commonly). In all patients a venous angioma of the leptomeninges and less often, a choroidal angioma, and ipsilateral glaucoma is present. The facial and leptomeningeal angioma are usually ipsilateral, but both can be bilateral. Pial angiomatosis more frequently occurs in the occipital region, but it can be localized anywhere and can involve an entire hemisphere or even be bilateral. The extent of lesions that affect the facial skin, eyes, and central nervous system vary between patients, and in some cases only a single-organ system may be affected.[1] Cases of SWS exist without the facial port-wine stain.

Associated common neurological symptoms include seizures, hemiparesis or hemiplegia, visual field deficits, headaches, stroke-like events (SLEs), and learning disabilities. The degree of disability associated with SWS varies significantly between patients and some may remain seizure free with no neurological deficits while others may present with severe intractable epilepsy, profound neurological deficits, and developmental delay.[2] Migraines can also be very problematic in these children as well.[3]

Seizures are usually the presenting neurologic symptom. Roughly 70% of patients with epilepsy have their first seizure within the first year of life. In about 20%, the onset of seizures is between the ages of 1 and 3 years but may vary from birth to 23 years of age.[4,5] Early seizures are triggered by fever in about one-third of patients, and are often long lasting, usually consisting of unilateral status epilepticus. Seizures are focal in most of the cases with frequent secondary generalization.[6–8] Status epilepticus, occurring as prolonged clonic seizures, is reported in 50% of cases, and less commonly, infantile spasms, and myoclonic seizures.[6,9] Bilateral leptomeningeal involvement is correlated with an earlier seizure onset and a poorer developmental prognosis.[10]

In one series of 77 patients with SWS, 39% evidenced a clustering pattern of severe seizures separated by prolonged periods (months to years) of seizure freedom.[11] The clusters can be problematic and require benzodiazepines or hospitalization to treat status epilepticus. The prolonged recovery period is similarly problematic in regards to making decisions about when to proceed with epilepsy surgery.[11]

Hemiplegias of SWS often appear after an episode of serial seizures or unilateral status epilepticus that generally occurs during the first year of life.[6] Therefore, they are acquired hemiplegias that closely resemble those observed in the hemiconvulsion–hemiplegia–epilepsy (HHE) syndrome. Temporary hemiplegia or hemiparesis that is not preceded by epileptic seizures is also observed. Some have referred to these manifestations as "SLEs" or "stroke-like events." Their timing with respect to seizures can be difficult, and therefore may represent a subtle postictal phenomenon. However, they are often treated with aspirin to theoretically reduce frequency.[12] One recent retrospective study found that the median number of seizures was also reduced from 3 to 1 episode per month ($p = 0.002$) with aspirin use.[13]

Approximately 60% of SWS patients present with psychomotor retardation of variable degree, and profound mental retardation is present in 32.5%.[4,14,15] Early onset of seizures and severity of the epilepsy represent the most important contributing factors. Anticonvulsant medications may also play a role, especially with multidrug regimens that are typical in children with SWS.

Ocular manifestations include glaucoma in 28%–70% of cases.[16–18] Glaucoma may be present at birth but can develop at any age, even in adults. Glaucoma is bilateral in almost half of bilateral facial angioma patients. Contralateral glaucoma is relatively rare in patients with SWS. This appears anecdotally to be more common when the port-wine stain involves the upper eyelid.

► DIAGNOSTIC WORKUP

The presence of a port-wine stain at birth may lead to a suspicion of SWS, although in most cases neurological deficits are absent (Fig. 33–1).

Neuroimaging is the investigation of choice when SWS is suspected. Head computerized tomography (CT) scan will often demonstrate the double contour

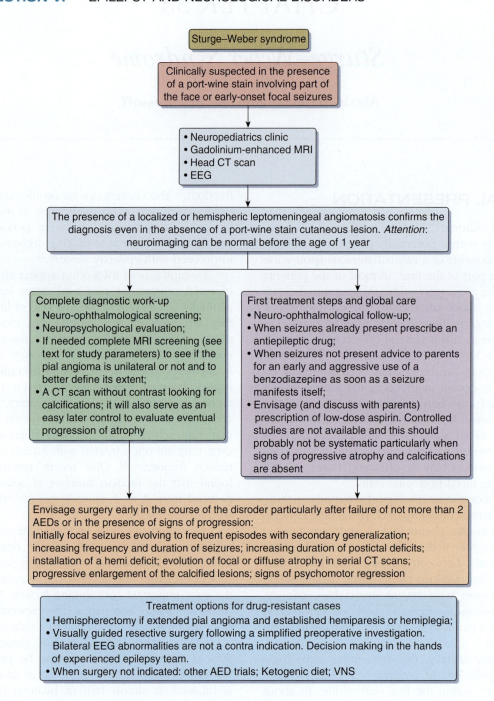

Figure 33–1. Diagnostic and treatment algorithm.

"train-track," intracranial calcifications. It can also demonstrate localized or hemispheric atrophy. In the neonatal period, CT scan can also detect an increase in the cerebral density of the affected hemisphere. Gadolinium-enhanced magnetic resonance imaging (MRI) is the best modality for demonstrating the presence of a leptomeningeal angiomatosis. Both CT and MRI may initially be normal and subsequently reveal abnormalities after 1 year of age. Therefore, there may be some value to waiting on neuroimaging in an asymptomatic infant with a port-wine stain.

Determining whether the pial angioma is strictly unilateral and its extent is crucial when discussing epilepsy surgery indications. In most Gadolinium-enhanced studies, MRI demonstrates the angioma, but should be performed at least 3 weeks after an episode of status epilepticus to avoid intracortical leakage due to blood–brain barrier alterations which do not correlate well with the extent of the angioma.[19] Both short echo and long repetition time and/or echo-time studies should be performed. In addition, gradient-echo sequences are helpful for demonstrating the presence of micro-calcifications.[20] One report suggests that postcontrast FLAIR imaging and time-of-flight MR venography may be more sensitive for detecting the leptomeningeal angioma,[21,22] and magnetic resonance spectroscopy and susceptibility-weighted imaging may detect abnormalities not be seen on standard MRI with contrast.[23,24] In addition, most children with SWS have an enlarged ipsilateral choroid plexus, which may assist in diagnosis.

Video-electroencephalography (V/EEG) is often obtained after the child with SWS develops seizures but is generally of limited diagnostic value. The interictal EEG shows nonspecific focal or unilateral depression of the background activity over the area of the leptomeningeal angiomatosis. Polymorphic delta slowing is the next most common EEG abnormality, and, when unilateral, correctly lateralizes the angiomatosis.[6,25] Focal epileptiform abnormalities are uncommon in infants, even in those with frequent seizures. Bilateral epileptiform abnormalities occur early in cases with bilateral lesions, but usually do not appear until after 3 years of age in cases with unilateral lesions.[26,27] Quantitative EEG has emerged as a method of determining asymmetry in children with SWS, but remains investigational.[28]

The diagnosis of SWS is clinically evident in a child presenting with seizures. However, in some cases, the pial angiomatosis occurs without a facial angioma, and, in others, the pial angioma may be bilateral, while the facial nevus is unilateral.[2,29]

Neuropsychological evaluation is indicated early in the course of the disorder. It serves as a reference for future decisions, particularly in cases with potentially surgically treatable epilepsy. Neuro-ophthalmological screening should complete the diagnostic workup. Children with SWS should be regularly followed in a pediatric neurology department with extensive experience in epilepsy care and epilepsy surgery.

▶ TREATMENT

Global care of SWS patients is symptomatic and accordingly should focus on treatment of seizures, glaucoma and the facial angioma, and utilize physical and occupational therapy as well as school support (Fig. 33–1). For this reason, children often benefit from a multidisciplinary team that can address all of these comorbidities. Glaucoma can be problematic and may require trabeculectomy, even at a young age.[30] Behavioral problems occur frequently in children with SWS, with one series reporting 31% with mood disorder, 25% with disruptive behavior, and 25% with adjustment disorder.[31] In this same series, a left frontal and parietal leptomeningeal angioma was associated with higher risk of disruptive behavior.[31] Children with psychiatric features of SWS should be treated with appropriate medication and adapted therapies.

Low-dose aspirin is reported to reduce stroke-like episodes by improving blood flow and preventing potential thrombus formation;[12] however, it is controversial whether this is appropriate for young children[13,32] and controlled studies are not available. Many centers will start children on a low dose of aspirin, typically 3 mg/kg per day.[13] Reye syndrome in children with SWS has not been reported to our knowledge, but there can be a slightly increased risk of bruising and bleeding.[13]

The risk of prolonged seizures or episodes of status epilepticus being the first neurological manifestation is highest in the first 2–3 years of life. A small case-controlled prospective study[33] suggested that presymptomatic treatment with phenobarbital might be helpful. However, a larger randomized prospective trial would be necessary before such an approach can be generally recommended. Furthermore, in most children with SWS decisions regarding which anticonvulsant to start, at what dose, and for what duration remain arbitrary. The initial management should be similar to current practices for other children at risk for prolonged seizures disorders: advice to parents for an early and aggressive use of a benzodiazepine as soon as a seizure manifests itself. Although topiramate has an inherent risk of glaucoma, it does not seem to be problematic in children with SWS already at risk, and may even be helpful for the migraines reported by many children.

Epilepsy is reported to be benign in as many as a quarter of patients in one study[34] and could be controlled with antiepileptic drugs in 40%–50% of patients in others.[4,6] All available antiepileptic drugs (AEDs) for the control of focal and/or generalized seizures are indicated but controlled studies are not available.

Patients with SWS and epilepsy should be considered as potential candidates to a surgical treatment early in the course of the disorder, especially if seizures continue and progression is suspected. Progression of the disease process should be suspected when initially focal seizures evolve to frequent episodes with secondary generalization or when the frequency of episodes with a postictal deficit increases. Sometimes this can be due to exacerbation of partial seizures by anticonvulsants such as oxcarbazepine or carbamazepine, as has been reported.[35] Other signs suggesting progression may include increasing duration of postictal hemideficits over time, evolution of focal or diffuse atrophy in serial head CT scans, and progressive enlargement of the calcified lesions.[6,25] General principles of pediatric epilepsy surgery in lesional cases fully apply to SWS children, also considering that the timing of surgery is important if cognitive deterioration is to be avoided. Timing of surgery can be quite difficult, recognizing the clustering, intermittent pattern in a significant number of children with SWS.[11,36]

Hemispherectomy (functional or anatomical) is the approach of choice in children with an extended hemispheric pial angiomatosis and an established hemiparesis or hemiplegia. The decision is often more difficult for those children with a diffuse unilateral angiomatosis and episodes of prolonged postictal and only transitory hemiparesis. In these cases, and in the absence of objective selection criteria, timing of surgery remains controversial as it is the physicians' experience that will allow the best possible evaluation of the risk that transitory deficits will unavoidably lead to a permanent motor deficit while, in the meantime, intellectual impairments will be irreversibly established. A total number of 90 patients with SWS having benefited from hemispherectomy is reported in the literature (45 patients between 1979 and 2002; 32 patients in the 2002 survey by Kossoff et al; 8 patients in the 2007 series by Bourgeois et al; 4 patients by Maton et al[37] and 1 by Andrade et al.[38] Outcomes range from 33%–100% seizure-free response rates. In the Kossoff et al[39] survey although the complication rate was somewhat high (47%), the seizure-free rate was 81% (26/32). Interestingly, early literature[8] suggested that early surgery was predictive of higher intelligence quotient (IQ) postoperatively. The 2002 study[39] found the opposite trending that there was a higher rate of seizure freedom with an older age and seizure-freedom somewhat more likely to lead to normal cognition. However, the mean age of hemispherectomy in the latter cohort was still overall young (mean 2.7 years), so "early" surgery before adolescence is probably advised. Available knowledge on developmental plasticity should also be taken into consideration when discussing the most appropriate timing for extensive neurosurgery.

When pial angiomatosis is circumscribed to a limited area of the cortex the outcome of *resective surgery* (lesionectomy, lobectomy, or circumscribed cortical resection) is also reported to be quite good.[5,6,8,25,27,34,40,41] Selection criteria for surgical candidates are similar to other lesional epilepsies, mainly depending upon a benefit-risk evaluation of the functional and anatomic characteristics of the cortex involved. The series by Bourgeois et al[5] of 27 patients found that 11/19 (58%) with focal resections became seizure free, mostly after complete resection. Arzimanoglou et al[25] reported similar results in a group of 14 patients who underwent selective resection. All seven patients who had complete lesionectomy became seizure free while those with only partial resection had recurrent seizures. A recent publication[37] reported the association of cortical development abnormalities in children with SWS.

The number of cases reported with focal resections is relatively small at this time therefore there does not exist any evidence-based recommendations at this time. However, available data suggests that in cases with a unilateral, focal leptomeningeal angiomatosis a *simplified preoperative investigation* followed by a visually guided lesionectomy, with or without intraoperative electrocorticography, is sufficient in the majority of cases.[2,29] The presence of bilateral EEG abnormalities or generalized seizures is not a contraindication to surgery but careful screening within a comprehensive epilepsy surgery program is mandatory. Decision making for cases with bilateral angiomatosis is much more difficult[26,42,43] and no controlled studies are available.

Dietary therapy has been proposed for children with SWS, in a manner similar to other children with intractable epilepsy. The likelihood of seizure freedom is probably low, as typically children with focal, surgically approachable epilepsy tend to do slightly worse than other children treated with the ketogenic diet.[44] Children with SWS have been treated with the modified Atkins diet in a single pilot series.[45] In this series of five children aged 4–18 years, all maintained ketosis, had some seizure reduction (three of five with greater than 50% reduction in seizures), and no increase in SLEs due to dehydration or increased cholesterol risk.[45] Further studies are warranted. This is probably a very reasonable option as well for children with SWS that are having a cluster of seizures or secondary generalization (e.g., atonic- or absence-type seizures).

Vagus nerve stimulation is another treatment option for patients with intractable epilepsy, perhaps not candidates for epilepsy surgery. To our knowledge, its use for SWS specifically has not been published.

▶ CONCLUSIONS

In summary, children with SWS represent a unique population with epilepsy and other comorbidities, which can be very amenable to aggressive, multidisciplinary care. As soon as the diagnosis is suspected, they should be under the care of a pediatric neurologist and in liaison with a team experienced in epilepsy care.

REFERENCES

1. Roach ES. Neurocutaneous syndromes. *Pediatr Clin North Am* 1992;39(4):591–620.
2. Arzimanoglou A, Guerrini R, Aicardi J. *Aicardi's Epilepsy in Children.* Philadelphia: Lippincott, Williams & Wilkins, 2004; 3rd edn.
3. Kossoff EH, Hatfield LA, Ball KL, Comi AM. Comorbidity of epilepsy and headache in patients with Sturge–Weber syndrome. *J Child Neurol* 2005;20(8):678–682.
4. Sujansky E, Conradi S. Outcome of Sturge–Weber syndrome in 52 adults. *Am J Med Genet* 1995a;57(1):35–45.
5. Bourgeois M, Crimmins DW, de Oliveira RS, Arzimanoglou A, Garnett M, Roujeau T, Di Rocco F, Sainte-Rose C. Surgical treatment of epilepsy in Sturge–Weber syndrome in children. *J Neurosurg* 2007;106(1 Suppl):20–28.

6. Arzimanoglou A, Aicardi J. The epilepsy of Sturge–Weber syndrome: clinical features and treatment in 23 patients. *Acta Neurol Scand Suppl* 1992;140:18–22.

7. Ogunmekan AO, Hwang PA, Hoffman HJ. Sturge–Weber-Dimitri disease: role of hemispherectomy in prognosis. *Can J Neurol Sci* 1989;16:78–80.

8. Hoffman HJ, Hendrick EB, Dennis M, Armstrong D. Hemispherectomy for Sturge–Weber syndrome. *Childs Brain* 1979;5:233–248.

9. Fukuyama Y, Tsuchiya S. A study on Sturge–Weber syndrome. Report of a case associated with infantile spasms and electroencephalographic evolution in five cases. *Eur Neurol* 1979;18:194–209.

10. Boltshauser E, Wilson J, Hoare RD. Sturge–Weber syndrome with bilateral intracranial calcification. *J Neurol Neurosurg Psychiatry* 1976;39(5):429–435.

11. Kossoff EH, Ferenc L, Comi AM. An infantile-onset, severe, yet sporadic seizure pattern is common in Sturge–Weber syndrome. *Epilepsia* 2009;50(9):2154–2157.

12. Maria BL, Neufeld JA, Rosainz LC, Drane WE, Quisling RG, Ben-David K, Hamed LM. Central nervous system structure and function in Sturge–Weber syndrome: evidence of neurologic and radiologic progression. *J Child Neurol* 1998;13(12):606–618.

13. Bay MJ, Kossoff EH, Lehmann CU, Zabel TA, Comi AM. Survey of aspirin use in Sturge–Weber syndrome. *J Child Neurol* 2011;26(6):692–702.

14. Pascual-Castroviejo I, Díaz-Gonzalez C, García-Melian RM, Gonzalez-Casado I, Muñoz-Hiraldo E. Sturge–Weber syndrome: study of 40 patients. *Pediatr Neurol* 1993;9(4):283–288.

15. Pascual-Castroviejo I, Pascual-Pascual SI, Velazquez-Fragua R, Viaño J. Sturge–Weber syndrome: study of 55 patients. *Can J Neurol Sci.* 2008;35(3):301–307.

16. Cibis GW, Tripathi RC, Tripathi BJ. Glaucoma in Sturge–Weber syndrome. *Ophthalmology* 1984;91(9):1061–1071.

17. Sullivan TJ, Clarke MP, Morin JD. The ocular manifestations of the Sturge–Weber syndrome. *J Pediatr Ophthalmol Strabismus* 1992;29(6):349–356.

18. Sujansky E, Conradi S. Sturge–Weber syndrome: age of onset of seizures and glaucoma and the prognosis for affected children. *J Child Neurol* 1995b;10:49–58.

19. Benedikt RA, Brown DC, Walker R, Ghaed VN, Mitchell M, Geyer CA. Sturge–Weber syndrome: cranial MR imaging with Gd-DTPA. *AJNR Am J Neuroradiol* 1993;14(2):409–415.

20. Kuzniecky RI, Jackson GD. *Magnetic Resonance in Epilepsy.* New York: Raven Press, 1995.

21. Griffiths PD, Coley SC, Romanowski CA, Hodgson T, Wilkinson ID. Contrast-enhanced fluid-attenuated inversion recovery imaging for leptomeningeal disease in children. *AJNR Am J Neuroradiol* 2003;24(4):719–723.

22. Juhasz C, Chugani HT. An almost missed leptomeningeal angioma in Sturge–Weber syndrome. *Neurology* 2007;68(3):243.

23. Batista CE, Chugani HT, Hu J, Haacke EM, Behen ME, Helder EJ, Juhász C. Magnetic resonance spectroscopic imaging detects abnormalities in normal-appearing frontal lobe of patients with Sturge–Weber syndrome. *J Neuroimaging* 2008;18(3):306–313.

24. Hu J, et al. MR susceptibility weighted imaging (SWI) complements conventional contrast enhanced T1 weighted MRI in characterizing brain abnormalities of Sturge–Weber Syndrome. *J Magn Reson Imaging* 2008;28(2):300–307.

25. Arzimanoglou AA, Andermann F, Aicardi J, Sainte-Rose C, Beaulieu MA, Villemure JG, Olivier A, Rasmussen T. Sturge–Weber syndrome: indications and results of surgery in 20 patients. *Neurology* 2000;55(10):1472–1479.

26. Chevrie JJ, Specola N, Aicardi J. Secondary bilateral synchrony in unilateral pial angiomatosis: successful surgical treatment. *J Neurol Neurosurg Psychiatry* 1988;51:663–670.

27. Rosen I, Salford L, Starck L. Sturge–Weber disease—neurophysiological evaluation of a case with secondary epileptogenesis, successfully treated with lobe-ectomy. *Neuropediatrics* 1984;15:95–98.

28. Ewen JB, Kossoff EH, Crone NE, Lin DD, Lakshmanan BM, Ferenc LM, Comi AM. Use of quantitative EEG in infants with port-wine birthmark to assess for Sturge–Weber brain involvement. *Clin Neurophysiol* 2009;120(8):1433–1440.

29. Gupta A. Epilepsy in the setting of neurocutaneous syndromes. In: *Wyllie's Treatment of Epilepsy.* Philadelphia: Lippincott Williams & Wilkins, 2011; pp. 375–382.

30. Sharan S, Swamy B, Taranath DA, Jamieson R, Yu T, Wargon O, Grigg JR. Port-wine vascular malformations and glaucoma risk in Sturge–Weber syndrome. *J AAPOS* 2009;13(4):374–378.

31. Turin E, Grados MA, Tierney E, Ferenc LM, Zabel A, Comi AM. Behavioral and psychiatric features of Sturge–Weber syndrome. *J Nerv Ment Dis* 2010;198(12):905–913.

32. Greco F, Fiumara A, Sorge G, Pavone L. Subgaleal hematoma in a child with Sturge–Weber syndrome: to prevent stroke-like episodes, is treatment with aspirin advisable? *Childs Nerv Syst* 2008;24(12):1479–1481.

33. Ville D, Enjolras O, Chiron C, Dulac O. Prophylactic antiepileptic treatment in Sturge–Weber disease. *Seizure* 2002;11(3):145–150.

34. Erba G, Cavazzuti V. Sturge–Weber syndrome: natural history and indications for surgery. *J Epilepsy* 1990;3:287–291.

35. Ewen JB, Comi AM, Kossoff EH. Myoclonic-astatic epilepsy in a child with Sturge–Weber syndrome. *Pediatr Neurol* 2007;36(2):115–117.

36. Arzimanoglou A. The surgical treatment of Sturge–Weber syndrome with respect to its clinical spectrum. In: Tuxhorn I, Holthausen H, Boenigk H (eds), *Paediatric Epilepsy Syndromes and their Surgical Treatment.* London: John Libbey, 1997, pp. 353–363.

37. Maton B, Krsek P, Jayakar P, Resnick T, Koehn M, Morrison G, Ragheb J, Castellano-Sanchez A, Duchowny M. Medically intractable epilepsy in Sturge–Weber syndrome is associated with cortical malformation: implications for surgical therapy. *Epilepsia* 2010;51(2):257–267.

38. Andrade DM, McAndrews MP, Hamani C, Poublanc J, Angel M, Wennberg R. Seizure recurrence 29 years after hemispherectomy for Sturge Weber syndrome. *Can J Neurol Sci* 2010;37:141–144.

39. Kossoff EH, Buck C, Freeman JM. Outcomes of 32 hemispherectomies for Sturge–Weber syndrome worldwide. *Neurology* 2002;59(11):1735–1738.

40. Ito M, Sato K, Ohnuki A, Uto A. Sturge–Weber disease: operative indications and surgical results. *Brain Dev* 1990; 12:473–477.

41. Hoffman HJ. Benefits of early surgery in Sturge–Weber syndrome. In: Tuxhorn I, Holthausen H, Boenigk H (eds), *Paediatric Epilepsy Syndromes and their Surgical Treatment.* London: John Libbey, 1997; pp. 364–370.

42. Alkonyi B, Chugani HT, Karia S, Behen ME, Juhász C. Clinical outcomes in bilateral Sturge–Weber syndrome. *Pediatr Neurol* 2011;44(6):443–449.

43. Jiruska P, Marusic P, Jefferys JG, Krsek P, Cmejla R, Sebronova V, Komarek V. Sturge–Weber syndrome: a favourable surgical outcome in a case with contralateral seizure onset and myoclonic-astatic seizures. *Epileptic Disord* 2011;13(1):76–81.

44. Stainman RS, Turner Z, Rubenstein JE, Kossoff EH. Decreased relative efficacy of the ketogenic diet for children with surgically approachable epilepsy. *Seizure* 2007;16(7):615–619.

45. Kossoff EH, Bosarge JL, Comi AM. A pilot study of the modified Atkins diet for Sturge–Weber syndrome. *Epilepsy Res* 2010;92(2–3):240–243.

CHAPTER 34

Epilepsy Associated with Chromosomal Disorders

Kette D. Valente

► OVERVIEW

Many chromosomal anomalies are associated with childhood-onset epilepsy with distinctive features. Accurate electroclinical delineation helps identify chromosomal anomalies in infants classified with *cryptogenic* epilepsy. Chromosomal disorders carry distinct risks of recurrence making accurate classification important for proper genetic counseling.

Chromosome anomalies may result from abnormalities in number or structure. Abnormalities of chromosome number include polyploidy and autosomal and sex chromosome aneuploidy. Aneuploidy refers primarily to "monosomy" (the presence of only one copy of a chromosome in an otherwise diploid cell) and "trisomy" (three copies of a chromosome). Abnormalities of chromosome structure consist primarily of translocations (interchange of genetic material between nonhomologous chromosomes); deletions (caused by a chromosome break and subsequent loss of genetic material); and duplications (i.e., partial trisomy of genetic material).[1] The classic belief that karyotype is sufficient to rule-out chromosomal anomalies applies only to chromosomal anomalies related to number. Structural anomalies do not fit this scenario and often require more detailed investigation. Therefore, for some syndromes, it is important to first recognize the disorder clinically in order to facilitate correct genetic testing.

This chapter summarizes some of the relevant aspects of epilepsy, electroencephalography (EEG) and genetic data that may guide the identification of chromosomal disorders in early postnatal life, when the phenotype does not confer the diagnosis.

► CHROMOSOME 1

1p36 DELETION

The 1p36 deletion syndrome is a disorder with multiple congenital anomalies and mental retardation characterized by growth delay, epilepsy, congenital heart defects, a characteristic facial appearance, and precocious puberty[2,3] (Fig. 34–1).

Monosomy 1p36 is a contiguous gene syndrome considered to be the most common subtelomeric microdeletion syndrome, with an estimated prevalence is 1–5.000. 1p36 deletions account for 0.5%–1.2% of idiopathic mental retardation.[3]

CLINICAL DIAGNOSIS

PHENOTYPE

The most common features include suggestive facial traits (epicanthus, straight eyebrows, deep-set eyes, midface hypoplasia, broad nasal root/bridge, long philtrum, and pointed chin), microbrachycepahly, large late-closing anterior fontanelle, posteriorly rotated low-set abnormal ears (Fig. 34–2). In addition, motor-delay hypotonia, moderate to severe mental retardation, growth delay, sensorineural deafness, and eye/visual abnormalities with visual inattentiveness, epilepsy, brachy/camptodactyly, and/or short fifth finger(s) are also observed. The majority of patients have heart defects, and some present with a rare congenital cardiomyopathy that results from failure of myocardial development during embryogenesis (noncompaction cardiomyopathy). Associated malformations include central nervous system (CNS) and skeletal and renal abnormalities and abnormal genitalia, Affected patients have abusive behavior, hypotonia, and developmental delay with poor or absent speech.[3–7]

ELECTROCLINICAL FEATURES

Epilepsy occurs in approximately 50%–75% of patients.[2,3,5,8] Seizures begin in infancy or early childhood (mean age of 3 months) with tonic, tonic–clonic, myoclonic, and partial motor seizures. At a mean age of 5 months, seizures may evolve into infantile spasms (IS) (40%–45%) with a hypsarrhythmic pattern.[5]

Epilepsy evolves with a wide variety of seizure types, including tonic–clonic seizures, IS, partial seizures—complex and simple—and myoclonic and atypical absence seizures.[9]

Epilepsy presents two patterns of clinical outcome: (1) patients experience few seizures in infancy and (2) have a normal electroencephalogram. After transient therapy with antiepileptic drugs, there are no seizure recurrences until after the age of 1 year.

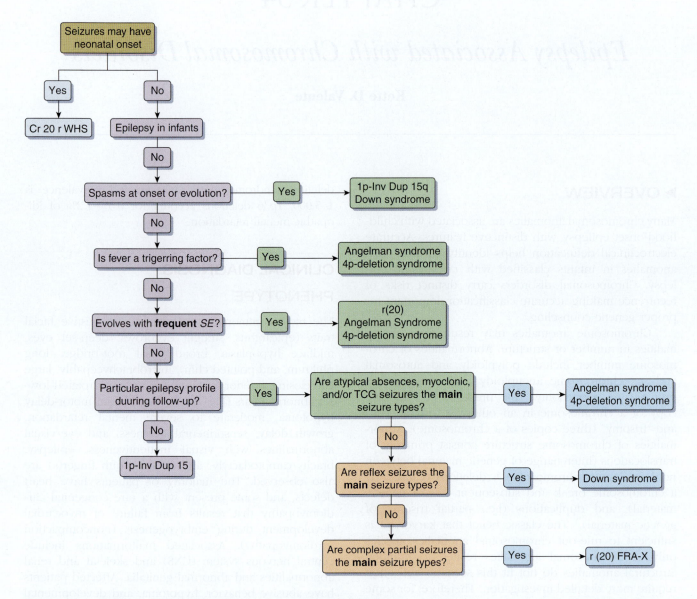

Figure 34–1. Epilepsy characterization in chromosomal disorders.

Patients may also experience more severe epilepsy starting in early life with an abnormal EEG and difficult-to-control epilepsy.

DIAGNOSIS

Monosomy 1p36 may result from terminal deletions or interstitial deletions at various sizes and different breakpoints[10] on chromosome 1 or more complex rearrangements.[11] Conventional cytogenetic studies may not detect all rearrangements, particularly ones on derivative chromosomes. To date, the parental origin of this anomaly is controversial.[10,11] Standard cytogenetics, fluorescence in situ hybridization (FISH) of the subtelomeric regions or array comparative genomic hybridization are used for diagnosis.

TREATMENT

Early treatment of IS is mandatory for better clinical outcome.[3] According to Bahi–Boulisson,[5] spasms with or without hypsarrhytmia (West syndrome) may be refractory to vigabatrin but respond well to corticosteroids. The epilepsy may evolve toward different types of seizures. Treatment is related to seizure type, although medically refractory epilepsy is common.[3,9]

GENOTYPE–PHENOTYPE CORRELATION

Although haploinsufficiency of the potassium channel beta-subunit (KCNAB2) is thought to be responsible for intractable seizures in some cases of 1p36-deletion

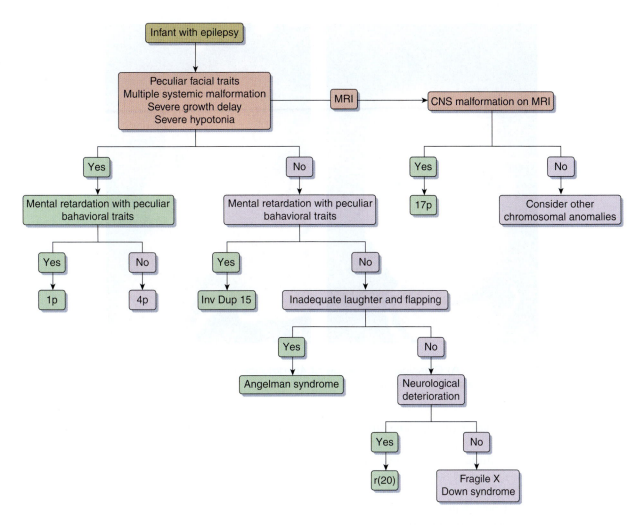

Figure 34–2. Diagnostic evaluation based on epilepsy associated to clinical findings.

syndrome,[12] this was not found in 3 of 11 patients by by Kurosawa et al.[8] Therefore, further investigation of the 1p36 region may be necessary to allow identification of the genes responsible for the 1p36-deletion syndrome.

► CHROMOSOME 4

4p DELETION: WOLF–HIRSCHHORN SYNDROME AND PITT–ROGER–DANKS SYNDROME

Wolf–Hirschhorn syndrome (WHS) is characterized by severe growth retardation and mental defect, microcephaly, "Greek helmet" facies, and closure defects (cleft lip or palate, coloboma of the eye, and cardiac septal defects).

Molecular analysis reveals that the Wolf–Hirschhorn and Pitt–Roger–Dank syndromes which were, previously regarded to be distinct clinical entities, result from the absence of similar, if not identical, genetic segments

and the observed clinical differences likely result from allelic variation in the remaining homolog.[13]

4p deletion is an uncommon disorder with an estimated incidence of 1 per 50,000–20,000 births and a sex ratio of 2 females to 1 male.[1,14–16]

CLINICAL DIAGNOSIS

PHENOTYPE

Cases of the 4p-deletion syndrome may be subdivided into "classical" and "mild" forms. Only the minimal diagnostic criteria are expressed in milder cases. The minimal diagnostic criteria are: severe mental retardation; hypotonia; marked growth retardation and failure to thrive; epilepsy; and microcephaly with Greek warrior helmet face (Fig. 34–3)[17] In the classical cases, systemic manifestations such as closure defects (cleft lip or palate, coloboma of the eye, and cardiac septal defects) occur.[17] Epilepsy in this disorder often has a favorable prognosis and a good outcome is a frequent finding; prenatal onset growth deficiency followed by

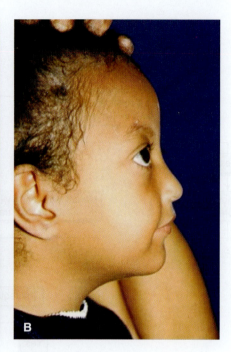

Figure 34–3. (**A**) Classical phenotype of 4p-deletion with microcephaly with Greek warrior helmet face.

short stature and slow weight gain, skeletal anomalies, heart lesions, abnormal tooth development, and hearing loss are common findings in classical cases. Structural CNS anomalies occur in 80%. Global developmental delay of varying degrees is present in all patients, although almost 50% will walk either alone or with support. Hypotonia is a feature in virtually all patients.[18]

EPILEPSY

The existence of a characteristic electroclinical profile in 4p- is recognized clinically and the high frequency of generalized epilepsy is a prominent feature. Epilepsy represents a major clinical challenge in WHS patients but may have a good prognosis.

Prevalence

There is a high frequency of epilepsy in this syndrome, ranging from 80%–90%.[18] For this reason, epilepsy is as an important criterion for clinical diagnosis and may be especially helpful in cases with a milder phenotype.

Age of Onset

Seizures typically begin within the first 3 years of life.[18,19] The age of onset ranges from 5 to 23 months, with a peak incidence from 9 to 10 months.[20] Neonatal onset is rare but may occur in patients with larger deletions.[18,20] Generalized seizures are most frequent at onset. Partial motor seizures (unilateral clonic or tonic), with or without secondary generalization, are also common at onset. The first seizure may be triggered by fever[19] which may evolve to *status epilepticus* (SE). Tonic spasms, complex partial seizures,[18] and myoclonic seizures, evolving to SE are less frequent.[21]

Seizure Types

There is a wide range of seizure types in the 4p-syndrome including: generalized tonic–clonic seizures (GTC) seizures, tonic spasms, myoclonic seizures, atypical absences variably associated with eyelid myoclonia, eye deviation and perioral jerks, partial motor seizures, and complex partial seizures.[9,18,21,22]

Generalized epilepsy is more frequent,[18,19,23,24] with myoclonic, atypical absences, and GTC being the most frequently encountered.[19,20] Atypical absences tend to occur after the first year of life and may be accompanied by a myoclonic component involving the eyelids and hands.[18] Partial motor seizures or "unilateral convulsive seizures" are also frequent.[19,25] An association between convulsive (generalized or unilateral) seizures, atypical absences, and segmental myoclonic seizures has also been described.[18,25]

Status Epilepticus and Epilepsy Aggravated by Fever

Two distinguishing features of this syndrome are (1) the presence of epilepsy aggravated by fever and SE and

(2) their frequent recurrence in some patients.[9,20,23,26] *Status epilepticus* may occur in 40% of patients, occasionally facilitated by fever and tending to disappear by ages 3–8 years. In early life, SE occurs despite adequate treatment.[18] All seizure types may occur during episodes of SE and the recognition of nonconvulsive episodes is often challenging. A predominance of myoclonic SE has been reported.[19] Myoclonic and atypical absence SE may persist for days or weeks accompanied by impairment of consciousness and remained underdiagnosed.

SE may be associated with hemiparesis or death.[21] The use of sodium bromide is particularly effective for preventing SE. The mean age of last SE in patients receiving sodium bromide was significantly younger than that in those not treated with sodium bromide.

Fever or even moderate temperatures may trigger the first seizure Furthermore, seizure worsening during febrile episodes is frequent and may lead to SE. These events may be recurrent in some patients.[19,20,26]

Evolution of Epilepsy

The first year of life is typically characterized by generalized or unilateral motor seizures. Subsequently, absence seizures accompanied by eyelid myoclonia appear between ages 1 and 5 years.[16,19,20] Epilepsy often remits after a period of daily disabling seizures during early childhood. Therefore, the prognosis of epilepsy is favorable for both seizure control and evolution despite the initial course.[20,23]

▶ DIAGNOSIS

EEG FEATURES

The EEG in the 4p- syndrome may demonstrate several characteristic findings, especially during childhood (Fig. 34–4).[20] Features frequently reportedinclude:

1. Presence of sharp-wave transients superimposed on a background of diffuse, high-voltage 3- to 4-Hz slow-wave discharges[22,27] (Fig. 34–5A).
2. Posterior discharges characterized by high amplitude sharp theta activity in the posterior head regions or repetitive spikes[22] (Fig. 34–5B).

These patterns share some similarity with the EEG patterns observed in patients with Angelman syndrome (AS).

GENETIC TESTING

The 4p-depletion syndrome is associated with a hemizygous deletion of the distal short arm of chromosome 4 (4p16.3) (Table 34–1). It is unclear whether a single locus is involved in the phenotype. One locus that may contribute to the phenotypic features of WHS and the allelic and milder Pitt–Rogers–Danks syndrome is the WHS candidate-1 gene (WHSC1).[28] There is evidence that the *HOX7* gene may be involved in determining the WHS phenotype. Wright et al (1999) characterized a novel gene in the 165-kb critical region in 4p16.3, which they designated WHS candidate-2 (WHSC2). It is considered a contiguous gene syndrome,

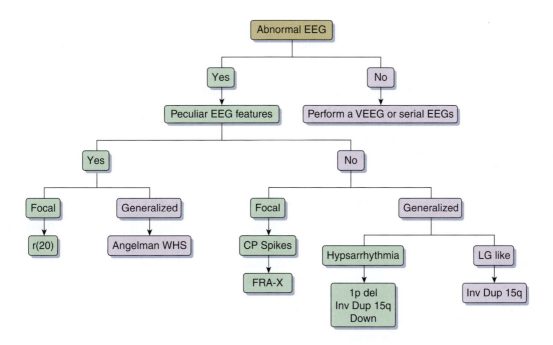

Figure 34–4. EEG features in chromosomal disorders.

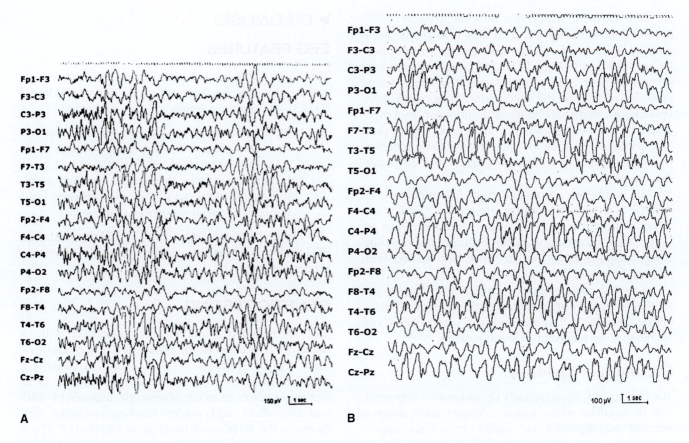

Figure 34–5. (**A**) Sharp–wave transients superimposed on a background of diffuse, high-voltage 3- to 4-Hz slow-wave discharges. (**B**) Posterior discharges characterized by high-amplitude sharp theta activity over the posterior regions.

since no single gene deletions or intragenic mutations have been shown to confer the full WHS phenotype.[29]

De novo deletions occur in 8% of patients (preferentially paternally derived) and in 13% of cases are secondary to familial translocation (often maternally derived). The size of the deletion varies from cytogenetically visible deletions to undetectable cytogenetic deletions. The diagnosis is based on standard cytogenetics in approximately 50%. FISH can be used to detect deletions of 4p16.3, the critical region for the phenotype.[30]

The testing strategy to confirm the clinical diagnosis requires (www.ncbi.nlm.nih.gov):

1. Conventional cytogenetic studies to detect large deletions and more complex cytogenetic rearrangements (ring chromosome, unbalanced chromosome translocations).
2. FISH analysis to detect smaller deletions involving the WHSCR.
3. Genome-wide chromosomal microarray analysis to detect deletions involving the WHSCR or imbalances resulting from more complex arrangements associated with 4p16.3 deletion (unbalanced translocations).

▶ **TABLE 34–1.** SUMMARY OF TESTING USED IN WOLF–HIRSCHHORN SYNDROME

Test Type		Rearrangement Detected	Mutation Detection Frequency by Test Type[1]
Cytogenetic analysis		Deletion or other complex rearrangements leading to deletion of 4p16.3	~50%–60%
	FISH	Deletion of WHSCR in 4p16.3	>95%
Deletion/duplication analysis[2]	Targeted to 4p16.3	Deletion of WHSCR in 4p16.3	>95%
	Chromosomal microarray analysis	Extent of deletion of 4p16.3 or other complex rearrangements leading to deletion of 4p16.3	>95%

▶ TREATMENT

Early diagnosis and treatment of atypical absences and myoclonic seizures is mandatory. In general, seizures in patients with the 4p- syndrome are not refractory and seizure control is possible with sodium valproate and phenobarbital.[18,23] Ethosuximide is also reportedly effective.[18] Benzodiazepines may be used as add-on therapy.[23]

▶ GENOTYPE–PHENOTYPE CORRELATION

There is a strong genotype–phenotype correlation in 4p syndrome.[16,17,31,32] The characteristic facial phenotype is less pronounced in patients with a smaller deletion, and microcephaly is not observed in patients with certain cryptic unbalanced translocations.[16] Therefore, there is also a correlation between deletion size and severity of epilepsy. Global improvement occurs over time.[18]

The mortality rate for patients with the 4p- syndrome correlates with deletion size and overall risk of death in de novo deletion cases. Approximately 35% of patients die during the first 2 years of life, and survival into adulthood is rare. Shannon et al[33] studied 159 cases of WHS and estimated a minimum birth incidence of 1 in 95,896. The crude infant mortality rate was 23 of 132 (17%), and in the first 2 years of life the mortality rate was 28 of 132 (21%).

▶ CHROMOSOME 15 DISORDERS

ANGELMAN SYNDROME

AS is a neurogenetic disorder with multiple genetic mechanisms involving the maternal chromosome 15q11–1q13. Estimates of the prevalence of AS range from 1:10,000 to 1.2000[34–37] and is similar to Rett syndrome (1.12.000), suggesting that AS remains underdiagnosed.

▶ CLINICAL FEATURES

PHENOTYPE

AS is characterized by severe mental retardation, speech disorder, stereotyped jerky movements, and a peculiar behavioral profile characterized by a happy disposition and outbursts of laughter. Eighty to ninety percent of patients manifest epilepsy and abnormal electroencephalographic patterns which may be used as diagnostic criteria, and become important when the phenotype is not suggestive enough, as in infants. Other features such as hyperactivity, hypopigmentation, ataxia, sleep disorder, and peculiar facial traits (macrostomia, wide-spaced teeth, prognathism, and macrognathism) have variable occurrence, ranging from 20% to 80%.[38–40]

EPILEPSY

Prevalence

Epilepsy in AS patients ranges from 80%[39] to 90%.[41] There is evidence that different genetic groups may present different profiles, with distinct degrees of severity, and that a more severe form of epilepsy occurs in patients with the deletion.[41] Patients with the deletion have a higher prevalence, estimated at close to 100%.[41–43]

Although less frequently documented and reported, there are variations regarding prevalence and seizure type. The prevalence ranges from 36.1%[42] to 75%[44] and is even higher when analyzing patients with the deletion (84.2%).[43]

Age of Onset

One of the most important aspects of AS is the late onset of the clinical phenotype, especially the diagnostic facial traits. However, in these developmentally delayed infants, epilepsy has an early onset,[42,43,45–47] preceding the clinical diagnosis in most patients, and may anticipate the diagnosis in children with developmental delay and early "cryptogenic" epilepsy. Epilepsy with a later onset (age 5) are encountered rarely.[42] Atypical absences and myoclonic seizures are the most frequent seizure types at onset.[42,43,45]

Seizure Types

Major seizure types include atypical absence, myoclonic, and GTC.[42,43]

All seizure types have been reported in AS but generalized seizures, especially atypical absences[42,43,45] and myoclonic seizures predominate.[46,48] Atypical absences and subtle myoclonic seizures are the most frequent seizure types documented by video-EEG (V-EEG), but not by parents who mostly report motor phenomena.[43] Atypical absences and myoclonic seizures may be prolonged events lasting weeks or months, reported as periods of decreased contact with the environment.[45]

Viani et al[49] reported complex partial seizures of occipital lobe origin as a frequent event, an observation not corroborated by others.[25,28,29] IS is reported rarely in AS.[45,49] Other less frequently reported seizure types are atonic, myoclonic absence, *hemigeneralized*, and partial.[41,44] It is possible that the frequency of myoclonic seizures, atypical absences, or even pure atonic seizures may be higher in AS patients.

Status Epilepticus and Epilepsy Aggravated by Fever

Seizure worsening during fever is as frequent as 52.6%[42,43,49] a high rate in comparison to age-matched controls. In some cases, fever triggers the first seizure[43,49] and may occur even with moderate temperatures.[43,48]

The higher incidence of SE in this syndrome may be related to the use of V-EEG monitoring to detect nonconvulsive status. By the same token, myoclonic status is higher in studies utilizing polygraphic recordings and back-averaging techniques.[46,48,49]

Evolution of Epilepsy

Patients with AS often evolve into a milder course of epilepsy with increasing age or less commonly achieve complete control.[42,43,48] Severity typically occurs during early life[42,43] and may improve during late childhood and puberty[44,46,50] or adulthood.[51]

There is little information on epilepsy in adults with AS. Atypical absences and myoclonic seizures may persist into adulthood.[41,51] Therefore, despite improvement in epilepsy severity, complete seizure control is obtained in approximately 30% of all patients.[43]

▶ **DIAGNOSIS**

The diagnosis of AS is based on phenotype, electroclinical profile and genetic data. The electroclinical profile may represent the only clue to diagnosis since the clinical phenotype is not relevant in early ages.

EEG PATTERNS

Suggestive EEG patterns were reported in AS[52,53] regarding morphology, burst duration, occurrence, frequency, amplitude, and distribution:

1. Delta patterns: Runs of generalized, rhythmic delta activity, usually with frontal emphasis, and of high amplitude, sometimes associated with epileptiform discharges (often more than 300 mV) (Fig. 34–6A).

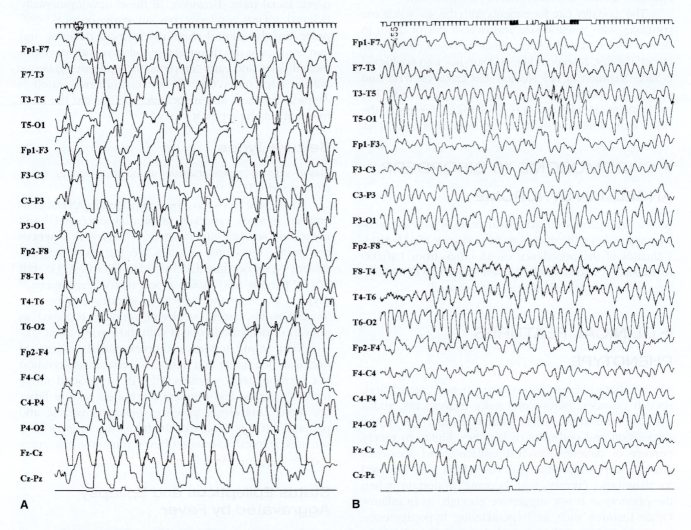

A   **B**

Figure 34–6. **(A)** Runs of generalized, rhythmic delta activity, usually with frontal emphasis, and of high amplitude, sometimes associated with epileptiform discharges. **(B)** High amplitude (about 200 mV), 4–6 Hz activity, generalized or over posterior regions, occupying most of the tracing. *(continued)*

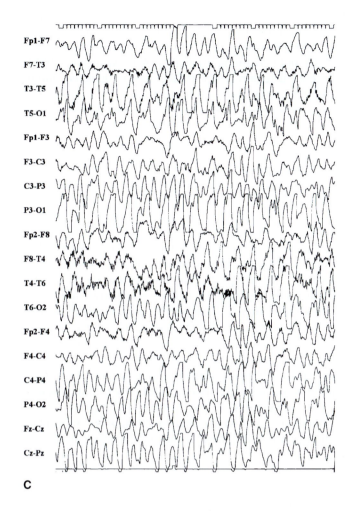

C

Figure 34–6. *(Continued)* **(C)** Spike and sharp waves mixed with high-amplitude 3–4 Hz activity, over posterior regions.

2. Theta patterns: High amplitude (about 200 mV), 4–6 Hz activity, generalized or over the posterior head regions, noted throughout the tracing (Fig. 34–6B).

3. Posterior discharges: Spike- and sharp-waves mixed with high amplitude 3–4 Hz activity over the posterior regions. These discharges are sometimes asymmetrical and occasionally triggered by passive eye closure (Fig. 34–6C).

The existence of a particular EEG profile, not a common finding in chromosomal disorders, is important to rule-out mimicking conditions such as Rett syndrome, alpha-thalassemia retardation syndrome (ATR-X), and Gurrieri syndrome. Symptom complexes include cerebral palsy, static encephalopathy, Lennox–Gastaut syndrome, autism spectrum disorder, pervasive developmental disorder, and mitochondrial disorders.[54]

GENETIC DIAGNOSIS

Four genetic mechanisms have been described in AS. These include deletion (del15q11–13),[55,56] paternal uniparental disomy,[57] imprinting center abnormality,[58] and *UBE3A* mutations,[59,60] all of which affect the maternal chromosome 15 (q11–13), a known imprinted region. Maternal del15q11–13, characterized by the loss of one part of the chromosome, occurs in 75%–80%.[61] Uniparental disomy or the inheritance of two alleles with the same parental origin, in this case from the father, is detected in 1%–3%.[62] Imprinting center abnormalities (ICAs) occur in 2%–5%[63] and here, although there is a biparental inheritance of chromosome 15, both chromosomes have a paternal expression, owing to a mutation in the imprinting center. Approximately 8% of all AS patients demonstrate the *UBE3A* mutation that determines loss of function of the gene encoding a ubiquitin protein ligase. The remaining 12%–15%, in spite of the absence of a detectable genetic mechanism, are considered AS patients with the diagnosis based on clinical and EEG grounds. Recurrence risk is distinct for each group.[64] Therefore, identification of AS patients is mandatory due to implications in genetic counseling.

DNA methylation analysis identifies approximately 80% of individuals with AS and is typically the first test ordered. If DNA methylation analysis is normal, *UBE3A* sequence analysis is the next appropriate diagnostic test.

▶ TREATMENT

Although, *UBE3A* dysfunction is seen as the cause of AS, *GABA* genes may have a contributory role in the phenotype,[65,66] especially in epilepsy. It may be postulated that the good therapeutic response to valproate, phenobarbital, and clonazepam, regardless of seizure type, observed in our series and in parents' questionnaires,[67] may be attributed to GABAergic receptor deletion.

Benzodiazepines are also effective, which may be explained by the decrease in benzodiazepine receptor density in 60%–80% of AS patients.[68] However, vigabatrin, which is also a GABAergic drug, is not effective.[43] The ability of vigabatrin to increase gamma-aminobutyric acid (GABA) without enhancing GABAergic receptor function may help to explain its failure to control seizures in AS. Seizure aggravation may occur with vigabatrin, carbamazepine, and oxcarbazepine.[43] The ketogenic diet,[43] topiramate,[69] and ethosuximide[70] improve epilepsy in small series of AS patients with refractory epilepsy. Levetiracetam has been used in refractory nonconvulsive status.[71]

▶ GENOTYPE–PHENOTYPE CORRELATION

There is evidence that patients with the AS deletion have a more severe clinical phenotype compared to patients without deletion.[41]

Valente et al[43] reported that AS patients with the deletion have a high prevalence of early-onset epilepsy that is typically medically refractory. In addition, seizure onset usually preceded clinical diagnosis based on phenotype, and could be used as an element for earlier diagnosis. Proper characterization of epilepsy in AS may be an important diagnostic tool, as the epilepsy is stereotyped with the presence of atypical absences, myoclonic seizures, epilepsy aggravated by fever, and *SE* during infancy and early childhood. We believe that AS should be considered in the differential diagnosis of developmentally delayed infants with severe, generalized cryptogenic epilepsy. The importance of breakpoints (size of the deletion) on the severity of epilepsy in patients with deletion remains undetermined, although it seems to determine the severity of clinical phenotype.[72]

INV DUP (15)

Inv dup (15) is the most common disease in the group of extrastructurally abnormal chromosomes (ESACs) or small supernumerary chromosomes. The Swedish survey of ESACs in 39–105 consecutive prenatal diagnoses (1994) demonstrated a total prevalence of 0.8 per 1000 ESACs (0.3–0.4 per 1000 for familial and 0.4–0.5 per 1000 for de novo ESACs cases).[73] The prevalence of inv dup (15) in ESACs, studied in a nationwide screening program,[74] showed that inv dup (15) was confirmed in 46.3% by FISH analysis.

The prevalence of large inv dup (15q) is estimated at 1:30.000, with a sex ratio of 1.[75] The small inv dup (15q), not containing the Prader–Willi syndrome (PWS)/AS critical region (PWS/ASCR), goes undetected due to the absence of phenotypic expression.

▶ CLINICAL DIAGNOSIS

PHENOTYPE

Most cases are characterized by mental and growth retardation, epilepsy, and mild dysmorphisms associated with behavioral findings. Hypotonia occurs in all cases and is associated with moderate to profound dysmorphism include downslanting palpebral fissures, epicanthal folds, deep-set eyes, low-set and/or posteriorly rotated ears, high arched palate, broad nose, anteverted nares; fifth finger clinodactyly, and unusual dermatoglyphics characterized by partial second to third toe syndactyly. These features are rarely useful diagnostic findings at an early age (Fig. 34–7).[74–82]

The behavioral profile, a key diagnostic feature, is characterized by poor social interaction, stereotyped movements, and the purposeless use of objects. Affected patients have difficulties sustaining eye contact and respond to simple commands with gesticulation. Language is echolalic and repetitive, with a tendency to repeat short and simple meaningless phrases. These behavioral patterns are regarded as signs of pervasive developmental disorder or atypical autism.[76]

ELECTROCLINICAL PROFILE

The prevalence of epilepsy is unknown, and ranges widely from 50%–100%.[78,83–85] This difference may be partially

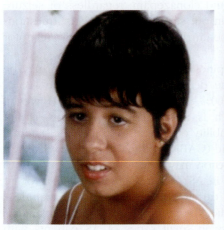 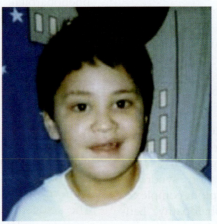 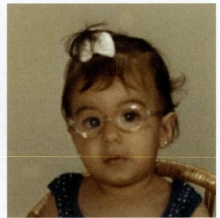

Figure 34–7. Inv dup (15q) patient with downslanting palpebral fissures, epicanthal folds, deep-set eyes, low-set and/or posteriorly rotated ears, broad nose, anteverted nares. These traits are not useful for the diagnoses at an early age.

explained by the fact that epilepsy may be a main reason for referral and diagnosis in some series.[77,78,83]

Age of Onset

The age of onset ranges from 6 months to 9 years.[76,78,79,82,86] Seizures usually begin in infancy (from 6 months to 1 year), and rarely in neonates.[77–79,81,83,86] Early seizure onset may be accompanied by IS.[77,78,86]

IS are one of the only similarities observed, since seizure type and evolution differ greatly among patients.[77,78,83,86] Although epilepsy is common in chromosomal disorders including inv dup (15), IS tends to be unusual and for this reason may be an important marker for this syndrome.[81–83,86]

Seizure Type

There is a clear predominance of generalized and refractory epilepsy, in inv dup (15) (18–23), and the presentation often resembles the Lennox–Gastaut syndrome with tonic, atonic, atypical absences, myoclonic, and GTC.[76,78,85,87–90] Myoclonic absence seizures,[83,91,92] sometimes induced by emotion have also been described. Partial epilepsy may evolve into nonconvulsive SE.[77,83]

Epilepsy may begin in childhood, as the *Lennox–Gastaut-like* syndrome[76] or evolve into a *Lennox–Gastaut-like* syndrome following a long period of refractory epilepsy with early onset.[77]

▶ DIAGNOSIS

EEG FEATURES

It is difficult to categorize EEGs as they typically present distinct features. Battaglia et al (1997)[76] described in detail the EEG findings during wakefulness and sleep. They include high-amplitude fast activity resembling recruiting rhythms and large amplitude generalized slow sharpspike-wave complexes lasting 2–20 seconds. Hypsarrhytmia was described in very young patients.

GENETIC DATA

The proximal region of chromosome 15q is predisposed to a wide range of structural rearrangements. Deletions of this region may result in PWS and AS, whether paternally or maternally derived.[93] Additional copies of the Prader–Willi–Angelman syndrome critical region (PWACR) may occur as supernumerary marker chromosomes, referred as to inv dup (15).[79,94–96] Inv dup (15) can thus be classified into two major groups according to size, determined by the presence or absence of PWACR, that have different phenotypic consequences.[79,95,97,98] Small inv dup (15), not containing PWACR, seem to have no phenotypic effects.[95,98] On the other hand, large inv dup (15) usually contain two

maternally derived extra copies of the q11–13 region and are associated with abnormal phenotypes.[79,81]

▶ TREATMENT

Most patients are medically refractory[76] but easy-to-control epilepsy cases have been reported.[77,87] Buoni et al[83] described a concomitant improvement of the seizures and EEG features with antiepileptic drugs, but the persistence of abnormal EEGs despite good seizure outcome suggests caution before discontinuing therapy.[77]

▶ GENOTYPE–PHENOTYPE CORRELATION

In some chromosomal disorders, the presence of one specific mechanism, such as deletion in AS or size of the deletion in 4p- determine loss of larger genetic material and correlate with a more severe electroclinical profile. In inv dup (15), the discrepancy between the mild phenotype and the severe chromosomal abnormality further supports the hypothesis that the breakpoint site is contributory to inv dup phenotype rather than the size of the chromosomal abnormality.[81] By the same token, Chifari et al[87] described two patients with large deletions and mild epilepsy. Therefore, the electroclinical heterogeneity in this syndrome may also be associated with the breakpoint and PWACR dosage, rather than the difference in the extension of the duplicated segment.

CHROMOSOME 20

Ring 20 Chromosome Syndrome

Cr 20r is a rare chromosomal anomaly with psychomotor delay and behavioral disorder that is associated with a distinctive electroclinical profile.[99,100]

▶ CLINICAL DIAGNOSIS

PHENOTYPE

Acquired psychomotor delay and behavioral disturbances, usually diagnosed as pervasive developmental disorder are the main clinical diagnostic features. The most consistent dysmorphic feature is microcephaly but others may not occur or appear late. Development may be normal or mildly delayed, followed by cognitive and behavioral decline after seizure onset.[101]

EPILEPSY

Epilepsy is the hallmark of this disease, with seizures occurring in virtually all cases. Onset is usually associated with cognitive regression and may occur up to age 17 years; neonatal onset is rare.[99] Most data in r(20) address epilepsy features in adolescence and adult life, demonstrating the long-time lag from the age at onset to diagnosis.[102] Epilepsy usually occurs as nonconvulsive status.[99,102–104] *Typical* seizure phenotypes in the classical presentation of this syndrome include.

NONCONVULSIVE STATUS EPILEPTICUS

Frequent seizures consist of a prolonged confusional state, speech difficulties, and complex automatisms, with or without motor seizures, and an ictal EEG pattern characterized by runs of long-lasting bilateral paroxysmal high-voltage slow waves with occasional spikes over the frontal lobes.[104–106]

Complex partial seizures of frontal onset with ictal terror or hallucinations and loss of consciousness, oroalimentary automatisms, and hypertonia are also common.[104]

NOCTURNAL FRONTAL LOBE SEIZURES

Characterized predominantly by subtle stretching, turning, or rubbing movements accompanied by highly characteristic bursts of diffuse but frontally dominant high-voltage fast activity. These events resemble physiological arousal behavior[107] and represent a spectrum of characteristic minimal to moderate motor signs, identified by VEEG as "subtle nocturnal seizures" (SNSs).[107] Nocturnal frontal lobe seizures (NS) have been identified as a possible cause of neurological deterioration.[107]

Motor seizures are the main seizure type in neonates.[99] According to Ville et al,[99] the interictal EEG shows a diffusely slow background activity and the ictal EEG demonstrates rhythmic theta activity affecting the temporo-occipital areas. A frontal localization of EEG abnormalities and nonconvulsive status epilepticus (NCSE) has not been reported. In childhood onset before age 7 years, seizures consisting of terror and hallucinations may cause misdiagnosis as a psychiatric disorder.[99] These events may be accompanied by motor manifestations and automatisms, and are usually brief. The EEG, from ages 4 to 5 years, shows 1–2 Hz delta slow waves and spike-and-wave activity, predominantly in the frontal areas.[99]

▶ DIAGNOSIS

EEG

The interictal EEG in r(20) is highly characteristic and consists of normal or near-normal background with trains or bursts of rhythmic sharply contoured theta waves in the frontocentral areas which may have a notched appearance. EEG features are not influenced by eye opening, level of vigilance, or intravenous injection of diazepam.[101]

The ictal EEG demonstrates characteristic slow and sharp waves. The slow waves are (1) usually synchronous high-voltage slow waves with or without a spike component predominantly in the frontal and frontopolar areas, (2) may change in frequency every several seconds, (3) continue for long periods, and (4) easily spread diffusely. The sharp waves are 5–6 Hz irregular and diffuse discontinuous sharp waves that sometimes appear predominantly in the centroparietal area. The clinical seizure pattern and EEG findings are similar in the 24 published cases.[108]

GENETIC TESTING

Ring chromosomes are caused by a break on both sides of the centromere. The extremes of the segment are subsequently united, but possibly accompanied by loss of genetic material.[109,110] Karyotyping should be performed looking at, at least, 100 mitoses, since the percentage of lymphocytes carrying the chromosome rearrangement may be low.[111]

The breakdown point of the chromosome locus of fusion between the deleted short and long arms in the ring chromosome- is p13q13 or p13q13.3 or p13q13.33.[104,112] The loss of telomeric material on both arms of chromosome 20 is usually identified by FISH.[110] Cases with a mosaicism for r20 have also been observed. Most cases are sporadic, but a few are familial.[101]

▶ TREATMENT

Epilepsy in r(20) is often refractory.[99] Progressive worsening of both clinical and EEG features over a long period has been reported.[113] Nonconvulsive *SE* is the hallmark of his syndrome and it is believed to be caused by dopaminergic dysfunction.[114] The study of Inoue et al[104] revealed frequent seizures consisting of a prolonged confusional state with speech difficulties and complex automatisms, with or without motor seizures, and an ictal EEG pattern of long-lasting bilateral paroxysmal high-voltage slow waves with occasional spikes. These episodes may not be distinguished from the baseline behavior and may precede other seizure types for years before being recognized as a seizure. It is usually refractory to treatment and related to neuropsychological deterioration, representing a major concern in this disease. Fatal nonconvulsive status in r(20) has been described.[103]

Nonconvulsive status in r(20) is more resistant than nonconvulsive status in other disorders such as Lennox–Gastaut syndrome, epilepsy with continuous spike-waves during slow-wave sleep and other forms of symptomatic generalized epilepsy. During status, continuous intravenous infusion of midazolam is effective and safe and can be used as first-line therapy.[115] Alternative therapeutic options include intravenous immunoglobulin, corticotrophin, and vagus nerve stimulation.[102,116]

► PHENOTYPE–GENOTYPE CORRELATION

A relationship between epilepsy severity and the percentage of mitoses is controversial.[104] There is evidence that 100% of cells affected by ring chromosome 20 are associated with earlier and more severe epilepsy.[99] Epilepsy severity as well as cognitive deterioration seems to correlate with the number of affected cells; however, this data needs further corroboration.

TRISOMY 21 (DOWN SYNDROME)

Down syndrome (DS) is the most common chromosomal disorder and cause of congenital mental retardation, with an approximate incidence of 1:650–800 births. In 95% of cases the cause of the syndrome is a nondisjunction of chromosomes 21 during meiosis; 4% of cases are caused by a trisomy originating from an unbalanced translocation. The risk of trisomy 21 increases with maternal age;[117,118] the causes of this association are unknown.

► CLINICAL DIAGNOSIS

Growth retardation, hypotonia, mental retardation of variable degree, flat facies with brachycephaly and upward-slanted eyes, epicanthal folds, small ears, speckling of the iris (Brushfields' spots), simian creases, and hypogonadism are characteristic features. Individuals with DS often have major congenital cardiac malformations (30%–40% in some studies), particularly the atrioventricular canal, and gastrointestinal malformations, such as duodenal stenosis or atresia, imperforate anus, and Hirschsprung disease. Leukemia [both acute lymphoblastic leukemia (ALL) and acute myeloid leukemia (AML)] and leukemoid reactions have an increased incidence in DS.[119]

Estimates of the relative risk of certain disorders range from 10 to 20 times the normal population; in particular, acute megakaryocytic leukemia occurs 200 to 400 times more frequently in DS than in the chromosomally normal population.[120] Ninety percent of all DS patients have significant conductive hearing loss.[121] Patients with DS develop the neuropathologic hallmarks of Alzheimer disease at an early age.[122] Characteristic senile plaques and neurofibrillary tangles are present in the brain of all individuals with DS over age 40 years.[123] The triplication of the amyloid precursor protein gene (*APP*, 104760) may explain this phenomenon; several mutations in the *APP* gene have been described.

DS is caused by the triplicate state (trisomy) of all or of a critical portion of chromosome 21. Therefore, many genes are involved in the phenotype. In particular, transient myeloproliferative disorder and megakaryoblastic leukemia of DS are associated with mutations in the *GATA1* gene (OMIM 305371) in conjunction with trisomy 21. The origin of free trisomy 21 is: (1) Errors in meiosis that lead to trisomy 21 are overwhelmingly of maternal origin; only about 5% occur during spermatogenesis. (2) Most errors in maternal meiosis occur in meiosis I at a mean maternal age of 32 years (the mean maternal age of the general population is approximately 27 years). Thus, meiosis I errors account for 76%–80% of maternal meiotic errors and 67%–73% of all instances of free trisomy 21. (3) Maternal meiosis II errors constitute 20%–24% of maternal errors and 18%–20% of all cases of free trisomy 21. Mean maternal age is also advanced between 31 and 34 years. (4) In rare families with paternal nondisjunction, most errors occur in meiosis II. The mean maternal and paternal ages are similar to the mean reproductive age in western societies. (5) In 5% of trisomic individuals, the supernumerary chromosome 21 appears to result from an error in mitosis. In these cases, there is no advanced maternal age and there is no preference for which chromosome 21 is duplicated.[124]

► EPILEPSY

Children with DS have an increased susceptibility to seizures in early life; superimposed systemic illness increases the likelihood of seizures. The prevalence ranges from 1.4% in childhood but increases to 12.2% in adults over 35 years.[125,126] There is a biphasic distribution with two peaks of incidence infancy (first year of life)[127,128] and the third decade.[129–132] The second peak may be related to other comorbidities observed in the syndrome, such as hypoxic-ischemic injury as a consequence of congenital heart disease in children, and dementia in adults. When epilepsy occurs in the first year of life, later onset is observed in patients without a structural abnormality.[128]

The presence of a structural abnormality may determine the presence of partial epilepsy in symptomatic cases. The most common seizure types are IS with hypsarrhythmia[128] and reflex epilepsy. Other seizure types include: partial seizures, myoclonic seizures, and GTC.

In *adults*, over 35 years, there is a high frequency of epilepsy in patients with DS and dementia. Epilepsy usually occurs years after the first signs of mental deterioration (113). Main seizure types were GTC, and more rarely partial complex and myoclonic (generalized and focal). Myoclonic senile dementia is rare.[129] In most late-onset DS epilepsy patients, seizures appeared to be infrequent but intractable;[129,130,133] however, no precise indication of seizure severity is available.

▶ TREATMENT

There is no recommended therapeutic regime for IS in DS. Remission is usually obtained with conventional antiepileptic drugs such as ACTH,[128] steroids,[134] and vigabatrin.[135] In most studies, IS is easy-to-control and syndrome other forms of refractory epilepsy are rare.[133–136] An exception to this rule is the occurrence of IS in DS determined by hypoxic insults.[128] In general, the evolution of epilepsy is favorable. The outcome of 252 children and adolescents with DS shows that 40% become seizure free.[133]

▶ EEG

EEG abnormalities are unspecific and are related to the type of epilepsy in each patient (i.e., hypsarrhythmia in infants with IS).

Silva et al (1996)[134] presented a detailed analysis of ictal and interictal EEG characteristics in 14 patients with DS without a brain lesion followed from 19 months to 14 years. Patients presented typical and symmetrical hypsarrhythmia, with recurrence of the hypsarrhythmic pattern after a cluster of spasms. The administration of diazepam improved the EEG without evidence of focal activity.

▶ PHENOTYPE–GENOTYPE CORRELATION

Approximately 1% of DS patients are mosaics for a normal and a trisomic cell line. These patients show a less severe phenotype. The observation of a few patients with a partial duplication of 21q and features suggestive of DS has allowed mapping of a DS critical region to 21q22.3 that, if triplicated, results in the phenotypic characteristics of the syndrome.[137,138]

FRAGILE-X

The fragile-X syndrome has an approximate incidence of 1/1500 males[139] and is the most common chromosomal abnormality associated with heritable mental retardation. Both males and females may be affected, but the phenotype is notably more severe in males. It is estimated that 1:1000 (see reference [140]) to 1:259 (see reference [141]) females are carriers.

▶ CLINICAL DIAGNOSIS

Fragile-X syndrome accounts for about one-half of cases of X-linked mental retardation and is the second most common cause of mental impairment after trisomy 21.[141]

Fragile-X mental retardation is characterized by moderate to severe mental retardation, macroorchidism, and distinct facial features, including long face, large ears, and prominent jaw.[142–145] Some patients exhibit a pervasive developmental disorder with autistic behavior.[146]

▶ GENETIC DATA

Fragile-X syndrome is caused by a mutation in the *FMR1* gene. In most cases, the disorder is caused by an unstable expansion of a CGG repeat in the *FMR1* gene and abnormal methylation, which results in suppression of FMR1 transcription and decreased protein levels in the brain.[147]

The X-chromosome of patients affected with this syndrome includes a fragile site at Xq27.3, when cells are grown in a folic-deprived medium. The condition results from a dynamic mutation in heritable unstable DNA (88), because of variation in the copy number of a trinucleotide repeat p(CCG)n within the *FMR1* gene. This fragile site is termed FRAXA.

A second site of fragility, symbolized FRAXE was identified in patients with the cytogenetic changes of fragile X syndrome (300624) but without the characteristic molecular changes (FMR1-mutation negative), Sutherland and Baker (1992).[148] A second gene was identified in this region, Xq28, called *FMR2*, that is transcribed distally from the CpG island at FRAXE and is downregulated by repeat expansion and methylation.[149,150] Patients with FMR2 have mental retardation that is milder than in FRAXA. There are no other clinical similarities with patients with FRAXA. The disorder has an unusual mode of inheritance. About 20% of males who carry the mutation are clinically and cytogenetically normal (normal transmitting males). About 30% of female carriers have mental impairment. Transmission through families is consistent with an X-linked semidominant condition.

▶ EPILEPSY

The prevalence of epilepsy ranges from 25% (see reference [151]) to 40% (see reference [152]) in males.

Musumeci et al[153] analyzed 192 male Fra-X patients and found a prevalence of 18.2%. Some studies[154,155] point to a high frequency of epilepsy (5%–7.8%) and EEG abnormalities (Lasctochkina et al, *citado em* Singh et al, 1999) even in women with the pre-mutation. Epilepsy occurs in the first decade of life in Fra-X. In one study,[153] age of seizure onset was between 2 and 9 years.

Fra-X patients present a variety of seizure types probably related to its heterogeneous clinical pheno-type. The main seizure types are: complex partial sei-zures, GTC, and partial seizures with motor phenomena (unilateral).[153] Febrile seizures are sporadic and occur in 7.1% of patients. The polymorphism of seizure types does not constitute a characteristic epilepsy pattern. Sei-zures occur before the age of 15 and disappear in the second decade of life. Refractory epilepsy is rare. Most studies suggest that epilepsy is responsive to conven-tional antiepileptic drugs.[153,156]

▶ EEG

A characteristic EEG abnormality frequently described in Fra-X and recognized as a "marker" of this condi-tion consists of bi- or triphasic spikes of medium to high amplitude, usually localized over the central or centrotemporal regions. They are occasionally found

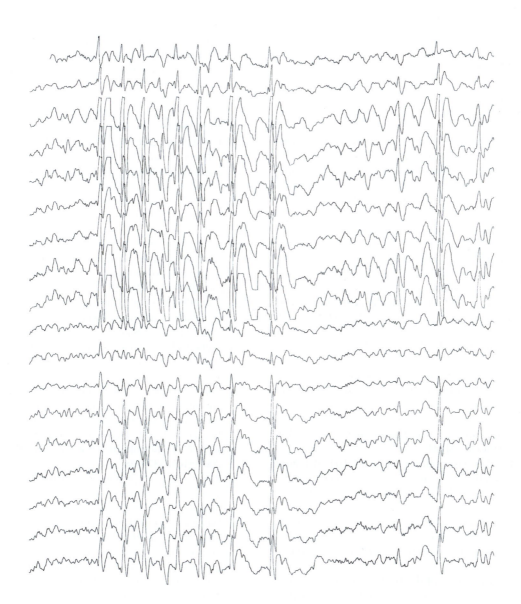

Figure 34–8. EEG abnormality in Fra-X consists of biphasic sharp waves of medium to high amplitude, usually localized over the central or centrotemporal regions, activated by sleep, as seen in benign childhood epilepsy with centro-temporal spikes.

over the posterior regions or as multifocal independent foci. Discharges may be isolated or occur in brief sequences, rarely associated with spike-and-wave complexes and activated by sleep, as seen in benign childhood epilepsy with centrotemporal spikes. (Fig. 34–8). This pattern occurs in up to 50% of patients and appears age related in its expression. Discharges typically disappear in the second decade of life.[153,156]

► PHENOTYPE–GENOTYPE CORRELATION

Clinical variability in seizure type may be a function of the great variability of amplification of the trinucleotide repeat among patients.[157]

REFERENCES

1. Battaglia A, Guerrini R. Chromosomal disorders associated with epilepsy. *Epileptic Disord* 2005;7(3):181–192.
2. Battaglia A. Del 1p36 syndrome: a newly emerging clinical entity. *Brain Dev* 2005;27(5):358–361.
3. Battaglia A. et al. Further delineation of deletion 1p36 syndrome in 60 patients: a recognizable phenotype and common cause of developmental delay and mental retardation. *Pediatrics* 2008;121(2):404–410.
4. Slavotinek A, Shaffer LG, Shapira SK. Monosomy 1p36. *J Med Genet* 1999;36(9):657–663.
5. Bahi-Buisson N, et al. Spectrum of epilepsy in terminal 1p36 deletion syndrome. *Epilepsia* 2008;49(3):509–15.
6. Shapira SK, et al. Chromosome 1p36 deletions: the clinical phenotype and molecular characterization of a common newly delineated syndrome. *Am J Hum Genet* 1997;61(3):642–650.
7. Shaffer LG, Heilstedt HA. Terminal deletion of 1p36. *Lancet* 2001;358(Suppl):S9.
8. Kurosawa K, et al. Epilepsy and neurological findings in 11 individuals with 1p36 deletion syndrome. *Brain Dev* 2005;27(5):378–382.
9. Battaglia A, Carey JC. Wolf–Hirschhorn syndrome and the 4p-related syndromes. *Am J Med Genet C Semin Med Genet* 2008;148C(4):241–243.
10. Wu YQ, et al. Molecular refinement of the 1p36 deletion syndrome reveals size diversity and a preponderance of maternally derived deletions. *Hum Mol Genet* 1999;8(2):313–321.
11. Heilstedt HA, et al. Physical map of 1p36, placement of breakpoints in monosomy 1p36, and clinical characterization of the syndrome. *Am J Hum Genet* 2003;72(5):1200–1212.
12. Heilstedt HA, et al. Loss of the potassium channel beta-subunit gene, KCNAB2, is associated with epilepsy in patients with 1p36 deletion syndrome. *Epilepsia* 2001;42(9):1103–1111.
13. Wright TJ, et al. Wolf–Hirschhorn and Pitt–Rogers–Danks syndromes caused by overlapping 4p deletions. *Am J Med Genet* 1998;75(4):345–350.
14. Lurie IW, et al. The Wolf–Hirschhorn syndrome. I. Genetics. *Clin Genet* 1980;17(6):375–384.
15. Battaglia A, et al. Karyotype/phenotype correlations in duplication 4q: evidence for a critical region within 4q27–28 for preaxial defects. *Am J Med Genet A* 2005;134(3):334–337.
16. Battaglia A, Filippi T, Carey JC. Update on the clinical features and natural history of Wolf–Hirschhorn (4p-) syndrome: experience with 87 patients and recommendations for routine health supervision. *Am J Med Genet C Semin Med Genet* 2008;148C(4):246–251.
17. Zollino M, Neri G. Genotype-phenotype correlations in Wolf–Hirschhorn syndrome. *Eur J Hum Genet* 2001;9(2):150.
18. Battaglia A, et al. Spectrum of epilepsy and electroencephalogram patterns in Wolf–Hirschhorn syndrome: experience with 87 patients. *Dev Med Child Neurol* 2009;51(5):373–380.
19. Sgro V, et al. 4p(-) syndrome: a chromosomal disorder associated with a particular EEG pattern. *Epilepsia* 1995;36(12):1206–1214.
20. Battaglia A, Carey JC. Wright TJ. Wolf–Hirschhorn (4p-) syndrome. *Adv Pediatr* 2001;48:75–113.
21. Kagitani-Shimono K, et al. Epilepsy in Wolf–Hirschhorn syndrome (4p-). *Epilepsia* 2005;46(1):150–155.
22. Battaglia A, Carey JC. Seizure and EEG patterns in Wolf–Hirschhorn (4p-) syndrome. *Brain Dev* 2005;27(5):362–364.
23. Valente KD, et al. A study of EEG and epilepsy profile in Wolf–Hirschhorn syndrome and considerations regarding its correlation with other chromosomal disorders. *Brain Dev* 2003;25(4):283–287.
24. Battaglia A, et al. Natural history of Wolf–Hirschhorn syndrome: experience with 15 cases. *Pediatrics* 1999;103(4 Pt 1):830–836.
25. Battaglia D, et al. Electroclinical patterns and evolution of epilepsy in the 4p- syndrome. *Epilepsia* 2003;44(9):1183–1190.
26. Miller OJ, et al. Partial deletion of the short arm of chromosome no. 4(4p-): clinical studies in five unrelated patients. *J Pediatr* 1970;77(5):792–801.
27. Bergemann AD. Distinctive EEG patterns in patients with Wolf–Hirschhorn syndrome. *Dev Med Child Neurol* 2009;51(5):337–338.
28. Wright TJ, et al. A transcript map of the newly defined 165 kb Wolf–Hirschhorn syndrome critical region. *Hum Mol Genet* 1997;6(2):317–324.
29. Wright TJ, et al. Comparative analysis of a novel gene from the Wolf–Hirschhorn/Pitt-Rogers-Danks syndrome critical region. *Genomics* 1999;59(2):203–212.
30. Johnson VP, et al. FISH detection of Wolf–Hirschhorn syndrome: exclusion of D4F26 as critical site. *Am J Med Genet* 1994;52(1):70–74.
31. Wieczorek D, et al. Effect of the size of the deletion and clinical manifestation in Wolf–Hirschhorn syndrome:

analysis of 13 patients with a de novo deletion. *Eur J Hum Genet* 2000;8(7):519–526.

32. Maas NM, et al. Genotype-phenotype correlation in 21 patients with Wolf–Hirschhorn syndrome using high resolution array comparative genome hybridisation (CGH). *J Med Genet* 2008;45(2):71–80.

33. Shannon NL, et al. An epidemiological study of Wolf–Hirschhorn syndrome: life expectancy and cause of mortality. *J Med Genet* 2001;38(10):674–679.

34. Kyllerman M. On the prevalence of Angelman syndrome. *Am J Med Genet* 1995;59(3):405; author reply 403–404.

35. Petersen MB, et al. Clinical, cytogenetic, and molecular diagnosis of Angelman syndrome: estimated prevalence rate in a Danish county. *Am J Med Genet* 1995;60(3):261–262.

36. Fombonne E, et al. Prevalence of pervasive developmental disorders in the British nationwide survey of child mental health. *J Am Acad Child Adolesc Psychiatry* 2001;40(7):820–827.

37. Fombonne E, et al. Pervasive developmental disorders in Montreal, Quebec, Canada: prevalence and links with immunizations. *Pediatrics* 2006;118(1):e139–e150.

38. Williams CA, et al. Angelman syndrome: consensus for diagnostic criteria. Angelman Syndrome Foundation. *Am J Med Genet* 1995;56(2):237–238.

39. Williams CA, et al. Angelman syndrome 2005: updated consensus for diagnostic criteria. *Am J Med Genet A* 2006;140(5):413–418.

40. Zori RT, et al. Angelman syndrome: clinical profile. *J Child Neurol* 1992;7(3):270–280.

41. Minassian BA, et al. Angelman syndrome: correlations between epilepsy phenotypes and genotypes. *Ann Neurol* 1998;43(4):485–493.

42. Laan LA, et al. Evolution of epilepsy and EEG findings in Angelman syndrome. *Epilepsia* 1997;38(2):195–199.

43. Valente KD, et al. Epilepsy in patients with angelman syndrome caused by deletion of the chromosome 15q11–13. *Arch Neurol* 2006;63(1):122–128.

44. Sugimoto T, et al. Angelman syndrome in three siblings: characteristic epileptic seizures and EEG abnormalities. *Epilepsia* 1992;33(6):1078–1082.

45. Matsumoto A, et al. Epilepsy in Angelman syndrome associated with chromosome 15q deletion. *Epilepsia* 1992;33(6):1083–1090.

46. Guerrini R, et al. Cortical myoclonus in Angelman syndrome. *Ann Neurol* 1996;40(1):39–48.

47. Clayton-Smith J. Clinical research on Angelman syndrome in the United Kingdom: observations on 82 affected individuals. *Am J Med Genet* 1993;46(1):12–15.

48. Buoni S, et al. Diagnosis of Angelman syndrome: clinical and EEG criteria. *Brain Dev* 1999;21(5):296–302.

49. Viani F, et al. Seizure and EEG patterns in Angelman's syndrome. *J Child Neurol* 1995;10(6):467–471.

50. Buntinx IM, et al. Clinical profile of Angelman syndrome at different ages. *Am J Med Genet* 1995;56(2):176–183.

51. Laan LA, et al. Angelman syndrome in adulthood. *Am J Med Genet* 1996;66(3):356–360.

52. Valente KD, et al. Angelman syndrome: difficulties in EEG pattern recognition and possible misinterpretations. *Epilepsia* 2003;44(8):1051–1063.

53. Boyd SG, Harden A, Patton MA. The EEG in early diagnosis of the Angelman (happy puppet) syndrome. *Eur J Pediatr* 1988;147(5):508–513.

54. Williams CA, Lossie A, Driscoll D. Angelman syndrome: mimicking conditions and phenotypes. *Am J Med Genet* 2001;101(1):59–64.

55. Knoll JH, Nicholls RD, Lalande M. On the parental origin of the deletion in Angelman syndrome. *Hum Genet* 1989;83(2):205–207.

56. Magenis RE, et al. Is Angelman syndrome an alternate result of del(15)(q11q13)? *Am J Med Genet* 1987;28(4):829–838.

57. Nicholls RD, et al. Paternal uniparental disomy of chromosome 15 in a child with Angelman syndrome. *Ann Neurol* 1992;32(4):512–518.

58. Buiting K, et al. Inherited microdeletions in the Angelman and Prader-Willi syndromes define an imprinting centre on human chromosome 15. *Nat Genet* 1995;9(4):395–400.

59. Kishino T, Lalande M, Wagstaff J. UBE3A/E6-AP mutations cause Angelman syndrome. *Nat Genet* 1997;15(1):70–73.

60. Matsuura T, et al. De novo truncating mutations in E6-AP ubiquitin-protein ligase gene (UBE3A) in Angelman syndrome. *Nat Genet* 1997;15(1):74–77.

61. Williams CA, et al. Incidence of 15q deletions in the Angelman syndrome: a survey of twelve affected persons. *Am J Med Genet* 1989;32(3):339–345.

62. Engel E. Chromosome 15 uniparental disomy is not frequent in Angelman syndrome. *Am J Hum Genet* 1991;49(2):459–460.

63. Dittrich B, Buiting K, Horsthemke B. PW71 methylation test for Prader-Willi and Angelman syndromes. *Am J Med Genet* 1996;61(2):196–197.

64. Burger J, et al. Different mechanisms and recurrence risks of imprinting defects in Angelman syndrome. *Am J Hum Genet* 1997;61(1):88–93.

65. DeLorey TM, et al. Mice lacking the beta3 subunit of the GABAA receptor have the epilepsy phenotype and many of the behavioral characteristics of Angelman syndrome. *J Neurosci* 1998;18(20):8505–8514.

66. DeLorey TM, Olsen RW. GABA and epileptogenesis: comparing gabrb3 gene-deficient mice with Angelman syndrome in man. *Epilepsy Res* 1999;36(2–3):123–132.

67. Ruggieri M, McShane MA. Parental view of epilepsy in Angelman syndrome: a questionnaire study. *Arch Dis Child* 1998;79(5):423–426.

68. Odano I, et al. Decrease in benzodiazepine receptor binding in a patient with Angelman syndrome detected by iodine-123 iomazenil and single-photon emission tomography. *Eur J Nucl Med* 1996;23(5):598–604.

69. Franz DN, et al. Topiramate therapy of epilepsy associated with Angelman's syndrome. *Neurology* 2000;54(5):1185–1188.

70. Sugiura C, et al. High-dose ethosuximide for epilepsy in Angelman syndrome: implication of GABA(A) receptor subunit. *Neurology* 2001;57(8):1518–1819.

71. Weber P. Levetiracetam in nonconvulsive status epilepticus in a child with Angelman syndrome. *J Child Neurol* 2009;25:393–396.

72. Varela MC, et al. Phenotypic variability in Angelman syndrome: comparison among different deletion classes and between deletion and UPD subjects. *Eur J Hum Genet* 2004;12(12):987–992.

73. Blennow E, et al. Swedish survey on extra structurally abnormal chromosomes in 39 105 consecutive prenatal diagnoses: prevalence and characterization by fluorescence in situ hybridization. *Prenat Diagn* 1994;14(11):1019–1028.

74. Hou JW, Wang TR. Unusual features in children with inv dup(15) supernumerary marker: a study of genotype-phenotype correlation in Taiwan. *Eur J Pediatr* 1998;157(2):122–127.

75. Schinzel A, Niedrist D. Chromosome imbalances associated with epilepsy. *Am J Med Genet* 2001;106(2):119–124.

76. Battaglia A, et al. The inv dup(15) syndrome: a clinically recognizable syndrome with altered behavior, mental retardation, and epilepsy. *Neurology* 1997;48(4):1081–1086.

77. Valente KD, et al. Inv dup (15): is the electroclinical phenotype helpful for this challenging clinical diagnosis? *Clin Neurophysiol* 2006;117(4):803–809.

78. Battaglia A. The inv dup(15) or idic(15) syndrome: a clinically recognisable neurogenetic disorder. *Brain Dev* 2005;27(5):365–369.

79. Crolla JA, et al. Supernumerary marker 15 chromosomes: a clinical, molecular and FISH approach to diagnosis and prognosis. *Hum Genet* 1995;95(2):161–170.

80. Gillberg C, et al. Autism associated with marker chromosome. *J Am Acad Child Adolesc Psychiatry* 1991;30(3):489–494.

81. Robinson WP, et al. Clinical and molecular analysis of five inv dup(15) patients. *Eur J Hum Genet* 1993;1(1):37–50.

82. Webb T, et al. Clinical, A, cytogenetic and molecular study of ten probands with supernumerary inv dup (15) marker chromosomes. *Clin Genet* 1998;53(1):34–43.

83. Buoni S, et al. The syndrome of inv dup (15): clinical, electroencephalographic, and imaging findings. *J Child Neurol* 2000;15(6):380–385.

84. Borgatti R, et al. Pervasive developmental disorders and GABAergic system in patients with inverted duplicated chromosome 15. *J Child Neurol* 2001;16(12):911–914.

85. Borgatti R, et al. Relationship between clinical and genetic features in "inverted duplicated chromosome 15" patients. *Pediatr Neurol* 2001;24(2):111–116.

86. Bingham PM, et al. Infantile spasms associated with proximal duplication of chromosome 15q. *Pediatr Neurol* 1996;15(2):163–165.

87. Chifari R, et al. Mild generalized epilepsy and developmental disorder associated with large inv dup(15). *Epilepsia* 2002;43(9):1096–1100.

88. Kobayashi Y, Yoshino A. A case of inv dup (15) mosaic with mental retardation and symptomatic generalized epilepsy. *No To Shinkei* 1999;51(3):259–262.

89. Takeda Y, et al. Symptomatic generalized epilepsy associated with an inverted duplication of chromosome 15. *Seizure* 2000;9(2):145–150.

90. Torrisi L, et al. Rearrangements of chromosome 15 in epilepsy. *Am J Med Genet* 2001;106(2):125–128.

91. Elia M, et al. Myoclonic absence-like seizures and chromosome abnormality syndromes. *Epilepsia* 1998;39(6):660–663.

92. Aguglia U, et al. Emotion-induced myoclonic absence-like seizures in a patient with inv-dup(15) syndrome: a clinical, EEG, and molecular genetic study. *Epilepsia* 1999;40(9):1316–1319.

93. Knoll JH, et al. Angelman and Prader-Willi syndromes share a common chromosome 15 deletion but differ in parental origin of the deletion. *Am J Med Genet* 1989;32(2):285–290.

94. Browne CE, et al. Inherited interstitial duplications of proximal 15q: genotype–phenotype correlations. *Am J Hum Genet* 1997;61(6):1342–1352.

95. Leana-Cox J, et al. Molecular cytogenetic analysis of inv dup(15) chromosomes, using probes specific for the Prader-Willi/Angelman syndrome region: clinical implications. *Am J Hum Genet* 1994;54(5):748–756.

96. Roberts SE, et al. Characterisation of interstitial duplications and triplications of chromosome 15q11-q13. *Hum Genet* 2002;110(3):227–234.

97. Huang B, et al. Refined molecular characterization of the breakpoints in small inv dup(15) chromosomes. *Hum Genet* 1997;99(1):11–17.

98. Long FL, et al. Triplication of 15q11-q13 with inv dup(15) in a female with developmental delay. *J Med Genet* 1998;35(5):425–428.

99. Ville D, et al. Early pattern of epilepsy in the ring chromosome 20 syndrome. *Epilepsia* 2006;47(3):543–549.

100. Serrano-Castro PJ. Ring chromosome 20 epilepsy syndrome in children: electroclinical features. *Neurology* 2002;58(6):987; author reply 987.

101. Canevini MP, et al. Chromosome 20 ring: a chromosomal disorder associated with a particular electroclinical pattern. *Epilepsia* 1998;39(9):942–951.

102. Alpman A, et al. Ring chromosome 20 syndrome with intractable epilepsy. *Dev Med Child Neurol* 2005;47(5):343–346.

103. Jacobs J, et al. Refractory and lethal status epilepticus in a patient with ring chromosome 20 syndrome. *Epileptic Disord* 2008;10(4):254–259.

104. Inoue Y, et al. Ring chromosome 20 and nonconvulsive status epilepticus. A new epileptic syndrome. *Brain* 1997;120(Pt 6):939–953.

105. Petit J, et al. Non-convulsive status in the ring chromosome 20 syndrome: a video illustration of 3 cases. *Epileptic Disord* 1999;1(4):237–241.

106. Gonzalez-Delgado M, et al. Ring chromosome 20: a distinctive syndrome identifiable by electroclinical diagnosis. *Neurologia* 2004;19(4):215–219.

107. Augustijn PB, et al. Ring chromosome 20 epilepsy syndrome in children: electroclinical features. *Neurology* 2001;57(6):1108–1111.

108. Kobayashi K, et al. Characteristic EEG findings in ring 20 syndrome as a diagnostic clue. *Electroencephalogr Clin Neurophysiol* 1998;107(4):258–262.

109. Back E, et al. Familial ring (20) chromosomal mosaicism. *Hum Genet* 1989;83(2):148–154.

110. Brandt CA, et al. Ring chromosome 20 with loss of telomeric sequences detected by multicolour PRINS. *Clin Genet* 1993;44(1):26–31.

111. Roubertie A, Petit J, Genton P. Ring chromosome 20: an identifiable epileptic syndrome. *Rev Neurol (Paris)* 2000;156(2):149–153.

112. Garcia-Cruz D, et al. Ring-20-syndrome and loss of telomeric regions. *Ann Genet* 2000;43(3–4):113–116.

113. de Falco FA, et al. Electroclinical evolution in ring chromosome 20 epilepsy syndrome: a case with severe phenotypic features followed for 25 years. *Seizure* 2006; 15(6):449–453.

114. Bouilleret V, et al. Involvement of the basal ganglia in refractory epilepsy: an 18F-fluoro-L-DOPA PET study using 2 methods of analysis. *J Nucl Med* 2005;46(3): 540–547.

115. Nobutoki T, et al. Continuous midazolam infusion for refractory nonconvulsive status epilepticus in children. *No To Hattatsu* 2005;37(5):369–373.

116. Parr JR, et al. Epilepsy responds to vagus nerve stimulation in ring chromosome 20 syndrome. *Dev Med Child Neurol* 2006;48(1):80; author reply 80.

117. Allen EG, et al. Maternal age and risk for trisomy 21 assessed by the origin of chromosome nondisjunction: a report from the Atlanta and National Down Syndrome Projects. *Hum Genet* 2009;125(1):41–52.

118. Hook EB. Issues pertaining to the impact and etiology of trisomy 21 and other aneuploidy in humans; a consideration of evolutionary implications, maternal age mechanisms, and other matters. *Prog Clin Biol Res* 1989; 311:1–27.

119. Fong CT, Brodeur GM. Down's syndrome and leukemia: epidemiology, genetics, cytogenetics and mechanisms of leukemogenesis. *Cancer Genet Cytogenet* 1987;28(1):55–76.

120. Zipursky A. Transient leukaemia—a benign form of leukaemia in newborn infants with trisomy 21. *Br J Haematol* 2003;120(6):930–938.

121. Mazzoni DS, Ackley RS, Nash DJ. Abnormal pinna type and hearing loss correlations in Down's syndrome. *J Intellect Disabil Res* 1994;38(Pt 6):549–560.

122. Masters CL, et al. Amyloid plaque core protein in Alzheimer disease and Down syndrome. *Proc Natl Acad Sci USA* 1985;82(12):4245–4249.

123. Wisniewski HM, Rabe A. Discrepancy between Alzheimer-type neuropathology and dementia in persons with Down's syndrome. *Ann N Y Acad Sci* 1986;477:247–260.

124. Antonarakis SE, et al. Mitotic errors in somatic cells cause trisomy 21 in about 4.5% of cases and are not associated with advanced maternal age. *Nat Genet* 1993;3(2):146–150.

125. Tatsuno M, et al. Epilepsy in childhood Down syndrome. *Brain Dev* 1984;6(1):37–44.

126. Veall RM. The prevalance of epilepsy among Mongols related to age. *J Ment Defic Res* 1974;18(2):99–106.

127. Stafstrom CE. Epilepsy in Down syndrome: clinical aspects and possible mechanisms. *Am J Ment Retard* 1993;98(Suppl):12–26.

128. Stafstrom CE, Konkol RJ. Infantile spasms in children with Down syndrome. *Dev Med Child Neurol* 1994;36(7): 576–585.

129. Crespel A, et al. Senile myoclonic epilepsy of Genton: two cases in Down syndrome with dementia and late onset epilepsy. *Epilepsy Res* 2007;77(2–3):165–168.

130. Ferlazzo E, et al. Lennox–Gastaut syndrome with late-onset and prominent reflex seizures in trisomy 21 patients. *Epilepsia* 2009;50(6):1587–1595.

131. Goldberg-Stern H, et al. Seizure frequency and characteristics in children with Down syndrome. *Brain Dev* 2001;23(6):375–378.

132. Romano C, et al. Seizures in patients with trisomy 21. *Am J Med Genet Suppl* 1990;7:298–300.

133. Smigielska-Kuzia J, et al. Clinical and EEG features of epilepsy in children and adolescents in Down syndrome. *J Child Neurol* 2009;24(4):416–420.

134. Silva ML, et al. Early clinical and EEG features of infantile spasms in Down syndrome. *Epilepsia* 1996;37(10): 977–982.

135. Nabbout R, et al. Infantile spasms in Down syndrome: good response to a short course of vigabatrin. *Epilepsia* 2001;42(12):1580–1583.

136. Kajimoto M, et al. West syndrome associated with mosaic Down syndrome. *Brain Dev* 2007;29(7):447–449.

137. Delabar JM, Aflalo-Rattenbac R, Creau N. Developmental defects in trisomy 21 and mouse models. *Scientific WorldJournal* 2006;6:1945–1964.

138. Delabar JM, et al. Submicroscopic duplication of chromosome 21 and trisomy 21 phenotype (Down syndrome). *Hum Genet* 1987;76(3):225–229.

139. Webb TP, et al. Population incidence and segregation ratios in the Martin–Bell syndrome. *Am J Med Genet* 1986;23(1–2):573–580.

140. Blomquist HK, et al. Fragile X syndrome in mildly mentally retarded children in a northern Swedish county. A prevalence study. *Clin Genet* 1983;24(6):393–398.

141. Rousseau F, et al. Prevalence of carriers of premutation-size alleles of the FMRI gene—and implications for the population genetics of the fragile X syndrome. *Am J Hum Genet* 1995;57(5):1006–1018.

142. Pellissier MC, Voelckel MA, Mattei JF. Fragile X syndrome: current knowledge. *Pediatrie* 1992;47(11):743–750.

143. Schapiro MB, et al. Adult fragile X syndrome: neuropsychology, brain anatomy, and metabolism. *Am J Med Genet* 1995;60(6):480–493.

144. Shapiro LR. The fragile X syndrome—clinical overview. *Prog Clin Biol Res* 1991;368:3–14.

145. Mattei JF, et al. Mental retardation linked to fragility of chromosome X: current knowledge. *J Genet Hum* 1984;32(3):167–192.

146. Reiss AL, et al. Psychiatric disability associated with the fragile X chromosome. *Am J Med Genet* 1986;23(1–2):393–401.

147. Devys D, et al. The FMR-1 protein is cytoplasmic, most abundant in neurons and appears normal in carriers of a fragile X premutation. *Nat Genet* 1993;4(4):335–340.

148. Sutherland GR, Jacky PB, Baker EG. Heritable fragile sites on human chromosomes. XI. Factors affecting expression of fragile sites at 10q25, 16q22, and 17p12. *Am J Hum Genet* 1984;36(1):110–122.

149. Gu Y, et al. Identification of FMR2, a novel gene associated with the FRAXE CCG repeat and CpG island. *Nat Genet* 1996;13(1):109–113.

150. Gecz J, et al. Identification of the gene FMR2, associated with FRAXE mental retardation. *Nat Genet* 1996;13(1): 105–108.

151. Wisniewski KE, et al. Fragile X syndrome: associated neurological abnormalities and developmental disabilities. *Ann Neurol* 1985;18(6):665–669.

152. Pueschel SM, Herman R, Groden G. Brief report: screening children with autism for fragile-X syndrome and phenylketonuria. *J Autism Dev Disord* 1985;15(3): 335–338.

153. Musumeci SA, et al. Epilepsy and EEG findings in males with fragile X syndrome. *Epilepsia* 1999;40(8):1092–1099.

154. Loesch DZ, Hay DA. Clinical features and reproductive patterns in fragile X female heterozygotes. *J Med Genet* 1988;25(6):407–414.

155. Kluger G, et al. Epilepsy and fragile X gene mutations. *Pediatr Neurol* 1996;15(4):358–360.

156. Wisniewski KE, et al. The Fra(X) syndrome: neurological, electrophysiological, and neuropathological abnormalities. *Am J Med Genet* 1991;38(2–3):476–480.

157. Fu YH, et al. Variation of the CGG repeat at the fragile X site results in genetic instability: resolution of the Sherman paradox. *Cell* 1991;67(6):1047–1058.

CHAPTER 35

Hypothalamic Hamartoma and Gelastic Epilepsy

Yu-tze Ng

▶ OVERVIEW

Hypothalamic hamartomas (HHs) are congenital mass lesions in the region of the third ventricle and tuber cinereum. Their true prevalence is unknown and is approximated to be 1 in 100,000. This estimated prevalence appears high but may actually be an underestimate as the diagnosis is often missed or at least significantly delayed.[1]

Two "main" clinical syndromes are recognized: precocious puberty and intractable epilepsy, including gelastic (laughing) seizures. Gelastic seizures are usually followed by the development of other seizure types including tonic, tonic–clonic, and complex partial.[2] Predominantly gelastic seizures, but also all other seizure types are often extremely refractory to antiepileptic drugs (AEDs). Associated clinical problems with the intrahypothalamic (sessile) subtype include developmental retardation, cognitive decline, and psychiatric symptoms such as mood liability and rage behavior.[3] Pedunculated lesions, which hang inferiorly from the tuber cinereum, are most likely to cause central precocious puberty, although many patients have both clinical syndromes.

There are several classifications of HHs. Arita et al classified lesions into two types on the basis of magnetic resonance imaging (MRI) characteristics. These include (1) a parahypothalamic type in which the HH is attached to the floor of the third ventricle or is pedunculated (and associated with precocious puberty) and (2) a intrahypothalamic type in which the HH is enveloped by the hypothalamus and distorts the third ventricle (more commonly associated with gelastic epilepsy, with or without precocious puberty, mental retardation, and behavioral problems).[4] The sessile or intrahypothalamic types of HHs have a prominent intraventricular component and are strongly associated with gelastic epilepsy probably because of their juxtaposition to the body of the hypothalamus and central connections.

Various therapies to control seizures have met with only limited success. These include vagal nerve stimulation, gamma-knife therapy (probably most successful), stereotactic destruction of the lesion through radio frequency, and even GnRH analogue (standard treatment for precocious puberty).[5] Initially, only single-case reports and small series reported favorable seizure control after surgical resection of the HH.[6] Subsequently, two surgical techniques have proven to be beneficial, often leading to curative results in the treatment of HH patients. These include surgical resection via an anterior transcallosal interforniceal approach and an endoscopic transventricular approach.[7–9] Although complete resection of the HH is preferential, incomplete resection with presumed complete disconnection of the HH from its attachment to the hypothalamus can also achieve seizure freedom.

▶ CLINICAL FEATURES

EPILEPSY

Gelastic seizures are the hallmark of HH. Gelastic seizures were first described by Daly and Mulder in 1957.[10] They are usually quite brief, typically lasting less than 30 seconds, and more often lasting just a few seconds in duration. They may be associated with little or no change in consciousness, particularly early in the course. They are very frequent, up to multiple seizure events hourly in severely affected patients.

Gelastic seizures are characterized by bouts of laughter which may resemble but more commonly differ from the patients' usual laughter that are associated with a slight sensation and appearance of discomfort. A related seizure type may involve crying and/or facial contraction with an exaggerated grimace; these are referred to as dacrystic seizures. Affected patients may manifest both forms of the seizures or seizures with mixed features of both types. Autonomic features such as flushing, tachycardia, and altered respiration are commonly associated. Most (but not all) seizures are simple partial with preserved awareness that are typically brief (less than 30 seconds) and lack a postictal phase. Status gelasticus is the most severe form, defined as a prolonged cluster of gelastic seizures lasting longer than 20–30 minutes although these clusters may actually last for several hours up to days.[11]

At least 75% of patients with intrahypothalamic HH develop other types of seizures.[1] These include simple and complex partial seizures, atonic, tonic, atypical absence, and generalized tonic–clonic seizures. It is hypothesized that secondary epileptogenesis results from the constant electrical discharging from the HH activating distant epileptic foci and multiple seizure types. Hence many affected patients present with severe epileptic encephalopathy resembling the Lennox–Gastaut syndrome.[2] In many patients the encephalopathymay be more detrimental than the seizures themselves.

ENCEPHALOPATHY

Associated comorbidities include developmental delay, mental retardation, rage attacks, and psychiatric symptoms consistent with autism, attention deficit hyperactivity, and obsessive-compulsive disorders. Progression of epilepsy severity and interictal electroencephalographic (EEG) abnormalities may be accompanied by cognitive decline and worsening psychiatric impairment.[1] Conversely, psychiatric, behavioral, and cognitive improvement may occur after successful epilepsy surgery. There is a strong association between the comorbidities of refractory epilepsy, cognitive impairment, and behavioral disturbance.[1]

PALLISTER–HALL SYNDROME

Most patients with HH have a sporadic form of the disease, without family history or risk of recurrence, and without associated congenital anomalies. However, roughly 5% of the subset of patients with the intrahypothalamic subtype of HH have Pallister–Hall syndrome which includes anomalies such as postradial polydactly, bifid epiglottis, and imperforate anus.[8,12] It is an autosomal dominant disease, fully penetrant but with variable expressivities, and a high new mutation rate. Specifically, Pallister–Hall syndrome is caused by genomic mutations in the *Gli3* gene, a zinc-finger transcription factor in the intracellular signaling pathway for the sonic hedgehog protein.[13] Sporadic HH cases with a somatic mutation in Gli3, demonstrated in HH tissue, but not in blood, has now been reported.[14]

PRECOCIOUS PUBERTY

Precocious puberty is predominantly associated with the pedunculated forms of the HH occurring either in isolation or with epilepsy and cognitive and behavioral impairment. As we continue to learn more about the HH, it is clear that there is overlap between the clinical presentations given the different neuroanatomical locations and forms of the HH. For example, the sessile form may be associated with isolated precocious puberty while the pedunculated form may present only with seizures. It has recently been suggested that the presence of precocious puberty (at least among the subgroup of HH patients with epilepsy) correlates with poorer intellectual functioning.[15]

▶ DIAGNOSIS AND DIAGNOSTIC STUDIES

NEUROIMAGING

Other than clinical presentation (where the diagnosis is often missed for months or even years), the definitive diagnosis is made by neuroimaging. MRI is typically required as computerized tomography may only diagnose larger HHs due to poorer resolution and reduced visualization toward the base of the brain. A dedicated imaging protocol consisting of fine cuts through the hypothalamus in both the sagittal and coronal planes is helpful for diagnosing smaller HHs.

HHs demonstrate various intensities on MRI, that is, various combinations of hyperintensity, isointensity, or hypointensity compared to normal gray matter on either T1- or T2-weighted images; they rarely enhance with gadolinium.

Analysis of MRI findings for 72 patients revealed that most HHs were hypointense on T1 (74%) and hyperintense on T2-weighted (93%) images.[16] Intrahypothalamic extension was noted in nearly all cases (97%) with frequent displacement of the postcommisural fornix and hypothalamic gray matter anteriorly. The HH nestled was between the fornix, mamillary body, and mamillothalamic tract.

Another study of 14 HH cases showed correlation of MRI and MR spectroscopy with tumor glial content.[17] Hyperintensity of the T2-weighted MRI lesions and higher myoinositol (mI)/creatine (Cr) ratios on MR spectroscopy positively correlated with higher glial content (glial/neuronal fraction as determined by histopathology).

ELECTROENCEPHALOGRAPHY

Routine scalp video-EEG monitoring in patients with HHs does not localize correctly. Although many patients with HHs evidence dramatic interictal multifocal and generalized epileptiform discharges, others do not exhibit interictal discharges. Gelastic seizures may or may be accompanied by ictal discharges and patterns. Thus, the scalp video-EEG monitoring is often misleading for localizing seizure onset. Not uncommonly seizures localize to temporal or nontemporal regions rather than the midline deep HH.

A case series of seven patients with HHs undergoing focal corticectomy following intracranial EEG recordings resulted in no improvement in their epilepsy.[18] Figures 35–1 and 35–2 illustrate the scalp-EEG recordings of the onset of two different complex partial seizures with similar semiology. As can be clearly seen, the onset of one seizure appears to originate more often from the left temporal region (Fig. 35–1), while the other originated from the right temporal region

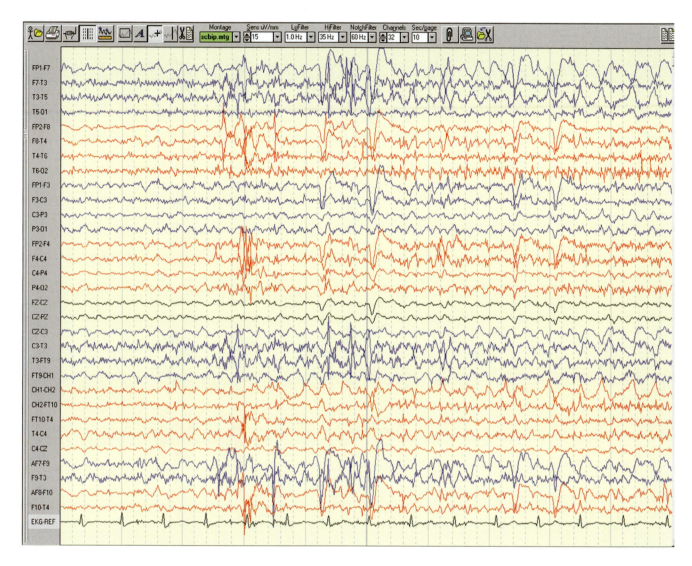

Figure 35–1. A seizure of a 24-year-old man with a hypothalamic hamartoma apparently originating from the left temporal region, albeit somewhat diffusely.

(Fig. 35–2). In addition, frequent, bilateral independent temporal lobe epileptiform discharges were noted. A HH was noted on MRI (Fig. 35–3) and endoscopic resection produced seizure freedom (Fig. 35–4).

Localization of the seizure types has been obtained predominantly by stereo video-EEG depth electrodes inserted into the hamartoma itself and ictal single-photon emission computed tomography.[19] These studies reveal that gelastic seizures but not generalized seizures originate from the HH. The origin of partial seizures and other seizure types is less clear, although they are clearly related to the HH.

HISTOPATHOLOGY

HH tissue is composed of abnormally distributed cytologically normal neurons and glia, including fibrillary astrocytes and oligodendrocytes.[20] Although neuronal elements predominate in most cases, a relative increase in astrocytic elements is seen with increasing age. Hence HHs differ from cortical dysplasia as atypical large ganglion-like balloon cells are almost never seen.

▶ TREATMENT

In the recent past, it was not even clear if the HH itself was responsible for the generation of seizures and epilepsy or if resection of the lesion would help seizures (Fig. 35–5). Despite accumulating evidence that the HH was responsible for the generation of gelastic seizures and other seizure types (either directly or via secondary epileptogenesis), safe approaches for resecting this deeply embedded tissue were not developed for several years. Currently two major neurosurgical approaches are commonly employed: the transcallosal

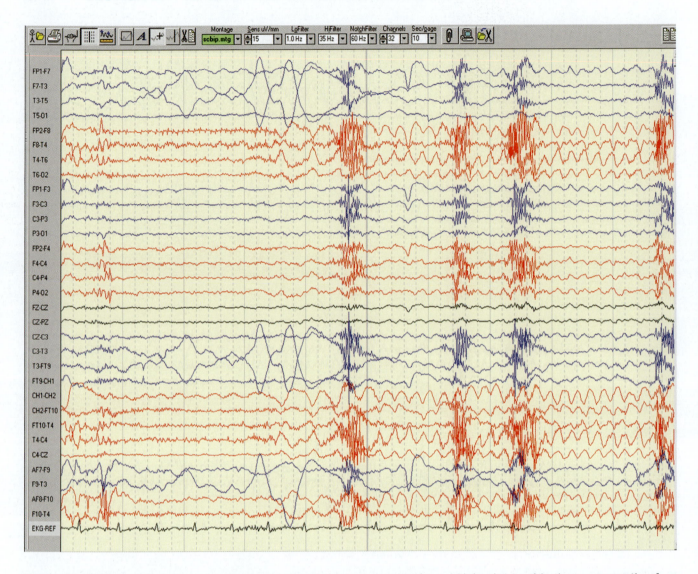

Figure 35–2. Scalp-electroencephalographic showing another complex partial seizure, this time apparently of right temporal onset in the same patient.

interforniceal approach and an endoscopic, transventricular approach.

ANTIEPILEPTIC DRUGS AND VAGUS NERVE STIMULATION

AEDs achieve limited success in the treatment of seizures in patients with HHs. In particular, gelastic seizures do not respond well to AEDs although there no specific drug study data is available.[1] Vagus nerve stimulation produced equivocal results in a series of six HH patients.[21] Many HH patients have had vagus nerve stimulators implanted with limited success and gone on to have successful HH resection. Similarly, many HH patients undergoing neurosurgery have failed treatment with the ketogenic diet although there are no specific studies evaluating the KGD and HH.[8,9]

RADIOSURGERY

Gamma-knife radiosurgery has been evaluated in preliminary results from a large study.[22] The median dose used at the marginal isodose was 17 Gy (range 13–26 Gy, mean 16.85) leading to 37% seizure freedom in 31 treated patients followed for more than 3 years.[22] Radiotherapy appears to be safe; the major side effect was transient poikilothermia in three patients.

Delay in efficacy after several months is an important issue in patients undergoing gamma-knife surgery. Gamma-knife radiosurgery is performed in patients with smaller type I lesions that are, deeply embedded in the hypothalamus and who can wait several months before surgery (i.e., the patient is not in status gelasticus).

More recently, treatment with interstitial radiosurgery with stereotactically implanted (125)I seeds was

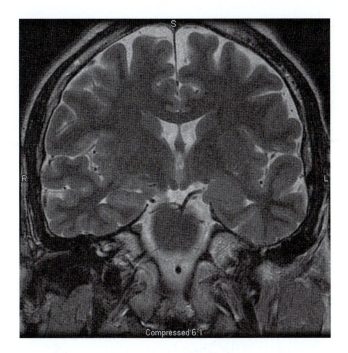

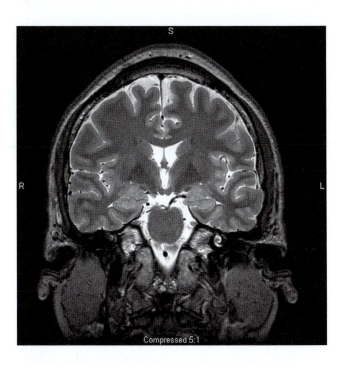

Figure 35–3. Patient's preoperative brain magnetic resonance imaging scan showing the left-sided attachment of his hypothalamic hamartoma to the hypothalamus and close proximity to the mammillary bodies.

Figure 35–4. His postoperative scan showing successful endoscopic resection of his hypothalamic hamartoma and resultant seizure freedom.

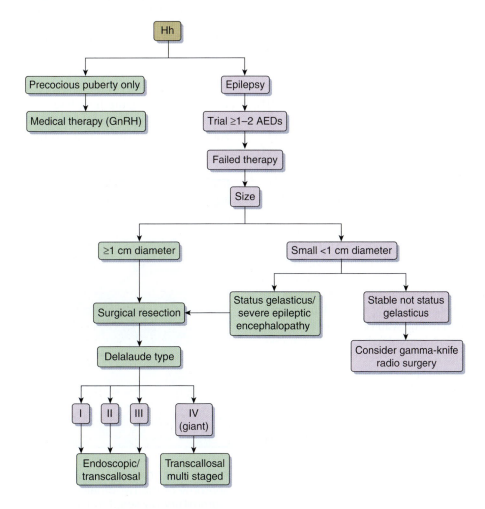

Figure 35–5. Management algorithm.

investigated.[23] At 24-month follow-up, only 12.5% of the patients were completely seizure free although 11 of 24 patients had at least a 90% reduction in seizures. Five patients developed brain edema and a few patients had cognitive dysfunction. Three of five patients with small (less than 10 mm diameter) HHs became seizure free with no significant complications after stereotactic radiofrequency thermocoagulation.[24]

SURGERY

Multiple surgical approaches and techniques have been used to resect HHs including: subfrontal, transsylvian, subtemporal, frontotemporal, pterional craniotomy, interhemispheric and translamina terminalis, and epidural subtemporopterygial approaches.[5] A combined approach from "above and below" has also been performed successfully.[25] Unfortunately, this approach is associated with high complication rates including capsular and thalamic infarcts (with associated hemiparesis), third nerve palsies and memory loss. More importantly, they often do not achieve adequate resection of the tumor and seizure activity persists.

Transcallosal Resection

Two major series of HH patients underwent transcallosal resection with very similar results. Rosenfeld (2001) was the first to describe the transcallosal, anterior interforniceal approach for the microsurgical resection of HH in five patients with refractory epilepsy.[6] A subsequent surgical method was performed utilizing a more anterior trajectory to minimize dissection and retraction of the columns of the fornix.[8] Surgery was performed with the patient's head rotated approximately 45° contralateral to the attachment side of the HH. This modification permits gravity to assist with the exposure of the corpus callosum and for the HH to "fall down" from its attachment to the hypothalamus (Fig. 35–6). This results in minimal retraction on the hemisphere. Once the corpus callosum is transected and the actual or potential space of the cavum septum pellucidum is traversed, the surgeon has an unobstructed view of the hamartoma, which is often attached to one wall of the third ventricle while the contralateral is uninvolved. Guided by frameless stereotaxis, the goal of the procedure is to remove all of the mass if possible (Fig. 35–7). At the end of the procedure, the pial surface above the interpeduncular cistern is identified.

The first large series of HH patients with intractable epilepsy was treated by an anterior transcallosal interforniceal approach. Fifty-two percent of 29 patients became seizure free and the complication rate was low ("Australian" series).[6,7]

Subsequently, the "Phoenix/American" experience with the transcallosal procedure in 26 patients resulted

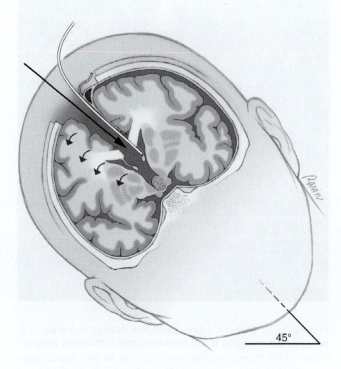

Figure 35–6. Transcallosal resection surgery performed with the head tilted to 45° to the side contralateral to the attachment of the hypothalamic hamartoma. ©Barrow Neurological Institute.

in a similar 54% seizure-freedom rate.[8] A further 35% and 24% of patients of the Phoenix and Australian series, who were not seizure free, had >90% reduction in their seizure frequency.[7,8] In addition, it was shown that seizure outcomes relate directly to the surgeon's ability to

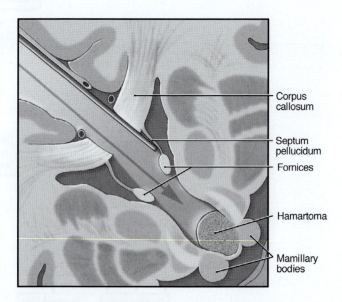

Figure 35–7. Closeup schematic diagram of the anatomy of the hypothalamic hamartoma to the mammillary bodies, fornices, and septum pellucidum. ©Barrow Neurological Institute.

remove the entire hamartoma.[8] Adverse events relating to transcallosal resection appear relatively modest in relation to seizure efficacy. A similar incidence of postoperative transient memory disturbance (56% vs. 48%) and long-term residual memory disturbance (8% vs. 13%) was noted in the Phoenix and Australian series.[7,8]

Parental perception of cognitive and behavioral postoperative changes was encouraging. Some cognitive improvement occurred in 65% of patients, and behavioral improvement was reported in 88% of patients.[8]

Endoscopic Resection

Most HH surgical procedures are endoscopic resections (except for "giant" or type IV or low-lying HHs). Surgery is performed under general anesthesia in a supine, head-up position. The preferred type of HH for neuroendoscopy is attached to only one wall of the hypothalamus (Fig. 35–8). Using frameless stereotactic guidance, the endoscope is placed into the lateral ventricle from the side opposite to the attachment of the HH. After the lateral ventricle is entered with the endoscope, the choroid plexus is followed to the foramen of Monro. The endoscope is then advanced to the foramen of Monro in a trajectory that approaches the level of the mammillary bodies. The initial disconnection is directed by the anatomic interface seen on MRI and defined by the frameless stereotaxis. With experience specific exclusion criteria can be identified. Patients with HHs

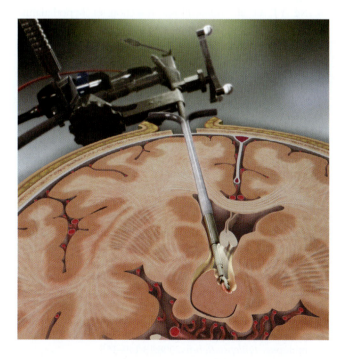

Figure 35–8. Schematic diagram of the endoscopic resection approach of the hypothalamic hamartoma from the side contralateral to the attachment and via the lateral ventricle and foramen of Monro. ©Barrow Neurological Institute.

lacking a clear interface with the hypothalamus within the third ventricle are excluded. Specifically, patients with masses filling the third ventricle are not candidates for endoscopic resection.

The largest described series of HH patients consisted of 37 patients with very frequent seizures, usually multiple types who underwent endoscopic resection.[9] Postoperative MRI demonstrated 100% resection of the HH from the hypothalamus in 12 patients. At latest follow-up [average 20.1 months (range 13–28 months)], 18 (48.6%) patients were seizure free, 26 (70.3%) patients had >90% reduction in their seizures, and another 8 (21.6%) of patients had 50%–90% seizure reduction. The most common short-term postoperative effects were transient, short-term memory problems in five patients (13.5%). However, this persisted in only three patients (8.2%). Other adverse reactions included mild, transient hemiparesis in four patients

Comparison of Endoscopic with Transcallosal Patients (Phoenix Group)

The size of the HH treated endoscopically (median 1.01 cm³, range, 0.13–11.7 cm³) was significantly smaller than that of HHs treated through the transcallosal approach (median 2.43 cm³; range, 0.41–15.7 cm³), $p = 0.0322$ by Satterthwaite t test. There was no difference between the efficacies of treatment in our patients who underwent a transcallosal approach compared to those who underwent endoscopic resection. In the transcallosal group, 54% were seizure free (vs. 49% of the endoscopic group) and the frequency of seizures was reduced more than 90% (vs. 70% of the endoscopic group), $p = 0.5136$ by χ^2-square test.[6] Postoperatively, the length of hospitalization for patients undergoing transcallosal resection (median 7.7 days, standard deviation [SD], 4.6 days) was significantly longer than the length of hospitalization for patients undergoing endoscopic resection (mean, 4.5 days; SD, 4.1; [$p = 0.0006$, Satterthwaite t test]). The long-term rates of short-term memory loss were comparable in patients regardless of their surgical treatment (transcallosal group, 2 of 26 patients; endoscopy group, 3 of 37 patients, $p = 1.0000$, Fisher exact test).

▶ SUMMARY

HHs are rare but significant congenital malformations of the inferior hypothalamus with typical triad of refractory mixed epilepsy and trademark gelastic seizures, precocious puberty, and cognitive/behavioral abnormalities. Once considered inoperable (epileptogenic) lesions, HH can, in fact, be surgically resected with a reasonable margin of safety. Resecting or radiating HH tissue with Gamma-knife radiosurgery requires a minimum of several months before significant improvements can be seen, a disadvantage of performing only Gamma-knife radiosurgery. In addition, to date only smaller HH lesions have/can be treated with gamma-knife radiosurgery.

No significant difference in the seizure-free rates after surgery between patients undergoing endoscopic (49%) compared to those undergoing transcallosal resection (54%) has been found.[9] Both rates are similar to other published results. Although each patient is reviewed on an individual basis, endoscopic resection of HH is favored by the Phoenix group. If the HH tumor is too large and attached bilaterally to the hypothalamus, transcallosal resection may be performed.

Two-thirds of the patients with complete (100%) endoscopic resection of an HH became seizure-free compared to 89% of the transcallosal patients.[9] Eighty-six percent of the endoscopic patients reported improvement in either cognition, behavior, or both. Epileptic encephalopathy, typically consisting of developmental delay/mental retardation and behavior with rage attacks, is an equally, if not more, devastating result of HH than seizures. The probability of improving these symptoms is another reason for advocating early surgical treatment of HHs.

The Phoenix group has "come full circle" with very recent successful results from ten patients with inferior plane of attachment who underwent orbitozygomatic rection.[26] Eight patients had >50% seizure reduction with four (40%) becoming seizure free.[26] There is ongoing debate as to whether HHs should be resected from below. There have been some anecdotal cases from elsewhere and locally with limited success following orbitozygomatic (inferior) resection hence opinions are divided.

Secondary epileptogenesis, in which the neocortex begins to generate seizures independently after a prolonged period of seizures generated by an HH, is a well-described phenomenon.[2] The associated "running down" phenomenon, which may represent the reversal of secondary epileptogenesis, was observed in two transcallosal series, 21% and 40% of the patients, respectively, had seizures in the intermediate to short-term postoperative period. However, eventually, they became seizure free.[7,8] This phenomenon was not observed in the patients treated endoscopically. Not one patient who had seizures in the short-term postoperative period became seizure free. The absence of immediate postoperative seizures was 23 times more likely to lead to long-term freedom from seizures than the presence of postoperative seizures.

▶ ACKNOWLEDGMENTS

Thank you to my good friend and colleague Dr Harold Rekate for helping write the neurosurgical treatment sections. He is the neurosurgeon who has performed all the HH surgeries for the Phoenix group, without whom our HH program would not be possible.

REFERENCES

1. Kerrigan JF, Ng YT, Chung S, Rekate HL. The hypothalamic hamartoma: a model of subcortical epileptogenesis and encephalopathy. *Sem Pediatr Neurol* 2005;12:119–131.
2. Freeman JL, Harvey AS, Rosenfeld JV, Wrennall JA, Bailey CA, Berkovic SF. Generalized epilepsy in hypothalamic hamartoma: evolution and postoperative resolution. *Neurology* 2003;60:762–767.
3. Berkovic SF, Andermann F, Melanson D, Ethier RE, Feindel W, Gloor P. Hypothalamic hamartomas and ictal laughter: evolution of a characteristic epileptic syndrome and diagnostic value of magnetic resonance imaging. *Ann Neurol* 1988;23:429–439.
4. Arita K, et al. The relationship between magnetic resonance imaging findings and clinical manifestations of hypothalamic hamartoma. *J Neurosurg* 1999;91:212–220.
5. Ng YT, Rekate HL, Kerrigan JF, Prenger E, Rosenfeld JV, Spetzler RF. Transcallosal resection of hypothalamic hamartoma: case report. *Barrow Quarterly* 2004;20:13–17.
6. Rosenfeld JV, Harvey AS, Wrennall J, Zacharin M, Berkovic SF. Transcallosal resection of hypothalamic hamartomas, with control of seizures, in children with gelastic epilepsy. *Neurosurgery* 2001;48:108–118.
7. Harvey AS, Freeman JL, Berkovic SF, Rosenfeld JV. Transcallosal resection of hypothalamic hamartomas in patients with intractable epilepsy. *Epileptic Disord* 2003;5:257–265.
8. Ng YT, et al. Transcallosal resection of hypothalamic hamartomas with intractable epilepsy. *Epilepsia* 2006;47:1192–1202.
9. Ng YT, et al. Endoscopic resection of hypothalamic hamartomas for refractory symptomatic epilepsy. *Neurology* 2008;70:1543–1548.
10. Daly DD, Mulder DW. Gelastic epilepsy. *Neurology* 1957;7:189–192.
11. Ng YT, Rekate HL. Coining of a new term, "Status Gelasticus". *Epilepsia* 2006;47:661–662.
12. Hall JG, et al. Congenital hypothalamic hamartoblastoma, hypopituitarism, imperforate anus and postaxial polydactyly—a new syndrome? Part I: clinical, causal, and pathogenetic considerations. *Am J Med Genet* 1980;7:47–74.
13. Kang S, et al. Linkage mapping and phenotypic analysis of autosomal dominant Pallister-Hall syndrome. *J Med Genet* 1997;34:441–446.
14. Craig DW, et al. Identification of somatic chromosomal abnormalities in hypothalamic hamartoma tissue at the GLI3 locus. *Am J Hum Genet* 2008;82:366–374.
15. Prigatano GP, et al. Intellectual functioning in presurgical patients with hypothalamic hamartoma and refractory epilepsy. *Epilepsy Behav* 2008;13:149–155.
16. Freeman JL, et al. MR imaging and spectroscopic study of epileptogenic hypothalamic hamartomas: analysis of 71 cases. *AJNR Am J Neuroradiol* 2004;25:450–462.
17. Amstutz DR, Coons SW, Kerrigan JF, Rekate HL, Heiserman JE. Hypothalamic hamartomas: correlation of MR imaging

and spectroscopic findings with tumor glial content. *AJNR Am J Neuroradiol* 2006;27:794–798.

18. Cascino GD, et al. Gelastic seizures and hypothalamic hamartomas: evaluation of patients undergoing chronic intracranial EEG monitoring and outcome of surgical treatment. *Neurology* 1993;43:747–750.

19. Ng YT, Kerrigan JF. Symptomatic seizures and epilepsy related to hypothalamic hamartomas. *Barrow Quarterly* 2004;20:18–22.

20. Coons SW, et al. The histopathology of hypothalamic hamartomas: study of 57 cases. *J Neuropathol Exp Neurol* 2007;66:131–141.

21. Murphy JV, Wheless JW, Schmoll CM. Left vagal nerve stimulation in six patients with hypothalamic hamartomas. *Pediatr Neurol* 2000;23:167–168.

22. Regis J, et al. Epilepsy related to hypothalamic hamartomas: surgical management with special reference to gamma-knife surgery. *Childs Nerv Syst* 2006;22:881–895.

23. Schulze-Bonhage A, et al. Outcome and predictors of interstitial radiosurgery in the treatment of gelastic epilepsy. *Neurology* 2008;71:277–282.

24. Homma J, et al. Stereotactic radiofrequency thermocoagulation for hypothalamic hamartoma with intractable gelastic seizures. *Epilepsy Res* 2007;76:15–21.

25. Gore PA, Nakaji P, Deshmukh V, Rekate HL. Synchronous endoscopy and microsurgery: a novel strategy to approach complex ventricular lesions. Report of three cases. *J Neurosurg* 2006;105(6 Suppl):485–489.

26. Abla AA, et al. Orbitozygomatic resection for hypothalamic hamartoma and epilepsy: patient selection and outcome. *Childs Nerv Syst* 2010;27:265–277.

CHAPTER 36

Hemispheric Disorders Associated with Cortical Malformation

Michael Duchowny

▶ OVERVIEW

Disorders of neurogenesis, neuronal maturation, and proliferation are responsible for many severe forms of childhood epilepsy. They may arise in discrete cortical areas or involve widespread brain regions in one or both cerebral hemispheres. While extensive unilateral involvement of one cerebral hemisphere is a relatively uncommon condition, the rare occurrence of a hemispheric malformation is associated with a high rate of morbidity and mortality. Affected children typically manifest cognitive delay, intractable epileptic seizures, and lateralized neurological deficits.

An awareness of the clinical presentations and management (Fig. 36–1) of this unusual group of disorders is an important part of pediatric epilepsy as the frequent association of unrelenting partial seizures and clinical deterioration may prove catastrophic in the first year of life. Prompt recognition of the various underlying causes and aggressive treatment, frequently surgical, are therefore essential.

▶ HEMIMEGALENCEPHALY

Hemimegalencephaly is a rare but clinically significant brain malformation characterized by the excessive growth of one cerebral hemisphere. Hemispheric asymmetry may present at birth but typically increases during the first year of life due to progressive hemispheric expansion. Affected infants often appear normal and their head circumference and shape appear unremarkable as the hemisphere enlarges. The classical signs of raised intracranial pressure, bulging fontanel, widening of skull sutures, and the "setting sun sign" are notably absent. Either cerebral hemisphere may be affected.

Three subtypes of hemimegalencephaly are now recognized.

ISOLATED HEMIMEGALENCEPHALY

In the isolated form, unilateral hemispheric enlargement is not associated with somatic hemicorporeal hypertrophy, cutaneous manifestations or other signs of systemic involvement.[1] Isolated hemimegalencephaly accounts for approximately half of all known hemimegalencephaly cases.[2] Its occurrence is typically sporadic with no known genetic pattern of inheritance.

SYNDROMIC HEMIMEGALENCEPHALY

The second form, syndromic hemimegalencephaly, is associated with one of several well-recognized developmental syndromes, mostly neurocutaneous disorders. All have known patterns of Mendelian inheritance, and systemic involvement is common. Syndromic disorders with hemimegalencephaly include the following disorders.

EPIDERMAL NEVUS SYNDROME

Affected patients manifest cutaneous epidermal nevi that are often unilateral. The linear nevus sebaceous of Jadassohn is commonly associated. Ocular and skeletal abnormalities are frequently noted.

HYPOMELANOSIS OF ITO

This neurocutaneous disorder presents with a linear area of depigmentaion variably associated with hemimegalencephaly ipsilateral or contralateral to the skin lesion. Both macrocephaly and callosal agenesis have been observed in affected children.

INCONTINENTIA PIGMENTI

A disorder characterized by irregular marbled or wavy linear cutaneous pigmentation caused by excess melanin deposition. Cavitary lesions in subcortical white matter and loss of cerebellar cortical neurons are common. Hemimegalencephaly has been described in a portion of patients.

NEUROFIBROMATOSIS-1

Although magalencephaly is particularly frequent in this disorder, hemimegalencephaly is unusual. Neurofibromatosis-1 occurs as an autosomal dominant disorder with frequent multiple organ involvement.

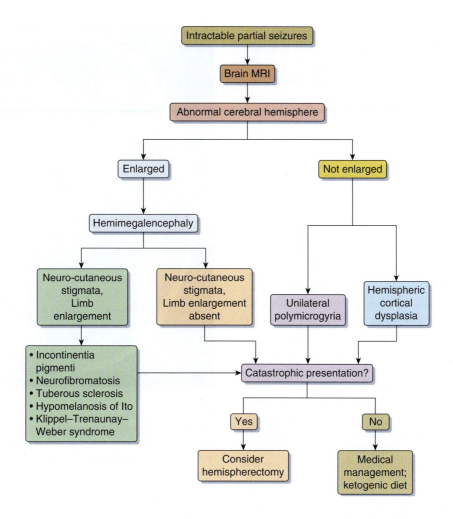

Figure 36–1. Management algorhythm: hemispheric disorders associated with cortical malformation.

KLIPPEL–TRENAUNAY–WEBER SYNDROME

Vascular nevi in conjunction with hemicorporeal enlargement of osseous and soft tissues characterize this unusual disorder. Contralateral or ipsilateral hemimegalencephaly has been described. Macrocephaly is common.

TUBEROUS SCLEROSIS COMPLEX

An association between tuberous sclerosis complex and hemimegalencephaly has been reported rarely.[3] Several overlapping histological features and the tendency for a portion of the hemisphere to calcify in both disorders has led to speculation that hemimegalencephaly may represent a more widespread expression of an underlying process also responsible for tuberous sclerosis.

TOTAL HEMIMEGALENCEPHALY

The third form, so-called "total" hemimegalencephaly, is the rarest subtype and is characterized by unilateral enlargement of the cerebellum and brainstem in con-

junction with ipsilateral hemisphere expansion. Total hemimegalencephaly occurs in either an isolated or syndromic form.

Gross inspection of the megalencephalic hemisphere reveals hemihypertrophy and polymicrogyria. Involvement is variable ranging from slight enlargement to growth of the hemisphere approaching almost twice normal size. Histological examination of hemimegalencephalic tissue demonstrates abnormal gyration, poor gray–white matter differentiation, dyslamination, neuronal cytoskeletomegaly, and subcortical and deep gray matter neuronal heterotopia.[4] The elements of abnormal cellular growth and cytomorphometry, including balloon cells, and a lack of cells in the mitotic cycle, suggest that hemimegalencephaly is primarily a disorder of neuroepithelial cell lineage and cellular growth; disordered neuronal migration may contribute to dyslamination but is probably secondary.[5]

Hemimegalencephaly presenting in infancy is often a severe disorder. There is classically a triad of symptoms—partial epilepsy, developmental regression, and hemiparesis. Seizures are often the first presenting sign and may occur on the first day of life. Partial seizures are extremely frequent with as many as 50 seizures daily. Secondary generalization is common. Antiepileptic drug therapy usually provides only limited relief and multidrug combinations are the rule in severely affected infants. Given the extremely high seizure frequencies, medical intractability can be determined rapidly in most cases.

While infants with hemimegalencephaly typically manifest pharmacoresistant seizures and global developmental delay, older children with the isolated subtype may exhibit a more benign presentation. Partial seizures are still encountered but are more easily controlled by conventional antiepileptic medications.

The diagnosis of hemimegalencephaly is made definitively on magnetic resonance imaging (MRI). Asymmetric enlargement of one cerebral hemisphere, dysplastic cortex, and unilateral deformation of the ventricular system are hallmarks of the disorder. An increased volume of white matter occurs relatively early in many patients. The midline is usually displaced laterally but there is no evidence of mass effect. The uninvolved hemisphere may appear small and distorted as a consequence of displacement. Computerized tomography typically demonstrates extensive areas of calcification that may not be appreciated on MRI. The electroencephalogram (EEG) evaluation provides supportive evidence for unihemispheric involvement including asymmetric fast frequencies, decremental patterns, and high-amplitude epileptiform discharges.[6] Normal background features are typically absent (Fig. 36–2).

Virtually every conventional antiepileptic medication and corticosteroid therapy has been administered to patients with the early-onset severe form of hemimegalencephaly. Functional hemispherectomy remains the treatment of choice for affected patients who are pharmacoresistant.[7] This procedure should be performed by an experienced neurosurgeon as the megalencephalic hemisphere lacks standard anatomic landmarks and has an enlarged vasculature with increased vascular fragility. Gaining surgical access to a larger than normal hemisphere is also technically challenging. These factors contribute to higher surgical morbidity and mortality of hemispherectomy in patients with hemimegalencephaly.

Hemispherectomy provides remission or improvement of seizures in a high proportion of cases. Improved developmental milestones and speech development are attributable to the reorganization of functionality in the normal hemisphere.[8] Seizure persistence may result from incomplete tissue removal or subtotal disconnection of the hemisphere, or more rarely from seizures due to unrecognized or underappreciated neuropathological abnormalities in the contralateral hemisphere.[9]

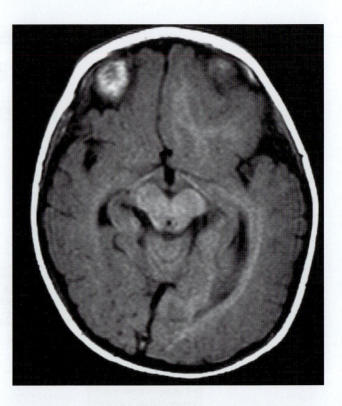

Figure 36–2. Hemimegalencephaly. Axial T1 WI of a 9-month-old girl with intractable right partial motor seizures. There is diffuse enlargement of the left cerebral hemisphere with dysplastic cortex and loss of the gray–white matter differentiation. Increased signal is noted in the left periventricular white matter. Abnormalities are seen diffusely throughout the left cerebral hemisphere. There are no focal lesions in the right cerebral hemisphere.

▶ UNILATERAL POLYMICROGYRIA

Polymicrogyria may present as a lateralized disorder with unilobar, multilobar, or hemispheric involvement. Perisylvian distribution is common but all brain regions may be affected. In a report of 20 patients with lateralized polymicrogyria, three quarters experienced seizures, contralateral hemiparesis, and cognitive delay.[10] Approximately 80% of seizures are partial while 20% are (secondarily) generalized. Multiple seizure patterns may coexist and the age of seizure onset is extremely heterogeneous. There is a significant trend for unilateral polymicrogyria to involve eloquent cortical regions, particularly sensorimotor cortex (Fig. 36–3).

A relationship between unilateral multilobar polymicrogyria and the syndrome of electrical status epilepticus during sleep (ESES) has been reported.[11] Affected children present in the first decade of life with multiple diurnal seizure types. Seizures usually remit before adolescence but the acquired neurocognitive impairment is often permanent. The unique occurrence of ESES in polymicrogyria but not other cortical

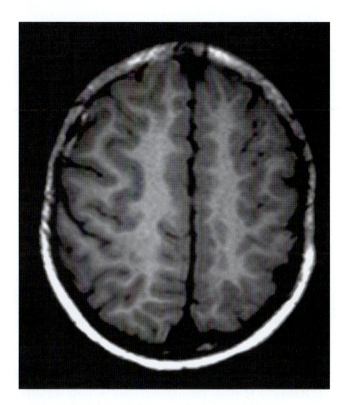

Figure 36–3. Hemispheric polymicrogyria. Axial T1 WI in a 5-year-old left-handed boy with history of congenital right hemiparesis and development delay who presented with refractory partial and secondary generalized epilepsy. There is diffuse polymicrogyria of the left hemisphere, compromising the frontal, temporal, and parietal lobes and to a much lesser degree the occipital lobe with decreased size of the left hemisphere. There is no signal abnormality in the white matter.

malformations suggests a special but as yet unknown predisposition of polymicrogyric cortex.

Treatment of seizures in patients with unilateral polymicrogyria generally consists of trials of standard antiepileptic drugs for partial epilepsy. Resection of the polymicrogyric hemisphere is much less likely to be performed given the favorable seizure prognosis and inconsistent neuropsychological outcome. A catastrophic presentation in early life often mandates serious surgical consideration.

▶ HEMISPHERIC CORTICAL DYSPLASIA

Cortical dysplasia may rarely present in a diffuse distribution throughout one cerebral hemisphere. This presentation is uncommon but, similar to unilateral polymicrogyria, often manifests in infancy with partial seizures, delayed cognitive development, and contralateral weakness. Higher grades of cortical dysplasia (Palmini type 2A and 2B) are

associated with lateralized neuroimaging findings, but low-grade dysplasia (Palmini 1A and 1B) may go undetected.

Seizures often present in the first year of life and are frequent, debilitating, and medically intractable, prompting early surgical consideration.

Hemispherectomy is indicated when there is extensive dysplastic involvement. A more conservative resection offers hope for minimizing functional compromise but often results in unsatisfactory seizure control. Hemispherectomy in infancy will optimize future recovery of function. Hemispherectomy has produced seizure freedom in two infants with Ohtahara syndrome (early infantile epileptic encephalopathy) and pharmacoresistant partial epilepsy.[12]

▶ OTHER UNILATERAL HEMISPHERIC MALFORMATIONS

Hemispheric malformations constitute a wide spectrum of disorders with variable expression. Intractable partial epilepsy may be caused by dysplastic tissue confined to

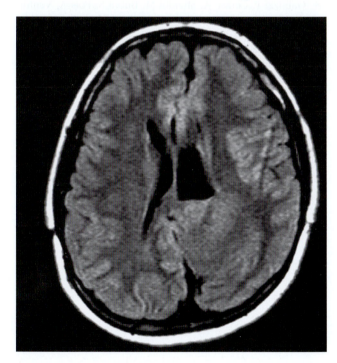

Figure 36–4. Hemispheric dysplasia and subcortical heterotopia. Axial T1 WI in a 13-year-old boy with paresthesias of the tongue, right arm, and right leg with "clawing" of the right hand. May smell burning rubber at onset or through the seizure, and may have a sensation of deja vu. There are extensive areas of cortical thickening and subcortical heterotopia in the left hemisphere compromising the temporal, parietal, and occipital lobes. Curvilinear areas of neuronal heterotopia are also identified in the temporal, parietal, and occipital lobes and in the left amygdala and hippocampal formation.

several lobes but not involving the entire hemisphere. Posterior quadrantic dysplasia or "hemihemimegalencephaly" has been reported in infants presenting with infantile spasms.[13]

Gray matter heterotopia may occur as localized nodules or in a more diffuse subcortical band-like pattern throughout the cerebral hemisphere. The heterotopic cortex is functionally active and evidences a metabolic profile on positron emission tomography (PET) that is similar to superficial cortex. Heterotopic tissue is capable of epileptogenesis and has been identified as the source of medically resistant partial seizures in patients being evaluated for surgical treatment (Fig. 36–4).

REFERENCES

1. Flores-Sarnat L. Hemimegalencephaly: part 1. Genetic, clinical and imaging aspects. *J Child Neurol* 2002;17:373–384.
2. Tinkle BT, et al. Epidemiology of hemimegalencephalaly: a case series and review. *Am J Med Genet* 2005;139:204–211.
3. Galluzzi P, Cerase A, Strambi M, Buoni S, Fois A, Venturi C. Hemimegalencephaly in tuberous sclerosis complex. *J Child Neurol* 2002;17:677–680.
4. Takashima S, et al. Aberrant neuronal development in hemimegalencephaly: immunohistochemical and golgi studies. *Pediatr Neurol* 1991;7:275–280.
5. Flores-Sarnat L, et al. Hemimegalencephaly part 2: neuropathology suggests a disorder of cellular lineage. *J Child Neurol* 2003;18:776–785.
6. Paladin F, et al. Electroencephalographic aspects of hemimegalencephaly. *Dev Med Child Neurol* 1989;31:377–383.
7. Vigevano F, et al. Hemimegalencephaly and intractable epilepsy: benefits of hemispherectomy. *Epilepsia* 1989;30:833–843.
8. Di Rocco C, et al. Hemimegalencephaly: clinical implications and surgical treatment. *Childs Nerv Syst* 2006;22:852–856.
9. Jahan R, Mischel PS, Curran JG, Peacock WJ, Shields DW, Vinters HV. Bilateral neuropathological changes in a child with hemimegalencephaly. *Pediatr Neurol* 1997;17:344–349.
10. Guerrini R, et al. Localized cortical dysplasia; good seizure outcome after sleep-related electrical status epilepticus. In: Guerrini R, Andermann F, Canapicchi R, Roger J, Zifkin B, Pfanner P (eds), *Dysplasias of Cerebral Cortex and Epilepsy*. Philadelphia, PA: New York: Lippincott-Raven, 1996, pp. 329–335.
11. Guerrini R, et al. Multilobar polymicrogyria, intractable drop attack seizures and sleep-related electrical status epilepticus. *Neurology* 1998;51:504–512.
12. Hamiwka L, et al. Hemispherectomy in early infantile epileptic encephalopathy. *J Child Neurol* 2007;22:41–44.
13. D'Agostino MD, et al. Posterior quandrantic dysplasia or hemi-hemimegalencephaly: a characteristic brain malformation. *Neurology* 2004;62:2214–2220.

CHAPTER 37

Rasmussen Syndrome

Yvonne Hart and Christian G. Bien

► OVERVIEW

Rasmussen syndrome (RS) or Rasmussen encephalitis (chronic encephalitis and epilepsy) was first described by Rasmussen et al in 1958.[1] It is an unusual condition typically developing in childhood, and is characterized by the occurrence of refractory partial epilepsy, often with *epilepsia partialis continua* (EPC), associated with progressive hemiparesis and cognitive impairment. Changes of unilateral hemispheric atrophy are seen on neuroimaging.

► CLINICAL PRESENTATION

Based on the largest available patient series, the "average" RS patient can be described as follows: he or she (there is no gender predominance in RS) starts experiencing intractable unilateral focal motor seizures or temporal lobe seizures at the age of 6 years. Later on, when the inflammatory process spreads across the affected hemisphere, new seizure semiologies indicating new epileptogenic areas are observed. EPC, that is, more or less continuous myoclonic twitching of the distal extremities or the face, is frequent. Within a few months of epilepsy onset there is a progressive loss of neurological function associated with one hemisphere, typically hemiparesis, hemianopia, and (if the dominant side is affected) aphasia.[2,3]

Serial brain magnetic resonance imaging (MRI) shows focal cortical and subcortical signal increase on T2 and fluid attenuated inversion recovery (FLAIR) images followed by progressive, centrifugal hemiatrophy of the cerebral hemisphere contralateral to the affected side of the body. The initial changes are usually peri-Sylvian; a frequent early MRI feature is volume loss of the head of the ipsilateral caudate nucleus.[4,5] After a year or so, the main decline remits, and there is a residual stage of stable neurological deficit and cerebral hemiatrophy. Seizure frequency remains high but is lower than in the "acute stage."[3] In reality, this "average" or "typical" RS patient is uncommon. Due to the complexity of potential symptoms, the presentation of RS can take a variety of different forms.

LESS COMMON PRESENTATIONS OF RS

Since the original description of RS, other presentations have been recognized. Although RS typically develops in children, a similar presentation has been described in adults.[6–8] although the course is often slower and less severe. Villani et al distinguished two phenotypes in adults: an "epileptic" form characterized by focal motor epilepsy refractory to antiepileptic drug treatment, and a "myoclonic" form with EPC and/or unilateral cortical myoclonus (focal or multifocal).

Although secondary spread of seizures to the contralateral side, or a minor degree of contralateral atrophy is sometimes seen in patients with RS, true bilateral involvement in the form of bilateral inflammation has only rarely been described,[9,10] and no case of subsequent spread to the opposite side has been reported following the successful surgical treatment of unilateral RS.[11] The bilateral nature of RS is usually apparent within 13 months of onset of the disorder.

Dual pathology, in which there is a second cerebral abnormality such as cortical dysplasia, vascular abnormality, or tuberous sclerosis, occurs in approximately 10% of patients,[12] leading to speculation that a breach in the blood-brain barrier may play a part in the genesis of the disease. Recent observations suggest that otherwise typical RS may occur in patients with delayed seizure onset,[13] or in the absence of seizures.[14] In a few patients, movement disorders including hemiathetosis and hemidystonia have been described in addition to EPC.[15,16]

► DIAGNOSIS

The most characteristic and unique feature of RS is the progressive unilateral loss of function and hemispheric atrophy occurring over several months or years. This acute stage is followed by a stable residual stage. Prior to the acute stage, a nonspecific prodromal period with less frequent seizures and occasional mild neurological deficit may be observed.[3]

Given the rarity of the syndrome, it is difficult to distinguish "typical" from "atypical" cases. To standardize the diagnosis of RS, a European consensus panel

▶ **TABLE 37–1.** DIAGNOSTIC CRITERIA FOR RASMUSSEN SYNDROME

Part A:		
1.	Clinical	Focal seizures (with or without epilepsia partialis continua) and unilateral cortical deficit(s)
2.	EEG	Unihemispheric slowing with or without epileptiform activity and unilateral seizure onset
3.	MRI	Unihemispheric focal cortical atrophy and at least one of the following: Gray or white matter signal T2/FLAIR hyperintense signal Hyperintense signal or atrophy of the ipsilateral caudate head
Part B:		
1.	Clinical	Epilepsia partialis continua or progressive[a] unilateral cortical deficit(s)
2.	MRI	Progressive[a] unihemispheric focal cortical atrophy
3.	Histopathology:	T-cell-dominated encephalitis with activated microglial cells (typically, but not necessarily forming nodules) and reactive astrogliosis Numerous parenchymal macrophages, B cells or plasma cells or positive signs of viral infections (viral inclusion bodies or immunohistochemical demonstration of viral protein) exclude the diagnosis of RE

Rasmussen syndrome can be diagnosed if either all three criteria of part A or two out of three criteria of B are present. Check first for the features of part A, then, if these are not fulfilled, of part B.

[a]'Progressive' means that at least two sequential clinical examinations or MRI studies are required to meet the respective criteria. To indicate clinical progression, each of these examinations must document a neurological deficit, and this must increase over time. To indicate progressive hemiatrophy, each of these MRIs must show hemiatrophy, and this must increase over time.

From Bien CG, Granata T, Antozzi C, et al. Pathogenesis, diagnosis and treatment of Rasmussen encephalitis: a European consensus statement. *Brain* 2005;128:454.

recently proposed formal diagnostic criteria[17] which are given in Table 37–1.

NEUROIMAGING

As in many other brain disorders, MR imaging is a diagnostic mainstay in suspected cases. Within the first 4 months after disease onset, most patients exhibit unilateral enlargement of the inner and outer cerebrospinal fluid (CSF) compartments, most marked in the insular and peri-insular regions. Atrophy of the head of the ipsilateral caudate nucleus is a typical feature of hemispheric atrophy. T2 and FLAIR signals are focally enhanced in cortical and subcortical regions, or both.

Serial MRIs reveal that during the acute stage regions of signal increase spread across the affected hemisphere leaving behind further atrophic areas.[4,5] A typical MRI course is shown in Figure 37–1. Other modern neuroimaging techniques including positron emission tomography (PET), single-photon emission computed tomography (SPECT), and magnetic resonance spectroscopy (MRS) cannot adequately define the inflammatory nature of the condition but may help confirm the unihemispheric nature in suspected early RS cases.

EEG

Pathological electroencephalography (EEG) changes in RS are characterized by polymorphic delta waves over the affected hemisphere, mainly in a centrotemporal distribution. Epileptiform abnormalities are frequent and not infrequently evolve into (subclinical) electrographic seizures. During disease evolution, initially impoverished background activity shows further flattening. Contralateral asynchronous slow waves and epileptiform discharges occur in the majority of patients.[18] Later, they may be more frequent than the ipsilateral abnormalities (which may falsely rise the suspicion of "bilateral disease").[19] As in other conditions, EPC in RS is not always accompanied by rhythmic EEG discharges on surface EEG.[20]

LABORATORY TESTS

The serum test for GluR3 antibodies, published in the mid 1990s,[21] can no longer be regarded as a useful diagnostic method. These antibodies are neither specific nor sensitive for the disease.[22–24] CSF cell counts and protein content are normal in 50% of examinations. In the remainder, moderately elevated cell counts (16–70 cells/μL, predominantly lymphocytes), and moderately increased protein concentrations (50–100 mg/dL) are observed.[25] Oligoclonal bands are an inconsistent finding ranging from 0% to 67% in three small series.[18,26,27] Therefore, standard CSF tests are insufficient to exclude or confirm the diagnosis of RE. In combination with serological tests, they can exclude central nervous system (CNS) infection by a known neurotropic agent.

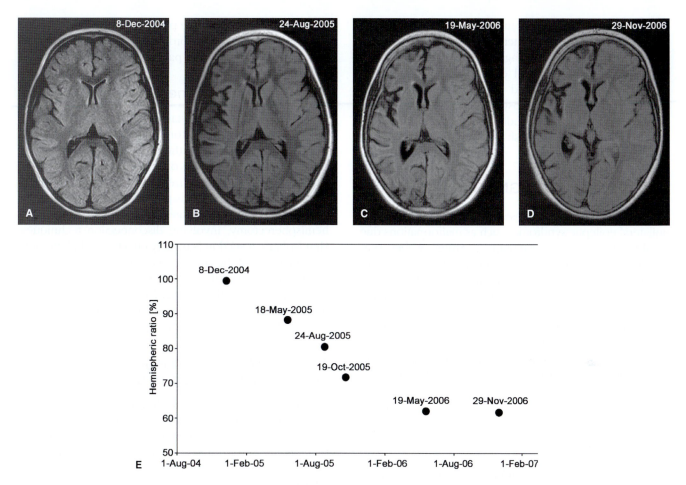

Figure 37–1. Serial brain MRI and course of cerebral atrophy in a patient with Rasmussen syndrome. (**A–D**) Serial axial fluid attenuated inversion recovery MR images in Rasmussen syndrome (RS). Symptoms of RS started in August 2004 when this girl was 8 years 10 months old. In parallel to the increasing right-sided cerebral hemiatrophy, motor function of the left-sided extremities deteriorated. Note the progressive enlargement of the right-sided sulci, the shrinkage of the subcortical white matter and the dilatation of the right anterior horn of the ventricle that progressively "replaces" the head of the ipsilateral caudate nucleus. Apparently, **C** and **D** represent the residual stage. The girl has a left-sided hemiparesis, the lower extremity is more strongly affected than the upper one. The authors thank PD Dr. H. Urbach, University of Bonn, Dept. of Radiology/ Neuroradiology, Bonn, Germany, for providing MR images. (**E**) Graphical depiction of the progressive course of hemispheric atrophy indicated by the "Hemispheric ratio" (HR). This measure indicates the relative size of the affected hemisphere compared to the unaffected one. A value of 100% means that the hemispheres are of equal size; values <100% indicate hemiatrophy. The HR is determined by planimetric quantitative assessment of axial and coronal MRI slices including the Sylvian fissure. The ratio of the pixels of the affected and the unaffected hemisphere is computed for the selected coronal and axial slices, and the mean of these two values is calculated and given in percent. (For a detailed description of the procedure, see reference [3])

BRAIN BIOPSY

As evident from Table 37–1, the diagnosis of RS rests either on a characteristic combination of features on cross-sectional, noninvasive assessment (part A criteria), or the demonstration of the progressive nature of the condition (part B criteria, 1 and 2). Only in cases in which neither can be clearly demonstrated, is brain biopsy (part B criteria, 3) indicated. This situation usually occurs in patients with very recent onset of clinical symptoms suggestive of RS (e.g., EPC) who lack other typical features. Such a patient may profit from early

conclusive diagnosis because subsequent initiation of long-term immunotherapy (see later) may prevent irreversible loss of brain tissue and function. If there are no contraindications, open biopsy of the meninges, gray and white matter is preferable. Stereotactic biopsies are more likely to yield falsely negative results due to sampling error. Even in open brain biopsy, extensive evaluation of serial sections may be necessary.

The biopsy should be taken from a noneloquent area with increased T2/FLAIR signal on MRI.[4] Alternatively, abnormal areas identified on PET or SPECT scans may be biopsied.[28] Frontal or temporal biopsies are more often positive because of a gradient of inflammatory intensity from anterior to posterior cortical areas.[29] The differential diagnosis on biopsy is small and includes: chronic viral encephalitides,[30] paraneoplastic encephalitis,[31,32] and nonparaneoplastic limbic encephalitis.[33] If brain biopsy results are inconclusive, further clinical and MRI studies (e.g., every 6 months) may be required to establish the progressive nature of the condition.

DIFFERENTIAL DIAGNOSES

The major alternative diagnoses include noninflammatory unilateral epileptic syndromes such as malformations due to abnormal cortical development, Sturge–Weber syndrome, stroke, hemiconvulsion-hemiplegia-epilepsy syndrome, and tumors including gliomatosis cerebri. Rarely, other causes of EPC must be excluded, particularly metabolic disorders (mitochondrial encephalomyopathy, lactic acidosis, and stroke-like episodes, renal, or hepatic encephalopathy) or inflammatory conditions (vasculitis, HIV, Russian spring summer meningoencephalitis, and several others). An inclusive list is provided in a recent consensus statement.[17]

▶ TREATMENT

CRITERIA FOR STARTING TREATMENT

Treatment in RS in general has two aims: first, to reduce (or potentially eliminate) the epileptic seizures, and secondly, to counteract the progressive tissue loss during the acute disease stage in order to improve the functional long-term outcome of the patients (Fig. 37–2).

Antiseizure Treatment

Antiepileptic drugs are started at seizure onset, but seizures are often refractory to treatment, and these drugs have no effect on the underlying course of the disease. Until recently the only treatment demonstrated to halt the course of the disease has been hemispherectomy. The anatomical hemispherectomies originally performed have now been largely superseded by functional hemispherectomy, involving disconnection techniques. Hemispheric resection is usually effective in halting both the seizures and the progressive cognitive deterioration, albeit sometimes at the cost of increased limb weakness in patients with early disease. More focal resections are usually unsuccessful, leading to an improvement in seizure control only in the short term, if at all.

Treatment Directed Against Hemispheric Cerebral Degeneration

Existing data indicate that in RS brain cells degenerate as a consequence of chronic inflammatory processes. Therefore, immunosuppressive or immunomodulatory treatments are promising candidates to prevent tissue loss and improve the functional long-term outcome of affected individuals. Several treatment approaches have been reported in case reports or small, usually uncontrolled patient series, mostly with beneficial effects. As

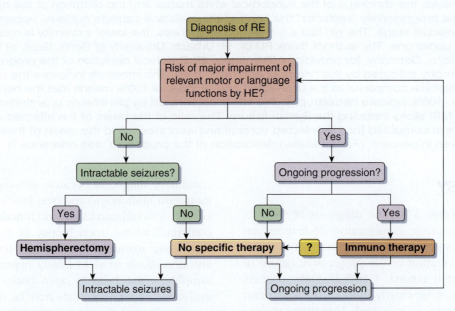

Figure 37–2. Therapeutic approach to a patient with Rasmussen syndrome (From Bien CG, Granata T, Antozzi C et al. Pathogenesis, diagnosis and treatment of Rasmussen encephalitis: a European consensus statement. *Brain* 2005;128:454).

judged from these studies, most positive experience exists with long-term corticosteroids[9,34,35] intravenous immunoglobulins (IVIGs),[34–36] plasmapheresis or protein A immunoabsorption,[35,37,38] and tacrolimus.[39]

OPTIMAL TREATMENT REGIMEN

The majority of RS patients suffer from epileptic seizures. Therefore, anticonvulsive pharmacotherapy is usually indicated, appropriate drugs for the seizure type being tried. Epilepsy due to RS is often refractory to treatment and EPC is notoriously difficult to control: it is important to avoid excess treatment, and particularly polytherapy with multiple antiepileptic drugs, with their associated adverse effects, particularly sedation.[40]

Injections of botulinum toxin may be helpful in the management of involuntary movements and localized myoclonus associated with RS.[41,42] If intractable seizures persist, the option of hemispherectomy should be considered and the potential benefit (high chance of seizure freedom) should be weighed against the expected deficits. Most centers would not perform this operation in patients with functional fine finger movements or patients with language representation within the affected hemisphere. However, if the condition or its treatment causes such severe impairments that the expected benefits of surgery appear to outweigh the likely deficits, hemispherectomy may be offered.

In those patients in whom hemispherectomy is thought inappropriate long-term immunotherapy is indicated if the condition is still progressive (as judged by the clinical and neuroradiological course over the last 6–12 months). There is insufficient evidence to recommend any specific regimen, and the following suggestions, therefore, describe the most frequently reported "successful" regimens. In general, the tolerability and the effect of long-term immunotherapy should be evaluated every 6 to 12 months. If the disease progresses during this time in the form of additional neurological deficits or increasing cerebral hemiatrophy, the treatment should be changed. If treatment is successful, as evidenced by halting of the disease progression, it is unclear when immunotherapy may be discontinued. It would be reasonable to continue treatment until the patient's condition has been stable for at least 2–3 years.

Long-Term Corticosteroids

A suggested schedule is to start with three boluses of intravenous methylprednisolone at a dose of 400 mg/m[2] body surface on alternate days for 6 days, followed by oral prednisone or prednisolone, starting at a dose of 2 mg/kg body weight daily.[9,34] The oral dose is tapered slowly over a period of several months according to the clinical response. Thereafter, monthly boluses

of 400 mg methylprednisolone/m[2] are administered. The usual recommendations regarding surveillance of patients receiving long-term steroid treatment should be followed (regular tests for arterial hypertension, hyperglycemia, glaucoma, electrolyte disturbances, etc.;[43] and medical prophylaxis of gastric ulcer and osteoporosis depending on the patient's age.[44–46]) Steroid boluses have been observed to sharply reduce seizure frequency in patients with an exacerbation of epilepsy.[35]

Long-Term IVIG

Initially, a total dose of 1.2–2.0 g/kg body weight[34] is administered over a period of two to five successive days. Thereafter, monthly doses of 0.4 g/kg[9] or 2.0 g/kg (over 2–5 days[35]) are given. A combination of long-term steroid therapy with long-term IVIG administration has been recommended.[34] Most positive results with IVIG have been achieved in adult RS patients.[47,48]

Plasmapheresis/Protein A Immunoadsorption

Plasmapheresis cycles are performed at a frequency of three to six single volume exchanges on consecutive or alternate days, repeated every 2–8 weeks.[35,37] Selective periodic immunoadsorption with protein A has been used as a long-term therapy with positive results in adolescent-adult onset patients.[38] Plasmapheresis or protein A immunoadsorption improves neurological function and seizure frequency in some patients during the weeks following the intervention, which can be repeated with future treatments.[35]

Tacrolimus

In a series of seven RS patients, the effect of the T-cell specific immunosuppressant tacrolimus (given as capsules) was investigated using motor performance and seizure frequency plus a surrogate marker of the RE disease process (the quantification of hemispheric tissue loss assessed on serial MRIs). The results were compared with a control group of 12 historical untreated patients. The tacrolimus patients had a superior outcome with regard to neurological function and progression rate of cerebral hemiatrophy on MRI, but no better seizure outcome. Also, their cognitive outcome was surprisingly good (only one patient deteriorated). Treatment was well tolerated.[39]

The following dosing recommendations are based on our personal experience (Bonn epilepsy centre): Similar to tacrolimus use in organ transplantation, we aim at trough levels of 12–15 ng/mL during the first 6 months of treatment (determined 12 hours after most recent intake of the drug). To achieve this blood level, we start with 0.5 mg/kg body weight in two divided doses in patients without enzyme inhibiting or inducing comedication. If an enzyme-inhibiting drug (valproic acid) is given in parallel, we start with 0.25 mg/kg. Coadministration of enzyme-inducing drugs often necessitates doses of >0.7 mg/kg. The first blood level is taken after 3–5 days and the dose is adjusted accordingly. Doses >15 ng/mL may cause reversible CNS side effects like dizziness, tremor, ataxia, and confusion. During months 7–12, we aim at blood trough levels of 8–12 ng/mL, thereafter 5–8 ng/mL. The compound should not be taken together with grapefruit juice because this may increase the blood levels. Tacrolimus should be taken one hour prior to the next meal or 2–3 hours after the last food intake; otherwise, there may be diminished absorption of the drug.

► PROGNOSIS

With regard to prognosis, patients appear to fall into two distinct groups.[3] "Type 1" patients are younger at onset, usually developing the condition before the age of 6 years. Typically the child is healthy prior to the onset of seizures. The acute phase of intractable focal motor or temporal lobe seizures is short, leading if untreated to the rapid development of hemiparesis and other neurological deficits. Hemispherectomy may become necessary to control seizures and halt the progression of the condition. "Type 2" patients are typically older at onset (usually adolescents or adults) and have a milder, more prolonged, disease course. Hemiparesis is rare, and hemispheric atrophy less marked than in type 1 cases.

REFERENCES

1. Rasmussen T, Olszewski J, Lloyd-Smith D. Focal seizures due to chronic localized encephalitis. *Neurology* 1958;8:435.
2. Oguni H, Andermann F, Rasmussen TB. The syndrome of chronic encephalitis and epilepsy. A study based on the MNI series of 48 cases. *Adv Neurol* 1992;57:419.
3. Bien CG, et al. The natural history of Rasmussen's encephalitis. *Brain* 2002;125:1751.
4. Bien CG, et al. Diagnosis and staging of Rasmussen's encephalitis by serial MRI and histopathology. *Neurology* 2002;58:250.
5. Chiapparini L, et al. Diagnostic imaging in 13 cases of Rasmussen's encephalitis: can early MRI suggest the diagnosis? *Neuroradiology* 2003;45:171.
6. Gray F, et al. Chronic localised encephalitis (Rasmussen's) in an adult with epilepsia partialis continua. *J Neurol Neurosurg Psychiatry* 1987;50:747.
7. Hart YM, et al. Chronic encephalitis and epilepsy in adults and adolescents: a variant of Rasmussen's syndrome? *Neurology* 1997;48:418.
8. Villani F, et al. Adult-onset Rasmussen's encephalitis: anatomical-electrographic-clinical features of 7 Italian cases. *Epilepsia* 2006;47:41.
9. Chinchilla D, et al. Reappraisal of Rasmussen's syndrome with special emphasis on treatment with high doses of steroids. *J Neurol Neurosurg Psychiatry* 1994;57:1325.
10. Tobias SM, et al. Bilateral Rasmussen encephalitis: postmortem documentation in a five-year-old. *Epilepsia* 2003;44:127.
11. Larionov S, et al. MRI brain volumetry in Rasmussen encephalitis: the fate of affected and "unaffected" hemispheres. *Neurology* 2005;64:885.
12. Hart YM, et al. Double pathology in Rasmussen's syndrome: a window on the etiology? *Neurology* 1998;50:731.
13. Korn-Lubetzki I, et al. Rasmussen encephalitis with active inflammation and delayed seizures onset. *Neurology* 2004;62:984.
14. Bien CG, et al. Slowly progressive hemiparesis in childhood as a consequence of Rasmussen encephalitis without or with delayed-onset seizures. *Eur J Neurol* 2007;14(4):387–390.
15. Frucht S. Dystonia, athetosis, and epilepsia partialis continua in a patient with late-onset Rasmussen's encephalitis. *Mov Disord* 2002;17:609.
16. Bhatjiwale MG, et al. Rasmussen's encephalitis: neuroimaging findings in 21 patients with a closer look at the basal ganglia. *Pediatr Neurosurg* 1998;29:142.
17. Bien CG, et al. Pathogenesis, diagnosis and treatment of Rasmussen encephalitis: a European consensus statement. *Brain* 2005;128:454.
18. Granata T, et al. Rasmussen's encephalitis: early characteristics allow diagnosis. *Neurology* 2003;60:422.
19. Andrews PI, McNamara JO, Lewis DV. Clinical and electroencephalographic correlates in Rasmussen's encephalitis. *Epilepsia* 1997;38:189.
20. So N, Gloor P. Electroencephalographic and electrocorticographic findings in chronic encephalitis of the Rasmussen type. In: Andermann F (ed), *Chronic Encephalitis and Epilepsy. Rasmussen's syndrome.* Boston: Butterworth-Heinemann, 1991; p. 37
21. Rogers SW, et al. Autoantibodies to glutamate receptor GluR3 in Rasmussen's encephalitis. *Science* 1994;265:648.
22. Wiendl H, et al. GluR3 antibodies: prevalence in focal epilepsy but no specificity for Rasmussen's encephalitis. *Neurology* 2001;57:1511.
23. Mantegazza R, et al. Antibodies against GluR3 peptides are not specific for Rasmussen's encephalitis but are also present in epilepsy patients with severe, early onset disease and intractable seizures. *J Neuroimmunol* 2002;131:179.
24. Watson R, et al. Absence of antibodies to glutamate receptor type 3 (GluR3) in Rasmussen encephalitis. *Neurology* 2004;63:43.
25. Oguni H, Andermann F, Rasmussen TB. The natural history of the syndrome of chronic encephalitis and epilepsy: a study of the MNI series of forty-eight cases. In: Andermann F (ed), *Chronic Encephalitis and Epilepsy. Rasmussen's syndrome.* Boston: Butterworth-Heinemann, 1991; p. 7.
26. Grenier Y, Antel JP, Osterland CK. Immunologic studies in chronic encephalitis of Rasmussen. In: Andermann F (ed), *Chronic Encephalitis and Epilepsy. Rasmussen's Syndrome.* Boston: Butterworth-Heinemann, 1991; p. 125.

27. Dulac O, et al. High-dose steroid treatment of epilepsia partialis continua due to chronic focal encephalitis. In: Andermann F (ed), *Chronic Encephalitis and Epilepsy. Rasmussen's Syndrome.* Boston: Butterworth-Heinemann, 1991; p. 193.

28. Lee JS, et al. Patterns of cerebral glucose metabolism in early and late stages of Rasmussen's syndrome. *J Child Neurol* 2001;16:798.

29. Pardo CA, et al. The pathology of Rasmussen syndrome: stages of cortical involvement and neuropathological studies in 45 hemispherectomies. *Epilepsia* 2004;45: 516.

30. Booss J, Esiri MM. *Viral Encephalitis in Humans.* Washington, D.C.: ASM Press, 2003.

31. Farrell MA, et al. Chronic encephalitis associated with epilepsy: immunohistochemical and ultrastructural studies. *Acta Neuropathol Berl* 1995;89:313.

32. Bernal F, et al. Immunohistochemical analysis of anti-Hu-associated paraneoplastic encephalomyelitis. *Acta Neuropathol (Berl)* 2002;103:509.

33. Bien CG, et al. Limbic encephalitis not associated with neoplasm as a cause of temporal lobe epilepsy. *Neurology* 2000;55:1823.

34. Hart YM, et al. Medical treatment of Rasmussen's syndrome (chronic encephalitis and epilepsy): effect of high-dose steroids or immunoglobulins in 19 patients. *Neurology* 1994; 44:1030.

35. Granata T, et al. Experience with immunomodulatory treatments in Rasmussen's encephalitis. *Neurology* 2003; 61:1807.

36. Villani F, et al. Positive response to immunomodulatory therapy in an adult patient with Rasmussen's encephalitis. *Neurology* 2001;56:248.

37. Andrews PI, et al. Plasmapheresis in Rasmussen's encephalitis. *Neurology* 1996;46:242.

38. Antozzi C, et al. Long-term selective IgG immunoadsorption improves Rasmussen's encephalitis. *Neurology* 1998; 51:302.

39. Bien CG, et al. An open study of tacrolimus therapy in Rasmussen encephalitis. *Neurology* 2004;62:2106.

40. Dubeau F, Sherwin AL. Pharmacologic principles in the management of chronic focal encephalitis. In: Andermann F (ed), *Chronic Encephalitis and Epilepsy. Rasmussen's Syndrome.* Boston: Butterworth-Heinemann, 1991; p. 179.

41. Lozsadi DA, Hart IK, Moore AP. Botulinum toxin A improves involuntary limb movements in Rasmussen syndrome. *Neurology* 2004;62:1233.

42. Browner N, Azher SN, Jankovic J. Botulinum toxin treatment of facial myoclonus in suspected Rasmussen encephalitis. *Mov Disord* 2006;21:1500.

43. Seth A, Aggarwal A. Monitoring adverse reaction to steroid therapy in children. *Indian Pediatr* 2004;41:349.

44. Brown JP, Josse RG. 2002 clinical practice guidelines for the diagnosis and management of osteoporosis in Canada. *CMAJ* 2002;167:S1.

45. Brown JJ, Zacharin MR. Proposals for prevention and management of steroid-induced osteoporosis in children and adolescents. *J Paediatr Child Health* 2005;41:553.

46. Ward LM. Osteoporosis due to glucocorticoid use in children with chronic illness. *Horm Res* 2005;64:209.

47. Leach JP, et al. Improvement in adult-onset Rasmussen's encephalitis with long-term immunomodulatory therapy. *Neurology* 1999;52:738.

48. Arias M, et al. Rasmussen encephalitis in the sixth decade: magnetic resonance image evolution and immunoglobulin response. *Eur Neurol* 2006;56:236.

SECTION VII
Status Epilepticus

CHAPTER 38

Convulsive Status Epilepticus

James J. Riviello Jr

▶ INTRODUCTION

Status epilepticus (SE) is a life-threatening medical emergency that requires prompt recognition and treatment. SE is not a specific disease but rather a manifestation of a primary central nervous system (CNS) insult or a systemic disorder with secondary CNS effects. Adherence is mandatory to the basic principles of neuroresuscitation, the A, B, and Cs, followed by a planned treatment protocol. Proper management requires the identification and treatment of the underlying cause in order to facilitate seizure control and prevent ongoing neurologic injury. Specific clinical and electrographic stages of SE have treatment implications and there are certain special circumstances that require immediate seizure control. This chapter focuses on the evaluation and treatment convulsive SE (CSE), including refractory SE (RSE).

▶ DEFINITION

SE is defined as more than 30 minutes of either continuous seizure activity or two or more sequential seizures without full recovery of consciousness in-between.[1] However, treatment starts before this duration. Lowenstein, Bleck, and Macdonald proposed an "operational definition" for treatment of generalized CSE in adults and older children (age >5 years): 5 minutes or more of either a continuous seizure, or two or more discrete seizures between which there is incomplete recovery of consciousness.[2] These principles apply to all ages.

SE is classified by seizure type, either partial (focal) or generalized as defined by the International Classification of Epileptic Seizures.[3] A modified system is based on semiology[4]: CSE or nonconvulsive SE (NCSE). NCSE occurs with either generalized (absence) or focal (partial complex) epilepsy, or as the end stage of CSE. SE is also classified by etiology: acute symptomatic, remote symptomatic, remote symptomatic with acute precipitant, progressive encephalopathy, cryptogenic, idiopathic, and febrile SE.[5]

CSE consists of continuous tonic and/or clonic motor activity, which may be asymmetric, overt, or subtle, with bilateral, although frequently asymmetrical, electroencephalogram (EEG) ictal discharges and altered consciousness[4,6] NCSEs or subtle CSEs have no obvious signs despite marked impairment of consciousness and bilateral EEG discharges,[6] and may evolve from convulsive SE or its apparent successful treatment. Pseudo-SE also occurs in children.[7,8]

▶ STAGES OF STATUS EPILEPTICUS

The clinical stages of SE are listed in Table 38–1.[9] The premonitory stage consists of confusion, myoclonus, or increasing seizure frequency; the early stage, continuous seizure activity; subtle CSE or NCSE may develop in the refractory stage. If identified, the premonitory stage is treated. We have delineated special circumstances in the early stage that require immediate seizure control (Table 38–2).[10] The transition stage is actually the time within the early stage when compensatory systems become overwhelmed, which marks the beginning of the late stage. This transition stage differs from patient to patient, depending on the circumstances. EEG stages correlate with the clinical stages[11] (Table 38–3). Antiepileptic drug (AED) treatment in the early stage controls

▶ **TABLE 38–1.** STAGES OF STATUS EPILEPTICUS[a]

Premonitory (prodromal)
Incipient (0–5 min)
Early stage (5–30 min)
Transition stage (from the early to the late, or established, stage)
Late, or established, stage (30–60 min)
Refractory stage (greater than 60–90 min)
Postictal stage

[a]Data from references[9] and.[10]

▶ **TABLE 38–3.** EEG STAGES OF STATUS EPILEPTICUS

1. Discrete seizures with interictal slowing
2. Waxing and waning of ictal discharges (the merging stage)
3. Continuous ictal discharges
4. Continuous ictal discharges punctuated by flat periods
5. Periodic epileptiform discharges (PEDS), on a flat background

From Treiman DM, Walton NY, Kendrick C. A progressive sequence of electroencephalographic changes during generalized convulsive status epilepticus. *Epilepsy Res* 1990; 5:49–60.

seizure activity better than when given later.[11] However, not every defined stage occurs in an episode of SE.[12]

▶ PATHOPHYSIOLOGY

Initially, brain compensatory mechanisms, especially hypertension with increased cerebral blood flow (CBF), may prevent neuronal injury. Lothman outlined the systemic and brain metabolic alterations that occur with prolonged SE[13]: hypoxemia, hypercarbia, hypotension, and hyperthermia, with decreased brain oxygen tension, a mismatch between the sustained increase in oxygen and glucose utilization and a fall in CBF and depletion of brain glucose and oxygen. Brain compensation requires adequate airway, breathing, circulation, and CBF and timelines assume that compensatory mechanisms remain intact during the incipient and early stages. However, a higher morbidity and mortality occurs with new-onset inpatient SE, suggesting already compromised compensatory mechanisms.[14] Experimental data also support earlier therapy. In an animal model, both diazepam and phenytoin prevented SE when administered early but efficacy decreased when

given later.[15] A loss of inhibitory GABA-A receptors[16] and a functional change in GABA-A receptors occurs[17,18] as the duration of partial SE increases. These findings have also been demonstrated in young animals.[19]

▶ EPIDEMIOLOGY

The incidence of SE in children ranges from 10 to 58/100,000 per year.[20–23] In population-based studies of children with epilepsy, the incidence of SE varies from 9.5% to 27%.[24–26] SE occurs in the very young, especially in those less than age 2 years, with 80% having an afebrile or acute symptomatic etiology.[27] In a study of seizure duration in 407 new onset seizures, two time distributions occurred: (1) 76% had mean seizure duration of 3.6 minutes and (2) 24% had a mean duration of 31 minutes. The longer the seizure lasted, the less likely it would stop within the next several minutes.[28] The American Academy of Neurology (AAN) practice parameter retrospectively analyzed 2093 children, excluding neonates, less than the age of 19 years from 20 studies.[29] The etiologic categories were assessed (Table 38–4). The occurrence of a remote symptomatic with an acute precipitant episode was low, but this category was not included in the majority of the studies. When included in the prospective London data,

▶ **TABLE 38–2.** SPECIAL CIRCUMSTANCES, EARLY STAGE

Postoperative patients, especially with cardiac surgery and neurosurgery
Head trauma, increased intracranial pressure, brain tumor, intracranial hematoma, subarachnoid hemorrhage
Stroke: ischemic and hemorrhagic
CNS infections (meningitis or encephalitis)
Organ failure, especially hepatic, or multisystem failure
Hyperthermia; malignant hyperthermia; hyperthyroidism
Metabolic disorders prone to develop increased intracranial pressure: diabetic ketoacidosis, organic acid disorders

From Riviello JJ. Status epilepticus in children. In: Drislane FW (ed), *Status Epilepticus: A Clinical Perspective*. Totowa: Humana Press, 2005, pp. 313–338.

▶ **TABLE 38–4.** CATEGORIES SE FROM AAN PRACTICE PARAMETER (*N* = 2093)

Acute symptomatic SE	548 (26%)
Remote symptomatic	695 (33%)
Remote symptomatic with an acute precipitant	17 (1%)
Progressive encephalopathy	57 (3%)
Febrile	471 (22%)
Cryptogenic (was idiopathic)	305 (15%)

From Riviello JJ, Ashwal Shirtz D, Glauser T, Ballaban-Gil K, Kelley K, Morton LD, Phillips S, Sloan E, Shinnar S. Practice parameter: diagnostic assessment of the child with status epilepticus (an evidence-based review): Report of the Quality Standards Subcommittee of the American Academy of Neurology and the practice committee of the Child Neurology Society. *Neurology* 2006;67:1542–1550.

▶ **TABLE 38–5. SE CATEGORIES IN NLSTEPSS** (*N* = 176)

Prolonged febrile seizure	56 (32%)
Acute symptomatic	30 (17%)
Remote symptomatic	29 (16%)
Acute on remote symptomatic	28 (16%)
Idiopathic epilepsy related	18 (10%)
Cryptogenic epilepsy related	3 (2%)
Unclassified	12 (7%)

From Chin RFM, Neville BGR, Peckham C, Bedford H, Wade A, Scott RC. Incidence, cause, and short-term outcome of convulsive status epilepticus in children: prospective, population-based study. *Lancet* 2006;368:222–229.

called acute on remote, this category was more frequent (Table 38–5).

The North London SE in childhood surveillance study (NLSTEPSS), the first prospective population-based study of CSE in children, identified and prospectively followed 176 children after an initial episode of SE[30] (see Chapter 61). The ascertainment adjusted incidence was between 17 and 23/100,000 per year. Ninety-eight were healthy prior to SE (56%) and 56 of these (57%) had a prolonged febrile seizure. The incidence of recurrence within 1 year was 16% and mortality was 3%. The age-adjusted incidence for acute symptomatic SE was 16.9% in those less than 1 year of age, 2.5% in those 1–4 years, and 0.1% in those 5–15 years of age. The incidence of an acute or remote (remote symptomatic with an acute precipitant) was 6%, 5.3%, and 0.7%, respectively. A prolonged febrile seizure occurred in 4.1/100,000, acute symptomatic causes in 2.2/100,000, remote symptomatic in 2.3/100,000, acute on remote in 2.1/100,000, idiopathic in 1.4/100,000, cryptogenic in 0.2/100,000, and unclassified in 1/100,000.

▶ ETIOLOGY AND PROGNOSIS

Prognosis depends on etiology, age, duration, and treatment adequacy. Etiology is a very important determinant of morbidity and mortality and the specific cause must be determined and treated in order to prevent ongoing neuronal injury and facilitate seizure control. The disorders causing the acute symptomatic category may require a specific therapy. In a classic study of 239 cases of pediatric SE by Aicardi and Chevrie, 113 cases were symptomatic and 126 were cryptogenic. In those with symptomatic SE, 63/113 (56%) had acute CNS insults, including treatable disorders such as bacterial meningitis, encephalitis, dehydration or electrolyte disorders, toxic ingestions, or subdural hematoma.[31] In those with cryptogenic SE, 67/126 (53%) were associated with fever (a prolonged, or complex, febrile seizure). In the later study by Maytal et al: 45/193 (23%)

were acute symptomatic and 45/193 (23%) were remote symptomatic.[32]

The Richmond Study included adults and identified different etiologies for children; the most common cause in adults was cerebrovascular disease (25.2%) whereas fever and infection (35.7%) were more common in children.[33] A recent medication change was a major precipitant of SE in all ages, accounting for 20% of cases in children and 19% in adults.

Acute symptomatic etiologies occur in 17%[30] to 23%[32] in two modern studies; the most common etiology is prolonged febrile seizures.[30] SE is more common in the very young, especially in those less than 2 years, with over 80% of young children having a febrile or acute symptomatic etiology.[27] In a population-based study of 226 children, acute bacterial meningitis (ABM) was the most frequent acute symptomatic etiology, followed by viral infections, metabolic disturbances, and head injury.[29] ABM was found in 17% of children with CSE and fever.[34]

Symptomatic SE has a maximum frequency and higher morbidity and mortality in the very young, occurring less frequently after 1 year of age.[35] Idiopathic SE is rare during the first several months, becoming more frequent after 6 months. In 31 infants less than 6 months of age, treatable causes included: infectious etiologies in 7%, 1 with pneumococcal meningitis; inborn errors of metabolism in 16%; electrolyte abnormalities in 16%, and trauma in 3%.[36] In a recent review, the short-term mortality was 3% to 5%,[37] the practice parameter mortality ranged from 4% to 11%.,[29] and the NLSTEPSS mortality was 3%.[30] The Maytal study had an overall mortality of 4%; occurring only in those with acute symptomatic or progressive symptomatic etiologies.[32] There were no deaths in a recent UK retrospective study of 137 children.[38] The Richmond study had an overall mortality of 6%.[35] When stratified by age, mortality within the first year was 17.8%, but in the first 6 months, mortality was 24% compared to 9% in infants aged 6–12 months. This difference was related to the higher incidence of symptomatic SE in the youngest children.[35]

With respect to morbidity, a Canadian study reported developmental deterioration in 34% of 40 children after a seizure duration of 30–720 minutes.[39] Speech delay has been reported after febrile SE.[40] Prolonged SE is associated with increased mortality reported as 1.8% in one study[41] a Dutch study of GCSE correlated outcome with treatment adequacy.[42]

▶ EVALUATION

The treatment of SE starts with attention to A, B, and Cs (Table 38–6). Diagnostic studies, obtained after stabilization, are guided by the history, examination, and

► **TABLE 38–6.** THE EVALUATION OF SE

Starts with the A, B, and C:
  Stabilize and maintain the airway
  Establish breathing (i.e., ventilation)
  Maintain the circulation
  Monitor the vital signs: pulse, pulse oximetry,
    respiratory rate, blood pressure, temperature

age, with a greater need to exclude treatable causes in the youngest children. Serum glucose should be rapidly checked to exclude hypoglycemia. CBC may be helpful for infection, although leukocytosis occurs from SE itself.

Electrolytes, calcium, phosphorus, and magnesium values may be helpful in children with vomiting and diarrhea.

Lumbar puncture (LP) to exclude meningitis must be considered in the febrile child, but LP is not absolutely necessary in every child, depending upon the clinical situation. If there is concern for increased intracranial pressure or a structural lesion, LP is deferred until neuroimaging is done, but antibiotics are given prior to LP, relying on cell count and bacterial cultures. A cerebrospinal fluid (CSF) pleocytosis may occur without infection, presumably due to a breakdown in the blood-brain barrier.[43] In one study, the highest CSF white blood cell count from SE alone (no acute insult) was $28/mm^3$.[44]

Low levels of AEDs, may be associated with SE. In one study of 51 children, AED levels were therapeutic in only 66%.[45] Neuroimaging is indicated for new onset SE, especially without a defined cause, or a prior history of epilepsy. The American Academy of Emergency Physicians (ACEP) and AAN practice parameter for neuroimaging in seizures recommended an[46] emergent (scan immediately) scan for new onset SE, or in a known epileptic not responding to treatment. However, it is critical that the child be stabilized before the scan.

A higher incidence of life-threatening lesions (hemorrhage, brain swelling, and mass effect) occurs with a first-time seizure or in a child with epilepsy and new focal deficits, persistent altered mental status, with or without intoxication, fever, recent trauma, persistent headache, cancer, or on anticoagulation. For pediatric seizures in general, a predisposing condition or focal seizure in a child less than 33 months has been associated with a high risk of an abnormal imaging study.[47] Magnetic resonance imaging is more sensitive but is rarely available for emergent studies, and computed axial tomography scan is adequate for life-threatening conditions. EEG is usually not indicated for the immediate treatment of CSE. However, an EEG can exclude NCSE or pseudo-SE.

In an adult study by DeLorenzo and colleagues, NCSE occurred in 14% of patients treated for CGSE.[48] In a study in children by Tay and colleagues, NCSE occurred in 5/19 following control of CSE; in 2 of these, NCSE occurred after treatment of CSE; and in 3, NCSE occurred after treatment of RSE.[49] In the Towne and colleagues study of mostly adults, NCSE was detected in 8% of all comatose patients[50]; the Tay study found NCSE in two children following an hypoxic-ischemic insult.[49]

The indications for emergency EEG include unexplained altered awareness (to exclude NCSE); neuromuscular paralysis for SE, which removes the convulsive movements by neuromuscular blockade; high-dose suppressive therapy (HDST) for RSE, or when there is no improvement or return to baseline mental status after controlling overt convulsive movements (to exclude NCSE).[51] The EEG is especially useful whenever the diagnosis is in doubt, especially for pseudoseizures.[52] In a study in children, 6 of 29 children admitted with CSE had pseudo-SE.[7]

The AAN practice parameter[29] reported the following abnormalities in children undergoing acute evaluation: abnormal electrolytes (6%), positive blood cultures (2.5%), CNS infection (2.8%), low AED levels (32%,) ingestion (3.6%), inborn error of metabolism (4.2%), epileptiform abnormalities (43%), and neuroimaging abnormalities (8%).

► **THERAPY FOR STATUS EPILEPTICUS**

Standard treatment guidelines are needed, but in a recent UK survey, only 12% had a planned protocol.[53] Phenobarbital, phenytoin, and the benzodiazepines, diazepam, and lorazepam have been the standard first-line agents. The adult VA Cooperative Study compared the efficacy of various first-line agents: lorazepam (0.1 mg/kg), phenobarbital (15 mg/kg), and diazepam (0.15 mg/kg) plus phenytoin (18 mg/kg) versus phenytoin alone (18 mg/kg).

Successful treatment was defined as control within 20 minutes. Treatment efficacy was similar with lorazepam (65%), phenobarbital (58%), and diazepam plus phenytoin (56%), whereas phenytoin alone had a lower efficacy (44%). However, this is likely related to the infusion time needed: 4.7 minutes with lorazepam versus 33 minutes with phenytoin alone.[54] Intravenous preparations of valproate and levetiracetam are now also available.

A four-step guideline has been devised and implemented in three UK centers Table 38–7[55] and the evidence-based treatment sequence for seizures/SE from Texas Children's Hospital is included[56] Fig. 38–1 Fosphenytoin is preferred over phenytoin because of hypotension, cardiovascular side effects, and soft tissue infiltration and injury.[57]

Three centers have analyzed their treatment protocols. Garr et al reported a 94% response to diazepam,

▶ **TABLE 38–7. TREATMENT GUIDELINES, BRITISH WORKING PARTY**

The steps are:
  (1) LZP, 0.1 mg/kg IV, or if no IV access, rectal DZP, 0.5 mg/kg
  After 10 minutes: (2) LZP, 0.1 mg/kg
  After 10 minutes: (3) PHT, 18 mg/kg, or if on PHT, Pb, 20 mg/kg and paraldehyde, 0.4 ml/kg
  After 20 minutes: consider pyridoxine for a child under 3 years of age
  (4) Thiopentone, 4 mg/kg, IV

From Appleton R, Choonara I, Martland T, Phillps B, Scott R, Whitehouse W. The status epilepticus working party. The treatment of convulsive status epilepticus in children. *Arch Dis Child* 2000; 83:415–419.

followed by phenytoin and paraldehyde.[58] Sixty nine (85%) responded to a single dose of diazepam (rectal in 41 and intravenous in 28). Many guidelines use a repeat benzodiazepine dose, but in this study, a repeat diazepam dose controlled seizures in only two additional children. Seizures ceased in five of ten children receiving combined paraldehyde and phenytoin; nine (11%) required ICU admission for persistent seizures and four for respiratory depression.

Eriksson and colleagues reported a 73% response to either IV or rectal diazepam, 16.5% then responded to either phenobarbital or fosphenytoin, and 11% needed barbiturate anesthesia.[59,60] Overall, the response rate to diazepam, another IV AED, or thiopental was 99%.[59] A Cochrane review found no evidence that lorazepam had a better efficacy than diazepam.[61] An audit of the treatment protocol from the NLSTEPSS study (N = 240), revealed that 32/147 (22%) cases were controlled by prehospital treatment (diazepam), 121/187 (65%) were controlled by first-line agents, 41/82 (50%) were controlled by second-line agents, and 41/82 required thiopentone.[62]

In a recent expert opinion consensus on the initial treatment of pediatric epilepsy, lorazepam was considered the drug of choice for all types of pediatric SE; rectal diazepam and fosphenytoin were also considered first-line agents for CSE.[63] The operational definition had suggested treatment after 5 minutes.[2] However, Eriksson and colleagues reported that a treatment delay became significant only after 30 minutes, and the response was related to etiology: no acute symptomatic case resolved spontaneously, whereas 52% of febrile seizures resolved spontaneously.[60]

Guideline time sequences are based on the assumption that brain compensatory mechanisms initially protect against neuronal injury. However, compensatory mechanisms may already be compromised in certain situations, the "special circumstances" of the early stage,

in which ongoing seizure activity requires immediate control: postoperative patients, especially after cardiac or neurosurgery, brain tumors, structural lesions or cerebral edema, CNS infections, organ failure, especially hepatic or multisystem organ failure, hyperthermia, or metabolic disorders with acidosis.[10] Safe infusion rates are recommended for these AEDs, whereas in these special circumstances, the safe infusion rate may be too long: for example, for fosphenytoin, the infusion time is approximately 7 minutes at a maximum rate of 150 mg/min for a 50 kg child. In a "special circumstance," if the seizure does not stop after lorazepam, an IV agent such as thiopental, propofol, or pentobarbital may be given for immediate seizure control. With hemodynamic instability, consider ketamine, or use the above agents and treat hypotension if it occurs. Propofol may also be used safely in the acute setting: Van Gestel and colleagues reported that propofol up to 5 mg/kg/h had better efficacy and less side effects that thiopental[64,65] but concern exists for prolonged therapy or for high infusion rates.[66]

▶ **SECOND-LINE AGENTS**

IV sodium valproate and levetiracetam are available and useful when first-line therapy fails, but are not Food and Drug Administration (FDA) approved for SE. The IV loading dose (LD) of VPA varies from 10 to 30 mg/kg.

A 20 mg/kg LD should achieve a level of 75 mg/L.[67] A study of safety and efficacy used a 25 mg/kg LD for SE, with a rate of 3 mg/kg/h.[68] Hypotension occurred in a child at a rate of 30 mg/kg/h (0.5 mg/kg/min).[69] A LD of 10–25 mg/kg over 30 minutes is used in neonates.[70]

The pharmacokinetic profile is similar for IV and oral levetiracetam[71] with no difference following an oral or IV dose of 500–1500 mg in adults.[72] In children, we have given a 10–30 mg/kg LD, over 30 minutes. For acute exacerbations of refractory epilepsy, we have used very high doses in nine children. The mean dose was 228 mg/kg per day. One child had increased seizures and no agitation or behavioral problems occurred.[73]

▶ **REFRACTORY STATUS EPILEPTICUS**

RSE occurs when seizures persist despite adequate treatment. By this time, the airway should be protected, ventilation controlled with intubation, the circulation maintained and transfer underway to the intensive care unit. The mortality in children with RSE varies from 16% to 43.5%[5,74,75] and etiology is important for prognosis.[5]

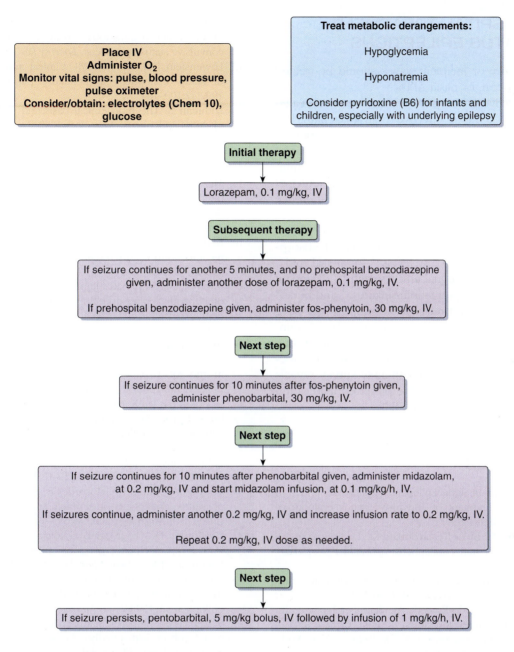

Figure 38–1. Antiepileptic drug treatment for seizures/status epilepticus: Texas Children's Hospital. Data from Initial Management of Seizures. Texas Children's Hospital Evidence-Based Guidelines. 2009, Summer. Evidence-based treatment for the initial management of seizures.

If convulsive activity stops but mental status does not improve, NCSE must be excluded.[48,49] Either an emergent EEG is done, if available; or if not available, empiric additional AEDs should be considered.

When SE persists for more than 30 minutes despite adequate doses of conventional AEDs, HDST with IV anesthetic agents should be employed. Pentobarbital, midazolam, high-dose pentobarbital, propofol, and thiopental are most commonly administered. There is controversy regarding the end point of HDST: should the clinical seizures or both the clinical and electrographic seizures be treated, or should the end point of treatment be EEG suppression?[76–78] Some authorities aim for a burst suppression pattern on EEG.[79,80]

▶ PREHOSPITAL TREATMENT OF STATUS EPILEPTICUS

The premonitory or incipient stages should be treated with rectal, buccal, or nasal AEDs.

A prospective prehospital treatment study revealed lorazepam to be more effective than diazepam.[81] A retrospective study of CSE in children ($N = 38$) showed that prehospital diazepam (0.6 mg rectal diazepam) resulted in a shorter duration (32 minutes vs. 60 minutes) and less seizure recurrence in the emergency department (58% vs. 85%), and there was no difference in intubation rates.[82]

Sublingual lorazepam[83] or intranasal or buccal midazolam can be given,[84] and rapid buccal absorption has been documented by levels.[85] Intranasal midazolam (0.2 mg/kg) has equal efficacy with IV diazepam (0.3 mg/kg) for prolonged febrile seizures,[86] and buccal midazolam (10 mg) and rectal diazepam (10 mg) have shown equal efficacy for seizures greater than 5 minutes.[85] These may be given by the intraosseous route. Another study shows that buccal midazolam was superior to IV diazepam.[87] A UK community survey reveals that buccal midazolam is now the preferred medication for the prehospital treatment of SE.[88]

REFERENCES

1. Working Group on Status Epilepticus, Epilepsy Foundation of America. Treatment of convulsive status epilepticus. *JAMA* 1993;270:854–859.
2. Lowenstein DH, Bleck T, Macdonald RL. It's time to revise the definition of status epilepticus. *Epilepsia* 1999;40:120–122.
3. Proposal for revised classification of epilepsies and epileptic syndromes. *Epilepsia* 1989;30:389–399.
4. Treiman DM, Delgado-Escueda AV. Status epilepticus. In: Thompson RA, Green RA, Green JR (eds), *Critical Care of Neurological and Neurosurgical Emergencies*. New York: Raven Press, 1980, pp. 53–99.
5. Sahin M, Menache C, Holmes GL, Riviello JJ. Outcome of severe refractory status epilepticus in children. *Epilepsia* 2001;42:1461–1467.
6. Treiman DM, DeGiorgio CM, Salisbury S, Wickboldt C. Subtle generalized convulsive status epilepticus. *Epilepsia* 1984;25:653.
7. Pakalnis A, Paolicchi J, Gilles E. Psychogenic status epilepticus in children: psychiatric and other risk factors. *Neurology* 2000;54:969–970.
8. Tuxhorn IEB, Fischbach HS. Pseudostatus epilepticus in childhood. *Pediatr Neurol* 2002;27:407–409.
9. Shorvon S. *Status Epilepticus: Its Clinical Features and Treatment in Children and Adults*. Cambridge: Cambridge University Press, 1994.
10. Riviello JJ. Status epilepticus in children. In: Drislane FW (ed), *Status Epilepticus: A Clinical Perspective*. Totowa: Human Press, 2005; pp. 313–338.
11. Treiman DM, Walton NY, Kendrick C. A progressive sequence of electroencephalographic changes during generalized convulsive status epilepticus. *Epilepsy Res* 1990;5:49–60.
12. Lowenstein DH, Aminoff MJ. Clinical and EEG features of status epilepticus in comatose patients. *Neurology* 1992;42:100–104.
13. Lothman E. The biochemical basis and pathophysiology of status epilepticus. *Neurology* 1990;40(Suppl 2):13–23.
14. Delanty N, French JA, Labar DR, Pedley TA, Rowan AJ. Status epilepticus arising de novo in hospitalized patients: an analysis of 41 patients. *Seizure* 2001;10:116–119.
15. Mazarati AM, Baldwin RA, Sankar R, Wasterlain CG. Time-dependent decrease in the effectiveness of antiepileptic drugs during the course of self-sustaining status epilepticus. *Brain Res* 1998;814:179–185.
16. Kapur J, Lothman EW, DeLorenzo RJ. Loss of GABAA receptors during partial status epilepticus. *Neurology* 1994;44:2407–2408.
17. Kapur J, Macdonal RL. Rapid seizure-induced reduction of benzodiazepine and Zn^{2+} sensitivity of hippocampal dentate granule cell GABAA receptors. *J Neurosci* 1997;17:7532–7540.
18. Jones DM, Esmaeil N, Maren S, Macdonald RL. Characterization of pharmacoresistance to benzodiazepines in the rat Li-pilocarpine model of status epielpticus. *Epilepsy Res* 2002;50:301–312.
19. Goodkin HP, Liu X, Holmes GL. Diazepam terminates brief but not prolonged seizures in young, naïve rats. *Epilepsia* 2003;44:1112–11090.
20. DeLorenzo RJ, et al. A prospective, population-based epidemiologic study of status epilepticus in Richmond, Virginia. *Neurology* 1996;46:1029–1035.
21. Coeytaux A, Jallon P, Galobardes B, Morabia A. Incidence of status epilepticus in French speaking Switzerland: (EPISTAR). *Neurology* 2000;55:693–697.
22. Hesdorffer DC, Logroscino G, Cascino G, Annegers JF, Hauser WA. Incidence of status epilepticus in Rochester, Minnesota, 1965–1984. *Neurology* 1998;50:735–741.
23. Wu YW, Shek DW, Garcia PA, Zhao S, Johnston SC. Incidence and mortality of generalized convulsive status epilepticus in California. *Neurology* 2002;58:1070–1076.
24. Sillanpaa M, Shinnar S. Status epilepticus in a population-based cohort with childhood-onset epilepsy in Finland. *Ann Neurol* 2002;52:303–310.
25. Berg AT, Shinnar S, Testa FM, Levy SR, Frobish D, Smith SN, Beckerman B. Status epilepticus after the initial diagnosis of epilepsy in children. *Neurology* 2004;66:1027–1034.
26. Stronk H, Geerts AT, van Donselaar CA, Boudewijn Peters AC, Brouwer OF, Peeters EA, Arts WF. Status epilepticus in children with epilepsy: Dutch study of epilepsy in childhood. *Epilepsia* 2007;48:1–8.
27. Shinnar S, Pellock JM, Moshe SL, Maytal J, O'Dell C, Driscoll SM, Alemany M, Newstein D, DeLorenzo RJ. In whom does status epilepticus occur: age-related differences in children. *Epilepsia* 1997;38:907–914.
28. Shinnar S, Berg AT, Moshe SL, Shinnar R. How long do new-onset seizures in children last? *Ann Neurol* 2001;49:659–664.
29. Riviello JJ, Ashwal Shirtz D, Glauser T, Ballaban-Gil K, Kelley K, Morton LD, Phillips S, Sloan E, Shinnar S. Practice Parameter: diagnostic assessment of the child

with status epilepticus (an evidence-based review): report of the Quality Standards Subcommittee of the American Academy of Neurology and the Practice Committee of the Child Neurology Society. *Neurology* 2006;67:1542–1550.

30. Chin RFM, Neville BGR, Peckham C, Bedford H, Wade A, Scott RC. Incidence, cause, and short-term outcome of convulsive status epilepticus in children: prospective, population-based study. *Lancet* 2006;368:222–229.

31. Aicardi J, Chevrie JJ. Convulsive status epilepticus in infants and children: a study of 239 cases. *Epilepsia* 1970; 11:187–197.

32. Maytal J, Shinnar S, Moshe SL, Alvarez LA. Low morbidity and mortality of status epilepticus in childhood. *Pediatrics* 1989;83:323–331.

33. DeLorenzo RJ, Towne AR, Pellock JM, Ko D. Status epilepticus in children, adults, and the elderly. *Epilepsia* 1992;33(Suppl 4):15–25.

34. Chin RFM, Neville BGR, Scott RC. Meningitis is a common cause of convulsive status epilepticus with fever. *Arch Dis Child* 2005;90:66–69.

35. Morton LD, Garnett LK, Towne AR, Waterhouse EJ, Brown AJ, Byers SF, Pellock JM, DeLorenzo RJ. Mortality of status epilepticus in the first year of life. *Epilepsia* 2001;42(Suppl 7): 164–165.

36. Bui TT, Delgado CA, Simon HK. Infant seizures not so infantle: first-time seizures in children under six months of age presenting to the ED. *Am J Emerg Med* 2002;20:518–520.

37. Raspall-Chaure M, Chin RFM, Scott RC. Outcome of paediatric status epilepticus: a systematic review. *Lancet Neurol* 2006;5:769–799.

38. Hussain N, Appleton R, Thorburn K. Aetiology, course and outcome of children admitted to paediatric intensive care with convulsive status epilepticus: a retrospective 5-year review. *Seizure* 2007;16:305–312.

39. Barnard C, Wirrell E. Does status epilepticus in children cause developmental deterioration and exacerbation of epilepsy? *J Child Neurology* 1999;14:787–794.

40. Van Esch A, Ramlal IR, van Steensel-Moll HA, Steyerberg EW, Derksen-Lubsen G. Outcome after febrile status epilepticus. *Dev Med Child Neurol* 1996;38:19–24.

41. Barry E, Hauser WA. Status epilepticus: the interaction of epilepsy and acute brain disease. *Neurology* 1993;43:1473–1478.

42. Scholtes FB, Renier WO, Meinardi H. Generalized convulsive status epilepticus: causes, therapy, and outcome in 346 patients. *Epilepsia* 1994;35:1104–1112.

43. Schmidley JW, Simon RP. Postictal pleocytosis. *Ann Neurol* 1981;9:81–84.

44. Barry E, Hauser WA. Pleocytosis after status epilepticus. *Arch Neurol* 1994;51:190–193.

45. Maytal J, Novak G, Ascher C, Bienkowski R. Status epilepticus in children with epilepsy: the role of antiepileptic drug levels in prevention. *Pediatrics* 1996;98: 1119–1121.

46. Greenberg MK, Barsan WG, Starkman S. Neuroimaging in the emergency patient presenting with seizure. *Neurology* 1996;47:26–32.

47. Sharma S, Riviello JJ, Harper MB, Baskin MN. The role of emergent neuroimaging in children with new-onset afebrile seizures. *Pediatrics* 2003:111;1–5.

48. DeLorenzo RJ, Waterhouse EJ, Towne AR, Boggs JG, Ko D, DeLorenzo GA, Brown A, Garnett L. Persistent nonconvulsive status epilepticus after the control of generalized convulsive status epilepticus. *Epilepsia* 1998; 39:833–840.

49. Tay SKH, Hirsch LJ, Leary L, Jette N, Wittman J, Akman CI. Nonconvulsive status epilepticus in children: clinical and EEG characteristics. *Epilepsia* 2006;47:1504–1509.

50. Towne AR, Waterhouse EJ, Boggs JG, Garnett LK, Brown AJ, Smith JR Jr, DeLorenzo RJ. Prevalence of nonconvuslive status epilepticus in comatose patients. *Neurology* 2000; 54:340–345.

51. Privitera MD, Strawsurg RH. Electroencephalographic monitoring in the emergency department. *Emerg Med Clin AM* 1994;12:1089–1101.

52. Thomas P. Status epilepticus: indications for emergency EEG. *Neurophysiol Clin* 1997;27:398–405.

53. Walker MC, Smith SJ, Shorvon SD. The intensive care treatment of status epilepticus in the UK. Results of a National Survey and recommendations. *Anaesthesia* 1995; 50:130–135.

54. Treiman DM, Meyers PD, Walton NY, Collins JF, Colling C, Rowan AJ, Handforth A, Faught E, Calabrese VP, Uthman BM, Ramsay RE, Mamdani MB. A comparison of four treatments for generalized convulsive status epilepticus. *N Eng J Med* 1998;339:792–798.

55. Appleton R, Choonara I, Martland T, Phillps B, Scott R, Whitehouse W. The status epilepticus working party. The treatment of convulsive status epilepticus in children. *Arch Dis Child* 2000;83:415–419.

56. Initial Management of Seizures. Texas Children's Hospital Evidence-Based Guidelines. 2009, Summer. Evidence based treatment for the initial management of seizures.

57. O'Brien TJ, Cascino GD, So EL, Hanna DR. Incidence and clinical significance of the purple glove syndrome in patients receiving intravenous phenytoin. *Neurology* 1998;51:1034–1039.

58. Garr RE, Appleton RE, Robson WJ, Molyneux EM. Children presenting with convulsions (including status epilepticus) to a paediatric accident and emergency department: an audit of a treatment protocol. *Dev Med Child Neurol* 1999;41:44–47.

59. Erikkson KJ, Koivikko MJ. Status epilepticus in children: aetiology, treatment and outcome. *Dev Med Child Neurol* 1997;39:652–658.

60. Erikssom E, Metsaranta P, Huhtala H, Auvinen A, Kuusela A-L, Koivikko M. Treatment delay and the risk of prolonged status epilepticus. *Neurology* 2005;65:1316–1318.

61. Appleton R, Martland T, Phillips B. Drug management for acute tonic–clonic convulsions including convulsive status epilepticus in children. *Cochrane Database Syst Rev* 2002;CD001905.

62. Chin RFM, Neville BGR, Peckham C, Wade A, Bedford H, Scott RC. Treatment of community-onset childhood convulsive status epilepticus: a prospective population-based study. *Lancet Neurol* 2008;7:696–703.

63. Wheless JW, Clarke DF, Carpenter D. Treatment of pediatric epilepsy, expert opinion, 2005. *J Child Neurol* 2005;20(Suppl 1):S1–S56.

64. Van Gestel JPJ, van Oud-Alblas HJ, Malingre M, Ververs FFT, Braum KPJ, van Nieuwenhuizen O. Propofol and

thiopental for refractory status epilepticus in children. *Neurology* 2005;65:591–592.

65. Schor NF, Riviello JJ. Treatment with propofol: the new status quo for status epilepticus? *Neurology* 2005;65:502–506.

66. Cornfield DN, Tegtmeyer K, Nelson MD, Milla CE, Sweeney M. Continuous propofol infusion in 142 critically ill children. *Pediatrics* 2002;110:1177–1181.

67. Hovinga CA, Chicella MF, Rose DF, Eades SK, Dalton JT, Phelps SJ. Use of intravenous valproate in three pediatric patients with nonconvulsive status epilepticus. *Ann Pharmacother* 1999;33:579–584.

68. Yu KT, Mills S, Thompson N, Cunanan C. Safety and efficacy of intravenous valproate in pediatric status epilepticus and acute repetitive seizures. *Epilepsia* 2003;44:724–726.

69. White JR, Santos CS. Intravenous valproate associated with significant hypotension in the treatment of status epilepticus. *J Child Neurol* 1999;14:822–823.

70. Alfonso I, Alvarez LA, Gilman J, Dunoyer C, Yelin K, Papazian O. Intravenous valproate dosing in neonates. *J Child Neurol* 2000;15:827–829.

71. Ramael S, Daoust A, Otoul C, Toublanc N, Troenaru M, Lu ZS, Stockis A. Levetiracetam intravenous infusion: a randomized, placebo-controlled safety and pharmacokinetic study. *Epilepsia* 2006;47:1128–1135.

72. Baulac M, Brodie MJ, Elger CE, Krakow K, Stockis A, Meyvisch P, Falter U. Levetiracetam intravenous infusion as an alternative to oral dosing in patients with partial-onset seizures. *Epilepsia* 2007;48:589–592.

73. Depositario-Cabacar DT, Peters J, Pong A, Roth J, Rotenberg A, Riviello JJ Jr., Takeoka M. High-dose intravenous levetiracetam for acute seizure exacerbation in children with intractable epilepsy. *Epilepsia* 2010;51:1319–1322.

74. Gilbert DL, Gartside PS, Glauser TA. Efficacy and mortality in treatment of refractory generalized convulsive status epilepticus in children: a meta-analysis. *J Child Neurol* 1999;14:602–609.

75. Kim SJ, Lee DY, Kim JS. Neurologic outcomes of pediatric patients treated with pentobarbital coma. *Pediatr Neurol* 2001;25:217–220.

76. Claassen J, Hirsch LJ, Emerson RG, et al. Treatment of refractory status epilepticus with pentobarbital, propofol, or midazolam: a systematic review. *Epilepsia* 2002;43:146–153.

77. Bleck TP. Management approaches to prolonged seizures and status epilepticus. *Epilepsia* 1999;40(Suppl 1):S59–S63.

78. Bleck TP. Refractory status epilepticus in 2001. *Arch Neurol* 2002;59:188–189.

79. Sahin M, Riviello JJ Jr. Prolonged treatment of refractory status epilepticus in a child. *J Child Neurol* 2001;16:147–150.

80. Kalviainen R, Eriksson K, Parviainen I. Refractory generalized convulsive status epilepticus. *CNS Drugs* 2005;19:759–768.

81. Alldredge BK, Gelb AM, Isaacs SM, Corry MD, Allen F, Ulrich S, Gottwald MD, O'Neil N, Neuhaus JM, Segal MR, Lowenstein DH. A comparison of lorazepam, diazepam, and placebo for the treatment of out-of-hospital status epilepticus. *N Engl J Med* 2001;345:631–637.

82. Alldredge BK, Wall DB, Ferriero DM. Effect on pre-hospital treatment of status epileptics in childhood. *Pediatr Neurol* 1995;12:213–216.

83. Yager JY, Seshia SS. Sublingual lorazepam in childhood serial seizures. *Am J Dis Child* 1988;142:931–932.

84. Holmes GL. Buccal route for benzodiazepines in treatment of seizures. *Lancet* 1999;353:608–609.

85. Scott RC, Besag FM, Neville BG. Buccal midazolam and rectal diazepam for treatment of prolonged seizures in childhood and adolescence: a randomized trial. *Lancet* 1999;20:623–626.

86. Lahat E, Goldman M, Barr J, Bistritzer T, Berkovitch. Comparison of intranasal midazolam with intravenous diazepam for treating febrile seizures in children: prospective randomized study. *BMJ* 2000;321:83–86.

87. Talukdar B, Chakrabarty B. Efficacy of buccal midazolam compared to intravenous diazepam in controlling convulsions in children: a randomized controlled trial. *Brain Dev* 2009;31:744–749.

88. Kimach VJ. Epic Clinical Network. The community use of rescue medication for prolonged epileptic seizures in children. *Seizure* 2009;18:343–346.

CHAPTER 39

Nonconvulsive Status Epilepticus

Shekhar G. Patil and Rod C. Scott

▶ INTRODUCTION

Status epilepticus is the most common neurological emergency in childhood and continues to be associated with significant mortality and morbidity. Although the main determinant of adverse outcome following status epilepticus is etiology, there continues to be concern that status epilepticus itself contributes to the outcome. Therefore, an understanding of the types of status epilepticus, the mechanisms, and frequencies of adverse outcomes and appropriate treatments is essential for defining strategies that aim to reduce morbidity associated with status epilepticus.

Status epilepticus is traditionally divided into convulsive and nonconvulsive forms. The aim of the current chapter is to provide an overview of nonconvulsive status epilepticus (NCSE) in terms of definition, clinical features, outcomes, treatments, and its relationship with epileptic encephalopathy. However, many of these aspects are not universally agreed and therefore there will also be discussion of the controversies surrounding NCSE.

▶ DEFINITION

In April 2004, a group of physicians with an interest in NCSE, representing a spectrum of opinion, met in Oxford[1] to discuss and debate the definition, diagnosis, and treatment of NCSE. There was no consensus on a specific definition and therefore the following broad definition was made; NCSE is a range of conditions in which electrographic seizure activity is prolonged and results in nonconvulsive clinical symptoms.

The International League Against Epilepsy suggest that status epilepticus should be defined as a seizure that shows no clinical signs of arresting after a duration encompassing the great majority of seizures of that type in most patients *or* recurrent seizures without interictal resumption of baseline central nervous system function. However, these definitions are not particularly useful in clinical practice as there is too much breadth; that is, what is prolonged?, and the definitions about clinical features are vague.

A time definition that is frequently used for NCSE is 30 minutes, which is the same as that commonly used to define convulsive status epilepticus. This construct appears to work for convulsive status epilepticus; after 30 minutes the seizure becomes self-sustaining, is more likely to cause brain injury and is associated with systemic decompensation, that is, hypotension, hypoglycemia, etc. However, the construct is less applicable to NCSE as 30 minutes may not describe a point following which there are potential pathophysiological changes that separate NCSE from short seizures with similar clinical manifestations.

The proposed definition from the Oxford meeting uses the term nonconvulsive clinical symptoms, which potentially means that any clinical feature (e.g., dizziness and headache) could be considered as a feature of NCSE if there were consistent electroencephalogram (EEG) features. The agreed component of the definition is that the features need to be associated with EEG abnormalities, but if any neurological symptom can be a manifestation of NCSE then many patients with neurological symptoms will require an EEG to rule out NCSE. It is likely that this is neither practical nor necessary.

Over the years, various authors have suggested definitions for the term NCSE and are inclusive of clinical changes such as impaired consciousness, and associated ictal electroencephalographic abnormalities, and response to treatment.[2-6] Most authors agree that alterations in the clinical state and associated plausible electroencephalographic changes should be the basis of the definition.[7] Clinical changes alone are not sufficient because these may be very subtle and sometimes hard to differentiate from normal behavior or nonepileptic medical disorders.[8] Therefore, at the current time, there is no universally accepted definition of NCSE, but the most consistent aspect of any proposed definition is the presence of electrical discharges continuing for a "prolonged" period of time.

▶ TYPES OF NCSE

NCSE in the adult population generally falls into two groups. The first consists of patients with generalized spike-wave discharge, often in the context of primary generalized epilepsy, known as absence status epilepticus. The second includes patients with focal epileptic discharges known as complex partial status epilepticus.

It is widely accepted that these two phenomena have differing clinical manifestations and outcomes, raising the issue as to whether NCSE can reasonably be considered a single entity. This issue is more difficult in children as the types of NCSE described in adults are less common in children, but frequent epileptic discharges that amount to NCSE in electrical terms are seen in other situations. Children with hypsarrhythmia,[9] Panayiotopoulos syndrome,[10,11] electrical status epilepticus in slow wave sleep (ESES),[12] benign Rolandic epilepsy, Landau–Kleffner syndrome (LKS), and Lennox–Gastaut syndrome may all meet electrical criteria but do not constitute a single pathophysiological entity.

► CLINICAL AND ELECTROGRAPHIC MANIFESTATIONS

There are many shared clinical features in absence and complex partial status epilepticus but the frequency of individual clinical features differ in either.

ABSENCE STATUS EPILEPTICUS

Patients with short absence seizures characteristically have complete loss of consciousness without recall of the event. However, in absence status epilepticus there is a spectrum in the degree of alteration of consciousness ranging from slight clouding, manifesting as difficulties in carrying out particular activities that are usually not problematic for the patient, to an epileptic stupor in which the patient is completely unresponsive. However, some degree of clouding of consciousness is almost universal in absence status epilepticus. Patients may also manifest motor phenomena[13] (myoclonus, atonia, blinking of eyelids, and pseudoataxia) and rarely psychiatric features including psychosis. Episodes may last hours or days and frequently terminate following a tonic–clonic convulsion. The majority of patients with absence status epilepticus have an existing diagnosis of absence epilepsy.[5]

There is a spectrum of electrographic abnormalities in patients with absence status epilepticus. The classical diagnostic pattern consists of continuous or near-continuous bilaterally synchronous and symmetrical spike-wave activity. The frequency of the discharges can be the typical 3 Hz spike and wave of a classical absence seizure,[14] or an atypical pattern with frequencies of 1.5–4 Hz.[14] In many patients, the EEG pattern is inconstant over time and the discharge frequency fluctuates.

COMPLEX PARTIAL STATUS EPILEPTICUS

The manifestations of complex partial status epilepticus are heterogeneous and typically consist of more than the patient's habitual focal seizure. Similar to absence status epilepticus, the seizures typically last for hours and occur most frequently in patients carrying a diagnosis of focal epilepsy.

Confusion is the cardinal manifestation of complex partial status epilepticus[15–19] and is more likely to be nonfluctuating than absence status epilepticus. Motor manifestations[15] are more obvious than in absence status epilepticus and include alterations in posture, unsteadiness, convulsive movements, and tonic spasms. There is a tendency to adversion and the patients may walk in circles; complex automatisms are more often seen in shorter seizures.[15] The patients may have behavioral changes including agitation, excitement, or psychomotor retardation and may have psychotic features. Speech patterns may be markedly abnormal and patients may become mute. In addition, there may be autonomic manifestations including pupillary dilatation, vomiting, borborygmi, and change in color.

Complex partial status epilepticus has very varied electroencephalographic manifestations.[2,14,16,19–21] Some patients have very few epileptic discharges and the EEG may not differ from the interictal state. Other ictal patterns include frequent (almost continuous) spike, spike-and-slow wave discharges, or desynchronizations that can be focal or more widespread. The most common anatomical location for focal discharges is the temporal lobe, although frontal lobe status epilepticus is not uncommon. Frontal lobe status epilepticus[22] may be associated with spike-wave discharges similar to absence status epilepticus.

Although these two types seem distinct there may be significant overlap in the clinical features[5,16–18,23] of absence[23,24] and complex partial types of NCSE. Fear, anxiety, irritability, and aggression are more frequent and also seen are automatisms, eye deviation, and nystagmus in those with complex partial NCSE. With both, complex partial seizures and absence NCSE total unresponsiveness, speech arrest, cyclic behavior, and stereotypic nonlateralized automatisms are common. Thus, these subtypes of NCSE may be difficult to distinguish on the basis of clinical features alone. As a rule, complex partial NCSE is more common in clinical practice than the absence type of NCSE.[17,25]

MANIFESTATIONS OF NCSE IN PEDIATRIC PRACTICE

Absence and complex partial status epilepticus in their purest forms are rare in childhood and NCSE in children is more typical of defined epilepsy syndromes. A variety of ictal manifestations that differ from adults have been described and include alterations in cognitive and behavioral status. Long-lasting epileptic EEG abnormalities may be observed in benign and severe epilepsy syndromes. Benign syndromes include

Panayiotopoulos syndrome and Benign–Rolandic epilepsy. The predominant clinical feature in Panayiotopoulos syndrome is ictal vomiting although other autonomic manifestations[11] such as color change, pupillary abnormalities, cardiorespiratory, and thermoregulatory alterations are also common. When these manifestations last at least 30 minutes they may be considered a form of NCSE.[11,26,27]

As with the adult forms of NCSE, treatment of the NCSE results in improvement in the EEG and a return of the child to their preictal state that in Panayiotopoulos syndrome is usually a return to normal. Children with benign Rolandic epilepsy[1] may have frequent Rolandic discharges in the EEG in sleep but there is seldom evidence for a clinical manifestation that could be considered to be status epilepticus, that is, the ictal clinical manifestations are usually short.

In a setting of acute change in behavior from a baseline as seen in developmentally normal children, NCSE may be relatively easy to diagnose because of the clear contrast between the two states and in presence of a clearly abnormal EEG. However, in children with severe epilepsy associated with learning and behavioral difficulties the diagnosis of NCSE is extremely difficult, and this is probably the most likely setting for NCSE in children.[28,29]

Severe syndromes in which there are epileptic discharges that may persist for at least 30 minutes include Ohtahara syndrome, West syndrome, Dravet syndrome, LKS, Lennox–Gastaut syndrome, and ESES; see Figure 39–1. The conditions are frequently referred to as epileptic encephalopathies although the terminology "encephalopathy with epilepsy" may be preferable, as the latter term does not imply that the observed encephalopathy is caused by epileptic discharges. The relationships between frequent epileptic discharges in the EEG and the clinical manifestations in the patients with these syndromes are not entirely clear. In these syndromes, there is often a complex interaction between the effects of the underlying etiology, the seizures, and the electrical abnormality such that it is not possible to discern individual effects.[29]

In West syndrome[9] there may be ongoing epileptic discharges (hypsarrhythmia) associated with functional deficits such as loss of normal visual behavior which could be considered as a clinical manifestation of NCSE. The infantile spasms are each short but may occur in clusters that last 30 minutes and it is uncertain whether this constitutes a separate manifestation of NCSE or is a form of convulsive status epilepticus.

In LKS the main clinical feature is loss of language although manifestations in other domains of functioning (motor, behavior, and learning) are common. However, in LKS, it is not clear whether these are ictal manifestations or a function of an associated encephalopathy. Successful treatment of the epileptic discharges may result in some recovery but it is not usually complete and occasionally there is an apparent response to treatment with little change in the EEG abnormality. In addition, there is no obvious relationship between the severity of the EEG abnormality and the clinical features. Similarly, in ESES, the EEG may be normal in the waking state, but it is in this state that the predominant clinical features of behavior and learning impairments are most common. It is in the sleep state that the EEG is consistent with NCSE.

Understanding the relationship between EEG abnormalities and ictal clinical manifestations is even more complex in children with Lennox–Gastaut syndrome and other encephalopathies with epilepsy. This is more glaring when we have a "boundary syndrome" in the classification scheme as suggested by Shorvon.[1] The term boundary syndrome includes cases of epilepsy with encephalopathy in which it is unclear as to the extent of contribution of the electrographic activity to the observed clinical impairment. This may induce a subjective bias to the diagnosis of NCSE in such a clinical setting.[9]

The EEG abnormality that may look like atypical absence status epilepticus may persist for many years. Clinical correlates include learning and behavioral impairments. In these children, it is often difficult to assess the baseline behavior because of the associated impairments and behavior may continue to worsen at a steady-state unrelated or independent of the EEG, so when it comes to defining change from baseline, it is a challenge to ascribe such changes to NCSE.[29]

Children with Lennox–Gastaut syndrome have periods when they lose further function and become unsteady, less responsive, and drool. They are sluggish, uncooperative, and often drowsy, walk with an unsteady gait and are known to have frequent falls.[1] These features are said to be descriptive of NCSE in children with learning and behavioral difficulties.[1,16,28,29] Periods of worsening may or may not be associated with a worsening of the EEG (see Figs. 39–2 and 39–3), but treatment as if this worsening was an episode NCSE may return the child to their previous state. If the background loss of function is considered to be NCSE then it is unclear what the period of worsening is other than "worse" NCSE. Thus, in the setting of encephalopathy with epilepsy dissecting NCSE from seizures/nonepileptic events may be difficult.

Niedermeyer and Fernandez-Torre regard NCSE as an extremely rare[7,30,31] phenomenon while others[32] regard NCSE to be common. It has been suggested that nearly a quarter of all cases of adult status epilepticus are NCSE[2,16] and our definitions are broadening to include more individuals with NCSE although the advantage in terms of biological understanding, prognosis, and treatment is not obvious.[9] Widening the definition of NCSE may result in more aggressive therapy

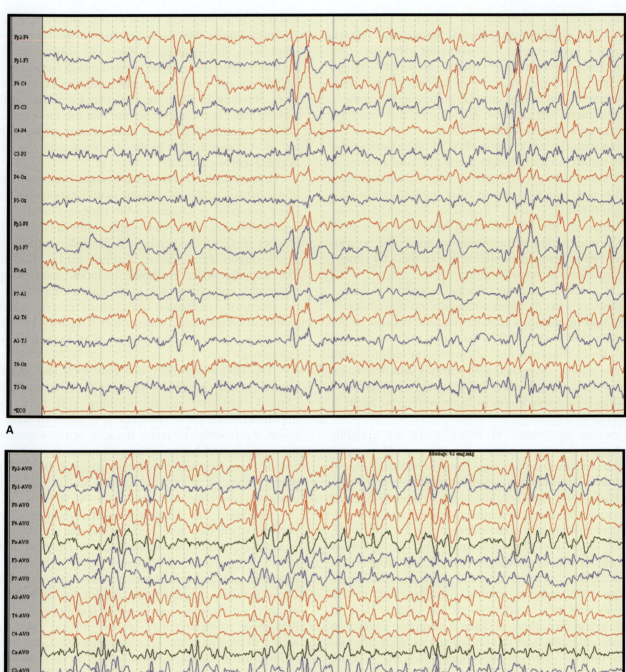

Figure 39–1. ESES. (**A**) EEG showing spike wave discharges just as the patient is getting drowsy. (**B**) EEG during slow wave sleep showing a flurry of discharges amounting to ESES.

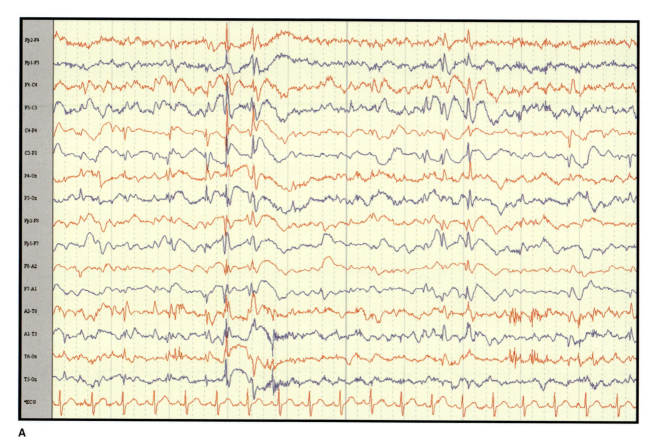

A

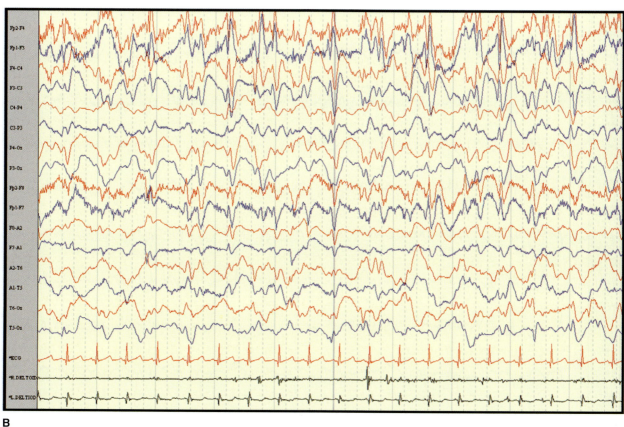

B

Figure 39–2. NCSE in a patient with LGS. (**A**) Interictal EEG in a 10-year-old boy with LGS. (**B**) EEG of the same patient during an episode of behavioral and cognitive change showing NCSE.

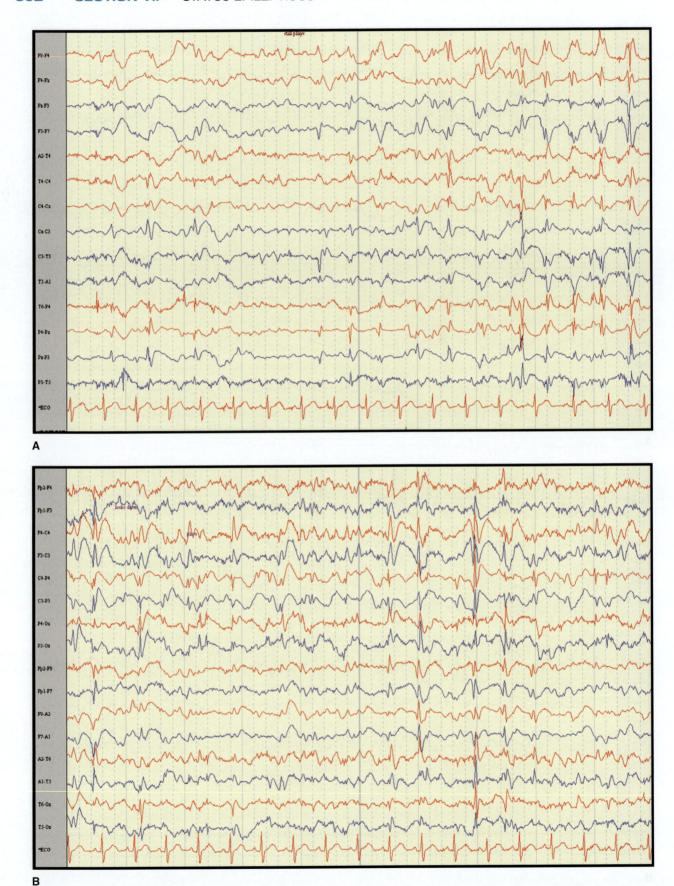

A

B

Figure 39–3. LGS—suspected NCSE. (**A**) Interictal EEG in an 8-year-old girl with LGS. (**B**) EEG of the same patient during an episode of behavioral/cognitive change leading to a suspicion of NCSE. However, the EEG does not show change from the baseline.

although evidence that this alters the long-term prognosis in children with for example encephalopathies with epilepsy is lacking.[27]

The diagnosis of NCSE[1,2,16,19,20] rests on the interpretation of the concurrent EEG. EEG interpretation itself can be difficult and distinction between ongoing epileptiform activity in children with encephalopathies with epilepsy and repetitive spike and wave or spike/sharp wave complexes may not be possible. However, a clear-cut acute deterioration in a premorbid normal child is usually reflected in the EEG. Accurate interpretation of what constitutes epileptiform activity is of utmost importance for a correct diagnosis of NCSE. Clearly defined and repetitive spike and slow wave complexes offer the most straightforward diagnosis, but other patterns[1,16] of "presumed seizure" activity such as rhythmic theta and delta waves may be challenging.

The concept of subtle generalized convulsive status epilepticus (sGCSE) has also been proposed as it may have important prognostic and therapeutic implications. sGCSE[1,2,16,19] is a clinical situation associated with ictal discharges on the EEG, with or without subtle convulsive movements such as rhythmic muscle twitches or tonic eye deviation and may occur in relation to an episode of GCSE[33] that is incompletely treated or in a comatose patient. The incidence of NCSE in comatose individuals is of particular interest. Some studies[34–36] quote a very high incidence of NCSE in coma, but its true incidence is uncertain. Kaplan[32] argues that epileptiform discharges in coma may be due to the underlying encephalopathy rather than true NCSE. A study in adults,[33] found less than 15% success in treatment of patients with subtle status epilepticus and their overall outcome was poor with a mortality of 65%. Even in the pediatric setting there is no consensus[36,37] regarding the true incidence of nonconvulsive status/seizures in children admitted to the intensive care unit with encephalopathy or an unexplained decreased level of consciousness. As a result of their poor response to conventional anticonvulsants and poor outcome, the European Federation of Neurological Societies (EFNS) guidelines[38] suggest using IV anesthetics early in management of sGCSE. However, there continues to be debate on whether sGCSE is pathophysiologically more similar to convulsive status epilepticus than to NCSE and therefore should not be considered to be a form of NCSE.

Practically speaking, clinicians faced with a patient with decreased level of consciousness and behavioral alterations should consider a possibility of NCSE. Resources may be an issue and one may need to rationalize the EEG requests. Features that may assist in the selection of patients requiring an urgent EEG include remote risk factors for seizures, oculomotor abnormalities, and seizure-like motor activity.[39,40]

NCSE is also associated with chromosomal disorders such as Angelman's syndrome[41,42] while prolonged atypical absences are seen in children with ring chromosome 20 syndrome.[43] Frequent NCSE may have effect developmental outcome of children with Angelman's syndrome.

▶ TREATMENT OF NCSE

As there is no consensus regarding the definition and precise nature of NCSE, it is difficult to suggest guidelines for its treatment. Several broad aspects of NCSE treatment need to be considered. These include the treatment of the epileptic discharges and encephalopathy, identification of precipitants, and management of comorbid impairments in cognition and behavior.

There are also limitations to the quality of the evidence for treatment of NCSE. Randomized controlled trials are usually considered to be the gold standard for deciding on whether a particular drug is effective. To date, there are no randomized controlled trials of treatments for NCSE. Large open trials with a clear definition of outcome provide useful information, but there are no trials of this type either. Therefore, anecdotal data forms the basis for choice of treatment.

Given the lack of studies evaluating therapy in NCSE, it is not surprising that there is little consensus on the most appropriate therapeutic strategies. This was highlighted in a recent study[44] evaluating the opinions of epileptologists and critical care neurologists who care for patients with complex partial status epilepticus. When asked how they would proceed after failure of first line therapy the responses ranged from further observation (20%) through use of another nonanaesthetizing antiepileptic agent (64%) to the use of general anesthesia (16%). The time that doctors were prepared to wait before instituting general anesthesia also varied considerably with 31% opting for general anesthesia within 30 minutes of onset of NCSE and 61% being prepared to wait for longer than 60 minutes. The parameter that most likely influences decision-making is the perception of NCSE's impact on brain injury. Kaplan[45] suggests that generalized NCSE does not cause lasting deficits, but debate persists regarding the morbidity of complex partial NCSE.

Benzodiazepines are first-line therapy for NCSE. Although intravenous benzodiazepines[46–48] is preferred, oral administration[49] is also effective and easier to administer. A single dose of oral benzodiazepines was effective in terminating NCSE in a study reported by Gastaut.[49] Diazepam is effective in 90%–100% of patients with NCSE in primary generalized epilepsy, but effectiveness diminishes to 15%–59% for Lennox–Gastaut syndrome and other epileptic encephalopathies. In practice a short course of benzodiazepines (e.g., clobazam three times a day for 3 days) is often administered because of a clinical impression that NCSE frequently recurs after a single dose (see Fig. 39–4).

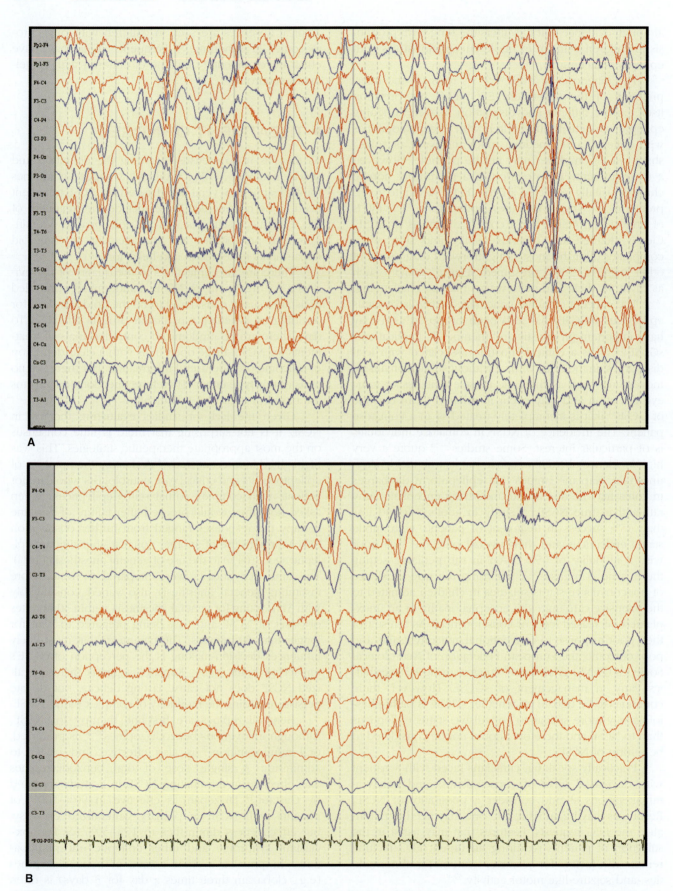

Figure 39–4. Response to benzodiazepines. (**A**) EEG of a 5-year-old boy during an episode of NCSE and before starting clobazam. (**B**) EEG of the same patient 36 hours later after receiving oral clobazam every 8 hours.

One needs to be somewhat cautious when using benzodiazepines for treatment of NCSE within the context of Lennox–Gastaut syndrome as they may induce NCSE.

NCSE in a setting of preexisting epilepsy or past history of status usually responds to first line anticonvulsants, that is, benzodiazepines in most situations, but even then recurrence is not unusual. On the other hand, *de novo* complex partial NCSE is known to be refractory to first line agents and usually requires other medications such as IV phenytoin or phenobaribitone[50,51] before the acute event is controlled.

Sodium valproate[52] is gaining in popularity although evidence supporting its use in NCSE is lacking; though certain characteristics of sodium valproate such as its availability for both oral and intravenous administration make it an attractive choice. In a study of 33 adults with NCSE,[50] 28 had complex partial NCSE and 5 had absence status, phenytoin was found to be effective in 80% of adult patients who mostly had complex partial status epilepticus. In addition, various other agents[53,54] such as levetiracetam, ketamine, acetazolamide have studied in case reports.

Treatment of some of the encephalopathies with epilepsy (e.g., LKS or ESES) using steroids[55–58] may reverse some of the clinical features but these children rarely achieve normal function. In other circumstances (e.g., Ohtahara syndrome or West syndrome), steroid treatment may effectively terminate seizures but there is little evidence that they alter long term developmental outcome except possibly in those children with infantile spasms and no identified underlying etiology.[59] In managing cases of complex partial NCSE due to a focal lesion long-lasting relief may be possible after surgery[60,61] to remove the focal lesion.

The cessation of ictal EEG activity and clinical symptoms may not rapidly reverse as in convulsive status epilepticus. Polytherapy[62,63] for epilepsy may occasionally induce an episode of NCSE. Besides antiepileptic drugs,[63–66] other agents[65–73] may provoke an episode of NCSE (Table 39–1).

Successful treatment of the discharges in NCSE does not necessarily result in return to baseline function and it may not be possible to eliminate all epileptic discharges. It is essential that any additional impairment are adequately characterized and that appropriate behavioral and educational interventions[74] are instituted, preferably using a multidisciplinary approach.

▶ OUTCOMES

While the outcome after convulsive status epilepticus is reasonably well described, the consequences of NCSE are far more poorly characterized and largely depend upon its clinical situation. Because there is no consensus in the definition of NCSE,[1] its true incidence is

▶ **TABLE 39–1. DRUGS PROVOKING NCSE**

Class of Drugs	Examples
Antiepileptic drug administration	Carbamazepine, phenytoin, phenobarbitone, tiagabine, vigabatrin, PR diazepam
Antiepileptic drug withdrawal	Benzodiazepines, replacement of sodium valproate with lamotrigine
Antibiotics	Cephalosporins
Antiasthma	Theophylline
Chemotherapeutic agents	Ifosamide
Medicines used in psychiatry	Lithium

unknown.[2,16,19,32] This has probably led to improper identification of cases or even failing to identify true NCSE resulting in a largely unknown outcome. Furthermore, a clear definition of the EEG patterns in NCSE has not been established making it challenging to correctly identify ictal EEG patterns.[45,75,76]

Patients with absence status epilepticus are likely to respond well to treatment; once the discharges have been treated the patient usually returns to their pre-NCSE state. There is no evidence that absence status epilepticus causes brain injury and is therefore considered to be a benign disorder. The consequences of complex partial status epilepticus are less clear and there remains considerable debate on whether complex partial status epilepticus can cause brain injury.[45,76–78] Clarification is of therapeutic importance as aggressive antiepileptic or neuroprotective[79] treatment is indicated to prevent potential brain damage. Shneker[80] et al studied 100 patients with NCSE and tried to prognosticate outcome based on associated comorbid conditions. They showed that underlying acute medical condition was the main cause of increased mortality rather than NCSE per se; patients with NCSE alone had a mortality of 3%.

Animal models[81–83] of limbic status epilepticus demonstrating damage to the mesial temporal structures support the hypothesis that complex partial status epilepticus could cause brain injury. However, these models also provide support for convulsive status epilepticus causing hippocampal injury. In humans, there is some evidence to suggest that convulsive status epilepticus can injure the hippocampus, but similar evidence relating to NCSE is lacking although complex partial status epilepticus in ambulatory patients has rarely been associated with measurable permanent neurologic deficit.[45,75,76]

The relationship between NCSE and the adverse neurological, cognitive, and behavioral outcomes of the encephalopathies with epilepsy is also unclear. There is an increasing body of opinion that frequent subclinical discharges that could amount to NCSE may result in permanent brain dysfunction and be the cause of the permanent encephalopathy seen in conditions like West syndrome, LKS, and Lennox–Gastaut syndrome. However, this can only be considered as hypothesis at this time as there are no data that strongly support this view. The alternative view that both the NCSE and the clinical features of encephalopathy are due to an underlying, currently unidentified, brain disorder is also hypothetical.

REFERENCES

1. Walker M, et al. Nonconvulsive status epilepticus: Epilepsy Research Foundation workshop reports. *Epileptic Disord* 2005;7(3):253–296.
2. Meierkord H, Holtkamp M. Non-convulsive status epilepticus in adults: clinical forms and treatment. *Lancet Neurol* 2007;6(4):329–339.
3. Mayeux R, Luders H. Complex partial status epilepticus: case report and proposal for diagnostic criteria. *Neurology* 1978;28:957–961.
4. Treiman DM, Delgado-Escueta AV. Complex partial status epilepticus. *Adv Neurol* 1983;34:69–81.
5. Tomson T, Lindbom U, Nilsson BY. Nonconvulsive status epilepticus in adults: thirty-two consecutive patients from a general hospital population. *Epilepsia* 1992;33:829–835.
6. Cockerell OC, Walker MC, Sander JW, Shorvon SD. Complex partial status epilepticus: a recurrent problem. *J Neurol Neurosurg Psychiatry* 1994;57:835–837.
7. Niedermeyer E, Ribeiro M. Considerations of nonconvulsive status epilepticus. *Clin Electroencephalogr* 2000;31:192–195.
8. Celesia GG. Modern concepts of status epilepticus. *JAMA* 1976;235:1571–1574.
9. Lux AL. Is hypsarrhythmia a form of non-convulsive status epilepticus in infants? *Acta Neurol Scand* 2007;115(4):37–44.
10. Shorvon S, Walker M. Status epilepticus in idiopathic generalized epilepsy. *Epilepsia* 2005;46(Suppl 9):73–79.
11. Panayiotopoulos CP. Autonomic seizures and autonomic status epilepticus peculiar to childhood: diagnosis and management. *Epilepsy Behav* 2004;5(3):286–295.
12. Tassinari CA, et al. The electrical status epilepticus syndrome. *Epilepsy Res Suppl* 1992;6:111–115.
13. Andermann F, Robb JP. Absence status. A reappraisal following review of thirty-eight patients. *Epilepsia* 1972;13(1):177–187.
14. Tay SK, Hirsch LJ, Leary L, Jette N, Wittman J, Akman CI. Nonconvulsive status epilepticus in children: clinical and EEG characteristics. *Epilepsia* 2006;47(9):1504–1509.
15. Shorvon S. Clinical forms of status epilepticus. In: Shorvon S (ed), *Status Epilepticus: Its Clinical Features and Treatment in Children and Adults.* Cambridge University Press, 1994; pp. 34–138.
16. Kaplan PW. The clinical features, diagnosis, and prognosis of nonconvulsive status epilepticus. *Neurologist* 2005; 11(6):348–361.
17. Tomson T, Svanborg E, Wedlund JE. Nonconvulsive status epilepticus: high incidence of complex partial status. *Epilepsia* 1986;27(3):276–285.
18. Cascino GD. Nonconvulsive status epilepticus in adults and children. *Epilepsia* 1993;34(Suppl 1):S21–S28.
19. Drislane FW. Presentation, evaluation, and treatment of nonconvulsive status epilepticus. *Epilepsy Behav* 2000; 1(5):301–314.
20. Granner MA, Lee SI. Nonconvulsive status epilepticus: EEG analysis in a large series. *Epilepsia* 1994;35:42–47.
21. Dan B, Boyd SG. Nonconvulsive (dialeptic) status epilepticus in children. *Curr Pediatr Rev* 2005;I:7–16.
22. Thomas P, Zifkin B, Migneco O, Lebrun C, Darcourt J, Andermann F. Nonconvulsive status epilepticus of frontal origin. *Neurology* 1999;52(6):1174–1183.
23. Snead OC III, Dean JC, Penry JK. Absence status epilepticus. In: Engel J Jr, Pedley TA (eds), *Epilepsy: A Comprehensive Textbook. Vol. 1.* Philadelphia: Lippincott-Raven, 1998; pp. 701–707.
24. Fujiwara T, Watanabe M, Nakamura H, Kudo T, Yagi K, Seino M. A comparative study of absence status epilepticus between children and adults. *Jpn J Psychiatry Neurol* 1988; 42(3):497–508.
25. Scholtes FB, Renier WO, Meinardi H. Non-convulsive status epilepticus: causes, treatment, and outcome in 65 patients. *J Neurol Neurosurg Psychiatry* 1996;61(1):93–95.
26. Ferrie CD, et al. Autonomic status epilepticus in Panayiotopoulos syndrome and other childhood and adult epilepsies: a consensus view. *Epilepsia* 2007;48(6):1165–1172.
27. Koutroumanidis M, Rowlinson S, Sanders S. Recurrent autonomic status epilepticus in Panayiotopoulos syndrome: video/EEG studies. *Epilepsy Behav* 2005; 7(3):543–547.
28. Stores G, Zaiwalla Z, Styles E, Hoshika A. Non-convulsive status epilepticus. *Arch Dis Child* 1995;73(2):106–111.
29. Hoffmann-Riem M, Diener W, Benninger C, Rating D, Unnebrink K, Stephani U, Ernst HP, Korinthenberg R. Nonconvulsive status epilepticus—a possible cause of mental retardation in patients with Lennox–Gastaut syndrome. *Neuropediatrics* 2000;31(4):169–174.
30. Niedermeyer E. Epileptic seizure disorders. In: Niedermeyer E, Lopes DA, Siva F (eds), *Electroencephalography: Basic Principles, Clinical Applications and Related Fields.* Philadelphia. PA: Lippincott, Williams & Wilkins, 2005; 5th edn: pp. 591.
31. Fernandez-Torre JL. Overuse of the term 'nonconvulsive status epilepticus'. *Clin Electroencephalogr* 2003;35:V.
32. Kaplan PW. Assessing the outcomes in patients with nonconvulsive status epilepticus: nonconvulsive status epilepticus is under diagnosed, potentially overtreated, and confounded by comorbidity. *J Clin Neurophysiol* 1999;16(4):341–352.
33. DeLorenzo RJ, et al. Persistent nonconvulsive status epilepticus after the control of convulsive status epilepticus. *Epilepsia* 1998;39(8):833–840.
34. Towne AR, et al. Prevalence of nonconvulsive status epilepticus in comatose patients. *Neurology* 2000;54(2): 340–345.
35. Jette N, Claassen J, Emerson RG, Hirsch LJ. Frequency and predictors of nonconvulsive seizures during continuous electroencephalographic monitoring in critically ill children. *Arch Neurol* 2006;63(12):1750–1755.

36. Hosain SA, Solomon GE, Kobylarz EJ. Electroencephalographic patterns in unresponsive pediatric patients. *Pediatr Neurol* 2005;32(3):162–165.

37. Saengpattrachai M, et al. Nonconvulsive seizures in the pediatric intensive care unit: etiology, EEG, and brain imaging findings. *Epilepsia* 2006;47(9):1510–1518.

38. Meierkord H, Boon P, Engelsen B, Gocke K, Shorvon S, Tinuper P, Holtkamp M. EFNS guideline on the management of status epilepticus. *Eur J Neurol* 2006; 13(5):445–450.

39. Husain AM, Horn GJ, Jacobson MP. Non-convulsive status epilepticus: usefulness of clinical features in selecting patients for urgent EEG. *J Neurol Neurosurg Psychiatry* 2003;74(2):189–191.

40. Khan RB, Yerremsetty PK, Lindstrom D, McGill LJ. Emergency EEG and factors associated with nonconvulsive status epilepticus. *J Natl Med Assoc* 2001;93(10):359–362.

41. Ohtsuka Y, et al. Relationship between severity of epilepsy and developmental outcome in Angelman syndrome. *Brain Dev* 2005;27(2):95–100.

42. Viani F, et al. Seizure and EEG patterns in Angelman's syndrome. *J Child Neurol* 1995;10(6):467–471.

43. Inoue Y, et al. Ring chromosome 20 and nonconvulsive status epilepticus. A new epileptic syndrome. *Brain* 1997; 120(Pt 6):939–953.

44. Holtkamp M, Masuhr F, Harms L, Einhaupl KM, Meierkord H, Buchhcim K. The management of refractory generalised convulsive and complex partial status epilepticus in three European countries: a survey among epileptologists and critical care neurologists. *J Neurol Neurosurg Psychiatry* 2003;74(8):1095–1099.

45. Kaplan PW. No, some types of nonconvulsive status epilepticus cause little permanent neurologic sequelae (or: "the cure may be worse than the disease"). *Neurophysiol Clin* 2000;30(6):377–382.

46. Tassinari CA, et al. Benzodiazepines: efficacy in status epilepticus. In: Delgado-Escueta AV, Wasterlain CG, Treiman DM, Porter RJ (eds), *Status Epilepticus: Mechanisms of Brain Damage and Treatment*. Vol. 34. New York: Raven Press, 1983; pp. 465–475.

47. Treiman DM, et al. A comparison of four treatments for generalized convulsive status epilepticus. Veterans Affairs Status Epilepticus Cooperative Study Group. *N Engl J Med* 1998;339(12):792–798.

48. Claassen J, Hirsch LJ, Emerson RG, Bates JE, Thompson TB, Mayer SA. Continuous EEG monitoring and midazolam infusion for refractory nonconvulsive status epilepticus. *Neurology* 2001;57(6):1036–1042.

49. Gastaut H, et al. Treatment of certain forms of status epilepticus by means of a single oral dose of clobazam. [French]. *Rev Electroencephalogr Neurophysiol Clin* 1984; 14:203–206.

50. Camacho A, et al. Nonconvulsive status epilepticus: experience in 33 patients. *[Spanish] Neurologia* 2001;16(9): 394–398.

51. Treiman DM, Walker MC. Treatment of seizure emergencies: convulsive and non-convulsive status epilepticus. *Epilepsy Res* 2006;68(Suppl 1):S77–S82.

52. Guerrini R. Valproate as a mainstay of therapy for pediatric epilepsy. *Paediatr Drugs* 2006;8(2):113–129.

53. Mewasingh LD, Sekhara T, Aeby A, Christiaens FJ, Dan B. Oral ketamine in paediatric non-convulsive status epilepticus. *Seizure* 2003;12(7):483–489.

54. Rupprecht S, Franke K, Fitzek S, Witte OW, Hagemann G. Levetiracetam as a treatment option in non-convulsive status epilepticus. *Epilepsy Res* 2007;73(3):238–244.

55. Lerman P, Lerman-Sagie T, Kivity S. Effect of early corticosteroid therapy for Landau–Kleffner syndrome. *Dev Med Child Neurol* 1991;33(3):257–260.

56. Sinclair DB, Snyder TJ. Corticosteroids for the treatment of Landau–Kleffner syndrome and continuous spike-wave discharge during sleep. *Pediatr Neurol* 2005;32(5): 300–306.

57. Robinson RO, Baird G, Robinson G, Simonoff E. Landau–Kleffner syndrome: course and correlates with outcome. *Dev Med Child Neurol* 2001;43(4):243–247.

58. Okuyaz C, Aydin K, Gucuyener K, Serdaroglu A. Treatment of electrical status epilepticus during slow-wave sleep with high-dose corticosteroid. *Pediatr Neurol* 2005;32(1):64–67.

59. Lux AL, et al. The United Kingdom Infantile Spasms Study (UKISS) comparing hormone treatment with vigabatrin on developmental and epilepsy outcomes to age 14 months: a multicentre randomised trial. *Lancet Neurol* 2005; 4(11):712–717.

60. Ng YT, Kerrigan JF, Rekate HL. Neurosurgical treatment of status epilepticus. *J Neurosurg* 2006;105(5 Suppl):378–381.

61. Ng YT, Kim HL, Wheless JW. Successful neurosurgical treatment of childhood complex partial status epilepticus with focal resection. *Epilepsia* 2003;44(3):468–471.

62. Ohtsuka Y, Sato M, Oka E. Nonconvulsive status epilepticus in childhood localization-related epilepsy. *Epilepsia* 1999; 40(7):1003–1010.

63. Loiseau P. Do antiepileptic drugs exacerbate seizures? *Epilepsia* 1998;39:2–4.

64. Perucca E, Gram L, Avanzini G, Dulac O. Antiepileptic drugs as a cause of worsening seizures. *Epilepsia* 1998; 39:5–17.

65. Skardoutsou A, Voudris KA, Vagiakou EA. Non-convulsive status epilepticus associated with tiagabine therapy in children. *Seizure* 2003;12(8):599–601.

66. Trinka E, et al. Non convulsive status epilepticus after replacement of valproate with lamotrigine. *J Neurol* 2002; 249(10):1417–1422.

67. Thomas P, Lebrun C, Chatel M. De novo absence status epilepticus as a benzodiazepine withdrawal syndrome. *Epilepsia* 1993;34(2):355–358.

68. Bellesi M, Passamonti L, Silvestrini M, Bartolini M, Provinciali L. Non-convulsive status epilepticus during lithium treatment at therapeutic doses. *Neurol Sci* 2006; 26(6):444–446.

69. Maganti R, Jolin D, Rishi D, Biswas A. Nonconvulsive status epilepticus due to cefepime in a patient with normal renal function. *Epilepsy Behav* 2006;8(1):312–314.

70. Martinez-Rodriguez JE, et al. Nonconvulsive status epilepticus associated with cephalosporins in patients with renal failure. *Am J Med* 2001;111(2):115–119.

71. Wengs WJ, Talwar D, Bernard J. Ifosfamide-induced nonconvulsive status epilepticus. *Arch Neurol* 1993;50(10): 1104–1105.

72. Marini C, Parmeggiani L, Masi G, D'Arcangelo G, Guerrini R. Nonconvulsive status epilepticus precipitated by carbamazepine presenting as dissociative and affective disorders in adolescents. *J Child Neurol* 2005;20(8):693–696.

73. Krieger AC, Takeyasu M. Nonconvulsive status epilepticus in theophylline toxicity. *J Toxicol Clin Toxicol* 1999; 37(1):99–101.

74. Pedro VM, Leisman G. Hemispheric integrative therapy in Landau–Kleffner syndrome: applications for rehabilitation sciences. *Int J Neurosci* 2005;115(8):1227–1238.

75. Kaplan PW. Nonconvulsive status epilepticus. *Neurology* 2003;61:1035–1036.

76. Kaplan PW. Prognosis in nonconvulsive status epilepticus. *Epileptic Disord* 2000;2(4):185–193.

77. Krumholz A. Epidemiology and evidence for morbidity of nonconvulsive status epilepticus. *J Clin Neurophysiol* 1999;16(4):314–322.

78. Drislane FW. Evidence against permanent neurologic damage from nonconvulsive status epilepticus. *J Clin Neurophysiol* 1999;16(4):323–331.

79. Fountain NB, Lothman EW. Pathophysiology of status epilepticus. *J Clin Neurophysiol* 1995;12(4):326–342.

80. Shneker BF, Fountain NB. Assessment of acute morbidity and mortality in nonconvulsive status epilepticus. *Neurology* 2003;61(8):1066–1073.

81. Krsek P, Mikulecka A, Druga R, Hlinak Z, Kubova H, Mares P. An animal model of nonconvulsive status epilepticus: a contribution to clinical controversies. *Epilepsia* 2001; 42(2):171–180.

82. Krsek P, et al. Long-term behavioral and morphological consequences of nonconvulsive status epilepticus in rats. *Epilepsy Behav* 2004;5(2):180–191.

83. Hosford DA. Animal models of nonconvulsive status. *J Cln Neurophysiol* 1999;16:306–313.

SECTION VIII
Comorbid Disorders

CHAPTER 40

Cognitive Deficits in Children with Epilepsy

Mary L. Smith, Anne Gallagher, and Maryse Lassonde

▶ INTRODUCTION

Cognitive problems among children with epilepsy are of paramount concern. Cognition includes a variety of skills such as intelligence, attention, learning, remembering, reasoning, judging, planning, and expressing and understanding language. One's proficiency in these processes can influence other aspects of function such as behavior and social skills. During development, the maturation of cognitive processes is protracted, extending from infancy though to adolescence, and for more complex aspects of cognition such as executive function, even into young adulthood. Thus, in youth with epilepsy, seizures occur during a long window of time that is essential for the development of basic and complex cognitive skills that form the core foundation for long-term educational, vocational, and interpersonal adaptation.[1]

Deficits in cognition are identified by children with epilepsy and their parents as a significant comorbidity. For example, in a study by Arunkumar et al,[2] parents of 80 children and adolescents with epilepsy were asked to list in order of importance their concerns about living with or caring for their children with epilepsy; children who were old enough to be interviewed were asked to express (independently of their parents) their own concerns about having epilepsy. For both parents and children, the second most common item identified was that of the cognitive effects of epilepsy. Their worries included learning disabilities, academic difficulties, poor attention and concentration, and impoverished memory.

▶ ONSET OF DEFICITS

Cognitive deficits appear to be present early on in the course of epilepsy and may even predate the onset of seizures. A study of children with idiopathic localization-related or primary generalized epilepsy approximately 10 months after seizure onset revealed a pattern of mild generalized cognitive difficulties.[3] It is thought that these deficits are related to structural brain anomalies. For example, in children evaluated soon after they experienced their first seizure, those with an abnormality detected on MRI performed more poorly on cognitive tasks than children without a significant brain abnormality.[4] These differences were widespread, and were found in the areas of intelligence, memory, language, processing speed, verbal learning and memory, and executive functions, with all these domains affected relatively equally. Cognitive deficits early in the course of epilepsy are especially pronounced in children with neurobehavioral comorbidities.[5]

The severity and duration of epilepsy are also important in determining the incidence and magnitude of cognitive deficits in children. There is evidence that childhood onset temporal lobe epilepsy is associated with adverse neurodevelopmental impact on both brain structure and function.[6] Patients with childhood onset seizures exhibited greater compromise across domains of cognitive performance and showed a substantial reduction in brain tissue volumes in extratemporal regions compared with patients with late onset temporal lobe seizures. Those patients with structural abnormalities at onset may be especially vulnerable to the long-term adverse effects of epilepsy.[4] Scores on neuropsychological tests were not related to EEG activity in children with recent onset epilepsy; however, in children with chronic epilepsy, the presence of slow wave activity was associated with memory impairment.[7] The authors speculated that the differences between the recent-onset and chronic samples represent a cumulative effect of neurophysiological abnormality on cognitive development.

► INTELLIGENCE

Although the majority of people with epilepsy have normal intelligence, the distribution of IQ scores is skewed toward lower values.[8–11] A study of 51 children with medically refractory epilepsy illustrated the wide range of cognitive functioning within this group.[12] The mean IQ was 84 (in the Low Average range, just over one standard deviation below the population mean of 100). The spread of IQ scores was considerable, spanning the Intellectually Deficient range (<1st percentile) to the Very Superior range (>99th percentile). In a community based sample of children followed for 10 years after diagnosis of epilepsy, 24% had IQs below the normal range.[13] In a study designed to document the occurrence of disabilities in an unselected population sample of children in Finland, 4–15 years of age, Sillanpaa[14] reported that the prevalence of epilepsy in the study population was 0.68%. Among the children with epilepsy, neurological deficit was found in 39.9%, the most frequent neurological impairments being mental retardation (31.4%), speech disorders (27.5%), and specific learning disorders (23.1%).

Even in individuals with normal intelligence, reports of deficits in specific aspects of neuropsychological functioning are common, particularly in the areas of attention and concentration, memory, executive function, and academic achievement. In this chapter, we review the evidence for problems in the areas of attention, memory, and executive function; we will also briefly address language function in children with epilepsy, although this area has not received as much research examination as the others. For each of these topics, we provide some practical suggestions to assist parents and teachers in the management of the cognitive dysfunction. These recommendations are not meant to be exhaustive. It must also be recognized that they will not apply to every child with epilepsy, as the patterns of cognitive strengths and weaknesses are quite individual. In the ideal situation, recommendations will be generated from an in-depth neuropsychological assessment of the child's abilities in multiple areas. We do not cover the area of academic achievement in any depth, as it is addressed in the chapter on "ADHD and Learning Disabilities" by Dunn and Bourgeois elsewhere in this book.

► ATTENTION

There is no clear and universally accepted definition of attention. One of the most explicit definitions comes from Lezac, Howieson, and Loring[15] who proposed that attention includes a collection of interrelated mechanisms underlying the organism's receptivity to stimuli and how it processes incoming excitation (whether internal or external). There are different kinds of attention. First, selective attention directs one's focus toward a target while ignoring nonrelevant stimulations. Sustained attention is the ability to maintain attention for a relatively long period of time in order to detect an infrequent event. Finally, divided attention is the capacity to share attentional resources into multiple and simultaneous stimuli. Based on the nature of the stimulus, attention is usually divided in terms of auditory and visual modalities. For instance, focusing on what a teacher is saying in a classroom refers to auditory attention whereas looking at graphics and figures on the blackboard would recruit visual attentional resources. Multiple cerebral regions are reported to be involved in attentional processing such as the reticular formation, prefrontal cortex, parietal regions, cingulum, and several cortical and subcortical networks.[14]

Attention deficits have been shown to be more frequent in the pediatric epilepsy population than in healthy children, or in other chronic pediatric ailments such as diabetes or heart disease.[17,18] Indeed, clinical studies report that 30%–40% of children with epilepsy also have attention deficit hyperactivity disorder (ADHD).[19,20] The reasons for this association are still unclear. Some hypothesis, such effects of antiepileptic medication, underlying neurodevelopmental vulnerability, effects of chronic seizures, and subclinical epileptiform activity on cognitive function and possible common genetic defect underlying both disorders, have been suggested.[21,22] Difficulties in sustaining attention are most consistently reported in the epilepsy literature.[23] For instance, children with absence seizures present with sustained attention deficits.[24] Patients with childhood absence epilepsy and juvenile myoclonic epilepsy (JME) have lower scores on sustained and selective attention tests than control participants.[25] Children with idiopathic generalized epilepsy exhibit significantly lower performance at visual and auditory attention tasks compared to healthy children.[26]

Data on attention profiles of different epilepsy types are variable. In fact, attention problems are not only associated with generalized epilepsy but also with focal epilepsy. For example, Pinton et al[27] showed impairments in children with benign childhood epilepsy with centrotemporal spikes (BECTS) compared to the normal age range. Hernandez et al[28] investigated attention capacities in children suffering from three different types of epilepsy (frontal lobe epilepsy, temporal lobe epilepsy, and generalized absence seizures). They showed that a deficit in sustained attention was present in all three groups compared to a control group of the same age and IQ. However, children with frontal lobe epilepsy presented significantly greater sustained attention deficits, and also visual attention problems, compared to the two other epileptic groups. Furthermore, in a questionnaire, parents of children with frontal lobe epilepsy described their child as more inattentive than parents of children with temporal lobe epilepsy or generalized absence seizures. Similarly, in a case study, Boone et al[29] described a 13-year-old girl with bilateral frontal foci who showed considerable fluctuation in auditory attention and working memory. Moreover, Jambaqué and Dulac[30] observed an important attention deficit on an auditory continuous performance task and a visual cancellation task in an 8-year-old boy with an epileptic focus in the right frontotemporal region. Impaired performance on the same auditory continuous performance task has also been reported for children with benign focal childhood epilepsy.[31] Children with frontal lobe epilepsy have more problems resisting interference from a distracter than do children with temporal lobe epilepsy or healthy children.[32] The fact that frontal lobe epilepsy is frequently associated to attention deficits might be explained by the significant involvement of the prefrontal cortex in attention control.[33] Attention deficits are commonly reported in patients with frontal lesions, and appear to be attributable to a difficulty ignoring irrelevant stimuli.[34] Although attention deficits seem to be frequently related to frontal epilepsy, the attention profile related to epilepsy involving other cerebral regions is heterogeneous, probably because there are multiple factors that can interfere with the neuropsychological portrait (antiepileptic medication, age at the onset, and duration of epilepsy, kind of seizures, and so on.).

Thus, attention skills seem to be vulnerable to various epileptic disorders. This cognitive function is also sensitive to some anticonvulsive medication. In some cases, attention problems seem to be elicited or exacerbated by antiepileptic drugs such as phenobarbital, benzodiazepines, topiramate, valproate, and vigabatrin[35] whereas lamotrigine does not seem to have any negative effects on attention.[36] Lamotrigine as an add-on therapy has even been reported in some cases to enhance attention, alertness, and emotional stability.[37] Furthermore, polypharmacotherapy has been reported to induce more attention and memory problems than monopharmacotherapy.[38] Bennett-Levy and Stores[39] showed that children who no longer took antiepileptic drugs and attended regular school displayed a decreased alertness compared to healthy classmates. However, those children still under antiepileptic therapy also presented a decreased alertness and scored lower than healthy children in concentration and mental processing measures. Based on these studies, the choice of the pharmacologi-

cal therapy is a concern and should be made considering possible cognitive side effects.

STRATEGIES FOR TREATMENT OF ATTENTIONAL DEFICITS

Attention deficits, without intellectual disability, constitute a significant predictor of academic difficulties in children with epilepsy.[40] Treatment and intervention plans thus are very important. Because better seizure control may be associated with cognitive improvement,[41] a first step is the reevaluation of seizure control through a review of the antiepileptic drug regime. Second, some studies have shown that surgery may improve attention skills,[42,43] presumably by a reduction of seizure frequency.[44] However, Smith et al[45] did not find any cognitive changes in children who underwent epilepsy surgery. Thus, while the possibility of surgery should be investigated for appropriate candidates, one must keep in mind that the benefits to attention or other cognitive functions may be minimal. Psychostimulant medication would also be an option that should be investigated by a physician. (*See Chapter of Dunn and Bourgeois in this book for a complete discussion on this topic*). However, a combination of pharmacologic and behavioral approaches has been shown to be the most effective with children presenting with attention deficits.

Cognitive rehabilitation methods can also be used to improve attention in children with epilepsy. Rehabilitation programs could be designed for each patient based on their environmental and familial context, diagnosis, neuropsychological assessment, and the attention component, which is particularly impaired. In a literature review on attention rehabilitation, Sturm and Leclercq[46] presented different attention retraining interventions that have been used with adult populations (brain injury, strokes, psychosis, and so on). The programs included computerized attention tasks or behavioral tasks in a laboratory setting and the duration of the intervention varied from a few weeks to 6 years. Most of them produced a significant enhancement of attention skills in neuropsychological tests, but the impact on daily life was not always clear. The authors concluded that attention retraining treatments must be specific to the deficient attention component (e.g., selective attention, sustained attention, or divided attention), because a lack of specificity could overload the attention system and then magnify the impairment.[47]

Improvement of attention skills after retraining has also been shown to improve other cognitive domains such as memory or executive functions,[48,49] probably because attention is an important element to their execution. Very few studies have been conducted on cognitive rehabilitation, however, and the populations under study, the protocols used and even the results are heterogeneous. To our knowledge, no study has yet been carried out on attention deficit rehabilitation in pediatric epilepsy, and only a few investigations have included adult epileptic patients.

In a case study, Gupta and Naorem[50] applied a neurorehabilitation program including cognitive retraining (attention, concentration, and memory), supportive therapy and relaxation therapy, to a 32-year-old man with epilepsy, and the results suggested that attention retraining and home intervention could provide substantial benefits to patients with epilepsy. The effectiveness of two methods used for rehabilitation of attention deficits, one aimed at retraining impaired cognitive function, and one aimed at teaching compensatory strategies, was evaluated in an adult population with focal epilepsy.[51] Both methods enhanced attention function and quality of life in this population compared to a waiting list control group. The compensatory method was more effective in improving quality of life, especially for patients with less education (≤11 years). The authors concluded that cognitive rehabilitation programs are effective for patients with focal epilepsy and attention problems and should be incorporated into comprehensive care programs.

Further research is needed before introducing attention rehabilitation programs as part of the regular clinical interventions with children with epilepsy. Nevertheless, some compensatory methods could readily be applied by parents and teachers. In this context, information concerning epilepsy and the child's abilities should be given early to parents and teachers.[52] Based on an interdisciplinary assessment, including neuropsychological assessment and questionnaires, an intervention plan and tailored recommendations can be established.

Level of education may be an essential part of rehabilitation of attention deficits. In a recent study conducted with adults presenting with JME, Pascalicchio et al[53] showed less severe cognitive deficits including attention problems in patients with a higher educational level (>11 years) than in patients who had a lower educational level (≤11 years). Conversely, the cognitive deficits may have limited the educational attainments; sustained attention deficits are predictive of academic failure, possibly even more so than memory dysfunction or socioeconomic status.[54] It is thus very important to provide strategies and create a favorable learning environment at home and at school to maximize school achievement.

Table 40–1 presents a list of some recommendations and advices that can be provided to parents and teachers with regard to attention problems.

► EXECUTIVE FUNCTIONS

Executive functions represent a cognitive construct that refers to the abilities necessary to maintain an appropriate problem-solving set for the attainment of future goals.[55] These abilities include planning, self-monitoring, organized search, concept formation, attention and impulse control[56] as well as working memory.[57] Executive dysfunction is associated with behavioral disturbance, social dysfunction, and reduced educational and occupational attainment,[15] and is frequently reported in the neuropsychological profile of children with epilepsy.[68]

The involvement of prefrontal cortex in executive functioning has been shown in a variety of studies of normal subjects and patients with lesions to the frontal lobes.[59] Frontal lobe epilepsy can also induce executive dysfunction[60] and may be more prone to elicit it than other types of focal epilepsy. Hernandez et al[61] compared the performance of children (aged between 8 and 16 years) with frontal lobe epilepsy, temporal lobe epilepsy, and generalized epilepsy on a battery of tests assessing executive functions. Children with frontal lobe epilepsy showed greater difficulties in planning, impulse control, mental flexibility, and complex motor sequence programming than children with other types of epilepsy. Younger children (8–12 years old) with frontal lobe epilepsy had greater "executive" deficits compared to the older ones (13–16 years old). They also showed limited lexical access in a verbal fluency task, a finding congruent with case studies. The 8-year-old child with frontal lobe epilepsy studied by Jambaqué and Dulac[30] showed impairment in verbal fluency, whereas the 13-year-old frontal lobe epilepsy patient described by Boone et al[29] did not. Young patients with frontal lobe epilepsy seem to have greater difficulties mobilizing their resources to initiate the verbal search. Thus, the impact of frontal lobe epilepsy on some executive functions may be greater when the frontal lobes are still at an early stage of development.

Compared to children with temporal lobe epilepsy or generalized epilepsy, children with frontal lobe epilepsy were also more sensitive to interference in a verbal learning test and showed greater working memory deficits.[28] Working memory refers to a capacity limited system that allows one to mentally manipulate information maintained in short-term memory. This memory function is very sensitive to interference and its perturbation is usually associated to a frontal dorsolateral cortex malfunctioning.[62] Working memory deficits and planning difficulties have also been documented in case studies of children with frontal lobe epilepsy.[29,30]

JME is a generalized epilepsy syndrome associated with thalamofrontal circuitry dysfunction[63] and structural thalamic and frontal abnormalities.[64] Pulsipher et al[64] recently reported that executive functioning of children with JME was significantly impaired compared to healthy control children and children with BECTS, which is not an epileptic syndrome specifically associated with frontal dysfunction.

Although deficits in executive functions are the hallmark of frontal lobe dysfunction, several studies have shown that children and adults suffering from

▶ **TABLE 40–1. RECOMMENDATIONS FOR PARENTS AND TEACHERS OF CHILDREN WHO PRESENT WITH ATTENTION DEFICITS**

For Parents
- Supply the children with a quiet area to study and do their homework while controlling visual and noisy distractions.
- Teach them how to prepare a proper working area to do their homework. For instance, show them to tidy away useless material before starting their work.
- Alternate intense working periods and moments of recreation.
- Use a blank sheet or turn down the working sheet in order to see one question at a time.
- Systematically encourage your children and give them your attention when they participate to activity for longer periods of time.
- If there is hyperactivity associated to the attention deficit, recommend a kinetic approach during the homework period using motor activity in the learning process. For example, make the children jump while learning multiplication tables or make them draw or manipulate objects related to the learning subject.

For Teachers
- Create an adapted school intervention plan to inform teachers and school management about the child's needs. A 6-month follow-up is advised.
- Keep frequent contacts (phone call once a month) among teachers, school staff, and parents.
- Withdraw a course that is not compulsory in the educational program in order to provide more time working on essential courses.
- Stay close to the child while providing explanations and use their material to give examples.
- Take away the class distracters as much as possible.
- Make the child participate actively in the classroom to maintain their attention.
- Establish a secret code with the children to catch their attention when they are unfocussed or to let the teacher know that they are not following anymore. For instance, the child could take a red pencil in their hand when they are lost in an explanation.
- Use the child's first name in examples.
- Use short instructions.
- Divide into segments long instructions or problems instead of presenting the whole information at the same time.
- Prepare for the child multiple short exams instead of a long evaluation, and distribute them over a few days.
- Assign a desk in front of the class, close to the teacher, and far from distracters (window, fan, door).
- The child may sit by a child who could help them and with whom they have a good relationship.
- If there is a hyperactivity associated to the attention deficit, the child can be appointed to bring things to the teacher's desk or to perform tasks that require them to go outside of the classroom (message, snack) making them move whenever it is possible.

temporal lobe epilepsy may present impairments that are similar to, albeit less severe than those seen in frontal lobe epilepsy patients on a number of "frontal" measures. Hernandez et al[61] found that a relatively high proportion (38%–50%) of children with temporal lobe epilepsy performed below age norms on tasks measuring motor coordination, verbal fluency, and mental flexibility. This finding is consistent with other studies. Children with temporal lobe epilepsy and hippocampal atrophy had below-normal performance on the Wisconsin Card Sorting Test (WCST), a test that purports to assess concept formation and mental flexibility.[65] These deficits may be due to the propagation of "neural noise" associated with epileptogenic discharges in medial temporal structures to neighboring extratemporal regions, notably the frontal cortex via a temporofrontal circuit.[66] Other studies also reported executive dysfunction in JME, idiopathic generalized epilepsy, and childhood absence epilepsy,[25,42,53,67] demonstrating that "frontal lobe" dysfunction may also be present in generalized epilepsies.

Only a few studies have been conducted to assess the presence of executive dysfunction related to antiepileptic drugs. In a prospective study, Hessen, Lossius, and Gjerstad[68] showed that withdrawal of antiepileptic drugs in a large group of seizure free epileptic adults on monotherapy is associated with a significant improved performance on executive function measures. While topiramate has been known to interfere with attention skills, it also affects executive functions such as working memory, inhibition, and verbal fluency in patients with epilepsy[69] and healthy volunteers.[70] A slight improvement of executive functioning after topiramate withdrawal in partial, especially temporal lobe epilepsy has been shown.[71] Considering that multiple executive function tests are often used to measure attention ability, this improvement could also be attributed, at least in part, to a gain of attention capacities. As suggested before, pharmacological therapy should be carefully chosen with regard to its possible cognitive side effects.

Considering that executive dysfunction has been shown to be a significant predictor of poor quality of life[72] and school achievement[73] in children with epilepsy, the treatment of executive function deficits is of considerable importance. Surgery is an alternative solution to medication in refractory epilepsy for appropriate patients, but it may interfere with cognitive functioning. However, data regarding postoperative deficits are inconsistent. Negative effects of frontal lobe epilepsy surgery have been reported on verbal fluency, design fluency, and mental flexibility tests in adults.[74] In contrast, Lendt et al[75] noted stable executive functioning a year after frontal lobe surgery in children.

STRATEGIES FOR TREATMENT OF EXECUTIVE FUNCTION DEFICITS

Cognitive rehabilitation may have the potential to enhance executive functioning in patients with epilepsy. To date, however, no study has been carried out on executive function rehabilitation and epilepsy and very few studies have been conducted with other clinical populations. Luria[76] was the first to propose a theoretical approach for executive problems improvement. He suggested that executive rehabilitation should be based on the replacement of the absent internal structure by an external guidance. Evans, Emslie, and Wilson[77] used external aids to improve initiation and organization in daily life activities (medication intake, plant watering, laundry, and bathing) in a 50-year-old woman with bilateral frontal lesions. They used a checklist and a *NeuroPage* (cellular telephone with an alphanumeric screen that sent a text message to the patient to inform her that she should start an activity) to provide an external cue to start an activity, to reduce potential distracters, and to prevent impulsive actions. Derouesné, Seron, and Lhermitte[78] successfully used an external regulation blurring technique and a preorganization and segmen-

tation strategy of an activity to enhance self-regulation capacity in neuropsychological tasks in patients with a frontal lesion. The rehabilitation was divided in six steps: (1) detailed oral instructions, (2) detailed written instructions, (3) less detailed oral instructions, (4) less detailed written instructions, (5) simple oral stimulation, and (6) no intervention. Cicerone and Wood[79] taught a self-instruction strategy to improve planning capacity in a 20-year-old man who suffered from traumatic brain injury. During the first training phase, the patient was instructed to verbalize out-loud a plan before and during the execution of the task. The second phase was similar but the participant was instructed to whisper the plan. The third step required to internally rehearse the instructions instead of loudly. This study shows that self-instruction strategies can be useful to alleviate planning and self-regulation problems, but specific training must also be provided to generalize the improvement to daily life tasks. Thus, a few studies have shown the positive impact of executive function rehabilitation but a major concern remains that of transferring the learning to other contexts and activities. Furthermore, more studies are needed to assess the efficacy of these techniques in epilepsy and to adapt them to children.

Table 40–2 presents some examples of recommendations that can be useful for parents and teachers of children presenting with executive functions deficits. Strategies adapted to each child can be developed and adjusted as a function of age and context.

▶ MEMORY

Memory refers to the capacity to store and retrieve information. It allows us to form lasting representations of our everyday lives, to remember events and people

---

▶ **TABLE 40–2. RECOMMENDATIONS FOR PARENTS AND TEACHERS OF CHILDREN WHO PRESENT WITH EXECUTIVE DYSFUNCTION**

For Parents
- Teach your child how to use a calendar and a diary.
- Teach them how to use an alarm watch that emits a sound when an important task has to be done.
- Define and write down in a notebook a step-by-step procedure related to tasks and activities they are performing frequently, and make this notebook available to them.
- Encourage your child to initiate tasks.
- Teach your child to divide an activity into multiple steps before initiating it.
- Before starting an activity, assist your child to establish and to prepare the equipment required and to define every step composing the activity.

For Teachers
- Use short instructions.
- Divide into segments long instruction or problems instead of presenting the whole information at the same time.
- In exercises or exams, highlight important instructions.
- Provide the child more time for exams and evaluations.
- Read out loud with them, or allow them to read out loud exam questions.
- Teach them some exam strategies (e.g., use a process of elimination with a multiple choice question, highlight important information, skip harder questions, and come back to them at the end).

in our present and past, and to learn the regularities in our worlds and adapt our behavior accordingly.[80] Memory can be affected by a number of other cognitive processes, such as attention, effort, self-monitoring, speed of information processing, and the use of strategies and organization.[15]

Memory problems are among the most common complaints of people with epilepsy. Thompson and Corcoran[81] conducted a survey of 760 individuals with epilepsy and asked about the frequency of everyday memory failures, such as forgetting where things have been put, of losing things, going back to check if one had done something that one had intended to do, and being unable to say a word, although that word was known and "on the tip of one's tongue." People with epilepsy not only endorsed a higher frequency of such events but also rated the nuisance arising from such memory failures as higher than did people without epilepsy. Of further interest was the finding that relatives rated the frequency of forgetting among their family members with epilepsy as higher than did the persons themselves, suggesting that people with epilepsy may forget how often they do forget.

This study by Thompson and Corcoran[81] was conducted with adults, and a comparable comprehensive survey has not been undertaken with children. However, qualitative studies based on interviews with children and teenagers revealed a number of themes that were consistent with the types of memory failures described by adults.[82,83] These youth complained of difficulty retaining learned material, whether it was very recently acquired or whether it had been learned some time in the past; this problem interfered significantly with progress in school. Similarly, they had difficulty with retaining instructions as they were being presented. Personal events from the recent and remote past were often forgotten, with some children complaining that they had little sense of their earlier childhood. Another theme that arose from their introspections was that they experienced marked difficulty with word finding, similar to the tip-of-the-tongue phenomena described by the adults in the Thompson and Corcoran[81] study. The youth were able to identify other factors that complicated their memory processing, namely the presence of seizures, antiepileptic drugs, fatigue, and difficulty with concentration and attention.

It is not surprising that problems in the realm of attention can affect memory; accurate and efficient encoding of material is essential for storage and later retrieval. The importance of attention for good memory in this population is supported by the finding that memory in children with epilepsy was significantly predicted by symptoms associated with inattention.[48,84]

In adults with epilepsy, memory impairments are described most often in association with temporal lobe seizures. In children, these deficits may be more widespread. Children with intractable temporal lobe epilepsy, frontal epilepsy, and absence epilepsy are at risk for memory disorders.[85] The severity of the deficits varied by syndrome; those with absence epilepsy were found to have mild problems, and those with temporal lobe epilepsy had the most severe difficulties.

Several investigators have reported memory deficits in children with epilepsy of temporal lobe onset, but the patterns of findings they observed differed across studies. Findings similar to those seen in adults have been documented in some studies, in that left temporal lobe seizure foci were associated with verbal memory deficits and right temporal lobe foci were associated with visuo-spatial deficits.[86–90] Others have found no differences between the effects of seizures arising from the left or right temporal lobes on memory performance across a variety of verbal and spatial tasks.[40,42,91–96] Children with hippocampal abnormality at the onset of their seizure disorder showed considerable variability in their neuropsychological profiles[4] as opposed to the more specific deficits in language and memory that have been documented in adults.[97]

To date, little work has been done on identifying whether certain aspects of memory are more problematic than others in children with epilepsy (e.g., whether learning, storage or retrieval might be more affected). As mentioned earlier, attention may play an important role in everyday memory in this population. Performance on memory tasks in pediatric epilepsy has been found to be influenced by attention, suggesting that there may be difficulties with the initial encoding of information.[96] Working memory is also important for the recognition and recall of information.[98] Children with left temporal lobe epilepsy have been described as having most difficulty with delayed recall of verbal information,[85] implying difficulty with retrieval or that memories are susceptible to rapid forgetting.

There is little research on the effects of AEDs on memory in children, although such effects have been demonstrated in adults. One drug on which data are available is topiramate that can result in forgetfulness and impaired memory and also in reduced attention and concentration, which could have secondary effects on memory.[99]

The research findings using standardized tests of memory are corroborated by youth self-report. In a qualitative study of children and adolescents with refractory epilepsy, 70% of the participants reported problems with learning and memory.[82] Memory deficits were identified as a significant impediment to progress in school, and also as having an impact on the youth's sense of self-worth, as some labeled themselves as "stupid" because of their struggles with learning and retaining their schoolwork. These young people identified a number of key factors that characterized their learning difficulties and that contribute to their deficits. They noted the need for frequent repetition due to the difficulty with registering new information as it is taught and because of rapid forgetting and trouble remembering even over the span of one day to the next. These observations speak to the importance of programming to lessen the impact of these memory deficits.

STRATEGIES FOR TREATMENT OF MEMORY DEFICITS

Cognitive rehabilitation programs have been used to address memory deficits in a variety of neurological disorders. Such programs typically include the use of environmental manipulations, the use technology such as palm-type computers, digital recorders, pagers or timers, and training in the use of strategies for encoding and retrieval of information.[100] Little work has been done with epilepsy[101] and the feasibility and utility of such programs in pediatric epilepsy is untested. Table 40–3 presents some recommendations and strategies that parents and teachers can implement.

Acetylcholinesterase inhibitors have been shown to improve memory functioning in diverse neurological conditions. Two studies have examined whether donepezil would improve memory in adults with epilepsy. One was an open-label study in which patients underwent neuropsychological testing before and 3 months following treatment with donepezil.[102] Results showed a significant improvement in word list learning; however, there was no control for placebo effects or assessment of mood or other aspects of cognition. A second study, designed to address these concerns, found that donepezil treatment was not associated with improvement in memory or other cognitive functions, mood, social functioning, or quality of life.[103] Comparable increases in self-rated memory functioning relative to baseline were evident during both the donepezil and placebo phases. No work on children has yet been done with this potential modality of treatment.

▶ LANGUAGE

Although there is not an extensive literature on language and pediatric epilepsy, studies show that many

---

▶ **TABLE 40–3. RECOMMENDATIONS FOR PARENTS AND TEACHERS OF CHILDREN WITH MEMORY DEFICITS**

For Parents and Teachers

- Increase attention. Children will not remember something that they did not pay attention to in the first place. Be sure the child's memory problems are not really attention problems.
- Be organized. Establish routines, keep things in the same places; these strategies will better enable children to know the when and where of activities and materials necessary for them.
- Suggest strategies. Look for memory tricks that can help the child. For example, when you teach left and right, have them hold up both hands in the shape of an L. The hand with the forward-facing L is the left one. To help them recall how to read a word with two consecutive vowels, tell them, "When two vowels go walking, the first does the talking."
- Get the details. Parents and teachers can have a long-term impact on memory development by including many questions and specifics in conversations with children about past events. When you talk about a recent movie, for instance, ask, "What was your favorite part?" or "What did the hero do?" Fill in the details if they cannot provide them.
- Break tasks into manageable parts. If the child has to memorize material, have them break the task down into parts, and work on the most difficult sections first.
- Enhance meaningfulness. Find ways to relate the content being discussed to the child's prior knowledge. Draw parallels to the child's own lives and interests. Bring in concrete, meaningful examples for children to explore so the content becomes more a part of their experience.
- Use hands-on activities. We remember content better when we experience it for ourselves.
- Use multiple modalities. For children with verbal memory problems, pictures can provide a memory advantage. Use pictures, photographs, illustrations, videotapes, or diagrams. Encourage children to create images, or "pictures in their heads." Conversely, children who have visual memory problems may benefit from the use of verbal or descriptive strategies.
- Increase the amount of repetition. Children remember information better if they have practice using it more frequently. Use lots of review in your teaching; do not simply finish one topic and then never mention it again. Remind the class, and have child's practice previous information frequently.
- Promote external memory. Many things that need to be remembered can be written down, a practice known as "external memory." Practices such as keeping an assignment notebook and maintaining a student calendar can be helpful in remembering to do things. Older children may be trained to use aids such as timers on watches that signal them to do specific events or to use palm pilots.
- Promote active thinking. Children retain information better if they actively think through new information, rather than simply repeating it.

For Teachers

- Evaluate the child's understanding of concepts in ways that do not rely solely on memory. For example, use projects and open-book tests instead of tests that emphasize memorization.

aspects of expressive language, receptive language, and written language may be affected. Children, aged 6–15 years, with cryptogenic or childhood absence epilepsy were found to have high rates of language impairments, and the proportion of children with such impairments increased with age.[104] In addition, the epilepsy-related psychiatric and demographic variables that predicted language performance varied by age.

A high proportion of children with seizures arising from the left hemisphere show impairments in language; these impairments are found even when there is evidence for cortical reorganization of language function resulting in bilateral or right hemisphere language representation.[105] Although impairments in language may be most prominent among children with left hemisphere abnormalities,[106,107] even children with frontal or temporal lobe seizure foci in the right hemisphere may have specific language difficulties.[106] In children with epilepsy and congenital hemiparesis, and in children with partial epilepsy, language difficulties were found not to show a clear effect of lateralization as related to the side of epileptiform discharges.[108] Among those samples, language impairments, including the auditory analysis of speech, understanding instructions, repeating words and nonword and rapid naming, were especially pronounced among children with congenital hemiparesis and chronic epilepsy, although children with newly diagnosed partial epilepsy were also worse than controls.[108]

Language function in pediatric epilepsy has also been studied with respect to the syndrome of BECTS. Despite the label of "benign," it has become apparent that this syndrome is associated with risk for neuropsychological impairment. Given that the EEG abnormalities are in the centrotemporal region, in areas close to the classic anterior (Broca's) and posterior (Wernicke's) language areas, research has been directed to understanding the consequences of BECTS for language function. BECTS has been associated with deficits in the understanding of words, retrieval of words, verbal fluency, phonological processing, and expressive grammar.[109–111]

Written language skills are also affected in BECTS; these children frequently have below average school performance and make errors on spelling and reading tasks that are similar to those shown by children with dyslexia.[112,113] Linguistic deficits were found throughout the course of epilepsy in BECTS; as the seizures resolve, some aspects may improve or disappear, but there is evidence that there are persistent deficits in children in remission, suggesting possible long-term effects.[109,114] In BECTS, language impairments are also not confined to children with spikes in the left hemisphere; children with right-sided spikes have been shown to have deficits relating to the semantic processing of words.[111]

Written language skills, such as reading, spelling, and writing may also be affected. In a study of reading skills, groups of children with temporal lobe epilepsy, frontal lobe epilepsy, or absence epilepsy were all found to be reading at levels approximately 2 years behind expectations.[115] Children in the frontal lobe group, and to a lesser extent, those in the absence group, had deficits on tasks related to phonological processing, whereas those with temporal lobe epilepsy did not differ from controls in this respect. An epileptogenic focus in the frontal lobe apparently affects the phonological underpinnings of reading. Children with temporal lobe epilepsy, particularly those with left-sided foci, may be disadvantaged in reading speed, accuracy, and comprehension.[107]

A study of thought disorder in children with epilepsy was informative of the range of language problems with which these children present.[116] Thought disorder is characterized by the impaired use of language to formulate and organize thoughts, poor use of cohesive elements, and poor use of strategies to correct errors during conversations. As a result, the listener has difficulty following the ideas the child is attempting to explain. Both complex partial seizures and primary generalized epilepsy with absence were associated with thought disorder, suggesting that epilepsy affects the normal maturation of children's discourse skills. Furthermore, difficulties in these aspects of language were associated with psychopathology, academic problems, low academic achievement, and poor peer interactions, although the relationships of these outcomes and age, sex, and seizure variables differed somewhat for the two types of epilepsy. Children who struggle to organize and express their ideas have difficulty in social situations, and are often rejected by their peers. The authors argued that deficits in complex aspects of language formulation are a component of the stigma, developmental disabilities, and comorbidities associated with pediatric epilepsy.

As reviewed earlier in the memory section, children with epilepsy often experience word finding problems, or the tip-of-the-tongue phenomenon. They often struggle to find the words to express their ideas, and as a result they may get stuck on a thought or use lengthy circumlocutions.[83] These difficulties frustrate the child and also the listener; peers in particular may not have the patience to wait for a sentence to be completed. These problems may be compounded by the slow processing speed that characterizes many children with epilepsy. They often require more time than is typical of children of their age to process and understand what is being said to them; similarly they require additional time to organize their thoughts for verbal or written output. Additionally, the memory problems reviewed earlier may have an impact on language development, and language use. One example is that the child may be disadvantaged with respect to the acquisition of new vocabulary. A second example is that of working memory that is necessary for holding onto our train of thought while we carry out other cognitive functions. Working memory is important

▶ **TABLE 40–4.** RECOMMENDATIONS FOR PARENTS AND TEACHERS OF CHILDREN WITH LANGUAGE IMPAIRMENTS

For Parents

- Engage your child in conversations every day—include new and interesting words in your conversation.
- Read to your child every day.
- When the book contains a new or interesting word, pause and define the word for your child.
- After reading the book, engage your child in a conversation about the book.
- Help build word knowledge by classifying and grouping objects or pictures while naming them.
- Help build your child's understanding of language by playing verbal games and telling jokes and stories.

For Parents and Teachers

- Use sounds to aid in word retrieval. Provide the first sound or syllable of the target word. With younger children, you may need to start with the syllable cue (*pum* for *pumpkin*) and then, as their retrieval skills improve, change to the first sound, not the letter name, (*p* for *pumpkin*). With older children who are able to read, you can give the letter cue (It starts with the letter *p*).
- Another strategy to assist in word finding is rhyming. For example, if a patient is having difficulty retrieving the word *door*, you could provide a cue by saying that the word they are looking for rhymes with *pour* or *four*.
- Speak at a slower pace and use natural pauses to divide the material into phrases and sentences.
- Allow your child time to process the information they hear, particularly with complicated information or directions.
- Stop to check for comprehension and allow for questions.
- Repeat, rephrase, or summarize when necessary.

For Teachers

- Determine whether the child has a specific language-based learning disability by referring the child for an appropriate assessment; provide the necessary academic program to address the nature of the learning disability.
- Help build language skills in class by playing oral and written word exercises and games.
- Teach students about the important, useful, and difficult vocabulary words before students read the text—will help remember the words and improve comprehension.
- Have students use newly taught vocabulary words often and in various ways both orally and in writing so they are better able to remember the words and their meanings.
- When the child is writing a test, check to ensure that they understand what the questions are asking.
- After giving oral directions to the class as a whole, provide additional directions to the child with epilepsy. When possible, give one direction at a time. Ask the child if they have understood what you want them to do; better still, ask them to repeat the directions.
- For children with slow processing speed, present information slowly and repeat when necessary. Reduce the amount of work you expect the child to complete within a specific amount of time (it may also be necessary to reduce expectations for the amount of assigned homework).

for communication tasks such as following conversations, processing a lessons being delivered by a teacher in the classroom, and reading comprehension. In each of these instances, one must hold temporarily in memory what has just been heard or read in order to integrate that information with what follows.

Treatments for epilepsy may have an impact on language function. Although the potential impact of antiepileptic medications on language has not been studied for the majority of drugs, there is evidence that topirimate can adversely affect verbal fluency.[117,118] Although much is known about language outcomes after epilepsy surgery in adults, there is minimal information on children. Four studies have documented no change in expressive, receptive, or written language function after temporal or frontal lobe resection,[42,45,75,106] and one has found an improvement in object naming after temporal lobectomy.[90]

TREATMENT STRATEGIES FOR LANGUAGE DEFICITS

There is no published information on specific approaches to treatment of the language disorders associated with pediatric epilepsy. Where appropriate, children should be referred for speech-language therapy.[119,120] Table 40–4 contains recommendations that may be of assistance to parents and teachers in helping children with language deficits.

▶ OTHER INFLUENCES ON COGNITIVE FUNCTION IN CHILDREN WITH EPILEPSY

A number of factors have been identified that can affect the child's cognitive ability in many of the domains described earlier. Consideration of these variables is necessary for proving the optimal environment for enhancing cognitive development and to allow the child to maximize their inherent cognitive skills.

FAMILY FACTORS

In a study of children with chronic epilepsy, Fastenau et al[121] examined the relation between neuropsychological function and academic achievement. Processes dependent on verbal reasoning, memory, and executive function were strongly related to achievement in reading, mathematics and writing. Psychomotor function was also predictive of performance on writing skills. Of interest, these effects were moderated by family factors. Children from supportive and organized homes suffered a lesser impact on academic achievement from the neuropsychological deficits than did children living in homes characterized as unsupportive and disorganized. These findings argue for the need for consideration of the family environment in understanding the outcomes of epilepsy. The authors recommend that interventions to increase structure, stability and provide emotional support be offered to families.

Oostrom et al[122,123] also documented the contribution of maladaptive parenting to the neuropsychological performance of children with idiopathic epilepsy. These effects were demonstrable in the first year after seizures started, and were still present among a subset of the children 3–4 years after diagnosis. In the approximately 20% of their sample in whom cognitive and behavioral problems were persistent, poor parenting, dysfunctional family situations, and prior existence of behavioral problems were overrepresented. These contextual factors had a stronger association with outcome than did etiology, seizure remission, or use of antiepileptic drugs. These results reinforce the need for social and family supports in addressing cognitive problems in children with epilepsy.

FATIGUE

Children with epilepsy may experience excessive fatigue because of seizures, interictal epileptogenic activity, side effects of antiepileptic medication, or nocturnal seizures. Children have described how this fatigue makes it difficult for them to think clearly and be available to participate in academic tasks or social activities.[82] Often they experienced this tiredness, sleepiness, and anergia as a continuous experience that at times was made worse by seizures. These excessive levels of fatigue mean that youth often need more hours of sleep than is typical for their age, which in an of itself reduces availability to participate in activities that provide normal learning opportunities. The tiredness and disrupted sleep associated with nocturnal seizures can lead to some of the disturbances described earlier such as restlessness, inattention, distractibility, and poor memory consolidation.

The school can assist children in managing the effects of fatigue on cognition by altering the schedule of classes. Perhaps the classes in which not as much attention, concentration, and new learning is needed can be scheduled for times when the child is more likely to be tired. It may be necessary to allow the child to start the school day at a later time in the morning. The school can provide a quiet place for the child to have naps if necessary during the day. Parents and teachers may need to alter the length of time that the child is expected to spend on any particular activity.

▶ CONCLUSIONS

As this review has shown, children with epilepsy may experience difficulties in one or more domains of cognitive function. Although a constellation of variables (age at seizure onset, type of syndrome, duration, severity of seizures, side effects of medication) may in some cases contribute to the emergence or severity of these deficits, recent research has shown that these difficulties may even be present prior to or soon after the onset of seizures. Cognitive problems can contribute to reduce quality of life throughout childhood and persisting into adulthood. They also play a major role in the determining the educational and occupational attainments of the person with epilepsy. Given that individuals with epilepsy may underachieve in these areas relative to predictions based on familial and sociodemographic variables, the cognitive deficits may contribute to the financial costs and burden of illness associated with epilepsy. Finally, these impairments can have an impact on children's self-esteem, and can contribute to their sense of being different from their peers. For all of these reasons, the recognition and management of cognitive problems in children with epilepsy should begin early in the course of the epilepsy.

REFERENCES

1. Seidenberg M, Berent S. Childhood epilepsy and the role of psychology. *Am Psychol* 1992;47:1130–1133.
2. Arunkumar G, et al. Parent- and patient-validated content for pediatric epilepsy quality-of-life assessment. *Epilepsia* 2000;41:1474–1484.
3. Hermann B, et al. Children with new-onset epilepsy: neuropsychological status and brain structure. *Brain* 2006;29(Pt. 10):2609–2619.
4. Byars AW, et al. The association of MRI findings and neuropsychological functioning after the first recognized seizure. *Epilepsia* 2007;48:1067–1074.
5. Hermann BP, et al. Growing up with epilepsy: a two year investigation of cognitive development in children with new onset epilepsy. *Epilepsia* 2008;49:1847–1858.
6. Hermann B, et al. The neurodevelopmental impact of childhood-onset temporal lobe epilepsy on brain structure and function. *Epilepsia* 2002;43:1062–1071.

7. Koop JI, et al. Neuropsychological correlates of electro-encephalograms in children with epilepsy. *Epilepsy Res* 2005;64:49–62.

8. Bourgeois BF, et al. Intelligence in epilepsy: a prospective study in children. *Ann Neurol* 1983;14:438–444.

9. Ellenberg JH, Hirtz DG, Nelson KB. Do seizures in children cause intellectual deterioration? *N Engl J Med* 1986;314:1085–1088.

10. Sillanpaa M. Children with epilepsy as adults: outcome after 30 years of follow-up. *Acta Paediatr Sc Suppl* 1990; 368:1–78.

11. Tarter RE. Intellectual and adaptive functioning in epilepsy. A review of 50 years of research. *Dis Nerv Syst* 1972; 33:763–770.

12. Smith ML, Elliott IM, Lach LM. Cognitive skills in children with intractable epilepsy: comparison of surgical and non-surgical candidates. *Epilepsia* 2002;43:631–637.

13. Berg AT, et al. Global cognitive function in children with epilepsy: a community based study. *Epilepsia* 2008; 49:608–614.

14. Sillanpaa M. Epilepsy in children: prevalence, disability, and handicap. *Epilepsia* 1992;33:444–449.

15. Lezac MD, Howieson DB, Loring DW. *Neuropsychological Assessment.* New York: Oxford University Press, 2004; 4th edn.

16. Posner M, Digirolamo G. Attention in cognitive neurosciences: an overview. In: Gazzaniga M (ed), *The New Cognitive Neurosciences.* Cambridge: MIT Press, 1996; pp. 623–631.

17. Carlton-Ford S, et al. Epilepsy and children's social and psychosocial adjustment. *J Health Soc Behav* 1995; 36:285–301.

18. Davies S, Heyman I, Goodman R. A population survey of mental health problems in children with epilepsy. *Dev Med Child Neurol* 2003;45:292–295.

19. Dunn DW, et al. ADHD and epilepsy in childhood. *Dev Med Child Neurol* 2003;45:50–54.

20. Hermann B, et al. The frequency, complications and aetiology of ADHD in new onset paediatric epilepsy. *Brain* 2007;130:3135–3148.

21. Hamoda HM, et al. Association between attention-deficit/hyperactivity disorder and epilepsy in pediatric populations. *Expert Rev Neurother* 2009;9(12):1747–1754.

22. Parisi P, et al. Attention deficit hyperactivity disorder in children with epilepsy. *Brain Dev* 2010;32(1):10–16.

23. Sanchez-Carpintero R, Neville BGR. Attentional ability in children with epilepsy. *Epilepsia* 2003;44:1340–1349.

24. McCarthy AM, Richman LC, Yarbrough D. Memory, attention, and school problems in children with seizure disorders. *Dev Neuropsychol* 1995;11:71–86.

25. Levav M, et al. Familial association of neuropsychological traits in patients with generalized and partial seizure disorder. *J Clin Exp Neuropsychol* 2002;24:311–326.

26. Henkin Y, et al. Cognitive function in idiopathic generalized epilepsy in childhood. *Dev Med Child Neurol* 2005;47:126–132.

27. Pinton F, et al. Cognitive functions in children with benign childhood epilepsy with centrotemporal spikes (BECTS). *Epileptic Disord* 2006;8:11–23.

28. Hernandez MA, et al. Attention, memory, and behavior adjustment in children with frontal lobe epilepsy. *Epilepsy Behav* 2003;4:522–536.

29. Boone KB, et al. Neuropsychological and behavioral abnormalities in an adolescent with frontal lobe seizures. *Neurology* 1988;38:583–586.

30. Jambaqué I, Dulac O. Syndrome frontal réversible et épilepsie chez un enfant de 8 ans. *Arch Fr Pédiatr* 1989;46:525–529.

31. Chevalier H, Metz-Lutz MN, Segalowitz SJ. Impulsivity and control of inhibition in benign focal childhood epilepsy. *Brain Cogn* 2000;43:86–90.

32. Auclair L, et al. Deficit of preparatory attention in children with frontal lobe epilepsy. *Neuropsychologia* 2005;43:1701–1712.

33. Fuster JM. Human neuropsychology. In: Fuster JM (ed), *The Prefrontal Cortex.* New York: Lippincott-Raven, 1997; pp. 1500–1584.

34. Mateer CA, Williams D. Effects of frontal lobe injury in childhood. *Developmental Neuropsychol* 1991;7:359–376.

35. Aldenkamp AP, De Krom M, Reijs R. Newer antiepileptic drugs and cognitive issues. *Epilepsia* 2003;44(Suppl 4): 21–29.

36. Glauser TA, et al. Childhood Absence Epilepsy Study Group. Ethosuximide, valproic acid, and lamotrigine in childhood absence epilepsy. *N Engl J Med* 2010;362(9): 790–799.

37. Prpic I, et al. Effect of lamotrigine on cognition in children with epilepsy. *Neurology* 2007;68:797–798.

38. Williams J, et al. The effects of seizure type, level of seizure control, and antiepileptic drugs on memory and attention skills in children with epilepsy. *Dev Neuropsychol* 1996;12:241–253.

39. Bennett-Levy J, Stores G. The nature of cognitive dysfunction in school children with epilepsy. *Acta Neurol Scand* 1984;66(Suppl 99):79–82.

40. Williams J, et al. Patterns of memory performance in children with controlled epilepsy on the CVLT-C. *Child Neuropsychol* 2001;7:15–20.

41. Aldenkamp AP, Arends J. The relative influence of epileptic EEG discharges, short nonconvulsive seizures, and type of epilepsy on cognitive function. *Epilepsia* 2004;45:54–63.

42. Lendt M, Helmstaedter C, Elger CE. Pre- and postoperative neuropsychological profiles in children and adolescents with temporal lobe epilepsy. *Epilepsia* 1999;40:1543–1550.

43. Cunningham C, et al. Epilepsy surgery in an 8-year-old boy with intractable seizures. *J Dev Behav Pediatr* 2010;31(3 Suppl):S79–S82.

44. Tomikawa M, et al. Neuropsychological changes after surgical treatment for temporal lobe epilepsy. *Epilepsia* 2001;42:4–8.

45. Smith ML, Elliott IM, Lach L. Cognitive, psychosocial and family function one year after pediatric epilepsy surgery. *Epilepsia* 2004;45:650–660.

46. Sturm W, Leclercq M. La revalidation des troubles de l'attention. In: Seron X, Van des Linden M (eds), *Traité de neuropsychologie clinique, Tome II.* Marseille: Solal, 2000; pp. 36–80.

47. Sturm W, et al. Do specific attention deficits need specific training? *Neuropsychol Rehabil* 1997;9:81–103.

48. Engle JA, Smith ML. Attention and material-specific memory in children with lateralized epilepsy. *Neuropsychologia* 2010;48:38–42.

49. Strache W. Effectiveness of two modes of training to overcome deficits of concentration. *Int J Rehabil Res* 1987;10:141–145.

50. Gupta A, Naorem T. Cognitive retraining in epilepsy. *Brain Inj* 2003;17:161–174.

51. Engelberts NH, et al. The effectiveness of cognitive rehabilitation for attention deficits in focal seizures: a randomized controlled study. *Epilepsia* 2002;43:587–596.

52. Bulteau C, Jambaqué I, Dellatolas G. Epilepsy, cognitive abilities and education, In: Jambaqué I, Lassonde M, Dulac O (eds), *Neuropsychology of Childhood Epilepsy.* New York: Kluwer Academic/Plenum Publishers, 2001; pp. 269–274.

53. Pascalicchio TF, et al. Neuropsychological profile of patients with juvenile myoclonic epilepsy: a controlled study of 50 patients. *Epilepsy Behav* 2007;10:263–267.

54. Williams J, et al. Factors associated with academic achievement in children with controlled epilepsy. *Epilepsy Behav* 2001;2:217–223.

55. Welsh MC, Pennington BF. Assessing frontal lobe functioning in children: views from developmental psychology. *Dev Neuropsychol* 1988;4:199–230.

56. Welsh MC, Pennington BF, Grossier DB. A normative-developmental study of executive function: a window on prefrontal function in children. *Dev Neuropsychol* 1991;7:131–149.

57. Petrides M, et al. Dissociation of human mid-dorsal from posterior dorsolateral frontal cortex in memory processing. *Proc Natl Acad Sci USA* 1993;90:873–877.

58. Parrish J, et al. Executive functioning in childhood epilepsy: parent-report and cognitive assessment. *Dev Med Child Neurol* 2007;49:412–416.

59. Riva D, et al. Neuropsychologic effects of frontal lobe epilepsy in children. *J Child Neurol* 2002;17:661–667.

60. Luton LM, Burns TG, Defillippis N. Frontal lobe epilepsy in children and adolescents: a preliminary neuropsychological assessment of executive function. *Arch Clin Neuropsychol* 2010;25(8):762–770.

61. Hernandez MA, et al. Deficits in executive functions and motor coordination in children with frontal lobe epilepsy. *Neuropsychologia* 2002;40:384–400.

62. Swartz BE, et al. Primary or working memory in frontal lobe epilepsy: an FDG-PET study of dysfunctional zones. *Neurology* 1996;46:737–747.

63. Moeller F, et al. Changes in activity of striato-thalamo-cortical network precede generalized spike wave discharges. *Neuroimage* 2007;39:1839–1849.

64. Pulsipher DT, et al. Thalamofrontal circuitry and executive dysfunction in recent-onset juvenile myoclonic epilepsy. *Epilepsia* 2009;50:1210–1219.

65. Igarashi K, et al. Wisconsin card sorting test in children with temporal lobe epilepsy. *Brain Dev* 2002;24:174–178.

66. Hermann B, Seidenberg M. Executive system dysfunction in temporal lobe epilepsy: effects of nociferous cortex versus hippocampal pathology. *J Clin Exp Neuropsychol* 1995;6:809–819.

67. Tian Y, et al. Attention networks in children with idiopathic generalized epilepsy. *Epilepsy Behav* 2010;19(3):513–517.

68. Hessen E, Lossius MI, Gjerstad L. Antiepileptic monotherapy significantly impairs normative scores on common tests of executive functions. *Acta Neurol Scand* 2009;119:194–198.

69. Fritz N, et al. Efficacy and cognitive side effects of tiagabine and topiramate in patients with epilepsy. *Epilepsy Behav* 2005;6:373–381.

70. Werz MA, et al. Subjective preference for lamotrigine or topiramate in healthy volunteers: relationship to cognitive and behavioural functioning. *Epilepsy Behav* 2006;8:181–191.

71. Kockelmann E, Elger CE, Helmstaedter C. Significant improvement in frontal lobe associated neuropsychological functions after withdrawal of topiramate in epilepsy patients. *Epilepsy Res* 2003;54:171–178.

72. Sherman EMS, Slick DJ, Eyrl KL. Executive dysfunction is a significant predictor of poor quality of life in children with epilepsy. *Epilepsia* 2006;47:1936–1942.

73. Hoie B, et al. Executive functions and seizure-related factors in children with epilepsy in western Norway. *Dev Med Child Neurol* 2006;48:519–525.

74. Risse GL, et al. Cognitive outcome in patients undergoing surgical resection of the frontal lobe. *Neurology* 1996;46:A213.

75. Lendt M, et al. Neuropsychological outcome in children after frontal lobe epilepsy surgery. *Epilepsy Behav* 2002;3:51–59.

76. Luria AR. *Restoration of Function After Brain Injury.* London: Pergamon Press, 1963.

77. Evans JJ, Emslie H, Wilson BA. External cueing systems in the rehabilitation of executive impairments of action. *J Int Neuropsychol Soc* 1998;4:399–408.

78. Derouesné J, Seron X, Lhermitte F. Rééducation de patients atteints de lesions frontales. *Rev Neurol* 1975;131: 677–689.

79. Cicerone KD, Wood JC. Planning disorder after closed head injury: a case study. *Arch Phys Med Rehabil* 1987;68: 111–115.

80. Banich MT. *Cognitive Neuroscience and Neuropsychology.* Boston: Houghton Mifflin Company, 2004; 2nd edn.

81. Thompson PJ, Corcoran R. Everyday memory failures in people with epilepsy. *Epilepsia* 1992;33(Suppl 6):S18–S20.

82. Elliott IM, Lach LM, Smith ML. "I just want to be normal". A qualitative study exploring how children and adolescents perceive the impact of intractable epilepsy on their quality of life. *Epilepsy Behav* 2005;7:664–678.

83. Smith ML, Elliott IM, Lach LM. Memory outcome after pediatric epilepsy surgery: objective and subjective perspectives. *Child Neuropsychol* 2006;12:151–160.

84. Kadis DS, et al. Cognitive and psychological predictors of everyday memory in children with intractable epilepsy. *Epilepsy Behav* 2004;5:37–43.

85. Nolan MA, et al. Memory function in childhood epilepsy syndromes. *J Paediatr Child Health* 2004;40:20–27.

86. Beardsworth ED, Zaidel DW. Memory for faces in epileptic children before and after brain surgery. *J Clin Exp Neuropsych* 1994;16:589–596.

87. Cohen M. Auditory/verbal and visual/spatial memory in children with complex partial epilepsy of temporal lobe origin. *Brain Cogn* 1992;20:315–326.

88. Fedio P, Mirsky A. Selective intellectual deficits in children with temporal lobe or centrencephalic epilepsy. *Neuropsychologia* 1969;3:287–300.

89. Jambaqué I, et al. Verbal and visual memory impairment in children with epilepsy. *Neuropsychologia* 1993;31:1321–1337.

90. Jambaqué I, et al. Memory functions following surgery for temporal lobe epilepsy in children. *Neuropsychologia* 2007;45:2850–2862.

91. Adams CBT, et al. Temporal lobectomy in 44 children: outcome of neuropsychological follow-up. *J Epilepsy* 1999;3(Suppl):157–168.

92. Hershey T, et al. Short-term and long-term memory in early temporal lobe dysfunction. *Neuropsychology* 1998;12:52–64.

93. Jocic-Jakubi B, Jovic NJ. Verbal memory impairment in children with focal epilepsy. *Epilepsy Behav* 2006;9:432–439.

94. Mabbott DM, Smith ML. Material-specific memory in children with temporal and extra-temporal lobectomies. *Neuropsychologia* 2003;41:995–1007.

95. Szabó CA, et al. Neuropsychological effect of temporal lobe resection in preadolescent children with epilepsy. *Epilepsia* 1998;39:814–819.

96. Williams J, Griebel ML, Dykman RA. Neuropsychological patterns in pediatric epilepsy. *Seizure* 1998;7:223–228.

97. Baxendale SA, et al. The relationship between quantitative MRI and neuropsychological functioning in temporal lobe epilepsy. *Epilepsia* 1998;39:158–166.

98. Smith ML, et al. The relationship of attention to memory in children with intractable epilepsy. *Epilepsia* 2001;42(Suppl 7):103.

99. Elterman RD, et al. A double-blind, randomized trial of topiramate as adjunctive therapy for partial-onset seizures in children. Topiramate YP Study Group. *Neurology* 1999;52:1338–1344.

100. Shulman MB, Barr W. Treatment of memory disorders in epilepsy. *Epilepsy Behav* 2002;3:830–834.

101. Aldenkamp AP, Vermeulen J. Neuropsychological rehabilitation of memory function in epilepsy. *Neuropsychological Rehabil* 1991;1:191–214.

102. Fisher RS, et al. A pilot study of donepezil for memory problems in epilepsy. *Epilepsy Behav* 2001;2:330–334.

103. Hamberger MJ, et al. A randomized, double-blind, placebo-controlled trial of donepezil to improve memory in epilepsy. *Epilepsia* 2007;48:1283–1291.

104. Caplan R, Siddarth P, Vona P, Stahl L, Bailey C, Gurbani S, Sankar R, Shields WD. Language in pediatric epilepsy. *Epilepsia* 2009;50(11):2397–2407.

105. Gleissner U, et al. Clinical and neuropsychological characteristics of pediatric epilepsy patients with atypical language dominance. *Epilepsy Behav* 2003;4:746–752.

106. Blanchette N, Smith ML. Language after temporal or frontal lobe surgery in children with epilepsy. *Brain Cogn* 2002;48:280–284.

107. Chaix Y, et al. Reading abilities and cognitive functions of children with epilepsy: influence of epileptic syndrome. *Brain Dev* 2006;28:122–130.

108. Kolk A, et al. Neurocognitive development of children with congenital unilateral brain lesion and epilepsy. *Brain Dev* 2001;23:88–96.

109. Monjauze C, et al. Language in benign childhood epilepsy with centro-temporal spikes. *Brain Lang* 2005;92:300–308.

110. Northcott E, et al. The neuropsychological and language profile of children with benign rolandic epilepsy. *Epilepsia* 2005;46:924–930.

111. Riva D, et al. Intellectual and language findings and their relationship to EEG characteristics in benign childhood epilepsy with centrotemporal spikes. *Epilepsy Behav* 2007;10:278–285.

112. Papavasiliou A, et al. Written language skills in children with benign childhood epilepsy with centrotemporal spikes. *Epilepsy Behav* 2005;6:50–58.

113. Staden U, et al. Language dysfunction in children with rolandic epilepsy. *Neuropediatrics* 1998;29:242–248.

114. Northcott E, et al. Longitudinal assessment of neuropsychologic and language function in children with benign Rolandic epilepsy. *J Child Neurol* 2006;21:518–522.

115. Vanasse CM, et al. Impact of childhood epilepsy on reading and phonological abilities. *Epilepsy Behav* 2005;7:288–296.

116. Caplan R, et al. Thought disorder: a developmental disability in pediatric epilepsy. *Epilepsy Behav* 2006;8:726–735.

117. Aldenkamp AP, et al. A multicenter randomized clinical study to evaluate the effect on cognitive function of topiramate compared with valproate as add-on therapy to cabamazepine in patients with partial-onset seizures. *Epilepsia* 2000;41:1167–1178.

118. Thompson PJ, Baxendale SA, Duncan JS, Sander JWAS. Effects of topiramate on cognitive function. *J Neurol Neurosurg Psychiatry* 2000;69:636–641.

119. Cirrin FM, Gillam RB. Language intervention practices for school-age children with spoken language disorders: a systematic review. *Lang Speech Hear Serv Sch* 2008;39:S110–S137.

120. Jitendra A, et al. What research says about vocabulary instruction for students with learning disabilities. *Exceptional Children* 2004;70:299–322.

121. Fastenau PS, et al. Neuropsychological predictors of academic underachievement in pediatric epilepsy: moderating roles of demographic, seizure, and psychosocial variables. *Epilepsia* 2004;45:1261–1272.

122. Oostrom KJ, et al. Not only a matter of epilepsy: early problems of cognition and behavior in children with "epilepsy only"—a prospective, longitudinal, controlled study starting at diagnosis. *Pediatrics* 2003;112(6 Pt 1):1338–1344.

123. Oostrom KJ, et al. Three to four years after diagnosis: cognition and behaviour in children with 'epilepsy only'. A prospective, controlled study. *Brain* 2005;128(Pt 7):1546–1555.

CHAPTER 41

Learning Disabilities and ADHD in Children with Epilepsy

David W. Dunn and Blaise F.D. Bourgeois

Children with epilepsy are at risk for cognitive disorders. They experience more academic underachievement and frequently suffer from impaired attention. These problems are found even in those children with epilepsy and a normal intelligence. In this chapter, we will concentrate on school-age children with epilepsy. We will review learning disorders (LD) and attention deficit hyperactivity disorder (ADHD). Additional information on mental retardation can be found in Chapters 27 and 28 and more information on cognitive problems in Chapter 33.

▶ LEARNING AND ADHD

Learning disorders and ADHD will be covered together for several reasons. First, both have significant impact on academic success. While LD quite obviously impacts school performance, ADHD in children with epilepsy may have a similarly negative effect on school performance. Williams et al[1] found that ADHD in children with epilepsy was a better predictor of academic difficulties than memory, socioeconomic status, or self-esteem. Second, LD and ADHD are frequently comorbid conditions. Approximately 30–35% of children with ADHD have LD.[2] Finally, these two problems initially may be difficult to distinguish. Attention deficit hyperactivity disorder may be mistaken for LD and vice versa. However, treatment of the two disorders is quite different.

Learning disorders must be distinguished from intellectual disability or mental retardation (MR). Intellectual disability is defined as a significantly below average intelligence with IQ scores of 70 or below on standardized, individually administered tests of cognitive function, impairment in multiple areas, and an onset prior to 18 years of age. The IQ score is used to delineate severity levels. Severity levels range from mild MR, with IQ scores of 50–70, to profound MR, with IQ score less than 20 or 25.[3]

Learning disorders, also called academic skills disorders or learning disabilities, have been defined in two somewhat different ways. The first is the discrepancy model that compares academic achievement to intelligence. In the current DSM-IV-TR, a diagnosis of learning disorders requires scores of achievement on a standardized, individually administered test that are below the level expected for the child's age, intelligence measured by psychoeducational testing, and education.[3] The disability must cause impairment and should not be explained by sensory deficits. Categories are reading disorder, mathematics disorder, disorder of written expression, and learning disorder not otherwise specified. Motor skills disorder and communication disorders are separate categories.

A second way of classifying learning disorder uses a below-average performance on a standardized measure of academic performance without regard for the child's intelligence. As an example, if a child had an IQ score 1.5 standard deviation (SD) below normal and a reading achievement score 1.5 SD below normal, the child would be considered to have a reading disorder. The distinction in definition of learning disorder is important practically in the determination of which child receives special education services in a school system.

Attention deficit hyperactivity disorder and problems with attention are similar and overlapping concerns but are not the same entities. Attention deficit hyperactivity disorder is a categorical (either present or absent) diagnosis defined by the presence of 6 of 9 symptoms of inattention and/or 6 of 9 symptoms of hyperactivity or impulsivity, starting before 7 years of age, causing impairment in two or more settings, and not better explained by other psychiatric disorders.[3] The diagnosis is made on the basis of history and questionnaires completed by parents, teachers, and occasionally the child or adolescent. In comparison, attention is a dimensional (existing on a continuum) psychological construct. It is measured by a variety of tests of problem solving, executive function, and performance. In children with epilepsy, deficits in sustained attention are particularly common.[4] Patients may have difficulties with attention without meeting criteria for ADHD and, in the unusual case of ADHD, predominantly hyperactive/impulsive type ADHD without impaired attention.

PREVALENCE OF LEARNING DISORDERS AND ADHD IN CHILDREN WITH EPILEPSY

We are aware of only one study that assessed the prevalence of learning disorder in children with epilepsy using the two separate definitions of learning disorder. Fastenau et al studied 173 children with epilepsy aged 7–15 years using an IQ screen and academic achievement testing.[5] Domains assessed were reading, mathematics, and written expression. Using the IQ achievement discrepancy definition, they found that 48% of the children could be labeled as having a learning disorder. When learning disorder was defined by an achievement test score 1 SD below the mean, 62% of the children met criteria for LD and, using 1.5 SD below the mean, 41% could be considered to have a learning disorder. Depending on the definition used, 13–32% had a reading disorder, 20–38% a mathematics disorder, and 35–56% a disorder of written expression.

Though the definitions varied, other groups also found higher rates of academic problems in children with epilepsy. Seidenberg et al[6] studied 122 children, 7–15 years of age, with an IQ of 70 or above. Using a definition of learning disorder as 1SD below expected for IQ, he found word recognition problems in 10.5% of boys and 10.1% of girls, spelling problems in 33.3% and 15.9%, mathematic difficulties in 28.1% and 31.9%, and reading comprehension impairment in 22.8% and 13%. Mitchell et al[7] also used the IQ discrepancy model in a study of 78 children 5–13 years of age with an IQ of 80 or above and found reading disorder in 16%, reading comprehension problems in 38%, spelling difficulty in 32%, mathematics disorder in 31% and below average general knowledge in 50%. Bailet and Turk[8] reported that 19% of children with epilepsy and a normal intelligence received special education services and 34% repeated a grade. Berg et al[9] found that 58% received special education services at some time during the 5 years after an initial seizure.

Attention deficit hyperactivity disorder is also found frequently in children and adolescents with epilepsy. Reported prevalence rates have varied substantially with rates of 0–77% found depending on study population and methods of determining problems with attention. One population-based study noted symptoms of ADHD in 44% of children with epilepsy.[10] Clinic-based studies utilizing DSM or other standard criteria commonly report symptoms of ADHD in 25–40% of children with epilepsy. Though not conclusive, there is some indication that ADHD, predominantly inattentive type is more common than ADHD combined type in children with epilepsy.[11]

RISK FACTORS

Just as epilepsy is a heterogeneous disorder with multiple different syndromes and levels of severity, the causes of academic problems are multiple and specific for the individual patient. Variables interact with some having more direct effects on learning and other moderating the effects of the primary variables. Central nervous system function, including neuropsychological deficits and seizure-related variables seem to have the most direct effect on academic function, while family factors and child response to illness have moderating effects. Family history of LD and/or ADHD should be significant. Biederman and Faraone[12] estimated a heritability of 0.76 for ADHD in the general population; however, family history is seldom assessed in studies of LD and ADHD in children with epilepsy.

Support for the importance of underlying CNS dysfunction causing both epilepsy and academic problems comes from studies of new-onset seizures, from the different effects of seizure syndromes, and from results of imaging studies. Three studies of new-onset seizures found that children with epilepsy were more likely than controls to have repeated a grade, required special education services, or scored lower on teacher ratings or school-based standardized tests prior to the diagnosis of epilepsy.[9,13,14] This suggests that underlying CNS dysfunction caused both seizures and academic difficulties. Both Nolan et al[15] and Berg et al[16] found that children with symptomatic or cryptogenic generalized epilepsy syndromes had more cognitive or adaptive problems than children with idiopathic generalized epilepsy syndromes or with partial epilepsies. Symptomatic and cryptogenic generalized epilepsies are more often associated with CNS dysfunction than other seizure syndromes. Byars et al[17] described an association between MRI abnormalities and deficits on neuropsychological testing in a sample of children with recent-onset seizures. Rantanen et al[18] described intellectual disability in 50% of children 3–6 years of age with epilepsy noting an association between intellectual disability and early age of onset, abnormal MRI, additional neurological deficits, and complicated epilepsy.

Seizure-related factors are an additional direct cause of academic problems. There is an overlap with CNS dysfunction as symptomatic generalized epilepsies are most strongly associated with learning disorders and these are the epilepsies most likely associated with underlying CNS structural damages. Other seizure related factors seem to have lesser impact on academic performance. Aldenkamp et al found an association of academic underachievement with localized and symptomatic generalized epilepsies.[19] In addition, frequent EEG discharges and antiepileptic drug (AED) polytherapy were associated with impaired vigilance. However, EEG discharges and AED polytherapy were associated with seizure syndrome, suggesting that seizure syndrome had the primary effect on academic performance. In a 3-year prospective study, there was no difference between reading and math scores of children with seizures and siblings at baseline, but the scores were lower in children with seizures than in siblings at 36 months.[20]

Academic performance problems are often attributed to AEDs though disentangling the effects of AEDs from seizure syndrome, seizure frequency, frequency of EEG discharges, and the behavioral and psychosocial responses to illness is difficult. When compared to placebo, many AEDs have adverse cognitive effects, but when compared to other AEDs, barbiturates and topiramate appear more likely to cause academic problems.[21] Polytherapy and elevated serum levels of AEDs also contribute to cognitive dysfunction. Even though adverse cognitive effects may be less likely with some of the newer AEDs, clinicians should monitor academic progress when starting any AED or increasing dosage as children may have their own unique idiosyncratic response to medication.

Family variables may contribute to LD. A family history of LD would be expected to be a significant variable, but this information frequently is missing in studies of academic problems in children with epilepsy. The home environment is important in learning. Mitchell et al[7] found that parental education and home environment were better predictors of academic difficulties than seizure related factors including duration and severity of seizures and AED exposure. Fastenau et al[22] found a moderating effect of family environment on academic achievement. Neuropsychological impairment had less negative impact on children in more supportive and organized families.

Risk factors for ADHD in children with epilepsy are similar to those found for LD. One population-based study found that ADHD, predominantly inattentive type, was a risk factor for subsequent new-onset seizures and another community-based study found elevated attention problem scores at the time of a first recognized seizure.[23,24] The presence of problems with attention prior to or at the onset of seizures suggests that CNS dysfunction is responsible for both seizures and impaired attention.

Both epidemiological and clinical studies have found that ADHD is more common in children with epilepsy plus additional neurological defects than in children with uncomplicated epilepsy.[25] Williams et al[26] reported fewer symptoms of ADHD in children with epilepsy and a normal MRI compared to those with an abnormal MRI.

Seizure related factors are less consistently associated with symptoms of ADHD. There are inconsistent reports of an association of seizure type and ADHD. Some studies found more symptoms in children with seizures localized to the frontal or temporal lobes, but others reported no relationship between seizure focus and symptoms of ADHD.[23,27] Frequent EEG discharges have been associated with slow processing speed, but seizure

syndrome was more directly associated with impaired attention.[19] The AEDs associated with impaired attention and hyperactivity are the barbiturates and topiramate. In a study of children with generalized absence seizures, more problems with attention were seen with valproic acid than with lamotrigine or ethosuximide.[28] There may be a limited negative effect of phenytoin, carbamazepine, and valproate on attention, though the individual child may react adversely to any of the AEDs.[29]

Family factors, other than a family history of ADHD, do not seem to contribute to the causation of ADHD, though an increased severity of symptoms of ADHD has been associated with dysfunction and discord in the family. In children with epilepsy, one study found an association between family disruption from the onset of seizures and slower speed of cognitive performance in children with epilepsy. However, these children with new-onset seizures did not have persistent problems with attention.[30]

ASSESSMENT (FIG. 41–1)

The initial step is recognition of the problem. In the preschool or school age child, a routine part of follow up in a comprehensive epilepsy clinic should include questions about developmental progress or academic performance. When the question of learning disorders is raised, the child should have a referral to the school system for psychoeducational assessment or to a psychologist for evaluation. The basic assessment of LD requires a test of intellectual ability and an array of academic achievement tests. These should be individually administered as group administered tests are much less reliable. In addition, tests of memory, language, attention and executive function are helpful (Table 41–1).

If the child has problems with attention, ADHD questionnaires should be completed by parents and teachers. Reports of problems in attention from the adolescent may be helpful, but reports from younger children are less valuable. Questionnaires specific for ADHD are especially helpful for diagnosis and follow up. Examples include the ADHD Rating Scale-IV[31] and the NICHQ Vanderbilt Assessment Scale.[32] Broad band questionnaires such as the Child Behavior Checklist[33] and the Behavior Assessment System for Children-2,[34] though less specific for ADHD, are valuable for detecting potential comorbid conditions such as depression or anxiety. Specific psychoeducational testing may be helpful but is not essential in the diagnostic evaluation. Children with epilepsy and ADHD have an increased prevalence of academic underachievement and neuropsychological deficits including prominent executive functioning difficulties.[35] Additional psychological assessment for LD is indicated if the child fails to show improvement in academic performance after appropriate treatment of ADHD (Table 41–2).

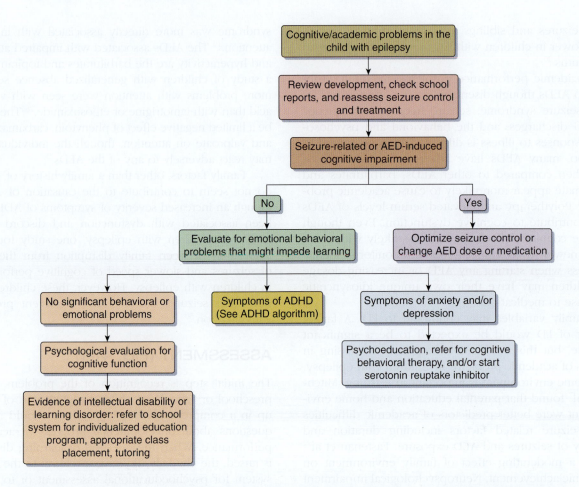

Figure 41–1. Differential diagnosis and evaluation of learning problems in children with epilepsy.

TREATMENT

Once LD or ADHD is suspected, the first step in both assessment and treatment is a review of the seizure control, AED therapy, and seizure etiology. If the child is having frequent nonconvulsive seizures, better

▶ **TABLE 41–1. STEPS IN THE EVALUATION AND TREATMENT OF LEARNING DISABILITY IN CHILDREN WITH EPILEPSY**

1. *Recognition:* Monitor development and school progress.
2. If learning problems found:
   a. *Assess seizure control:* Are recurrent seizures affecting cognition?
   b. *Review AEDs:* Are sedative medications interfering with cognition?
   c. *Reassess diagnosis:* Does the child have a progress disorder affecting cognition and causing seizures?
3. After neurological re-evaluation, if learning disability is present:
   a. Refer for psychoeducational assessment.
   b. Refer to school system for individualized educational plan (IEP).
   c. Refer to educational specialist for treatment of learning disorder.

seizure control may lead to improved cognitive function. Cognitive impairment due to AEDs can be addressed by modification in dosage of AED or by a change in medication. Cognitive decline may be a sign of a progressive neurological disorder requiring primary treatment.

A second step is to screen for emotional or behavioral problems that may be part of the differential diagnosis or comorbid with LD and ADHD. School failure may be an early sign of depression. Difficulty with concentration and restlessness are symptoms of ADHD, depression, and anxiety. Though rare in childhood, the psychosis associated with epilepsy often begins with social withdrawal and academic difficulties.

Once the neurological reevaluation is complete and the presence of a learning disorder is confirmed by psychological assessment, treatment shifts to the school system. A case conference at the child's school should determine the individualized educational plan for specific interventions to help remediate the LD. Tutoring or specialized after school educational interventions may be helpful for specific learning disabilities.

Specific treatment of ADHD should include behavioral components such as parent training and school interventions (Fig. 41–2). Pharmacological treatment for

▶ **TABLE 41–2.** STEPS IN THE ASSESSMENT AND TREATMENT OF ADHD IN CHILDREN WITH EPILEPSY

1. *Recognition:* Monitor school performance and behavior.
2. If symptoms of ADHD present:
   a. *Assess seizure control:* Are recurrent seizures affecting attention?
   b. *Review AEDs:* Could inattention or hyperactivity be due to AED?
   c. *Review psychiatric differential diagnosis:* Are there symptoms of autism, anxiety, or depression?
   d. Have ADHD questionnaires or rating scales completed by parents and teachers.
3. If symptoms are due to ADHD and not due to correctable seizure-related factors:
   a. Contact school to establish individualized educational plan (IEP).
   b. Instruct or refer parents for training in management of ADHD behaviors.
   c. If symptoms are causing impairment, start medication for ADHD.
4. Medication for ADHD in children with epilepsy:
   a. Start with methylphenidate (has most data for effectiveness).
   b. If not effective or has side effects, try amphetamines.
   c. If not effective or has side effects, use atomoxetine.
   d. Avoid bupropion and tricyclic antidepressants.
5. If medication started for ADHD:
   a. Monitor seizure control and AED levels.
   b. Monitor weight, height, blood pressure, and heart rate.
   c. Use rating scales completed by parent and teacher to assess effectiveness of medication.

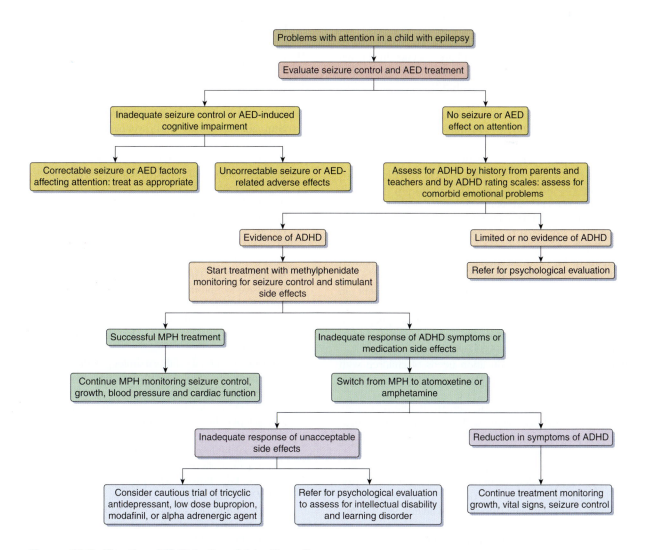

Figure 41–2. Treating ADHD in the child with epilepsy.

ADHD in children with epilepsy has been somewhat controversial. Information sheets from the manufacturers of all the stimulants recommend discontinuation of stimulants in the event of seizures. However, one double-blind placebo-controlled trial and several open label studies of methylphenidate for ADHD in children with epilepsy have shown that these medications are effective and that the risk of an increase in seizure frequency is small.[36] Modifications need to be made in the choice of nonstimulant medications for ADHD. Bupropion and the tricyclic antidepressants can lower the seizure threshold and should be used cautiously if at all. Atomoxetine has been effective for ADHD and has not increased the risk of seizures.[37] Atomoxetine should be considered when stimulants are not effective, cause side effects, or are unacceptable to parents.

REFERENCES

1. Williams J, et al. Factors associated with academic achievement in children with controlled epilepsy. *Epilepsy Behav* 2001;2:217–223.

2. Tannock R, Brown TE. ADHD with language and/or learning disorders in children and adolescents. In: Brown TE (ed), *ADHD Comorbidities. Handbook for ADHD Complications in Children and Adults.* Washington, DC: American Psychiatric Publishing, Inc., 2009; pp. 189–231.

3. American Psychiatric Association. *Diagnostic and Statistical Manual-IV-TR.* Washington, DC: American Psychiatric Association, 2000.

4. Sánchez-Carpintero R, Neville BGR. Attentional ability in children with epilepsy. *Epilepsia* 2003;44:1340–1349.

5. Fastenau PS, Shen J, Dunn DW, Austin JK. Academic underachievement among children with epilepsy: proportion exceeding psychometric criteria for LD and associated risk factors. *J Learning Disabilities* 2008; 41:195–207.

6. Seidenberg M, et al. Academic achievement of children with epilepsy. *Epilepsia* 1986;27:753–759.

7. Mitchell WG, et al. Academic underachievement in children with epilepsy. *J Child Neurol* 1991;6:65–72

8. Bailet LL, Turk WR. The impact of childhood epilepsy on neurocognitive and behavioral performance: a prospective longitudinal study. *Epilepsia* 2000;41:426–431.

9. Berg AT, et al. Special education needs of children with newly diagnosed epilepsy. *Dev Med Child Neurol* 2005; 47:749–753.

10. Turky A, Beavis JM, Thapar AK, Kerr MP. Psychopathology in children and adolescents with epilepsy: an investigation of predictive variables. *Epilepsy Behav* 2008;12: 136–144.

11. Dunn DW, Kronenberger WG. Attention-deficit hyperactivity disorder, attention problems, and epilepsy. In: Ettinger AB, Kanner AM (eds), *Psychiatric Issues in Epilepsy.* Philadelphia: Lippincott Williams & Wilkins, 2007; 2nd edn: pp. 272–285.

12. Biederman J, Faraone S. Attention-deficit hyperactivity disorder. *Lancet* 2005;366:237–248.

13. Schouten A, et al. School career of children is at risk before diagnosis of epilepsy only. *Dev Med Child Neurol* 2001;43:574–576.

14. McNelis AM, et al. Factors associated with academic achievement in children with recent-onset seizures. *Seizure* 2005;14:331–339.

15. Nolan MA, et al. Intelligence in childhood epilepsy syndromes. *Epilepsy Res* 2003;53:139–150.

16. Berg AT, et al. Longitudinal assessment of adaptive behavior in infants and young children with newly diagnosed epilepsy: influences of etiology, syndrome, and seizure control. *Pediatrics* 2004;114:645–650.

17. Byars AW, et al. The association of MRI findings and neuropsychological functioning after the first-recognized seizure. *Epilepsia* 2007;48:1067–1074.

18. Rantanen K, Eriksson K, Nieminen P. Cognitive impairment in preschool children with epilepsy. *Epilepsia* 2011;52: 1499–1505.

19. Aldenkamp AP, et al. Educational underachievement in children with epilepsy: a model to predict the effects of epilepsy on educational achievement. *J Child Neurol* 2005; 20:175–180.

20. Dunn DW, et al. Academic problems in children with seizures: relationships with neuropsychological functioning and family variables during the 3 years after onset. *Epilepsy Behav* 2010;19:455–461.

21. Bourgeois BFD. Determining the effects of antiepileptic drugs on cognitive function in pediatric patients with epilepsy. *J Child Neurol* 2004;19(Suppl 1):S15–S24.

22. Fastenau PS, et al. Neuropsychological predictors of academic underachievement in pediatric epilepsy: moderating roles of demographic, seizure, and psychological variable. *Epilepsia* 2004;45:1261–1272.

23. Hesdorffer DC, et al. ADHD as a risk factor for incident unprovoked seizures and epilepsy in children. *Arch Gen Psychiatry* 2004;61:731–736.

24. Austin JK, et al. Behavior problems in children prior to first recognized seizures. *Pediatrics* 2001;107:115–122.

25. Davies S, Heymann I, Goodman R. A population survey of mental health problems in children with epilepsy. *Dev Med Child Neurol* 2003;45:292–295.

26. Williams J, et al. The course of inattentive and hyperactive-impulsive symptoms in children with new onset seizures. *Epilepsy Behav* 2002;3:517–521.

27. Dunn DW, Austin JK, Harezlak J, Ambrosius WT. ADHD and epilepsy in childhood. *Dev Med Child Neurol* 2003; 45:50–54.

28. Glauser T, et al. Ethosuximide, valproic acid, and lamotrigine in childhood absence epilepsy. *N Engl J Med* 2010;362:790–799.

29. Loring DW, Meador KJ. Cognitive side effects of antiepileptic drugs in children. *Neurology* 2004;62:872–877.

30. Oostrom KJ, et al. Attention deficits are not characteristic of schoolchildren with newly diagnoses idiopathic or cryptogenic epilepsy. *Epilepsia* 2002;43:301–310.

31. DuPaul GJ, Power TJ, Anastopoulos AD, Reid R. *ADHD Rating Scale-IV: Checklists, Norms, and Clinical Interpretation.* New York: Guilford Press, 1998.

32. Wolraich ML, et al. Psychometric properties of the Vanderbilt ADHD Diagnostic Parent Rating Scale in a referred population. *J Ped Psychol* 2003;28:559–568.

33. Achenbach TM, Rescorla LA. *Manual for the ASEBA School-Age Forms & Profiles.* Burlington, VT: University of Vermont, Research Center for Children, Youth & Families, 2001.

34. Reynolds CR, Kamphaus RW. *BASC-2: Behavior Assessment System for Children.* Circle Pines, MN: AGS, 2004; 2nd edn.

35. Hermann B, et al. The frequency, complications and aetiology of ADHD in new onset paediatric epilepsy. *Brain* 2007;130:3135–3148.

36. Tan M, Appleton R. Attention deficit and hyperactivity disorder, methylphenidate, and epilepsy. *Arch Dis Child* 2005;90:57–59.

37. Wernicke JF, et al. Seizure risk in patients with attention-deficit-hyperactivity disorder treated with atomoxetine. *Dev Med Child Neurol* 2007;49:498–502.

CHAPTER 42

Depression and Anxiety Disorders in Children with Epilepsy

Bruce P. Hermann and Jana E. Jones

Children with epilepsy are at an increased risk for behavioral or psychiatric comorbidities.[1,2] Symptoms of depression, anxiety, and other behavioral difficulties (e.g., impulsivity, inattention) may be reported by the child, parent, teacher, or even the physician. It is increasingly evident that anxiety and depression are significant comorbidities among children with epilepsy.[3,4] If left unrecognized and untreated, psychiatric comorbidities may have an adverse psychosocial impact on the child in terms of academic and social development as well as family functioning as demonstrated in the general population. Psychiatric comorbidities in childhood can have long-term implications overflowing into adulthood impeding lifetime achievement and negatively impacting overall quality of life.

Contemporary psychiatric diagnostic systems (DSM [Diagnostic and Statistical Manual], ICD [International Classification of Diseases]) have only recently been used to comprehensively characterize the nature and type of these problems in children with epilepsy. There is minimal understanding of the additional complications caused by comorbid mental health disorders (e.g., cognitive problems, academic underachievement, increased health care utilization, adverse impact on family), and most striking is the lack of randomized controlled intervention trials to treat psychiatric comorbidities in youth with epilepsy with the exception of ADHD. Recently, research has indicated that epilepsy variables (i.e., seizure frequency, AEDs, and seizure type) are often not implicated in the occurrence of psychiatric comorbidities. This chapter will highlight the prevalence rates of anxiety and depression in children with epilepsy compared to children in the general population and review the current literature regarding recognition and treatment of anxiety and depression.

► EPIDEMIOLOGICAL EVIDENCE IN THE GENERAL POPULATION

Among children and adolescents in the general population, depression and anxiety disorders appear to be the most common psychiatric disorders[5] and represent a major public health problem.[6] The prevalence rates range from 4% to 24% for major depression and around 20% for all anxiety disorders including specific phobias (8%), social phobias (5%), GAD (4%), and all other anxiety disorders (3%).[5] Depression during childhood frequently occurs before, during, or after another psychiatric disorder;[7] as a result, if a child presents with a depressive disorder, another psychiatric disorder may be lurking in the shadows. Anxiety disorders in childhood and adolescence are risk factors for depressive disorders later in life.[8] Spady et al[9] reported that children and adolescents with psychiatric disorders in general had greater medical service usage compared to children with no psychiatric disorders. Increased direct costs associated include clinic visits, counseling, hospitalizations, prescription medications, and emergency room care. Increased indirect costs are attributable to reduced productivity, absenteeism from work and school, and suicide.[10] The majority of cost analyses have focused on adults. Greenberg et al[10] reported that in the United States anxiety disorders costs totaled $42.3 billion in 1990 dollars and half of these costs were for nonpsychiatric medical treatment. Anxiety disorders have been linked to academic difficulties, low self-esteem, peer relationship problems, and depression.[6] Anxiety and depression are significant disorders negatively impacting children and adolescents including those with epilepsy.

► EPIDEMIOLOGICAL EVIDENCE IN CHILDREN WITH EPILEPSY

Among children with epilepsy, the prevalence of psychopathology reportedly ranges from 16% to 77%.[4,11,12] There are no published population-based surveys to determine the prevalence of psychiatric comorbidity in children and adolescents with epilepsy in the United States.[2] Two major investigations were conducted in the United Kingdom (Fig. 42–1). Rutter[13] reported that 7% of the general population was identified with a mental health problem compared to 12% in children with nonneurological physical disorders, with significantly

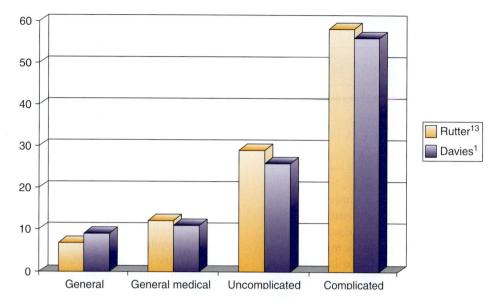

Figure 42–1. Psychiatric comorbidity in children with epilepsy.

higher rates in children with epilepsy, specifically, 29% in uncomplicated and 58% in complicated epilepsy. More recently, Davies et al[1] reported strikingly similar findings. Psychiatric disorders were found in 9.3% of the general population (based on DSM-IV criteria), and again there were marked differences in rates of psychiatric disorders among those children with uncomplicated compared to complicated epilepsy (26% vs. 56%).

Additionally, in Norway as part of an unselected population-based sample of adolescents age 13–16 years, Lossius et al[14] found higher rates of psychiatric symptoms in youth with epilepsy compared to adolescents without epilepsy. Among 10th graders with epilepsy, 40% reported borderline or abnormal scores on the Strength and Difficulties Questionnaire—Self-Report (SDQ-S)[15] compared to 13% of controls. The SDQ is a brief questionnaire that assesses common behavioral problems based on the DSM-IV and ICD diagnostic criteria in children and adolescents and can be completed by parents, teachers, and children who are between 11 and 16 years of age. Importantly, it was reported that adolescents with epilepsy who did not endorse psychiatric symptoms continued to report difficulties coping with daily life.

In summary, epidemiological studies indicated that youth with epilepsy have higher rates of psychiatric comorbidity compared to the general population as well as those with other disabilities (e.g., diabetes). Notably, children with epilepsy have not been compared to children with other neurological disorders, and as a result, it is unclear if higher rates of anxiety and depression only occur in children with epilepsy when compared to children with other neurological disorders.

There is also a large literature using broad spectrum self-report or parent/teacher report behavioral inventories (e.g., Child Behavior Checklist).[16] These studies have been consistent in indicating significantly more internalizing behavior problems (including anxiety and depression) than externalizing problems (e.g., ADHD, Conduct Disorder) in both observational and controlled study designs, the latter comparing children with epilepsy to healthy controls or other disease groups.[17,18] Rodenburg et al[19] conducted a review of the literature from 1970 (after the Isle of Wight study) to 2003 that included children with epilepsy between 4 and 21 years of age and utilized broadband measures (i.e., CBCL parent, teacher, and self-report) to identify rates of psychopathology. A meta-analysis was conducted on 46 studies including 2434 children with epilepsy. The authors reported that youth with epilepsy had higher rates of psychopathology in general compared to healthy controls and children with non-neurological chronic illness. In addition, it appeared that children with epilepsy experienced more internalizing than externalizing behavior problems. This is the opposite of what is reported in the general literature that indicates higher rates of externalizing disorders compared to internalizing disorders (23.0% v. 15%).[20]

Only a small number of studies have used contemporary research standard psychiatric interviews and diagnostic procedures to investigate rates of mental health problems in youth with epilepsy. Five studies, all quite recent, have demonstrated high rates of anxiety and mood disorders among children with epilepsy in selected populations (Table 42–1). Alwash et al[11] reported DSM-IV-based diagnoses in 101 Jordanian adolescents and young adults with epilepsy aged 14–24.

▶ **TABLE 42–1. PSYCHIATRIC COMORBIDITY— DSM AND ICD EVIDENCE**

	Depressive Disorder (%)	Anxiety Disorder (%)
Alwash et al[11]	77.2	48.5
Thome-Souza et al[21]	36.4	
Adewuya and Ola[22]	28.4	31.4
Caplan et al[3]	19.0	36.0
Jones et al[23]	22.6	35.8

They reported that 77.2% of the sample met criteria for depression and 48.5% met criteria for anxiety. Using the Kiddie Schedule for Affective Disorders and Schizophrenia (K-SADS), Thome-Souza et al[21] reported that among 78 children with epilepsy in Brazil, 36.4% met criteria for depression. Using the Diagnostic Interview Schedule for Children-IV (DISC-IV), a study of adolescents in Nigeria reported that 28.4% of the sample met criteria for depression and a third of the sample met criteria for an anxiety disorder.[22] Caplan et al[3] administered the K-SADS and reported that among 100 children with generalized or localization-related epilepsy aged 5–16 years, 57 (33%) met DSM-IV criteria for a mood or anxiety disorder, with anxiety especially common (36%). Most recently, Jones et al,[23] using the K-SADS as well, found that among 53 children with recent onset epilepsy 22.6% meet criteria for a depressive disorder and 35.8% met criteria for an anxiety disorder. While advancing the field by using current psychiatric research methodology and careful characterization of pediatric epilepsy syndromes, these studies often lack information regarding specific depressive and anxiety disorders or rates of other comorbid psychiatric disorders.

Table 42–2 summarizes investigations that have used self-report inventories to quantify the degree of depression in children with epilepsy and Table 42–3 summarizes investigations that have used self-report measures to measure symptoms of anxiety in youth with epilepsy. These studies were either observational or controlled (comparing children with epilepsy to controls). Ettinger et al[24] found significantly elevated rates of depressive and anxiety symptoms based on the Children's Depression Inventory (CDI) and Revised Child Manifest Anxiety Scale (RCMAS), respectively.

Elevated rates of anxiety were also reported by Williams et al.[25] In a controlled study of anxiety, Margalit and Heiman[26] reported that significantly more children aged 8–14 years with epilepsy had higher levels of trait anxiety compared to healthy controls. In another sample of 35 children and adolescents with epilepsy aged 9–18 years, Oguz et al[27] reported symptoms of anxiety to be higher in the epilepsy group compared to controls. Additionally, more symptoms of depression were found in the childhood epilepsy group compared to the controls based on the CDI. Elevated rates of trait anxiety were also found by other investigators.[12,28] In summary, studies utilizing self-report measures consistently report significantly elevated rates of depression and anxiety in youth with epilepsy compared to healthy controls. Most of these studies utilized health controls, and there are no studies using children with other neurological disorders as controls and only a few studies using other illness groups as controls (i.e., asthma, diabetes).

Frequently, there is an assumption that factors associated with seizures and their chronic course may increase the risk for psychiatric disorders. However, recently as part of a population-based study in Iceland, Hesdorffer et al[29] reported that depression and suicide were independent risk factors for unprovoked seizures in children and adolescents with epilepsy. In addition, Jones et al[23] reported that 45% of children with epilepsy who had a comorbid psychiatric disorder met criteria for the psychiatric disorder prior to the first recognized seizure. The presence of psychiatric or behavioral problems prior to the first seizure was first suggested by Austin and colleagues.[30] These findings indicate that there is a possibility of a preexisting neurobiological insult or abnormality. Further investigation of these findings is warranted to understand the factors involved in the expression of depression and anxiety in children and adolescents with epilepsy.

To summarize, the existing epidemiological, clinical DSM/ICD, and self-report literature consistently indicate that psychiatric comorbidity is elevated in youth with epilepsy relative to the general population. However, only a few studies have used contemporary classification systems. Uniformly, studies have not examined the major effect of the severity of the epilepsy (complicated vs. uncomplicated) revealed in epidemiological studies.

▶ **TABLE 42–2. DEPRESSION—SELF-REPORT-BASED EVIDENCE**

Self-Report Measure	Depression	Observational Studies
Ettinger et al[24]	CDI	26% elevated rates of depression
Dunn et al[17]	CDI	9.6% depressive disorders
		Controlled Studies
Oguz et al[27]	CDI	Significantly higher rates of depression in epilepsy vs. controls
Baki et al[28]	CDI	Significantly higher rates of depression in epilepsy vs. controls
Baker et al[12]	CDI	Significantly higher rates of depression in epilepsy vs. controls

▶ **TABLE 42–3.** ANXIETY—SELF-REPORT-BASED EVIDENCE

Self-Report Measure	Anxiety	Observational Studies
Ettinger et al[24]	RCMAS	16% elevated rates of anxiety
Williams et al[25]	RCMAS	23% elevated anxiety
		Controlled Studies
Margalit and Heiman[26]	STAI	Significantly higher trait anxiety in epilepsy vs. controls
Oguz et al[27]	STAI	Significantly higher state/trait anxiety in epilepsy vs. controls
Baki et al[28]	STAI	Significantly higher anxiety in epilepsy vs. controls
Baker et al[12]	SADS, LOI	Significantly higher levels of social anxiety and obsessive symptoms in epilepsy vs. controls

SADS, the social avoidance and distress scale; LOI, Leyton obsessional inventory; STAI, state trait anxiety inventory; RCMAS, revised manifest anxiety scale.

Additionally, these studies have not examined the co-occurrence among psychiatric disorders that would be expected (e.g., a diagnosis of depression *and* anxiety) and progression over time. There is little discussion regarding the additional burdens to family, cognition, and health care utilization beyond that associated with epilepsy alone.

▶ IDENTIFYING DEPRESSION AND ANXIETY IN YOUNG PATIENTS WITH EPILEPSY

As practitioners involved in the care of children with epilepsy, one important role for all practitioners is to evaluate the presence or absence of symptoms related to psychiatric comorbidity. Since the literature indicates there are high rates of depression and anxiety present in youth with epilepsy, it will be important to identify these children and determine if treatment is appropriate or if a referral for treatment should occur. There are many ways to evaluate and to measure symptoms of depression and anxiety, and a review of a few measures will follow.

Irritability, anger, and difficulties in school may indicate depression in children and adolescents. These children may have trouble making and keeping friends, leading to increased isolation and poor self-esteem. Children may also display increasing dependence, such as the appearance of separation anxiety, due to immature and maladaptive coping skills.[31] While assessing symptoms of depression, it should be noted if there is a family history of depression because a family history is a significant risk factor. As Salpekar and Dunn[32] indicated children with anxiety disorders may report discomfort in social situations. They may not want to go to the cafeteria for lunch or want to ride the bus to and from school. Additionally, children may report worrying throughout the day; they may worry about what others think about them; and they often cannot stop the worries to think about other things.

There are significantly higher rates of suicide ideation and attempts among children and adolescents with epilepsy compared to controls.[3] Suicide risk should be considered and assessed. This can be a difficult subject to discuss, but it is important to let the child or adolescent with epilepsy know that you are concerned about them as a whole person not just their seizures. Salpecker and Dunn[32] suggest a step-by-step approach to assess suicide risk utilizing similar lines of questioning: Do you sometimes feel so sad you wish you were never born or you wish you were not alive? Have you thought that you wanted to be dead? Have you thought about doing something to kill yourself?

There are a number of screening questionnaires that can be utilized to assess and identify comorbidities of depression and anxiety in children with epilepsy. There are broad-based instruments that can assess a number of domains and alert the clinician to potential problems, and these instruments have parent, teacher, and self-report versions.

CHILD BEHAVIOR CHECK LIST (CBCL)

The CBCL has a long history, and it has been extensively used in clinical and research settings. It was developed to assess behavior problems and social competencies in children aged 6–18.[16] It has been used to measure treatment outcomes. There are 118 items assessing behavioral and emotional problems. It includes general scales of internalizing and externalizing problems and provides more specific scales such as withdrawn, somatic, complaints, anxious/depressed, social problems, thought problems, attention problems, aggressive behavior, and delinquent behavior.

STRENGTHS AND DIFFICULTIES QUESTIONNAIRE (SDQ)

The SDQ is a relatively new screening instrument that briefly examines symptomatology, impairments, and burden of psychopathology for ages 4–16 with a self-report measure developed for ages 11–16.[15] It has been used in Europe and more recently in the United States as well as a number of other countries including Sweden, Germany, and Finland, and it has been translated into 40 different languages (www.sdqinfo.com). The SDQ has been reported to have strong correlations with CBCL and high internal consistency (Cronbach α) on the parent report—Total Differences Scale (0.82). There are five scales with five items in each scale for a total of 25 items, and the scales are as follows: emotional symptoms, conduct problems, hyperactivity inattention, peer relationship problems, and prosocial behavior. Additionally, there are five questions assessing impairment and burden related to the emotional and behavioral problems. This instrument was designed to reflect diagnostic criteria of the Diagnostic and Statistical Manual-IV (DSM-IV),[33] and the International Classification of Diseases 10th edition (ICD-10) (World Health Organization.[34]

Additionally, there are a number of questionnaires that assess symptoms of anxiety and depression independently. Here a two instruments that have been utilized in youth with epilepsy are presented.

THE CHILDREN'S DEPRESSION INVENTORY (CDI)

The CDI is comprised of 27 items designed to measure symptoms of depression in children ages 9 and up.[35] For each item, there are three statements and the child has to choose one statement that best describes him or her in the past 2 weeks. There are five subscales: negative mood, interpersonal problems, ineffectiveness, anhedonia, and negative self-esteem. It takes approximately 10 minutes to complete. Children who have a score greater than 65 are suspected to meet criteria for a diagnosis of depression.

MULTIDIMENSIONAL ANXIETY SCALE (MASC)

The MASC is a 39-item questionnaire assessing symptoms of anxiety in children ages 8–19.[36] The MASC can be completed in 10 minutes. The four subscales are as follows: physical symptoms, harm avoidance, social anxiety, and separation/panic. An overall Anxiety Disorders Index is tabulated and discriminates the most reliably between children with and without anxiety disorders. The MASC was normed and developed in the United States. It is reported to have excellent test/retest reliability, established factorial validity, strong sensitivity, and specificity.

REVISED CHILDREN'S MANIFEST ANXIETY SCALE (RCMAS)

The RCMAS is a 37-item questionnaire designed to assess anxiety in children ages 6–19.[37] It is completed by the child. All questions are in a yes/no format. There is a total anxiety score as well as three subscales: physiological anxiety, worry/oversensitivity, and social concerns/concentration. Higher scores indicate increased anxiety. This measure is reported to have good reliability and validity. It was normed on a large sample of school-aged children.

Self-report questionnaires can be useful tools to identify symptoms of depression and anxiety in children with epilepsy and ultimately inform the physician, neurologist, nurse, or other practitioners involved in patient care. Once identified a plan of action can be created to reduce or eliminate symptoms of anxiety or depression in youth with epilepsy.

▶ TREATMENT AND INTERVENTION STUDIES IN EPILEPSY

Despite awareness of the increased risk of mental health problems in youth with epilepsy, it is surprising to find that there are no psychological intervention studies aimed at treating cormorbid anxiety or mood disorders in children with epilepsy. There are no randomized controlled trials that demonstrate the valid use of psychotherapy in children and adolescents in epilepsy who also have depression and/or anxiety.[38]

Psychotherapy should be considered a treatment option that can be used independently or in conjunction with pharmacological treatments. Cognitive behavior therapy (CBT) is recommended for the treatment of depression in children and adolescents.[39] CBT focuses on problem-solving, developing coping mechanisms, and addressing cognitive distortions. Research indicates that CBT is efficacious in the treatment of major depression.

Randomized controlled trials of CBT have demonstrated that CBT is efficacious in reducing symptoms of anxiety in children and adolescents with treatment gains maintained at 1-year and 3-year follow-ups.[40] However, there has been no systematic examination of psychotherapeutic interventions in the treatment of anxiety disorders in children and adolescents with epilepsy. As in depression, more research is needed in psychotherapeutic and pharmacological treatment options for children and adolescents with epilepsy and comorbid anxiety disorders.

In the general pediatric literature, there are very few controlled medication treatment studies for children with psychiatric disorders and even fewer studies conducted with children with epilepsy and psychiatric comorbidities. In addition, children with seizures or other medical comorbidities are often excluded from randomized trials due to the fact that they have seizures.[32] For further discussion on this topic, see Dunn and Austin.[41]

▶ DISCUSSION

The majority of data reported in the literature is based on cross-sectional community-based studies primarily recruited from tertiary care centers. Only recently have structured psychiatric interviews been conducted and standard diagnostic criteria utilized. The majority of the studies do not report rates in each diagnostic category and rates of co-occurrence of psychiatric disorders (e.g., both depression and anxiety) are often ignored. Additionally, controls are not extensively utilized and children with other chronic illnesses or neurological disorders are often not utilized as controls. As discussed previously, studies have not examined the effect of severity of the epilepsy (complicated vs. uncomplicated). Despite the fact that there appears to be high rates of depression and anxiety among children with epilepsy, there continues to be no data evaluating interventions. Additionally there remains little examination of the additional burdens to family, cognition, and health care utilization beyond those associated with epilepsy alone. As a field, there is much more work to be done to understand, identify, and treat depression and anxiety in youth with epilepsy.

REFERENCES

1. Davies S, Heyman I, Goodman R. A population survey of mental health problems in children with epilepsy. *Dev Med Child Neurol* 2003;45:292–295.
2. Pellock JM. Defining the problem: psychiatric and behavioral comorbidity in children and adolescents with epilepsy. *Epilepsy Behav* 2004;5(Suppl 3):S3–S9.
3. Caplan R, et al. Depression and anxiety disorders in pediatric epilepsy. *Epilepsia* 2005;46:720–730.
4. Plioplys S, Dunn DW, Caplan R. 10-year research update review: psychiatric problems in children with epilepsy. *J Am Acad Child Adolesc Psychiatry* 2007;46:1389–1402.
5. Merikangas K, Avenevoli S. Epidemiology of mood and anxiety disorders in children and adolescents. In: Tsuang M, Tohen M (eds), *Textbook in Psychiatric Epidemiology.* New York: Wiley-Liss, Inc., 2002; 2nd edn: pp. 657–704.
6. Lépine JP. The epidemiology of anxiety disorders: prevalence and societal costs. *J Clin Psychiatry* 2002; 63(Suppl 14):4–8.
7. Pine DS, et al. The risk for early-adulthood anxiety and depressive disorders in adolescents with anxiety and depressive disorders. *Arch Gen Psychiatry* 1998;55: 56–64.
8. Zahn-Waxler C, Klimes-Dougan B, Slattery MJ. Internalizing problems of childhood and adolescence: prospects,

9. Spady DW, et al. Medical and psychiatric comorbidity and health care use among children 6 to 17 years old. *Arch Pediatr Adolesc Med* 2005;159:231–237.
10. Greenberg PE, et al. The economic burden of anxiety disorders in the 1990s. *J Clin Psychiatry* 1999;60:427–435.
11. Alwash RH, Hussein MJ, Matloub FF. Symptoms of anxiety and depression among adolescents with seizures in Irbid, Northern Jordan. *Seizure* 2000;9:412–416.
12. Baker GA, et al. Impact of epilepsy in adolescence: a UK controlled study. *Epilepsy Behav* 2005;6:556–562.
13. Rutter M, Graham P, Yule W. *A Neuropsychiatric Study in Childhood.* London: S.I.M.P./William Heineman Medical Books, 1970.
14. Lossius MI, et al. Psychiatric symptoms in adolescents with epilepsy in junior high school in Norway: a population survey. *Epilepsy Behav* 2006;9:286–292.
15. Goodman R. The extended version of the Strengths and Difficulties Questionnaire as a guide to child psychiatric caseness and consequent burden. *J Child Psychol Psychiatry* 1999;40:791–799.
16. Achenbach TM, Rescorla LA. *Manual for the ASEBA School-Age Forms and Profiles.* Burlington: University of Vermont, Research Center for Children, Youth and Families, 2001.
17. Dunn DW, Austin JK, Huster GA. Symptoms of depression in adolescents with epilepsy. *J Am Acad Child Adolesc Psychiatry* 1999;38:1132–1138.
18. Dunn DW, et al. Teacher assessment of behaviour in children with new-onset seizures. *Seizure* 2002;11:169–175.
19. Rodenburg R, et al. Psychopathology in children with epilepsy: a meta-analysis. *J Pediatr Psychol* 2005;30:453–468.
20. Costello EJ, et al. Prevalence and development of psychiatric disorders in childhood and adolescence. *Arch Gen Psychiatry* 2003;60:837–844.
21. Thome-Souza S, et al. Which factors may play a pivotal role on determining the type of psychiatric disorder in children and adolescents with epilepsy? *Epilepsy Behav* 2004;5:988–994.
22. Adewuya AO, Ola BA. Prevalence of and risk factors for anxiety and depressive disorders in Nigerian adolescents with epilepsy. *Epilepsy Behav* 2005;6:342–347.
23. Jones JE, et al. Psychiatric comorbidity in children with new onset epilepsy. *Dev Med Child Neurol* 2007;49:493–497.
24. Ettinger AB, et al. Symptoms of depression and anxiety in pediatric epilepsy patients. *Epilepsia* 1998;39(6):595–599.
25. Williams J, et al. Anxiety in children with epilepsy. *Epilepsy Behav* 2003;4:729–732.
26. Margalit M, Heiman T. Anxiety and self-dissatisfaction in epileptic children. *Int J Soc Psychiatry* 1983;29:220–224.
27. Oguz A, Kurul S, Dirik E. Relationship of epilepsy-related factors to anxiety and depression scores in epileptic children. *J Child Neurol* 2002;17:37–40.
28. Baki O, et al. Anxiety and depression in children with epilepsy and their mothers. *Epilepsy Behav* 2004;5:958–964.

pitfalls, and progress in understanding the development of anxiety and depression. *Dev Psychopathol* 2000;12:443–466.

29. Hesdorffer DC, et al. Depression and suicide attempt as risk factors for incident unprovoked seizures. *Ann Neurol* 2006;59:35–41.

30. Austin JK, et al. Behavior problems in children before first recognized seizures. *Pediatrics* 2001;107:115–122.

31. Plioplys S. Depression in children and adolescents with epilepsy. *Epilepsy Behav* 2003;4(Suppl 3):S39–S45.

32. Salpekar JA, Dunn DW. Psychiatric and psychosocial consequences of pediatric epilepsy. *Semin Pediatr Neurol* 2007;14:181–188.

33. American Psychiatric Association. *Diagnostic and Statistical Manual of Mental Disorders.* Text Revision. Washington, DC, American Psychiatric Association, 2000; 4th edn.

34. World Health Organization. *International Statistical Classification of Diseases and Related Health Problems.* Geneva, Switzerland: Who Press, 2010, 10th revision, edn.

35. Kovacs M. The children's depression, inventory (CDI). *Psychopharmacol Bull* 1985;21:995–998.

36. March JS, et al. The Multidimensional Anxiety Scale for Children (MASC): factor structure, reliability, and validity. *J Am Acad Child Adolesc Psychiatry* 1997;36:554–565.

37. Reynolds CR, Richmond BO. *Revised Children's Manifest Anxiety Scale.* Los Angeles: Western Psychological Services, 1985.

38. Ramaratnam S, Baker GA, Goldstein LH. Psychological treatments for epilepsy. *Cochrane Database Syst Rev* 2005; CD002029.

39. American Academy of Child and Adolescent Psychiatry. Practice parameters for the assessment and treatment of children and adolescents with depressive disorders. *J Am Acad Child Adolesc Psychiatry* 1998;37(10):63S–83S.

40. Kendall PC, et al. Therapy for youths with anxiety disorders: a second randomized clinical trial. *J Consult Clin Psychol* 1997;65:366–380.

41. Dunn DW, Austin JK. Differential diagnosis and treatment of psychiatric disorders in children and adolescents with epilepsy. *Epilepsy Behav* 2004;5(Suppl 3):S10–S17.

CHAPTER 43

Autism in Children with Epilepsy: Diagnosis and Treatment

Roberto Tuchman

Children with autism have higher rates of epilepsy than in the general population and children with epilepsy are at high risk of developing autism.[1,2] When epilepsy and autism coexist, the quality of life in these individuals is severely impacted.[3] Recognizing and diagnosing autism in children with epilepsy and understanding the treatment options is important for the comprehensive management of children with epilepsy. This chapter will focus on how to go about making the diagnosis of autism in children with epilepsy and on the treatment approach to children with epilepsy and autism.

▶ DIAGNOSIS

DIAGNOSING AUTISM IN CHILDREN WITH EPILEPSY (FIG. 43–1)

Autism-like epilepsy is a heterogeneous developmental disorder associated with many diverse etiologies and pathologies. The labels of autism spectrum disorders (ASD) or pervasive developmental disorders (PDD) are commonly used to describe individuals who have varying deficits in verbal and nonverbal communication, social skills, and a restricted repertoire of interests or repetitive behaviors (Table 43–1). Throughout this chapter, the term autism will be used to discuss this heterogeneous group of children.

The DSM-IV and ICD-10 systems provide a framework for the clinical diagnosis of autism and evidence-based guidelines have been established for the diagnosis of autism and related disorders.[4] From a research perspective the "gold-standard" for the diagnosis of autism are the Autism Diagnostic Observation System and the Autism Diagnostic Interview, which together provide both a structured detailed interview and an observation method to assess an individual's social ability, communication skills, and behavior objectively. A list of resources and references regarding the diagnosis and treatment for autism is available in Box 43–1.

The core clinical features that define autism and related disorders and differentiate it from other developmental disorders are a disturbance of social interaction, which may not be absolute. Social cognition is a complex concept and social behaviors will differ depending on the cognitive level and associated disabilities of a child. The defining features of the social cognitive deficits in children with autism include joint attention (defined as the behaviors used to share the experience of objects or events with others), disturbances in affect, impairments in imitation, impairments in the capacity for pretend play with objects or people and in the ability of individuals with autism to attribute beliefs to themselves and others (theory of mind).[5] How often social cognitive deficits exist in children with epilepsy is not known, but in adults with epilepsy mesial temporal epilepsy is associated with deficits in higher-order social cognition.[6]

In children with autism, reports of epilepsy range from 5% to 38.3%.[7] The large variations in reported rates of epilepsy in children with autism are dependent on the clinical characteristics of the subgroup of children with autism that is being studied. The common risk factors for both autism and epilepsy are genetics, mental retardation, and language regression.

Genetics

There are several gene disorders associated with both autism and epilepsy, for example, a susceptibility locus for autism has been found on chromosome 2 in the vicinity of the genes SCN1A and SCN2A, which are also susceptibility genes for seizures.[8] In some children who have epilepsy, mental retardation, and hypotonia in association with the autism phenotype cytogenetic abnormalities in chromosome 15 has been reported.[9] There is a recent description of a group of Amish children who develop intractable focal seizures in childhood with behaviors consistent with the autism phenotype in addition to having language regression and mental retardation. In this group of children, a homozygous mutation of contactin-associated protein-like 2 (CNTNAP2) has been found.[10]

Mental Retardation

Cognition is not part of the clinical criteria for the diagnosis of autism, but it co-exists with autism and is an important determinant of the well-established association

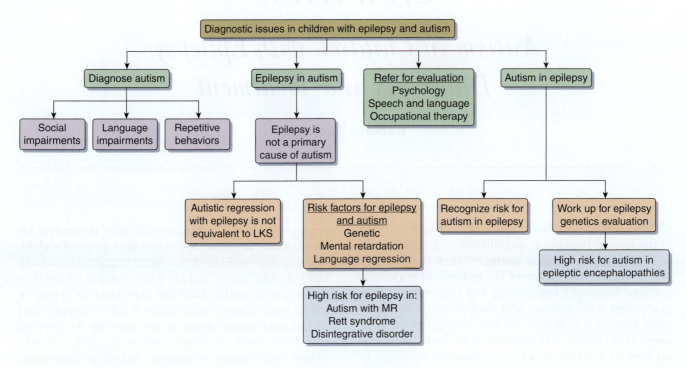

Figure 43–1. Diagnostic issues in children with epilepsy and autism.

between autism and epilepsy. Children with autism and severe mental retardation are at highest risk for developing epilepsy.[11] The two autism syndromes most likely to be associated with epilepsy, Rett and Childhood Disintegrative Disorder (CDD), are also the most likely to be associated with severe cognitive deficits.[12,13]

Language Regression

Language type and particularly regression in children with autism has been of particular interest to researchers investigating the relationship of autism and epilepsy. Regression or stagnation of language skills is reported by one-third of parents of children with autism and usually consists of the loss of a few words between 18 and 24 months, together with the appearance of autistic behaviors.[14] There has been significant controversy over the role of epilepsy in autistic regression. Recent studies suggest that language regression in isolation is different than the social and language regression that occurs in autism. Children with isolated language regression have a higher frequency of epileptiform discharges and

▶ **TABLE 43–1.** AUTISM SPECTRUM DISORDER CRITERIA

Behavioral Domain	More Likely in Lower Functioning Child with Autism	More Likely in Higher Functioning Child with Autism
Social	Gaze avoidance	Inappropriate affection
	Failure to respond when called	Lack of social or emotional empathy
	Failure to participate within groups	Impaired ability to make peer friendships
	Lack of awareness of others indifference to affection	Poverty of social skills
		Tend to be loners
Language	Failure to develop both expressive and receptive language skills	Abnormal melody
		Sing-song prosody
	Language is immature and characterized by echolalia, pronoun reversals, unintelligible jargon	Monotonous tone
		Inability to initiate or sustain an appropriate conversation
Repetitive behaviors	Resistance to change	Lack of symbolic play
	Insistence on certain routines	Repetition of certain words, phrases, or songs
	Attachments to objects	Focus on narrow topics such as train schedules, maps, or historical facts
	Fascination with parts and movement of objects	
	Lining up or manipulating the toys	
	Flapping, humming, rocking, running around in circles	

▶ **BOX 43–1.** **RESOURCES AND REFERENCES FOR DIAGNOSIS AND TREATMENT OF AUTISM**

American Psychiatric Association. *Diagnostic and Statistical Manual of Mental Disorders*. Washington, DC: American Psychiatric Association, 1994; 4th edn.

World Health Organisation. *International Classification of Diseases and Health Related Problems*. Geneva: World Health Organisation, 1992; 10th edn.

Rapin I. Autism. *NEJM* 1997;337(2):97–104.

Lord C, et al. The autism diagnostic observation schedule-generic: a standard measure of social and communication deficits associated with the spectrum of autism. *J Autism Dev Disord* 2000;30(3):205–223.

Ozonoff S, Goodlin-Jones BL, Solomon M. Evidence-based assessment of autism spectrum disorders in children and adolescents. *J Clin Child Adolesc Psychol* 2005;34(3):523–540.

Bryson SE, Rogers SJ, Fombonne E. Autism spectrum disorders: early detection, intervention, education, and psychopharmacological management. *Can J Psychiatry* 2003;48(8):506–516.

Centers for Disease Control. http://www.cdc.gov/ncbddd/dd/ddautism.htm.

American Academy Practice Guidelines for Autism. http://www.aan.com/professionals/practice/guidelines/guideline_summaries/Autism_Guideline_for_Clinicians.pdf.

National Autistic Society. http://www.nas.org.uk/.

National Institute of Health. http://health.nih.gov/result.asp/62.

National Research Council Educating Children with Autism. www.gao.gov/new.items/d05220.pdf.

Tuchman R, Rapin I (eds.). *Autism: A Neurological Disorder of Early Brain Development*. London: MacKeith Press, 2006.

seizures, than children with both language and autistic (social and behavioral) regression.[15] Neither epilepsy nor epileptiform discharges are a primary cause of autistic regression.[16]

Overlap of Epileptic Encephalopathies and Autism

There are rare case reports in the literature in which epilepsy can directly affect cognition and behavior or epileptic encephalopathies associated with behavioral and language regression and a behavioral phenotype similar to autism.[17] Landau–Kleffner syndrome (LKS) is the epileptic encephalopathy that is commonly confused with children with autism and regression who have an abnormal epileptiform EEG. The regression of language in LKS is more dramatic and the social deficits are less severe than in autistic regression. The age of regression in LKS is later, usually after 24 months and classically between ages 3 and 5 years when language is more clearly established. In addition, the EEG findings in children with LKS tend to be more dramatic than those reported in autistic regression.

Children with LKS commonly have Electrical Status Epilepticus during slow-wave Sleep (ESES), which is the EEG pattern present in several childhood syndromes associated with sleep-related epileptic encephalopathies with cognitive and language dysfunction.[18] The other epileptic encephalopathy associated with ESES is Continuous Spikes and Waves during slow-wave Sleep (CSWS). The majority of children with ESES, especially those with CSWS and Landau–Kleffner syndrome, have normal development prior to the onset of ESES, but almost all deteriorate cognitively and develop behaviors consistent with the autism phenotype during ESES.[19] The pattern of ESES is rare in children with autism and regression and is more likely to be found in children with childhood disintegrative disorder, in whom language and behavioral regression occurs between 3 and 6 years, and as late as age 10 years.[20]

Childhood disintegrative disorder overlaps with children with CSWS. Perez-Roulet and Deonna coined the term acquired epileptic frontal syndrome with CSWS for children who had cryptogenic or idiopathic partial epilepsy with a frontal focus and CSWS and normal prior development.[21–23]

Infantile spasms may also be associated with autism. Although all seizure types may exist in children with autism, infantile spasms as a seizure type is overrepresented in children with autism.[24] Children with infantile spasms are at high risk for developing autism.[25,26] The relationship between genetics, mental retardation, autism, epilepsy, and specifically the epileptic encephalopathies, such as infantile spasms is complex. For example, in children with tuberous sclerosis complex gene mutations may influence the development of autism directly.[27] However, the location of tubers in the temporal lobes, a history of infantile spasms, onset of seizures in the first 3 years of life, and temporal lobe epileptiform discharges all have a role in determining whether or not an individual with TSC develops autism.[28]

Children with autism and regression with or without epilepsy or with or without epileptiform discharges can and should be differentiated from children with an epileptic encephalopathy. The clinical implications of regression in children with epilepsy are different than the clinical implications of regression in autism. In children with epilepsy, especially with regression of language and behavior, the clinician needs to have a heightened awareness that the behavioral phenotype of autism may coexist. This is especially true in children with severe cognitive impairments and epilepsy and in those with epileptic encephalopathies where the association of autism and epilepsy is fairly robust.

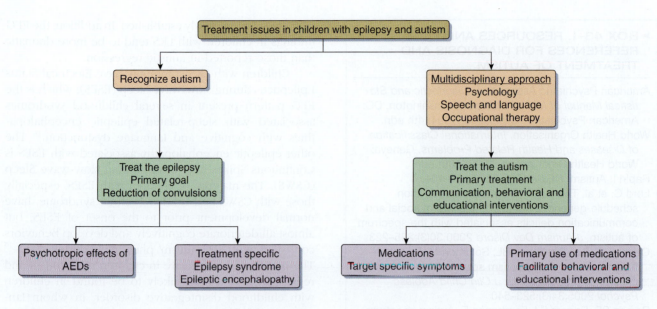

Figure 43–2. Treatment issues in children with epilepsy and autism.

▶ TREATMENT

TREATMENT OF AUTISM IN CHILDREN WITH EPILEPSY (FIG. 43–2)

Information on the effects of interventions in autism in general and in children with epilepsy and autism in specific is extremely limited. Neither pharmacological nor nonpharmacological interventions are a cure for autism. Appropriate behavioral management techniques, educational, and communication techniques form the basis of management of all children with autism (see appendix for resources on management of the child with autism). An interdisciplinary approach and referral to specialists in communication (speech and language pathologists), motor function (occupational therapists), psychology, and educators well versed in functional behavioral analysis and behavioral management techniques is an essential part of the management of all children with autism.

The primary use of pharmaceutical interventions in autism is the enhancement of communication, behavioral, and educational interventions. Medications also improve attention and reduce hyperactivity, repetitive behaviors, oppositional behaviors, agitation, aggression and self-injurious behavior promote sleep. There are no medications effective for social and communicative enhancement. A rather diverse array of medications, reflecting the heterogenous nature of autism and the multiple behaviors associated with this disorder, have been used in double-blind placebo-controlled trials in children with autism.[29]

The atypical antipsychotics that block postsynaptic dopamine and serotonin receptors and medications that modulate the serotonergic system, such as the selective

serotonin reuptake inhibitors (SSRI's), have had the largest positive impact in the treatment of autism.[30] The atypical antipsychotic risperidone, at least over a short-term period, seems to be an effective treatment of tantrums, aggression, or self-injurious behavior in children and adolescents with autism.[31] Specific serotonin reuptake inhibitors, such as fluoxetine, fluvoxamine, paroxetine, and setraline, have all been associated with improvements in repetitive thoughts and behaviors, self-injurious behavior, desire for sameness, and increased language use.[32] In general medication trials in children with autism have resulted in mixed results, have been used in small numbers of patients, and lack consistent replication. In addition, the extent of improvement with all pharmacological agents that have been used in children with autism is modest and the side-effect profiles of the medications limit their long-term use in autism.

Treatment of Epilepsy in Children with Autism

The treatment of the convulsions in children with autism is neither unusually difficult nor different from treatment for children with epilepsy without autism.[33] Antiepileptic drugs (AEDs) are administered widely to children with autism for two reasons: one is that children with autism have a high rate of convulsive disorders and the other is that AEDs are being used because children with autism often have or later develop symptoms and behaviors that in addition to those that qualify them for their primary diagnosis are also consistent with the diagnosis of affective disorders.

AEDs have been shown to have mood stabilizing effects as well as anxiolytic and antidepressant properties.

In determining which AED is appropriate to treat epilepsy in children with both epilepsy and autism, the potential effects on mood and behavior of the AED chosen, should be considered.[34,35]

There are several AEDs that have been reportedly useful in children with autism and epilepsy both for the convulsions and for behavior. There have been no controlled clinical trials on AEDs in children with autism and epilepsy and the studies done have been open-label trials that have included a small number of heterogenous children with autism and epilepsy.[36] The medications that have been investigated in case reports of children with epilepsy and autism include valproic acid, lamotrigine, levitiracetam, and topiramate in children with Rett syndrome. The benefit of one of these AEDs over the other cannot be determined from the limited data available. In children with intractable epilepsy and autism, aggressive treatment of the epilepsy has been suggested.[37,38] The limited data on the effects of epilepsy surgery in children with epilepsy and autism suggest that surgical intervention does not alter the symptoms of autism.[39] No general recommendations for the use of specific AEDs in children with epilepsy and autism can be made and the use of AEDs in children with autism and epilepsy should be individualized. Surgical intervention for children with epilepsy and autism should follow the guidelines for epilepsy surgery in children and the presence of autism does not alter in any specific way these recommendations.

In epilepsy syndromes whose outcome is associated with cognitive, language, and behavioral deficits, treating only the seizures is not adequate. Addressing the cognitive, language, and behavioral manifestations becomes an important component of the treatment of children with epilepsy and autism. Early recognition of autism in children with epilepsy can allow for prompt introduction of communication, behavioral, and educational interventions that can minimize the impact of autism and maximize the potential of children with epilepsy and autism.

REFERENCES

1. Steffenburg U, Hagberg G, Kyllerman M. Characteristics of seizures in a population-based series of mentally retarded children with active epilepsy. *Epilepsia* 1996;37(9):850–856.
2. Clarke DF, et al. The prevalence of autistic spectrum disorder in children surveyed in a tertiary care epilepsy clinic. *Epilepsia* 2005;46(12):1970–1977.
3. Danielsson S, et al. Epilepsy in young adults with autism: a prospective population-based follow-up study of 120 individuals diagnosed in childhood. *Epilepsia* 2005; 46(6):918–923.
4. Filipek PA, et al. Practice parameter: screening and diagnosis of autism. Report of the Quality Standards Subcommittee of the American Academy of Neurology and the Child Neurology Society. *Neurology* 2000;55(4):468–479.
5. Tuchman R. Autism. *Neurol Clin* 2003;21(4):915–932, viii.
6. Schacher M, et al. Mesial temporal lobe epilepsy impairs advanced social cognition. *Epilepsia* 2006;47(12):2141–2146.
7. Tuchman R, Rapin I. Epilepsy in autism. *Lancet Neurol* 2002;1(6):352–358.
8. Weiss LA, et al. Sodium channels SCN1A, SCN2A and SCN3A in familial autism. *Mol Psychiatry* 2003;8(2):186–194.
9. Battaglia A. The inv dup(15) or idic(15) syndrome: a clinically recognisable neurogenetic disorder. *Brain Dev* 2005;27(5): 365–369.
10. Strauss KA, et al. Recessive symptomatic focal epilepsy and mutant contactin-associated protein-like 2. *N Engl J Med* 2006;354(13):1370–1377.
11. Tuchman RF, Rapin I, Shinnar S. Autistic and dysphasic children. II: epilepsy. *Pediatrics* 1991;88(6):1219–1225.
12. Burd L, Fisher W, Kerbeshian J. Pervasive disintegrative disorder: are Rett syndrome and Heller dementia infantilis subtypes? *Dev Med Child Neurol* 1989;31(5):609–616.
13. Steffenburg U, Hagberg G, Hagberg B. Epilepsy in a representative series of Rett syndrome. *Acta Paediatr* 2001; 90(1):34–39.
14. Richler J, et al. Is there a 'regressive phenotype' of Autism Spectrum Disorder associated with the measles-mumps-rubella vaccine? A CPEA Study. *J Autism Dev Disord* 2006;36(3):299–316.
15. McVicar KA, et al. Epileptiform EEG abnormalities in children with language regression. *Neurology* 2005;65(1):129–131.
16. Tuchman R. Autism and epilepsy: what has regression got to do with it? *Epilepsy Curr* 2006;6(4):107–111.
17. Deonna T, Roulet E. Autistic spectrum disorder: evaluating a possible contributing or causal role of epilepsy. *Epilepsia* 2006;47(Suppl 2):79–82.
18. Jayakar PB, Seshia SS. Electrical status epilepticus during slow-wave sleep: a review. *J Clin Neurophysiol* 1991; 8(3):299–311.
19. Beaumanoir A, et al. (eds). *Continuous Spikes and Waves During Slow Sleep, Electrical Status Epilepticus During Slow Sleep, Acquired Epileptic Aphasia and Related Conditions.* London: John Libbey, 1995.
20. Rapin I. Autistic regression and disintegrative disorder: how important the role of epilepsy? *Semin Pediatr Neurol* 1995;2(4):278–285.
21. Roulet Perez E, et al. Mental and behavioural deterioration of children with epilepsy and CSWS: acquired epileptic frontal syndrome. *Dev Med Child Neurol* 1993;35(8):661–674.
22. Kyllerman M, et al. Transient psychosis in a girl with epilepsy and continuous spikes and waves during slow sleep (CSWS). *Eur Child Adolesc Psychiatry* 1996;5(4): 216–221.
23. Roulet Perez E, et al. Childhood epilepsy with neuro-psychological regression and continuous spike waves during sleep: epilepsy surgery in a young adult. *Eur J Paediatr Neurol* 1998;2(6):303–311.
24. Tuchman RF. Epilepsy, language, and behavior: clinical models in childhood. *J Child Neurol* 1994;9(1):95–102.
25. Riikonen R, Amnell G. Psychiatric disorders in children with earlier infantile spasms. *Dev Med Child Neurol* 1981; 23(6):747–760.
26. Askalan R, et al. Prospective preliminary analysis of the development of autism and epilepsy in children with infantile spasms. *J Child Neurol* 2003;18(3):165–170.

27. Smalley SL. Autism and tuberous sclerosis. *J Autism Dev Disord* 1998;28(5):407–414.

28. Bolton PF. Neuroepileptic correlates of autistic symptomatology in tuberous sclerosis. *Ment Retard Dev Disabil Res Rev* 2004;10(2):126–131.

29. Palermo MT, Curatolo P. Pharmacologic treatment of autism. *J Child Neurol* 2004;19(3):155–164.

30. King BH, Bostic JQ. An update on pharmacologic treatments for autism spectrum disorders. *Child Adolesc Psychiatr Clin N Am* 2006;15(1):161–175.

31. Jesner O, Aref-Adib M, Coren E. Risperidone for autism spectrum disorder. *Cochrane Database Syst Rev* 2007;(1):CD005040.

32. Posey DJ, et al. The use of selective serotonin reuptake inhibitors in autism and related disorders. *J Child Adolesc Psychopharmacol* 2006;16(1–2):181–186.

33. Gillberg C. The treatment of epilepsy in autism. *J Autism Dev Disord* 1991;21(1):61–77.

34. Di Martino A, Tuchman RF. Antiepileptic drugs: affective use in autism spectrum disorders. *Pediatr Neurol* 2001; 25(3):199–207.

35. Ettinger AB. Psychotropic effects of antiepileptic drugs. *Neurology* 2006;67(11):1916–1925.

36. Tuchman R. AEDs and psychotropic drugs in children with autism and epilepsy. *Ment Retard Dev Disabil Res Rev* 2004;10(2):135–138.

37. Nass R, et al. Outcome of multiple subpial transections for autistic epileptiform regression. *Pediatr Neurol* 1999; 21(1):464–470.

38. Neville BG, et al. Surgical treatment of severe autistic regression in childhood epilepsy. *Pediatr Neurol* 1997; 16(2):137–140.

39. Szabo CA, et al. Epilepsy surgery in children with pervasive developmental disorder. *Pediatr Neurol* 1999;20(5): 349–353.

CHAPTER 44

Treating Epilepsy in the Presence of Sleep Disorders

Paolo Tinuper, Francesca Bisulli, Federica Provini, James D. Geyer, and Paul R. Carney

► INTRODUCTION

Sleep disorders have an adverse impact on daily living for both children and their caregivers.[1] Sleep disturbance and lack of restful sleep can masquerade as a myriad of clinical problems, including inattention, depression, headache, and seizures. While most neurological disorders are well characterized during the waking state, descriptions of pathophysiology, signs and comorbidities are frequently poorly described during sleep. Physiologic changes associated with sleep can cause an alteration of signs and function during both REM (rapid eye movement) and non-REM (NREM) sleep. These changes may include alterations in muscle tone, central control of autonomic functions, and changes in cortical neurotransmitter system interaction and balance.

Epilepsy is also a disorder that affects every aspect of a child's cognitive, social, and emotional well-being. When these disorders coexist, they can be both challenging to identify and differentiate, and a burden to the young patient and their families.

This review is devoted to the relationships between epilepsy, sleep and its disorders. The effects of epilepsy on sleep architecture and the quality of children's sleep are reviewed. How sleep may affect epilepsy and the role of circadian rhythms is discussed next. Evidence regarding the relation between epilepsy and both childhood sleep breathing disorders and restless legs syndrome (RLS) is summarized. Finally, a discussion highlighting differences between epilepsy and the most common sleep disorders during childhood is provided. An outline of evaluation and treatment of the epileptic child with a sleep disorder ends this review.

PATHOPHYSIOLOGY OF SLEEP DISORDERS IN CHILDREN WITH EPILEPSY

Epilepsy and Sleep Architecture

Epilepsy has important effects on sleep and the sleep–wake cycle.[2] Alterations in total sleep, time sleep latency, and spontaneous awakenings have been demonstrated in epileptic children.[3] Epilepsy may affect both the quantity and the architecture of sleep. The effects of epilepsy on sleep vary depending on seizure type. In patients with primary generalized tonic–clonic seizures, the amount of REM sleep is decreased by 50%, while in those suffering from secondarily generalized seizures, it may be as low as 41%.[4,5] Infants with epileptic encephalopathies (hypsarrhythmia and Lennox–Gastaut syndrome)[6] also have decreased REM sleep as well as a decrease in total sleep time in a 24-hour period.[6–8] Prolonged sleep latency, an increase in the proportion of stages 1 and 2 NREM sleep, a decrease in the proportion of stages 3 and 4 NREM sleep, and an increase in the shifting between sleep stages have also been described.

Patients affected with childhood absence epilepsy and epilepsy with myoclonic absences do not show sleep disturbances.[9] Among patients with complex partial seizures, only in those suffering from multiple nocturnal seizures, as in nocturnal frontal lobe epilepsy (NFLE), the proportion of REM sleep significantly lowered.[10] Children with focal drug-resistant epilepsy studied with all-night polysomnography evidence a reduction of total sleep time, reduction of stage 2 and REM stage percentage and increase in first REM latency.[11,12] REM stage can also be reduced by 18%–12% in patients with daytime temporal lobe seizures.[13] Interestingly, patients with benign rolandic epilepsy have no associated sleep disorders.[14,15] Likewise, children with continuous slow spike waves of sleep have no associated sleep disorders.

Sleep Influences on Epilepsy

Sleep, on average, covers one third of the life span of a human being. Sleep tends to activate the EEG as delineated in Table 44–1. The relationship between sleep stages and ictal or interictal epileptiform discharges is well known,[16,17] the modulation of epileptiform paroxysms during sleep depending on the type of epilepsy and the different electrophysiological status characterizing NREM and REM stages. During drowsiness and the first stages of NREM sleep, EEG activity becomes more synchronized, thus facilitating the propagation of epileptiform discharges; muscular tone is diminished but preserved, permitting the clinical manifestation of the seizures. On the contrary, in REM sleep, when EEG activity is desynchronized and postural tone inhibited,

▶ **TABLE 44–1. ACTIVATION OF EEG DURING SLEEP**

Syndrome	Wake	Drowsy	NREM	REM	Arousal
Neonatal	+		Unknown		
West					+++
Lennox		+++	++		
Absence		++			
Myoclonic					+++
Partial		++	++		++

+, Mild; ++, Moderate; +++, Prominent.

the paroxysmal activity is inhibited. Interictal discharges of localization-related epilepsies tend to propagate during NREM sleep and become topographically restricted in REM stages. The thalamocortical volleys that physiologically evoke the K-complexes and spindles in NREM stages, drive burst-pause firing in cortical neurons, facilitating the occurrence of generalized discharges in primary generalized epilepsy.

Interictal epileptiform activity in the EEG occurs more frequently during NREM sleep than during wakefulness, and tends to be suppressed by REM sleep.[18]

Representative samples of sleep are very important in the evaluation of the pediatric epilepsy patient. In a significant percentage of children, epileptiform activity appears in the EEG recording only while the patient sleeps. Conversely, epileptiform activity in the EEG recording is rarely isolated to wakefulness.[19] Sleep deprivation is commonly used to increase the likelihood of obtaining a significant EEG recording in children. However, it is unclear whether this is best achieved by natural sleep, sedated sleep, or sleep deprivation[20] The existing literature supports a role for sleep deprivation, separate from the induction of sleep with a hypnotic agent, in activating epileptiform discharges.[20] A sleep-deprived patient is more likely to provide an adequate sleep tracking with activation of epileptiform discharges. Interestingly, it has been shown that sleep deprivation can increase the occurrence of epileptiform abnormalities in the waking portion of the EEG in a child who previously had a normal awake EEG.[21]

Both sleep and arousals may activate epileptiform discharges and facilitate seizures, and in several seizure disorders the occurrence of seizures is clearly state dependent.

Epilepsy Can Alter the Quality of Sleep and the Circadian Rhythms

Children with epilepsy have more sleep problems than siblings or healthy controls. In addition, children with active seizure disorders have more complaints than epileptic children who are seizure free. Children with idiopathic epilepsy have a greater incidence of parasomnias, bedtime difficulties, sleep fragmentation, and daytime drowsiness. Age is also a factor with younger children having more sleep problems than older children.[22] Zaiwalla and Stores[23,24] found that parents describe their children's sleep as "unrefreshing." The unrefreshing quality was associated with frequent physiologic arousals, daytime sleepiness, and lethargy. They also found increased incidence of parasomnias and sleep fragmentation in these children.[23] Rosen et al[2] observed a correlation between nighttime awakening and daytime problems in learning and behavior in children with epilepsy. Stores[24] examined 79 children with epilepsy and 73 age-matched controls. Epileptic children aged 5–16 years were found to have more frequent sleep disturbances than matched controls. These disturbances included poor sleep quality and anxiety about sleeping. There was also a correlation between seizure frequency and anxiety about sleeping. In younger children between the ages of 5 and 11 years, poor sleep quality was associated with daytime inattention. This correlation was not noted in the older group. For instance, Hunt and Stores[25] found significant sleep disruption in younger children with tuberous sclerosis and active epilepsy. Problems with daytime inattention were seen more frequently in children who were experiencing frequent nocturnal seizures.

Epilepsy can alter also circadian rhythms, in fact Fauteck et al[26] have demonstrated lack of melatonin variation in children with epilepsy and poor sleep and other studies have demonstrated improved sleep in developmentally disabled children with the use of melatonin.[27]

On the other hand, sleep fragmentation and the associated daytime sleepiness in children may cause an increase in seizure frequency and can produce difficulty in obtaining seizure control. Fountain et al[28] report an independent effect of sleep deprivation on epileptiform discharges from the activation observed during sleep. Patients with obstructive sleep apnea syndrome (OSAS) or restless leg syndrome may exhibit increased difficulty with seizure control secondary to sleep fragmentation produced by their sleep disorder. Patients with altered sleep patterns may also experience increased seizures. These sleep alterations may be secondary to behavioral problems associated with sleep onset. Central nervous system abnormalities that alter or interrupt circadian pathways may also affect sleep and seizure control.

Children with epilepsy underperform in achievement testing when compared with age and IQ-matched controls. It is hypothesized that underachievement in some children may in part be secondary to poor daytime alertness resulting from sleep fragmentation. Daytime sleepiness persisted in nine preadolescent children after discontinuation of anticonvulsant therapy despite seizure control. The persistence of daytime sleepiness in these children raises the question of an underlying increased sleep tendency in patients with epilepsy or the persistent effect of drugs on behavior after washout.

Anticonvulsants can improve sleep abnormalities by improving seizures decreasing microarousals and sleep fragmentation. Anticonvulsants can control seizures, which in turn may restore circadian rhythms and normalize sleep. Seizures cause change in circadian rhythms by means of propagation of discharges through the limbic system via the hypothalamus, producing alterations in melatonin, and/or direct effects on the suprachiasmatic nucleus. In addition, anticonvulsants may have a direct effect on sleep.

Epileptic Syndromes Related to Sleep

The most common epileptic disorders related to sleep are discussed later.

Epilepsy with grand mal (GTC) seizures on awakening is a particular form of generalized idiopathic epilepsy (GIE)[29] characterized by a frequent genetic trait, onset in late childhood, adolescence, and young adulthood. GTC seizures appear exclusively or predominantly after awakening or while relaxing.[30] After sleep deprivation and during early sleep stages or soon after awakening, the EEG may be diagnostic in revealing generalized spike-wave discharges.

In patients with myoclonic astatic epilepsy (Doose syndrome), tonic seizures, which present with 10–15 Hz spike series, occur almost exclusively during sleep.[31]

Infantile spasms also occur more frequently in the period that just precedes or follows from sleep, rarely occur during NREM sleep, and never during REM. The brief, generalized tonic seizures associated with Lennox–Gastaut syndrome occur more frequently in clusters upon awakening and during NREM sleep.[32]

Children with infantile spasms exhibit a hypsarrhythmia (West syndrome) in the awake EEG tracing. NREM sleep can alter this pattern with bursts of more diffuse polyspike-waves and more synchronous slow spike and waves. Spindles may be superimposed on a generalized low-amplitude tracing between bursts. Periods of bursts and low-amplitude activity may alternate, resembling burst-suppression pattern.[33] The hypsarrhythmic pattern may be completely suppressed in REM sleep, paradoxically normalizing the EEG.

Recently Kohyama et al[34] reported that, seizure control in children with infantile spasms could be predicted by an increase in the number of spontaneous horizontal eye movements associated with phasic chin muscle activity during REM sleep. Patients with a good response to valproate, clonazepam, and/or zonisamide had significantly fewer simultaneous phasic events than poor responders who subsequently required hormonal therapy.[34] In patients with good response to treatment, REM phasic activity was similar to controls. It was postulated that an increase in REM phasic activity suggests

loss of inhibition from the pons to the motor neurons controlling REM muscle atonia. During wakefulness, children with Lennox–Gastaut syndrome show a typical 2–2.5 Hz slow spike-wave pattern. However, during NREM sleep, frontally dominant bilateral rhythmic discharges with a frequency of about 10 Hz occur that are considered to be an essential feature of this syndrome, and which are sometimes, but not always accompanied by tonic seizures.

Juvenile Myoclonic Epilepsy (JME)[35] is another GIE in which the myoclonic jerks usually occur after awakening and are often precipitated by sleep deprivation. Interictal EEG tracings show generalized bursts of spike- and polyspike-and-wave complexes at 3–6 Hz that are facilitated by sleep deprivation, intermittent light stimulation, and awakening,[36] but usually disappear during both REM and NREM sleep.

Seizures in *benign epilepsy of childhood with centrotemporal spikes* (BECT) and *idiopathic* (with age-related onset), *localization-related epilepsies* are strongly activated by sleep. Typical EEG pictures show diphasic high-amplitude spikes followed by a slow wave localized on the centrotemporal areas. Activation of EEG abnormalities in drowsiness and sleep is typical and in about 30% of patients spikes appear only during sleep.[37,38] Spikes can remain unilateral but in about half of the cases they are bilateral synchronous or asynchronous, often shifting location in subsequent EEG recordings. Other uncommon EEG aspects are the coexistence of occipital spikes or generalized spike-and-wave discharges.

Seventy-five percent of children with Rolandic epilepsy have seizures exclusively during either daytime or nighttime sleep; while approximately 15% have seizures whether they are awake or asleep, and 10%–20% only experience seizures when awake. Not only are Rolandic seizures more likely to occur during sleep, but when nocturnal, are also typically longer and more likely to secondarily generalize.[33] Epilepsies with seizures occurring primarily during the day are rare and can be seen in young patients with benign epilepsy of childhood with occipital paroxysms.

The *Landau–Kleffner syndrome* (LKS),[39–41] a disorder characterized by an acquired speech disturbance (aphasia and auditory agnosia) occurring in previously age-appropriate children, is characterized on sleep EEG by almost continuous bitemporal paroxysmal activity. Disrupted executive and cognitive functions, more than language, leading to severe cognitive and behavioral disturbances are characteristic of *Continuous Spike and Waves during Sleep* (CSWS)[9,42] in which EEG paroxysmal activity accounts for at least 85% of sleep and predominates on both frontal areas. The EEG features of LKS and CSWS differ from those recorded in Lennox–Gastaut syndrome, in which sleep EEGs usually show polyspike-and-wave activity and bursts of low-amplitude fast activity related or not to tonic fits.

Localization-related seizures in lesional or cryptogeneic partial epilepsy may have a random occurrence. In some patients, irrespective of the clinical form, seizures may acquire a more regular circadian rhythm during the illness and appear preferentially or almost only during sleep and seizures can be induced by relative sleep deprivation in some patients with temporal lobe epilepsy.[43]

However, there is a peculiar form of partial epilepsy, *NFLE*, in which seizures appear almost exclusively during sleep.[44]

▶ HOT SPOTS IN THE DIFFERENTIAL DIAGNOSIS BETWEEN EPILEPSY AND SLEEP DISORDERS

Sleep disorders or sleep-related physiological events frequently coexist in patients with epilepsy and may mimic epileptic seizures. Prompt recognition of phenomena mimicking epilepsy is vital to prevent patients undergoing unnecessary and costly investigations, and clinicians instigating potentially harmful therapeutic regimens (Table 44–2). Furthermore, it is important to recognize these cases because treatment of the sleep

▶ TABLE 44–2. COMPLEX MOTOR PHENOMENA

Insomnia
Sleep-related breathing disorders
Hypersomnias of central origin
Circadian rhythm sleep disorders
Parasomnias: disorders of arousal (from NREM sleep); parasomnias usually associated with REM sleep; other parasomnias
Sleep-related movement disorders: restless legs syndrome; periodic limb movement disorder; sleep-related leg cramps; sleep-related bruxism; sleep-related rhythmic movement disorder; sleep-related movement disorder, unspecified; sleep-related movement disorder due to drug or substance; sleep-related movement disorder due to medical condition
Isolated symptoms, apparently normal variants, and unresolved issues: long sleeper; short sleeper; snoring; sleep talking; sleep starts (hypnic jerks); benign sleep myoclonus of infancy; propriospinal myoclonus at sleep onset; excessive fragmentary myoclonus
Other sleep disorders
Appendix A: sleep disorders associated with conditions classifiable elsewhere: fibromyalgia; sleep-related epilepsy; sleep-related headaches; sleep-related gastroesophageal reflux disease; sleep-related abnormal swallowing, choking, and laryngospasm

Modified from the International Classification of Sleep Disorders (ICSD), 2nd edn., excluding sleep disorders not common in children.

disorder may contribute to seizure control by decreasing sleep disruption.[14,45]

SLEEP-RELATED BREATHING DISORDERS

Sleep-disordered breathing problems represent an important category of pediatric sleep problems and encompass a wide spectrum of respiratory disorders occurring during sleep, ranging from primary snoring to OSAS. OSAS is characterized by repetitive episodes of upper airway obstruction or cessation of breathing during sleep, associated with blood oxygen saturation reduction and consequent arousals and sleep disruption.[46] The prevalence of pediatric OSAS is estimated at 1%–4% for children between the ages of 2 and 18. The symptoms of obstructive sleep apnea (OSA) in children differ from those seen in adults. Although daytime sleepiness and fatigue are reported in children, behavioral problems, hyperactivity, and neurocognitive deficits are much more common in children with sleep apnea compared to normal controls. Children with severe sleep-disordered breathing often have multiple respiratory obstructive episodes; when chronic, this pattern leads to sleep deprivation and excessive daytime sleepiness (EDS).[47] Pediatric OSAS can be confirmed with polysomnography. The severity of OSAS has been defined by use of apnea/hypopnea index (AHI) criteria alone. The criteria differ from adults, with an apnea index of more than one per hour considered abnormal.

Awakenings with feeling of suffocation and fear due to sleep apnea are common, with intense distress and may be mistaken for a nightmare, sleep terror, seizure, or panic attack, but obstructive apneas occur repeatedly during the night, compared to the typical single occurrence per night for nocturnal panic (a waking from sleep in a state of panic, defined as an abrupt and discrete period of intense fear or discomfort, accompanied by tachycardia, sweating, shortness of breath, chest pressure, and so on.).[48]

The typical cause of OSAS in children is enlarged tonsils and adenoids and for 70% of children symptoms of OSAS are alleviated by tonsillectomy and/or adenoidectomy.[49] For children who are overweight, weight loss is the recommended treatment. Craniofacial surgeries are also an option in selected children with anatomic abnormalities.

Finally, in children in whom tonsillectomy or adenoidectomy is contraindicated or unsuccessful, nasal continuous positive airway pressure (CPAP) may be appropriate.

NARCOLEPSY

Narcolepsy is a chronic neurologic disorder occurring in approximately 1 in 2000 persons that peak in the second decade of life. There is no significant gender difference but a significant ethnic difference as the disorder is more frequent in Japan. Symptoms include EDS with or without cataplexy (a bilateral loss of muscle tone, triggered by strong emotion such as laughter or crying with consciousness usually unaffected), hypnagogic hallucinations, sleep paralysis, and fragmented nighttime sleep.[46]

As sleepiness may be the only symptom in children, the diagnosis of narcolepsy may be more difficult in children and adolescents.[50] Narcolepsy is likely an under-recognized disorder in pediatric practice; 30% of adults report symptom onset before 15 years, perhaps 16% before 10 years of age, and possibly 4% before the age of 5.[51]

The symptoms of narcolepsy are frequently misdiagnosed as neurologic, psychiatric, or behavioral.[52–54] Diagnostic confusion arises because a lack of responsiveness due to excessive sleepiness is mistaken for epileptic absences and cataplexy is confused with a variety of seizures types. In young children, recognition of excessive sleepiness can be confounded by the occurrence of daytime naps in normal children. However, these should normally cease by the age of 3–4 years after which the reappearance of repeated napping is significant. The variety in the degree and distribution of loss of tone in cataplexy can therefore be mistaken for different types of focal and generalized epileptic seizures. A lack of responsiveness associated with tiredness can be confused with facial myoclonia associated with absences.

The identification of triggers for cataplexy (usually strong emotions such as laughter or crying) is important in differentiating these paroxysmal events. Home-video recording of events by parents can be more use than attempting to capture events in unfamiliar environments such as hospitals because a degree of familiarity with surroundings and a relatively relaxed state is often required for cataplexy to occur. The relative frequency of attacks, their relation to emotional experience, and preservation of consciousness are useful guides to genuine cataplexy. Polysomnography with a multiple sleep latency test (MSLT) may provide clear evidence of narcolepsy, but results are not always conclusive in children, and repeat studies might be necessary. Monozygotic twins are discordant for narcolepsy. Eighty-six percent of narcoleptics with definite cataplexy have HLA DQB1–0602 on chromosome 6, but greater than 99% of patients with these haplotypes are normal.

The recent findings of reduced or absent cerebrospinal fluid hypocretin in most cases of narcolepsy with cataplexy, mean that estimation of this neuropeptide may aid diagnosis.[55]

The current treatment recommendations for narcolepsy in children include education (with the family and the other individuals with whom the child interacts), sleep hygiene (appropriate sleep scheduling and daily naps), and pharmacological interventions. Modafinil (Provigil), a pro-alerting drug that is FDA approved for the treatment of narcolepsy in adults, can dramatically improve daytime sleepiness. If Modafinil proves ineffective, traditional stimulants such as methylphenidate, and dextroamphetamine may also be of benefit; anticholinergic drugs are useful to treat cataplexy.[56]

PARASOMNIAS

Parasomnias are considered benign phenomena, especially in children, and do not usually have a serious impact on sleep quality and quantity. They include disorders of arousal (arising from NREM sleep), parasomnias usually associated with REM sleep and other parasomnias.[46]

a. *Disorders of arousal* are common pediatric sleep disorders that tend to cease with development.[57] The three basic types of arousal disorders recognized in the ICSD-2 are confusional arousals, sleep terrors, and sleepwalking.

Confusional arousals, affecting up to 20% of children, are characterized by mental confusion and disorientation, relative unresponsiveness to environmental stimuli, and difficulty awakening the subject[58] (Fig. 44–1). These events present a difficult diagnostic problem since the confusion can resemble postictal confusion in a patient with seizures. They are sometimes associated with incontinence. *Sleep terrors*, affecting 1%–7% of children, are "arousals from slow-wave sleep accompanied by a cry or piercing scream and autonomic nervous system and behavioural manifestations of intense fear" generally lasting 1–5 minutes[46] (Fig. 44–2). Although appearing alert, the child typically does not respond when spoken to, and more forceful attempts to intervene may meet with resistance and increased agitation.

Sleepwalking, peaking by age 8–12 years,[57] is defined as "a series of complex behaviours (such as changes in bodily position, turning and resting on one's hand, playing with the sheets, sitting up in bed, resting on knees, etc.) that are usually initiated during arousals from slow-wave sleep and culminate in walking around with an altered state of consciousness and impaired judgment."[46]

During disorders of arousal, although children are asleep, they may appear awake (eyes open), but they may not recognize their parents and resist attempts to be comforted or soothed,

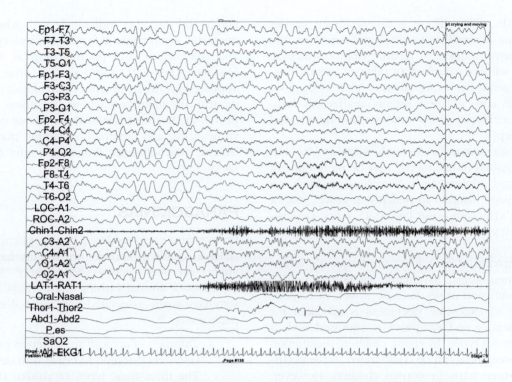

Figure 44–1. Confusional arousal with the patient sitting up and mumbling. Polysomnographic tracing during the event documents a delta–theta activity associated with increased muscle tone and change in respiratory and heart rates. (From Geyer J, Payne T, Carney P. Parasomnias. In: Geyer J, Payne T, Carney P (eds), *Atlas of Polysomnography*. Philadelphia: Lippincott Williams & Wilkins, 2010; 2nd edn: pp. 209–224.)

with attempts to wake the child often prolonging the event. Typical parasomnias resolve spontaneously with children rapidly returning to sleep, with no recollection of the event in the morning.

Disorders of arousal may be triggered by a variety of factors including sleep deprivation, a disruption to the sleep environment or sleep schedule, stress, febrile illness, medications, alcohol, emotional stress in susceptible individuals, or the presence of sleep-disordered breathing.[59] Disorders of arousal tend to occur in the first part of the night when NREM stages 3 and 4 predominate. Polysomnography during the events reveals a rhythmic, delta activity pattern, associated with a marked increase in muscle tone, and changes in respiratory and heart rates.

Parasomnias may mimic epileptic seizures, although historical features are very useful in distinguishing these disorders. Features that suggest a NREM parasomnia rather than seizures are a low rate of same-night recurrence of the episodes, long duration, appearance within the first few hours of sleep, (seizures may occur

throughout the night) and the characteristic motor pattern (parasomnias are not stereotypical and complex and repetitive behavior with abnormal movements, such as dystonic and dyskinetic postures, are absent).[60] Moreover, the clinical picture of arousal disorders (early age at onset, decrease in frequency, or disappearance after puberty) differs from NFLE that first occurs between ages 10 and 20 years, often persists into adulthood, and manifests with daytime complaints such as sleepiness (Fig. 44–3). Sleep terrors are also distinguished from nocturnal panic attacks by being followed by a quick return to sleep without recall of the event.[48]

Many parasomnias can be diagnosed on the basis of history-taking. Patients should be considered for video-EEG monitoring if events are stereotypic or repetitive, occur frequently (minimum one event per week), have not responded to medications, and the history is suggestive of potentially epileptic events.[61] Prompting the patient to make audio–video recordings at home with subsequent data analysis and comparison with the episodes recorded at the sleep

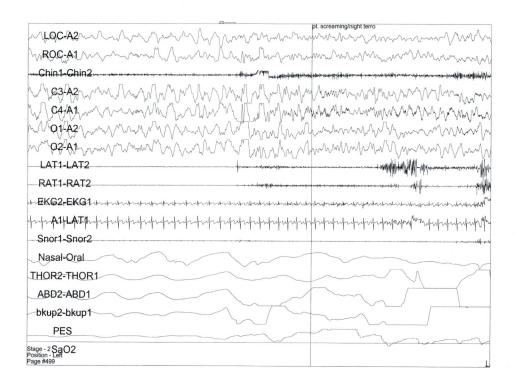

Figure 44–2. Sleep terror in a 7-year-old boy. The patient sits on his bed, open his eyes, touches the objects around him with the left hand looking around frightened, and then rapidly goes back to sleep. Polysomnographic tracing during the event documents a rhythmic delta activity, associated with increased muscle tone and marked increase of heart rate. (From Geyer J, Payne T, Carney P. Parasomnias. In: Geyer J, Payne T, Carney P (eds), *Atlas of Polysomnography*. Philadelphia: Lippincott Williams & Wilkins, 2010; 2nd edn: pp. 209–224.)

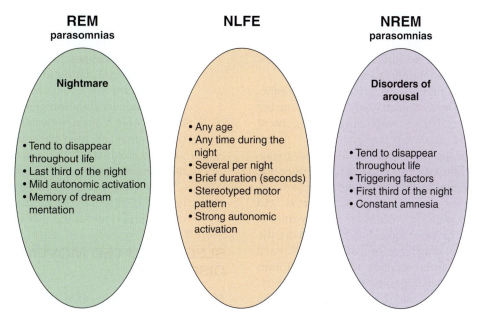

Figure 44–3. Typical features distinguishing nocturnal paroxysmal episodes. On the left REM-related parasomnias; on the right NREM phenomena. NFLS that can appear at any sleep stage, are in the center. In each field, only the distinctive clinical features of the phenomenon are listed.

laboratory may facilitate the diagnosis of arousal parasomnia.

Management includes reassuring parents that these episodes are a developmental phenomenon, harmless and they should not awaken their child who should be gently redirected back to bed without awakening. Every effort should be made to avoid any predisposing and triggering factors identified by a careful general medical and sleep history and polysomnography. Medications are rarely used to treat these sleep disorders but may be indicated if episodes are very frequent or when the child or others in the home are in danger of the behavior. In these cases imipramine or clonazepam at bedtime are beneficial in some patients.

b. REM parasomnias

Nightmares are "disturbing mental experiences that generally occur during REM sleep and often result in awakening."[46] They are common in young children, peaking at ages 3–6 years[62] and their frequency decreases with age. A careful sleep history that focuses on the time of night of fearful awakenings helps to distinguish REM-related nightmares from disorders of arousals: the distinctive features of a nightmare are the recall of a long, frightening dream, and clear orientation on awakening. The major distinction between nightmares and nocturnal panic is the stage of sleep: a panic attack is a NREM event usually occurring from stages NREM 2 to 3.[48]

The lack of motor behavior during the episodes and the absence of confusion on awakening, as well as the availability of detailed dream reports helps distinguish nightmares from nocturnal frontal lobe seizures.[60] In doubtful cases, video-polysomnography is indicated.

Sporadic nightmares are not worrisome, and require reassurance only, but recurrent nightmares or those with disturbing content may indicate excessive daytime stress.[63] Once the basis for the nightmares is discerned, measures should be taken to eliminate or reduce the child's exposure to the causative factor.

Recurrent isolated sleep paralysis is "an inability to perform voluntary movements at sleep onset or on awaking from sleep in the absence of a diagnosis of narcolepsy."[46] Each episode lasts from seconds to a few minutes and is usually accompanied by intense anxiety. Sleep paralysis should be differentiated from atonic seizures that occur during wakefulness and nocturnal panic attacks usually not associated with paralysis (patients typically sit up and/ or get out of bed).[48] Reassurance and education are the most useful treatment in isolated cases.

If the frequency of sleep paralysis is bothersome to patients, there is a suggestion that SSRIs may be of some benefit, likely because of their REM-suppressing properties.[64]

c. Other parasomnias

Sleep enuresis is "characterized by recurrent involuntary voiding during sleep." In primary sleep enuresis, recurrent involuntary voiding occurs at least twice weekly during sleep after age of 5 years.[46] The prevalence of primary nocturnal enuresis is approximately 30% of 4-year olds and is more common in boys than girls at all ages.[46] In secondary enuresis the patients, older than 5 years of age, have previously been consistently dry during sleep for at least 6 months. Epileptic seizures are excluded because in these cases enuresis is the only symptom and occurs without any motor phenomenon.

Primary nocturnal enuresis is a heterogeneous condition for which various causative factors have been identified, so the treatment could be a combination of noninvasive tools and only particular cases and motivated patients should receive a specific pharmacologic treatment.[65]

Sleep-related groaning (catathrenia) is an unusual sleep-related behavior characterized by an expiratory groaning noise occurring almost every night, mainly during REM sleep and in the second half of the night.[66–68] The noise occurs without any respiratory distress or concomitant motor phenomena; patients are unaware of their groaning, and upon awakening in the morning, do not recall anything particular about the night and feel restored. Affected patients have no overt neurological or respiratory diseases and during the groaning arterial oxygen saturation remains normal. Its predominant or exclusive occurrence during REM sleep, its duration (groaning usually lasts few seconds, often repeated in clusters), and the absence of any concomitant motor phenomena distinguish this nocturnal sound from moaning occurring during epileptic seizures.

Therapy remains problematic as patients usually decline any treatment because they are unconcerned about the problem.

SLEEP-RELATED MOVEMENT DISORDERS

Restless legs syndrome (RLS). Although the prevalence of RLS and periodic limb movement disorder (PLMD) is not well defined in the general pediatric population, it is worthy of discussion.[69] RLS is a sensorimotor disorder characterized by uncomfortable sensations usually involving only the legs that worsen in the evening and with long periods of inactivity (e.g., a long car ride or movie).[46,70] Sensations are often described as creepy-crawly or tingling feelings, temporarily alleviated by movement. These sensations are often confused with "growing pains." Patients, especially young children may have difficulty describing the symptoms. Children may get into trouble at school or at home because they have difficulty sitting still. RLS can also fragment sleep in children. EDS can be seen in association with RLS in adolescents. In younger children, Walters et al[71] have demonstrated an association with hyperactivity. In patients with epilepsy this phenomena, RLS, may be confused with their underlying seizure disorder.

Primary RLS is a genetic disorder with an autosomal dominant pattern. Secondary RLS, associated with a precipitating factor, is less common. Renal failure, iron deficiency, and diabetes may contribute to the restlessness.

PLMD commonly co-occurs with RLS but may also appear independently. Periodic limb movements in sleep (PLMS) are brief repetitive movements or jerks, lasting 0.5–5 seconds and occurring every 5 to 90 seconds, in a sequence of four or more movements, especially during sleep stages 1 and 2. PLMD occurs when PLMS occur during more than five per hour of sleep in a patient with sleep-related complaints such as sleep disturbance or daytime fatigue.[46]

Dopamine agonist therapy is the mainstay of RLS treatment in adults. No agents have been FDA approved for treatment of RLS in children. Use of simple nonpharmacological therapies may be of some benefit including teaching the child to visualize an activity or simply allowing the child to move the legs. Teachers should be informed of the condition and the fact that it is not a form of attention deficit disorder should be emphasized. Symptoms may be caused by an underlying iron or vitamin deficiency and supplementing with iron, vitamin B_{12}, or folate (as indicated) may be sufficient to relieve symptoms in these specific cases.

Sleep bruxism or teeth-grinding is "an oral activity characterized by grinding or clenching teeth during sleep, usually associated with sleep arousals" which, when long-lasting, can cause significant tooth wear.[46] Sleep bruxism occurs most commonly in children aged 3–12 years, without any sex prevalence, and then decreases throughout life; in many cases patients are unaware of the jaw movements.[72] Polysomnographic recordings demonstrate that bruxism occurs in all stages of sleep but is most common during NREM, especially stages 1 to 2 of sleep, in the absence of associated abnormal EEG activity.

Nocturnal faciomandibular myoclonus is a recently described hypnic phenomenon whose relationship with sleep bruxism is still a matter of debate. It is characterized by nocturnal myoclonic jerks involving the masseter, orbicularis oculi, and oris muscles.[73] These abnormal movements can trigger nocturnal awakenings due to painful tongue biting and bleeding sometimes leading to the misdiagnosis of tongue biting due to an epileptic seizure. The detailed description of the episodes, collected from a bed partner or other observer helps establish the correct diagnosis. However, rhythmic jaw movements could be a semiological feature of epileptic seizures such as temporal lobe attacks, but in these cases, the movements represent a more diffuse oroalimentary behavior, and are often preceded by an arising gastric aura accompanied by other motor automatisms not limited to the face.[74] There is no specific treatment for sleep bruxism: each subject has to be individually evaluated and treated. The three management alternatives are dental, pharmacological, and psychobehavioral therapy.[75]

Sleep-related rhythmic movement disorders (RMD) are "repetitive, stereotyped, and rhythmic motor behaviours (not tremors) occurring predominantly during drowsiness or sleep and involving large muscle groups"[46] (Fig. 44–4). They comprise head-banging, head-rolling, and body-rocking. The rhythmic behaviors are generally benign and self-limiting in normal children: they are common in infancy dropping to 5% by the age of 5 years.[76] Episodes are not only restricted to sleep–wake transition and occur more frequently in wake and stages NREM 1 and 2 but also in REM and slow-wave sleep.[77] Movements typically occur at a frequency of 0.5–2 times per second and events last 5–15 minutes. Children are usually nonresponsive during the episodes and do not recall the events on awakening.[77] Although sleep-related epilepsy is a diagnostic consideration, the characteristic movements make epilepsy far less likely. Also, unlike epilepsy, patients usually can arrest waking movements on request. The behaviors only rarely result in a significant complaint (interference with normal sleep or daytime function, or self-inflicted bodily injury requiring medical treatment). Pharmacological treatment is therefore rarely necessary. In severe cases, RMD episodes respond favorably to clonazepam at low doses.[78]

ISOLATED SYMPTOMS, APPARENTLY NORMAL VARIANTS, AND UNRESOLVED ISSUES

Sleep talking is defined as talking during sleep "with varying degrees of comprehensibility."[46] It can arise from both slow-wave sleep and REM sleep. Although considered the most frequent parasomnia, sleep talking is usually without consequences and is rarely a reason for consultation.

Sleep starts, also known as *hypnagogic* or *hypnic jerks,* are bilateral, sudden, brief, nonperiodic jerks, mainly affecting the legs or arms, just before sleep onset. The jerks are associated with a subjective feeling

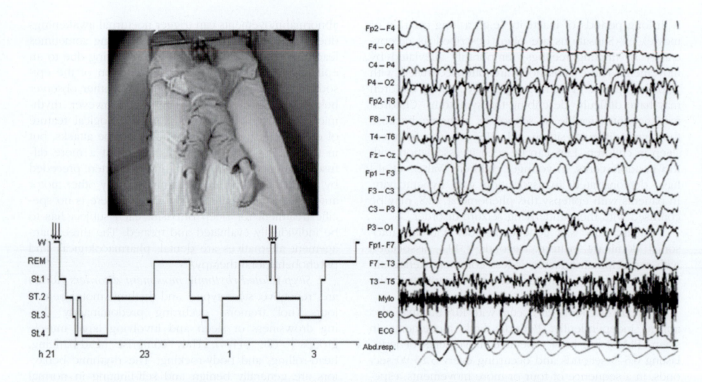

Figure 44–4. Sleep-related rhythmic movement disorders (head-banging) in a 10-year-old boy. The patient presents repetitive, stereotyped, and rhythmic head movements characterized by forcible banging the head back and down into the pillow. Polygraphic tracing (right of the figure) shows the typical artefact due to the movements. The episodes appear during the sleep–wake transition and during infrasleep wakefulness as shown in the excerpt of the hypnogram (bottom of the figure). Mylo, mylohyoideus muscle; EOG, electroculogram; Abd. Resp., abdominal respiration.

of falling, or a sensory flash, or a hypnagogic dream.[46] Sleep starts are a common and normal phenomenon occurring in persons of both sexes and all ages with a prevalence of 70%. Although usually a single contraction, they may be so severe as to be a true sleep disorder like sleep onset insomnia.[46] The characteristics of sporadic, isolated, brief jerks, usually associated with psychosensory experience and mainly present during drowsiness will differentiate sleep starts from epileptic clonias that are always associated with EEG spike-wave discharges of varying complexity. Repetitive sleep starts are described in epileptic children with spastic-dystonic diplegia and cognitive deficits.[79] In most cases, reassurance that sleep start is a normal phenomenon provides sufficient reassurance. If drugs are necessary to treat cases of severe sleep disturbance and daily drowsiness, benzodiazepine appears to be the drug of choice.

Benign sleep myoclonus of infancy (BSMI) is a non-epileptic paroxysmal disorder characterized by repetitive myoclonic jerks during NREM sleep in the early life of healthy newborns.[80–82] BSMI is characterized by rhythmic or arrhythmic, generalized or sometimes segmental jerks, involving one limb or one side of the body, which typically appear during NREM sleep. They frequently occur in clusters, lasting 20–30 minutes, and

terminate ending with awakening unremarkable and psychomotor development is normal.

According to ICSD-2, the following criteria are necessary for diagnosis: repetitive myoclonic jerks involving the whole body, trunk or limbs; onset in early infancy, typically birth to 6 months of age; the movements occur only during sleep and stop abruptly and consistently with arousal. In addition, the movements can be precipitated by rocking during sleep.[83] The syndrome is usually sporadic; only a few familial cases have been reported in the literature.[84] No medication is required.

Propriospinal myoclonus (PSM) at sleep onset is a distinctive form of spinal myoclonus characterized by violent muscle jerks arising from axial muscles (in the neck or trunk), which extends up and down to the rostral and caudal muscles along the propriospinal pathways intrinsic to the cord.[85] In many cases, PSM shows a striking relationship with vigilance level, as it typically occurs during postural and mental rest, particularly when patients try to fall asleep giving rise to a severe and persistent insomnia.[86] The time of occurrence of the jerks (confined to the wake–sleep transition or to intrasleep arousals), the frequent recurrence of the jerks and suppression of the motor phenomena by mental and sensory stimuli are the features that distinguish PSM from epileptic phenomena. Clonazepam (0.5–2 mg) can reduce muscular jerks and make sleep more restful. Opiates are also effective but carry the risk of dependence.[86]

Excessive fragmentary myoclonus (EFM) consists in an abnormal intensification of the physiologic hypnic myoclonia. It is characterized by brief involuntary arrhythmic asynchronous and asymmetric brief twitches involving various body areas. They occur throughout the night, including relaxed wakefulness and all sleep stages.[87] Patients are usually unaware of the twitch-like movements, which may be present during wakefulness or sleep. In many cases, EFM is diagnosed strictly as an incidental finding on polysomnographic recording that demonstrates recurrent and persistent very brief (75–150 ms) EMG potentials in various muscles occurring asynchronously and asymmetrically in a sustained manner without clustering; more than five potentials per minute are sustained for at least 20 minutes of NREM sleep stages.

If severe, EFM may disturb sleep onset and sleep continuity.[88] EFM is readily distinguished from epileptic seizures by its atypical motor patterns (minor movements of the fingers and toes or twitching of the corners of the mouth) and prolonged persistence throughout the night across all sleep stages. Pharmacological treatment is rarely required.

SLEEP DISORDERS ASSOCIATED WITH CONDITIONS CLASSIFIABLE ELSEWHERE

Sleep-related gastroesophageal reflux disease is caused by symptoms and/or signs related to the reflux of gastric acid or intestinal bile contents onto the esophageal mucosa. The most common and essentially pathognomonic symptoms of gastroesophageal reflux (GER) are heartburn and regurgitation.[89] Chronic acid reflux is often associated with frequent arousals during sleep. According to ICSD-2 diagnostic criteria "the patient complains of recurrent awakenings from sleep with shortness of breath or heartburn or a sour bitter taste in the mouth upon awakening from sleep or sleep-related coughing or choking or awakening from sleep with heartburn." Polysomnography and esophageal pH monitoring demonstrate gastroesophageal reflux during sleep with associated arousal.

► EVALUATION AND TREATMENT OF THE EPILEPTIC CHILD WITH A SLEEP DISORDER

The proper identification and treatment of common sleep disorders is an essential part of the overall evaluation and management of children with epilepsy. A sleep history is the essential tool to evaluate sleep problems and involves a thorough review of the child's 24-hour routine, focusing on bedtime habits, nighttime behaviors, nap and daytime behavior. All behaviors and activities need to be evaluated for appropriateness for the child's age and time of day, recognizing the opportunity to make beneficial changes to restore optimal sleep for both child and family. Nighttime behaviors after sleep onset such as parasomnias and symptoms of OSA (snoring, gasping, breathing pauses, and restless sleep) should also be assessed. A sleep diary can be helpful in delineating the exact sleep pattern. Table 44–3 provides an outline for a sleep history in children.

Insufficient sleep syndrome remains a major problem for adolescents. In addition, there is a growing body of literature stating that adolescents have some degree of delayed sleep phase syndrome, which leads to early morning sleepiness and insufficient sleep. School start times, extra curricular activities, and peer pressure contribute to a chronic state of sleep deprivation, placing most adolescent patients at risk for activation of their seizure disorder. Regular sleep habits must be recommended by physicians and enforced by parents.

Patients with epilepsy frequently complain of daytime sleepiness, usually considered an unavoidable adverse effect of antiepileptic therapy. Nevertheless in patients with persistent hypersomnia, particularly if on AED monotherapy or with low serum drug concentrations and well-controlled seizures, primary sleep disorders should be suspected.[90] Study of these patients by video-EEG polysomnography or home video may be indicated.[13] Evaluation of sleep with polysomnography should be performed with extended EEG montages in children with epilepsy to correlate arousal with seizures and interictal activity. Monitoring for sleep-related breathing disorders, RLS, or parasomnias should also be performed. Therapy should be directed at resolving any sleep disorder observed, as improved seizure control might result. Adenotonsillectomy remains the initial therapy for obstructive apnea and upper airway resistance syndrome. CPAP should be reserved for those patients who fail adenotonsillectomy. Anticonvulsant monotherapy should be attempted whenever possible to minimize the side effects of sedation. Less sedating anticonvulsants should be used as primary anticonvulsant therapy avoiding barbiturates, benzodiazepines, and topiramate.

► HOW TREATMENT OF SLEEP DISORDERS AFFECTS SEIZURES

It is well documented that the treatment of an underlying sleep disorder and improvement of sleep hygiene benefits not only daytime sleepiness but also seizure control. An example is the beneficial effect on seizure

► **TABLE 44–3. COMPONENTS OF SLEEP HISTORY**

Bedtime
Associated routines and rituals?
Lights-out time?
Time until asleep?
Sleep onset
Sudden awakening?
Hypnogogic hallucinations?
Uncomfortable sensations?
Uncontrolled movements?

Nighttime behavior
Arousals?
When do arousals occur?
How frequently do arousals occur?
Behaviors associated with arousals?
Does the child have difficulty falling asleep?
Abnormal movements or sounds during the night?
Does the child snore or have apnea? Is there enuresis or encopresis?
Does the child bite the tongue or is there blood on the bedclothes?
What position does the child sleep in? Is the child restless?

Morning awakening
When does the child awaken?
Now long does it take for the child to be alert? Is the child refreshed?
Is their sleep paralysis?
Are there abnormal movements at arousal?
Is there early morning headache, nausea, or vomiting?

Daytime behavior
Is the child sleepy during the day?
When does this sleepiness manifest?
Does the child nap during the daytime?
How long is the nap?
Length of time to fall asleep?
Does the nap refresh?
What is the child's behavior upon awakening after nap?

General concerns
Duration of the problem?
Is the source of concern related to the problem; the child, parent and/or school?
Family and/or personal stress?
Is there drug or alcohol use?
Excessive caffeine use?
Is the child depressed?

frequency that some authors obtain surgically treating children with OSA,[5,91] without changes in the drug regimen. Resolution of chronic sleep deprivation, improvement in cerebral hypoxemia, and reduction in arousals from sleep have been postulated to be the reason whereby treatment of a sleep disorder improves seizure control, even if the exact mechanism is unknown.[92]

On the other hand, sleep problems in young children may present with hyperactivity or behavioral problems rather than excessive somnolence. Recognition of the paradoxical response of hyperactivity as the result of EDS is central to the pediatric patient evaluation.

Insomnia has frequently been reported in children with epilepsy and may be caused by different situations. Children with epilepsy may become disabled that will lead to "behaviourally" induced circadian rhythm problems because the patient may choose their own sleep hours if inactive. Nighttime fears may affect children with epilepsy as well, especially if they have nocturnal seizures. Also, parents may feel anxious about leaving the child alone in the room.[93] Abnormal sleep habits have also been reported in children with epilepsy: longer sleep latency, shorter total sleep time, more nocturnal awakenings, less willingness to go to sleep, and greater tendency to fall asleep in places other than bed compared to age-matched controls.[94]

Modulation of Circadian Rhythms Can Alter Epilepsy

For children with epilepsy who complain of insomnia or others sleep disorders, melatonin may represent a good therapeutic choice by improving sleep structure and hence the quality of life.[94] Melatonin has recently been used in a number of children to improve sleep and seizure control. Fautek et al[26] found improved sleep in 8 out of 10 children studied. In responders seizures decreased from 8 to 12 seizures per day to 1 to 2 seizures per day. Sleep behavior improvements included marked decrease in nighttime awakenings, increased quality of sleep, early awakenings, and less daytime naps. A recent randomized controlled study coadministered melatonin with valproate that was perceived to improve the sleep score of patients with epilepsy.[95]

Melatonin administration in another placebo-controlled trial on children and adolescents with mental retardation with or without epilepsy was shown to improve the sleep pattern.[96] Melatonin has also been shown to normalize sleep behavior and favorably influence the underlying epilepsy as well.[97] The effect of melatonin may be consequent to its primary role as a modulator of circadian rhythms or to the direct effect of melatonin as a neuroactive substance. Melatonin has been reported to have both proconvulsant and anticonvulsant effects in animals and in neurologically disabled children.[98]

Improvement in seizure control is observed with melatonin with a dosage of 5–10 mg administered 1 hour prior to bedtime. Sleep improvement is described in all children to date with improved seizure control. This is especially relevant since exogenous melatonin has hardly any serious side effects. Further randomized controlled trials are necessary before recommending routine use of melatonin.

Finally, the majority of sleep disorders do not need pharmacological treatment. Behavioral therapy and regular sleeping habits may reduce the problem to some extent in many cases (see Table 44–4).

▶ HOW TREATMENT OF SEIZURES AFFECTS SLEEP

Not only seizures but also antiepileptic drugs (AEDs) may contribute to sleep disorders and adversely affect sleep. For example, in a patient predisposed to OSA, barbiturates and benzodiazepines may worsen the frequency of apneas and hypopneas by reducing the muscle tone of the upper airways and increasing the arousal threshold. Similarly AEDs that are associated with weight gain (i.e., VPA) may worsen OSA. Avoiding these agents in patients with untreated OSA may be advisable, especially if alternative AEDs are available.

Clinicians may base their AED choice not only on the epilepsy syndrome but also on its effects on coexisting sleep disorders and complaints (Table 44–5).

Somnolence and diurnal sedation are among the most common side effects of AEDs especially in patients on polytherapy.[94,99] Whether it is epilepsy itself or AEDs that cause abnormal sleep architecture is difficult to determine. This adverse effect on sleep is especially relevant to the AED effect on cognitive

▶ TABLE 44–4. TREATMENT OF SLEEP DISORDERS

Sleep Disorder	Treatment
Obstructive	Tonsillectomy and/or adenoidectomy
Sleep apnea syndrome	Weight loss
	Continuous positive airway pressure
Narcolepsy	Education
	Sleep hygiene
	Pharmacological interventions: modafinil (for excessive daytime sleepiness) and anticholinergic drugs (for cataplexy)
Disorders of arousal	Parental education and reassurance
	Avoidance of exacerbating factors
	Safe sleep environment
	Medication rarely used
Nightmares	If sporadic: reassurance only
	If chronic or posttraumatic: cognitive-behavioral techniques
Recurrent isolated sleep paralysis	Reassurance and education
	If frequent: SSRIs may be of some benefit
Sleep enuresis	Noninvasive tools after identification of causative factors (drinking and voiding chart; alarms in reduced bladder capacity cases)
	Only in particular cases and motivated patients: specific pharmacologic treatment (desmopressin)
Sleep-related groaning (catathrenia)	Patients usually decline any treatment
Restless legs syndrome and periodic limb movement disorder	Benzodiazepine
	Dopaminergic drugs
	Gabapentin
Sleep bruxism	Each subject has to be individually evaluated and treated
	Three strategies:
	• dental
	• pharmacological (benzodiazepines, muscle relaxant, L-dopa, β-adrenergic antagonist)
	• psychobehavioral (relaxation, biofeedback, training programs, hypnosis)
Sleep-related rhythmic movement disorders	Treatment is unnecessary
	Ensure that children are safe and protected from injury
	In severe forms: clonazepam at low doses
Sleep talking	Pharmacological treatment is unnecessary
Sleep starts	Pharmacological treatment is unnecessary
	In severe cases: benzodiazepines
Benign sleep myoclonus of infancy	Pharmacological treatment is unnecessary
Propriospinal myoclonus at sleep onset	Clonazepam
	Opiates?
Excessive fragmentary myoclonus	Pharmacological treatment is unnecessary

▶ **TABLE 44–5. PRACTICAL GUIDELINES FOR CHOICE OF AED IN PRESENCE OF SLEEP DISORDERS**

	CBZ	PB PRI	ETS	VPA	VGV	BDZ	GBP	LTG	PHT
Insomnia	+	+		+		+	+	−	
Obstructive sleep apnea syndrome	−			−		−			
Narcolepsy	−					−		+	
Disorders of arousal						+			
Nightmares						+			
Restless legs syndrome and periodic limb movement disorder						+	+		
Bruxism						+			
Propriospinal myoclonus						+			
Excessive fragmentary myoclonus						+			
Sleep-related rhythmic movement disorders, Sleep talking; Sleep starts, Benign sleep myoclonus of infancy; Sleep paralysis Sleep enuresis; Catathrenia						These disturbances do not need treatment			

functions. It is likely that cognitive effects of AEDs on memory and concentration are related to drug effect on the central nervous system mediating arousal rather than the specific effect on cognitive functions.

Ideally, the AED chosen to treat epilepsy should have least effect on sleep. This may not be always possible.

AEDs have been shown to have a variety of effects on sleep and daytime vigilance. However, the literature is confounded by significant methodological variations across studies, including composition of the study population, dose, timing, and duration of treatment and failure to control for seizures and concomitant AEDs. Much of the available literature on the older AEDs comes from animal studies, but with the use of newer anticonvulsants in other neurologic and psychiatric conditions, new data are becoming available on patients exposed to AEDs for the first time.

It has been shown that anticonvulsants can improve seizure control by stabilizing sleep.[15,100] Although it is certainly possible that part of the improved sleep seen with the use of anticonvulsants may be the result of the suppression of seizures, it seems clear that AEDs also affect sleep independently of their antiepileptic effect. They may also cause state-dependent seizures to become dispersed randomly during the sleep/wake cycle.[101]

a. Effect of AEDs on sleep architecture

In general, many of the traditional AEDs can reduce sleep latency and sleep fragmentation, delay REM onset, or decrease the percentage of time spent in REM sleep.[100] The effects of specific AEDs on sleep architecture are discussed in Table 44–6.

Phenytoin. With chronic phenytoin use, most investigators have found a shortened sleep latency, an increase in stages 1 and 2, a small decrease in REM sleep, and increased arousals.[102,103]

Carbamazepine. Carbamazepine is the most extensively studied AED. In general, most studies have shown decreased sleep latency, increased total sleep time, decreased fragmentation, and improved sleep continuity.[102–105]

Valproate. Most studies have found no notable alteration of sleep by valproate that appears to promote a more normal distribution of REM sleep during the night, and can also stabilize the sleep cycle.[102,106]

Ethosuximide. Few studies are available describing the effects of ethosuximide. Most studies show an increase in stage 1 of NREM sleep with a concomitant decrease in stage 3, an increased number of awakenings, and an increase in the percentage of REM.[102,103]

Phenobarbital. Multiple studies are available concerning the effects of phenobarbital on sleep. Phenobarbital in chronic treatment shortened sleep latency and led to a reduction in body movements and arousals, increased total sleep time with a higher sleep efficiency.[103,107] It also caused a reduction in REM sleep and its abrupt withdrawal can cause a rebound of REM parasomnias. Usually phenobarbital may produce EDS, but in children paradoxical effects on sleep behavior with hyperactivity are noted.

Primidone. The effects on sleep of primidone are similar to those of phenobarbital.

Benzodiazepines. Most benzodiazepines have been described to cause a decrease in sleep latency and the number of arousals. This is accompanied by an increase in the percentage of stage 2 sleep, with a decrease in the amount of stages 3 and 4 NREM sleep. REM sleep latency is increased, with longer acting benzodiazepines causing a greater suppression of REM sleep.[108]

▶ **TABLE 44–6.** EFFECT OF AED ON SLEEP ARCHITECTURE

AED	Sleep Latency	Total Sleep Time	Sleep Fragmentation and Number of Arousals	Stages 1–2	Stages 3–4	REM
PHT	↓	NA	↑	↑	C	↓
CBZ	↓	↑	↓	NA	NA	↓
VPA	NA	=	NA	NA	↑	=
ETS	NA	NA	↑	↑	↓	↑
PB	↓	↑	↓	↑	=	↓
BDZ	↓	NA	NA	↑	↑	↓↓
LTG	↓ / =	↓ / =	↓	↑	↓	↑
GBP	NA	NA	↓	NA	↑	↑
VGV	=	=	=	NA	NA	NA

Legend, ↑ increase ↓↓ decrease; na, data not available; C, controversial.

Lamotrigine. Compared with the older AEDs, LTG seems to have less effect on disruption of sleep. The only significant effects of LTG treatment included an increase in stage 2 (light sleep) and a decrease in SWS (deep sleep). Although, it did not reach statistical significance, treatment with LTG was associated with a slight reduction in arousals and stage shifts and an increase in the number of REM periods without affecting sleep efficiency, suggesting a tendency for sleep to be less disrupted.[92] Other authors reported different effects of LTG on sleep with an increase in the percentage of REM sleep, and a decrease in the fragmentation of REM sleep usually present in epileptic patients. Overall, sleep was also more stable, with a decreased number of phase shifts.[109] There was no correlation between the increase in REM sleep and the decrease in spikes, leading investigators to believe that the sleep stabilizing effect of lamotrigine acts independently of its antiepileptic effect.

Another controversial point regarding LTG effects on sleep is insomnia of sufficient severity to require discontinuation or dose reduction. This adverse effect was reported in 6.4% of patients treated with LTG in a recent series of 109 subjects.[110] Difficulty initiating and maintaining sleep developed shortly after LTG was introduced, increased with dose escalation, and resolved quickly with discontinuation or dose reduction. Symptoms developed at a mean daily dose of 286 mg (100–500). Based on these data, we believe that LTG may be less disruptive to sleep than the older AEDs. Because sleep fragmentation reduces seizure threshold in some individuals, these changes may contribute to the anticonvulsant effects of the drug.

Gabapentin. In general, patients on GBP show a subjective improvement in sleep.[108] An increase in the percentage of REM sleep, and a prolonged duration of REM periods, and a decreased number of awakenings have been observed in epileptic patients treated with GBP.[111]

Vigabatrin. Vigabatrin as add-on therapy showed no difference in sleep latency, total sleep time, or number of awakenings without improvement in daytime sleepiness.[112]

b. Effect of VNS on sleep

Vagus nerve stimulation (VNS), a nonpharmacological therapy for epilepsy involving intermittent stimulation of the left vagus nerve peripherally, may decrease daytime sleepiness in epilepsy patients documented by MSLTs performed 3 months after VNS treatment was initiated (mean sleep latency from 6.4 to 9.8 minutes).[113] However, VNS may also contribute to decreases in respiratory airflow and effort during sleep and exacerbate OSA via central and peripheral mechanisms.[114]

▶ SUMMARY

The pediatric patient presents challenges both in the manifestations and in the diagnosis of their sleep problems. Seizure syndromes unique to childhood, such as infantile spasms, Lennox–Gastaut syndrome, benign rolandic and occipital epilepsies, and JME are sleep and circadian dependent. The varied presentation and clinical manifestations of sleep-related breathing disorders in children makes diagnosis more challenging. The use of melatonin as a modulator of circadian rhythms holds promise for improving seizure control, but controlled clinical trials are necessary. Treatment of sleep apnea in patients with generalized epilepsies appears to offer improved seizure control and daytime functioning, but formal trials confirming this observation are lacking.

► ACKNOWLEDGMENTS

We thank Lucia T. Carney-Manubens and Stephenie C. Dillard, M.D. for assistance with the manuscript, the University of Florida Sleep Laboratory, the Alabama Neurology and Sleep Medicine Sleep Program, and the University of Michigan Sleep Laboratory.

We thank Prof. Antonia Prarmeggiani for patients' images, Elena Zoni for graphic production, and Anne Collins for editing the manuscript.

REFERENCES

1. Carney PR, Berry RB, Geyer JD. *Clinical Sleep Disorders.* Philadelphia: Lippincott Williams & Wilkins, 2005; 1st edn.

2. Rosen I, Blennow G, Risberg AM, Ingvar DH. Quantitative evaluation of nocturnal sleep in epileptic children. In: Sterman MB, Shouse MN, Passouant P (eds), *Sleep and Epilepsy.* New York: Academic, 1982; pp. 397–409.

3. Sterman MB, Shouse MN, Passouant P (eds). *Sleep and Epilepsy.* New York: Academic, 1982.

4. Besset A. Influence of generalized seizures on sleep organization. In: Sterman MB, Shouse MN, Passouant P (eds), *Sleep and Epilepsy.* New York: Academic, 1982; pp. 339–346.

5. Carney PR, Kohrman MH. Relation between epilepsy and sleep during infancy and childhood. In: Bazil CW, Malow BA, Sammaritano MR (eds), *Sleep and Epilepsy: The Clinical Spectrum.* Amsterdam: Elsevier Science BV, 2002; pp. 359–372.

6. Horita H, Khumagai K, Mackawa K. Overnight polygraphic study of Lennox–Gastaut syndrome. *Brain Dev* 1987;9: 627–635.

7. Hrachovy RA, Frost JD, Kellaway P. Sleep characteristics in infantile spasms. *Neurology* 1981;31:668–694.

8. Plouin P, et al. Enregistrement ambulatoire de l'EEG pendant 24h dans les spasmes infantiles epileptiques. *Rev EEG Neurophysiol Clin* 1987;17:309–318.

9. Tassinari CA, Bureau M, Dravet C, Dalla Bernardina B, Roger J. Epilepsy with continuous spikes and waves during slow sleep. In: Roger J, Dravet C, Bureau M, Dreifuss FE, Wolf P (eds), *Epileptic Syndromes in Infancy, Childhood and Adolescence.* London: John Libbey, 1992; pp. 245–256.

10. Baldy-Moulinier M. Temporal lobe epilepsy and sleep organization. In: Sterman MB, Passouant P (eds), *Sleep and Epilepsy.* New York: Academic Press, 1982; pp. 347–359.

11. Nunes ML, Ferri R, Arzimanoglou A, Curzi L, Appel C, Costa da Costa J. Sleep organization in children with partial refractory epilepsy. *J Child Neurol* 2003;18:763–766.

12. Maganti R, Sheth RD, Hermann BP, Weber S, Gidal BE, Fine J. Sleep architecture in children with idiopathic generalized epilepsy. *Epilepsia* 2005;46:104–109.

13. Bazil CW, Castro LHM, Walczak TS. Reduction of rapid eye movement sleep by diurnal and nocturnal seizures in temporal lobe epilepsy. *Arch Neurol* 2000;57:363–368.

14. Clemens B, Oláh R. Sleep studies in benign epilepsy of childhood with rolandic spikes: I. Sleep pathology. *Epilepsia* 1987;28:20–23.

15. Shouse MN, Martins da Silva A, Sammaritano M. Circadian rhythm, sleep and epilepsy. *J Clin Neurophysiol* 1996;13:32–50.

16. Shouse MN, Martins da Silva A. Chronobiology. In: Engel J, Pedley TA (eds), *Epilepsy: A Comprehensive Textbook.* Philadelphia: Lippincott-Raven, 1997; pp. 1917–1927.

17. Shouse MN, Martins da Silva A, Sammaritano M. Sleep. In: Engel J, Pedley TA (eds), *Epilepsy: A Comprehensive Textbook*, Philadelphia: Lippincott-Raven, 1997; pp. 1929–1942.

18. Billiard M. Epilepsies and the sleep–wake cycle. In: Sterman MB, Shouse MN, Passouant P (eds), *Sleep and Epilepsy.* New York: Academic, 1982; pp. 269–285.

19. El-Ad B, Neufeld MY, Korczyn AD. Should sleep EEG record always be performed after sleep deprivation? *Electoencephalogr Clin Neurophysiol* 1994;90:313–315.

20. Degen R, Degen HE, Reker M. Sleep EEG with or without sleep deprivation? Does sleep deprivation activate more activity in patients suffering from different types of epilepsy? *Eur Neurol* 1987;26:51–59.

21. Pratt KL, et al. EEG activation of epileptics following sleep deprivation: a prospective study of 114 cases. *Electroencephalogr Clin Neurophysiol* 1968;24:11–15.

22. Cortessi F, Gionnotti F, Ottaviano S. Sleep problems and behavior in childhood idiopathic epilepsy. *Epilepsia* 1999; 40:1557–1565.

23. Zaiwalla Z. Sleep abnormalities in children with epilepsy. *Electroencephalogr Clin Neurophysiol* 1989;72:29.

24. Stores G. Confusions concerning sleep disorders and the epilepsies in children and adolescents. *Br J Psychiatry* 1991;158:1–7.

25. Hunt A, Stores G. Sleep disorders and epilepsy in children with tuberous sclerosis: a questionnaire based study. *Dev Med Child Neurol* 1994;136:108–115.

26. Fauteck J, Schmidt H, Lerchl A, Kurlemann G, Wittkowski W. Melatonin in epilepsy: first results of replacement therapy and first clinical results. *Biol Signals Recept* 1999;8:105–110.

27. Jan IE, Freeman RD, Fast DK. Melatonin treatment of sleep–wake cycle disorders in children and adolescents. *Dev Med Child Neurol* 1999;41:491–500.

28. Fountain NB, Kim JS, Lee SI. Sleep deprivation activates epileptiform discharges independent of the activating effects of sleep. *J Clin Neurophysiol* 1998;15:69–75.

29. Commission on Classification and Terminology of the ILAE. Proposal for revised classification of epilepsies and epileptic syndromes. *Epilepsia* 1989;30:389–399.

30. Janz D, Wolf P. Epilepsy with grand mal on awakening. In: Engel J, Pedley TA (eds), *Epilepsy: A Comprehensive Textbook.* Philadelphia: Lippincott-Raven, 1997; pp. 2347–2354.

31. Doose H. Myoclonic astatic epilepsy of early childhood. In: Roger J, et al (eds), *Epileptic Syndromes in Infancy, Childhood and Adolescence.* London: John Libbey, 1992; pp. 103–114.

32. Beaumanoir A, Dravet C. The Lennox–Gastaut syndrome. In: Roger J, et al (eds), *Epileptic Syndromes in Infancy,*

Childhood and Adolescence. London: John Libbey, 1992; pp. 115–132.

33. Bourgeois B. The relationship between sleep and epilepsy in children. *Semin Pediatr Neurol* 1996;3:29–35.

34. Kohyama J, et al. REM sleep components predict the response to initial treatment of infantile spasms. *Epilepsia* 1999;40:992–996.

35. Wolf P. Juvenile myoclonic epilepsy. In: Roger J, Dravet C, Bureau M, Dreifuss FE, Wolf P (eds), *Epileptic Syndromes in Infancy, Childhood and Adolescence*. London: John Libbey, 1992; 2nd edn: pp. 313–328.

36. Wolf P, Goosses R. Relation of photosensitivity to epileptic syndromes. *J Neurol Neurosurg Psychiatr* 1986;49:1368–1391.

37. Holmes GL. Rolandic epilepsy: clinical and electroencephalographic features. *Epilepsy Res Suppl* 1992; 6:29–43.

38. Blom S, Heijbel J. Benign epilepsy of children with centrotemporal EEG foci. Discharge rate during sleep. *Epilepsia* 1975;16:133–140.

39. Landau WM, Kleffner FR. Syndrome of acquired aphasia with convulsive disorder in children. *Neurology* 1957;7:523–530.

40. Hirsch E, et al. Landau–Kleffner syndrome: a clinical and EEG study of five cases. *Epilepsia* 1990;31:756–767.

41. Deonna T, Roulet E. Acquired epileptic aphasia (AEA): definition of the syndrome and current problems. In: Beaumanoir A, Bureau M, Deonna T, Mira L, Tassinari CA (eds), *Continuous Spike and Waves During Slow Sleep Electrical Status Epilepticus During Slow Sleep*. London: John Libbey, 1995; pp. 37–45.

42. Smith MC. Landau–Kleffner syndrome and continuous spike and waves during slow sleep. In: Engel J, Pedley TA (eds), *Epilepsy: A Comprehensive Textbook*. Philadelphia: Lippincott-Raven, 1997; pp. 2367–2377.

43. Rains P, Veres J. Correlations between night sleep duration and seizure frequency in temporal lobe epilepsy. *Epilepsia* 1993;34:574–579.

44. Provini F, Plazzi G, Tinuper P, Vandi S, Lugaresi E, Montagna P. Nocturnal frontal lobe epilepsy. A clinical and polygraphic overview of 100 consecutive cases. *Brain* 1999;122:1017–1031.

45. Gastaut H, et al. Childhood epileptic encephalopathy with diffuse slow spike-waves (otherwise known as "petit mal variant") or Lennox syndrome. *Epilepsia* 1966; 7:139–179.

46. ASDA (ed). *The International Classification of Sleep Disorders: Diagnostic and Coding Manual*. Westchester, IL: American Academy of Sleep Medicine, 2005; 2nd edn.

47. Guilleminault C, Billiard M, Montplaisir J, Demerit WC. Altered states of consciousness in disorders of daytime sleepiness. *J Neurol Sci* 1976;26:377–393.

48. Craske MG, Tsao JCI. Assessment and treatment of nocturnal panic attacks. *Sleep Med Rev* 2005;9:173–184.

49. Marcus CL. Sleep-disordered breathing in children. *Am J Resp Crit Care* 2001;164:16–30.

50. Ohayon MM, et al. How age influences the expression of narcolepsy. *J Psychosom Res* 2005;59:399–405.

51. Challamel MJ, et al. Narcolepsy in children. *Sleep* 1994;17: S17–S20.

52. Zeman A, Douglas N, Aylward R. Narcolepsy mistaken for epilepsy. *BMJ* 2001;322:216–218.

53. Macleod S, Ferrie C, Zuberi SM. Symptoms of narcolepsy in children misinterpreted as epilepsy. *Epileptic Disord* 2005;7:13–17.

54. Stores G. The protean manifestations of childhood narcolepsy and their misinterpretation. *Dev Med Child Neurol* 2006;48:307–310.

55. Mignot E, Chen W, Black J. On the value of measuring CSF hypocretin 1 in diagnosing narcolepsy. *Sleep* 2003;26: 646–649.

56. Ivanenko A, Tauman R, Gozal D. Modafinil in the treatment of excessive daytime sleepiness in children. *Sleep Med* 2003;4:579–582.

57. Ohayon MM, Guilleminault C, Priest RG. Night terrors, sleepwalking, and confusional arousals in the general population: their frequency and relationship to other sleep and mental disorders. *J Clin Psychiatry* 1999;60: 268–276.

58. Broughton RJ. Sleep disorders: disorders of arousal? *Science* 1968;159:1070–1078.

59. Guilleminault C, Palombini L, Pelayo R, Chervin RD. Sleepwalking and sleep terrors in prepubertal children: what triggers them? *Pediatrics* 2003;111:17–25.

60. Tinuper P, et al. Movement disorders in sleep: guidelines for differentiating epileptic from non-epileptic motor phenomena arising from sleep. *Sleep Med Rev* 2007;11: 255–267.

61. Kushida CA, Littner MR, Morgenthaler T, Alessi CA, Bailey D, Coleman J Jr, Friedman L, Hirshkowitz M, Kapen S, Kramer M, Lee-Chiong T, Loube DL, Owens J, Pancer JP, Wise M. Practice parameters for the indications for polysomnography and related procedures: an update for 2005. *Sleep* 2005;28:499–521.

62. Leung AK, Robson WL. Nightmares. *J Natl Med Assoc* 1993;85:233–235.

63. Adair RH, Bauchner H. Sleep problems in childhood. *Curr Probl Pediatr* 1993;23:147–170.

64. Koran LM, Raghavan S. Fluoxetine for isolated sleep paralysis. *Psychosomatics* 1993;34:184–187.

65. Lottmann HB, Alova I. Primary monosymptomaic nocturnal enuresis in children and adolescents. *Int J Clin Pract Suppl* 2007;155:8–16.

66. Vetrugno R, Provini F, Plazzi G, Vignatelli L, Lugaresi E, Montagna P. Catathrenia (nocturnal groaning): a new type of parasomnia. *Neurology* 2001;56:681–683.

67. DeRoeck J, Van Hoof E, Cluydts R. Sleep-related expiratory groaning: a case report. *Sleep Res* 1983;12: 237.

68. Pevernagie D, Boon P, Mariman A, Verhaeghen D, Pauwels R. Vocalization during episodes of prolonged expiration: a parasomnia related to REM sleep. *Sleep Med* 2001;2:19–30.

69. Meltzer LJ, Mindell JA. Sleep and sleep disorders in children and adolescents. *Psychiatr Clin N Am* 2006; 29:1059–1076.

70. Allen R, et al. Restless legs syndrome: diagnostic criteria, special considerations, and epidemiology. A report from the restless legs syndrome diagnosis and epidemiology workshop at the National Institutes of Health. *Sleep Med* 2003;4:101–119.

71. Walters A, et al. Restless legs syndrome in childhood and adolescence. *Pediatr Neurol* 1994;11:241–245.

72. Kato T, Thie N, Montplaisir J, Lavigne G. Bruxism and orofacial movements during sleep. *Dent Clin North Am* 2001;45:657–684.

73. Vetrugno R, et al. Familial nocturnal facio-mandibular myoclonus mimicking sleep bruxism. *Neurology* 2002a; 58:644–647.

74. Meletti S, Cantalupo G, Volpi L, Rubboli G, Magaudda A, Tassinari CA. Rhythmic teeth grinding induced by temporal lobe seizures. *Neurology* 2004;62:2306–2309.

75. Bader G, Lavigne G. Sleep bruxism: an overview of an oromandibular sleep movement disorder. *Sleep Med Rev* 2000;4:27–43.

76. Chisholm T, Morehouse RL. Adult head-banging: sleep studies and treatment. *Sleep* 1996;19:343–346.

77. Mayer G, Wilde-Frenz J, Kurella B. Sleep related rhythmic movement disorder revisited. *J Sleep Res* 2007;16:110–116.

78. Manni R, Tartara A. Clonazepam treatment of rhythmic movement disorders. *Sleep* 1997;20:812.

79. Fusco L, Pachatz C, Cusmai R, Vigevano F. Repetitive sleep starts in neurologically impaired children: an unusual non-epileptic manifestation in otherwise epileptic subjects. *Epileptic Disord* 1999;1:63–67.

80. Coulter DL, Allen RJ. Benign neonatal sleep myoclonus. 1982;39:191–192.

81. Resnick TJ, Moshe SL, Perotta L, Chambers HJ. Benign neonatal sleep myoclonus: relation to sleep state. *Arch Neurol* 1986;43:266–268.

82. Di Capua M, Fusco L, Ricci S, Vigevano F. Benign neonatal sleep myoclonus: clinical features and video-polygraphic recordings. *Mov Disord* 1993;8:191–194.

83. Alfonso I, et al. A simple maneuver to provoke benign neonatal sleep myoclonus. *Pediatrics* 1995;96:1161–1163.

84. Cohen R, Shuper A, Straussberg R. Familial benign neonatal sleep myoclonus. *Pediatr Neurol* 1996;5:334–337.

85. Brown P, Thompson PD, Rothwell JC, Day BL, Marsden CD. Axial myoclonus of propriospinal origin. *Brain* 1991;114:197–214.

86. Montagna P, Provini F, Plazzi G, Liguori R, Lugaresi E. Propriospinal myoclonus upon relaxation and drowsiness. A cause of severe insomnia. *Mov Disord* 1997; 12:66–72.

87. Broughton R, Tolentino MA. Fragmentary pathological myoclonus in NREM sleep. *Electroencephalogr Clin Neurophysiol* 1984;57:303–309.

88. Vetrugno R, Plazzi G, Provini F, Liguori R, Lugaresi E, Montagna P. Excessive fragmentary hypnic myoclonus: clinical and neurophysiologic findings. *Sleep Med* 2002;3: 73–76.

89. Richter JE. Extraesophageal presentations of gastroesophageal reflux disease. *Semin Gastrointest Dis* 1997;8:75–89.

90. Foldary-Schaefer N. Sleep complaints and epilepsy: the role of seizures, antiepileptic drugs and sleep disorders. *J Clin Neurophisiol* 2002;19:514–521.

91. Koh S, Ward SL, Lin M, Chen LS. Sleep apnea treatment improves seizure control in children with neurodevelopmental disorders. *Pediatr Neurol* 2000;22: 36–39.

92. Foldvary N, Perry M, Lee J, Dinner D, Morris HH. The effects of lamotrigine on sleep in patients with epilepsy. *Epilepsia* 2001;42(12):1569–1573.

93. Rodriguez AJ. Pediatric sleep and epilepsy. *Curr Neurol Neurosci Rep* 2007;7:342–347.

94. Aneja S, Gupta M. Sleep and childhood. *Indian J Pediatr* 2005;72:687–690.

95. Gupta M, Aneja S, Kohli K. Add-on melatonin improves quality of life in epileptic children on valproate monotherapy: a randomized, double-blind, placebo-controlled trial. *Epilepsy Behav* 2004;5:316–321.

96. Coppola G, Iervolino G, Mastrosimone M, La Torre G, Ruiu F, Pascotto A. Melatonin in wake–sleep disorders in children, adolescents and young adults with mental retardation with or without epilepsy: a double-blind, crossover placebo-controlled trial. *Brain Dev* 2004;26: 373–376.

97. Peled N, Shorer Z, Peled E, Pillar G. Melatonin effect on seizures in children with severe neurologic deficit disorders. *Epilepsia* 2001;42:1208–1210.

98. Sheldon SH. Proconvulsant action of oral melatonin in neurologically disabled children. *Lancet* 1998;351: 1254.

99. Foldvary N. Sleep and epilepsy. *Curr Treat Options Neurol* 2002;4:129–135.

100. Touchon J, et al. Sleep organization and epilepsy. In: Degen R, Rodin EA (eds), *Epilepsy, Sleep and Sleep Deprivation*. Amsterdam: Elsevier, 1991; pp. 73–81.

101. Kellaway P, Frost JD, Mizrabi EM. Ethosuximide effcct on thalamic oscillation mechanisms, spindles and generalized 3-Hz spike-and wave bursts [abstract]. *Ann Neurol* 1991;30:293.

102. Declerck AC, Wauquier A. Influence of antiepileptic drugs on sleep patterns. In: Degen R, Rodin EA (eds), *Epilepsy, Sleep and Sleep Deprivation*. Amsterdam: Elsevier, 1991; 2nd edn: pp. 153–162.

103. Wolf P, Röder–Wanner UU, Brede M. Influence of therapeutic phenobarbital and phenytoin medication on the polygraphic sleep of patients with epilepsy. *Epilepsia* 1984;25:467–475.

104. Manni R, Galimberti CA, Zucca C, Parietti L, Tartara A. Sleep patterns in patients with late onset partial epilepsy receiving chronic carbamazepine therapy. *Epilepsy Res* 1990;7(1):72–76.

105. Obermayer WH, Benca RM. Effects of drugs on sleep. *Neurol Clin* 1996;14:827–840.

106. Findji J, Catani P. The effects of valproic acid on sleep parameters in epileptic children: clinical note. In: Sterman MB, Shouse MN, Passouant P (eds), *Sleep and Epilepsy*. New York: Academic Press, 1982; pp. 395–396.

107. Barzaghi N, et al. Time-dependent pharmacodynamic effects of phenobarbital in humans. *Ther Drug Monit* 1990;11:661–666.

108. Ehrenberg B. Importance of sleep restoration in co-morbid disease: effect of anticonvulsants. *Neurology* 2000;54(Suppl 1):S33–S37.

109. Placidi F, Diomedi M, Scalise A, Marciani MG, Romigi A, Gigli GL. Effect of anticonvulsants on nocturnal sleep in epilepsy. *Neurology* 2000;54(Suppl 1):S25–S32.

110. Sadler M. Lamotrigine associated with insomnia. *Epilepsia.* 1999;40(3):322–325.

111. Placidi F, Diomedi M, Scalise A, Silvestri G, Marciani MD, Gigli GL. Effect of long-term treatment with gabapentin on nocturnal sleep in epilepsy. *Epilepsia* 1997;38(Suppl 8): 179–180.

112. Bonanni E, et al. A quantitative study of daytime sleepiness induced by carbamazepine and add-on vigabatrin in epileptic patients. *Acta Neurol Scand* 1997;95:193–196.

113. Malow BA, Edwards J, Marzec M, Sagher O, Fromes G. Effects of vagus nerve stimulation on respiration during sleep: a pilot study. *Neurology* 2000;55:1450–1454.

114. Malow BA, Edwards J, Marzec M, Sagher O, Ross D, Fromes G. Vagus nerve stimulation reduces daytime sleepiness in epilepsy patients. *Neurology* 2001;57: 879–884.

CHAPTER 45

Impact of Comorbidities on Health Outcomes

David Friedman and Frank G. Gillaim

The World Health Organization defines health as "a state of complete physical, mental, and social well-being and not merely the absence of disease or infirmity."[1] In the past, measures of success in treating medical illness have been thought of in terms of freedom of disease or identifiable quantifiable endpoints, such as serum glucose, systolic blood pressure, or seizures.[2] However, recently, there has been an emergence of interest in measuring health-related quality of life (HRQOL), a valid and significant indicator of health in patients with disease. This idea has been studied over the past decade and applied to develop reliable and valid measures of function and well-being for use in patients with epilepsy.[3] This concept especially pertains to chronic epilepsy, where though many treating clinicians focus on treating the ictal phenomenon of the disease, namely seizures, the disease itself carries a multitude of clinically relevant interictal comorbidities that affects patients' overall HRQOL.

Indeed, this concept is not specifically inclusive to adults, as the negative impact on quality of life in children is common, and typically manifests with impaired social functioning, peer relationships, self-esteem, mood, and academic performance.[4-7] In addition, epilepsy can have a negative impact on not only the many aspects of a child's life but also on his or her family as well.[6,8-10] Issues with subjective health status can be especially challenging for children living with epilepsy, because the maturation of a healthy self-identity is recognized as a fundamental task in a child's development.[11]

There has been increased focus concerning HRQOL and epilepsy in children over the past decade. Most of these studies used various standardized measures to systematically investigate the various aspects that contribute to HRQOL.[12-22] However, many studies did not analyze qualitative measures, and were thus unsuccessful in investigating subjective health status by direct exploration of children's views.[23]

This review will examine the contribution and impact of different forms of comorbidity on overall health status in children in epilepsy. We will discuss neuropsychiatric comorbidity, medication effects, seizure burden, and outcomes of epilepsy surgery pertaining to overall HRQOL.

▶ IMPACT OF DEPRESSION IN CHILDREN WITH EPILEPSY

Depression is the most common comorbid psychiatric disorder in patients with epilepsy.[24] Extensive literature has indicated that depression is a frequent complication of chronic epilepsy.[25-29] However, symptoms of psychological distress are often unrecognized by clinicians treating children with epilepsy.[28,29] There are a variety of potential causes of depression in children with epilepsy. For example, depression may be reactive and secondary to being diagnosed with a chronic, debilitating condition.[30] Psychosocial factors, such as perceived social stigma and parental overprotection might be related to psychopathology, but there is little empirical research on this topic and the findings are inconsistent.[31] Studies have shown that psychiatric problems may exist prior to the identification of the diagnosis of epilepsy in children, and therefore are likely due to underlying pathophysiological disturbances of the disease.[32,33] Indeed, associations have been made between underlying brain dysfunction occurring in patients with epilepsy with depression.[34-38] Different forms of psychiatric comorbidity have also been shown to be associated with different types of epilepsy in children.[39,40] For instance, thought disorder and hyperactivity are linked with different forms of localization-related epilepsy,[41] while both Axis I disorders and personality disorders are associated with juvenile myoclonic epilepsy.[42]

Epilepsy and behavior have a complex association. Particular attention should be paid to the temporal relationship of psychiatric symptoms with seizure occurrence. Psychopathology can accordingly be classified as either ictal (due to the clinical properties during the seizure), peri-ictal (clinical manifestations preceding or following the seizure), or interictal (symptoms occurring independent of seizure occurrence).[43] Ictal depression has been associated with partial seizures of temporal origin.[44] The most common form of peri-ictal psychiatric symptoms encountered is that seen following a seizure, and have been identified in as many as 7% of patients.[45] Symptoms may include postictal psychosis or depression.

Postictal depression may persist as long as 2 weeks following the seizure.[46]

Interictal depression is by far the most common form of psychopathology in patients with epilepsy. It has a prevalence of up to 55% among adult patients with pharmacoresistant epilepsy.[47–49] Pediatric patients have lower rates of depression, ranging between 23% and 26%.[28,50] This may be secondary to the fact that diagnosing depression in children can be more challenging than in adults, irrespective of the patient having a diagnosis of epilepsy. Depression often manifests differently in children than adults. Children infrequently have depressive symptoms, and instead may express multiple somatic complaints. Children with mood disorders often display symptoms of irritability rather than depression, and may carry more than one psychiatric diagnosis, such as attention-deficit disorder, depressive disorder, and language disorders, further clouding the proper identification of the disorder.[51] It may be for this reason that though recent studies have revealed a strong negative correlation between mood status and overall HRQOL in adults,[28,47–49,52,53] there is a paucity of literature linking poor subjective health status with mood disorders in children with epilepsy.

Children with epilepsy were found to be consistently behaviorally disturbed and demonstrated lower self-esteem when compared to children with diabetes.[54] However, this was not reported to be associated with HRQOL. Older adolescents reporting poor HRQOL were more likely to perceive a greater negative impact on life and general health, and had more negative attitudes toward epilepsy than younger patients.[18]

Though interictal comorbid depression and epilepsy is not as common in childhood, it has a substantial effect on HRQOL. Systematic screening for depression facilitates treatment with psychotropic medications or psychotherapy, potentially improving comprehensive care.

▶ IMPACT OF ATTENTION DEFICIT HYPERACTIVITY DISORDER (ADHD) IN CHILDREN WITH EPILEPSY

Attention deficit hyperactivity disorder (ADHD) affects approximately 3%–7% of all children in the general population.[55,56] ADHD has a negative impact on personal and social functioning, given the relationship of ADHD with learning difficulties, school failure, poor peer relationships, as well as accompanying mood, anxiety, and conduct disorders, potentially leading to adverse effects on occupational attainment.[57–59]

Symptoms resembling those of ADHD were first reported in 8% of children with epilepsy over 50 years ago, described as an interictal "hyperkinetic syndrome."[60] The prevalence of ADHD in the epilepsy population in recent studies has varied widely, depending on the samples studied and the measures for ADHD used. In studies of children with chronic epilepsy, 28%–39% had symptoms of hyperactivity and impulsivity.[61,62] Forty-two percent were reported to have problems with attention.[63] These studies, however, did not use the standard diagnostic criteria for ADHD.

More recent studies of patients with chronic epilepsy using established measures for ADHD found a striking difference with regards to the symptoms of ADHD in primary ADHD and ADHD in children with epilepsy. The inattention component of ADHD has been found to be more prevalent than hyperactivity impulsive types, with 24%–40% and 2%–18%, respectively.[64,65] The likely explanation for the higher prevalence of the inattention subtype of ADHD in children with epilepsy is the epilepsy-specific neurologically based risk factors for disturbances in attention in these particular patients. These include the pathophysiological disturbances accounting for interictal cognitive dysfunction in patients with epilepsy, as well as medication effects.[66–68]

Patients with epilepsy and ADHD have a two- to fourfold increase in poor HRQOL, indicating that the symptoms of ADHD have substantial effects on patients, with significant implications on overall subjective health status.[65] These findings are similar to other studies investigating the effect of ADHD on HRQOL in patients without epilepsy.[69–71] Once again, this study found that inattention was the main symptom in the children with epilepsy and ADHD. The fact that ADHD has a negative effect on HRQOL has particularly relevant clinical implications, namely screening and treatment of ADHD in this population.

Screening and treatment of ADHD in pediatric patients is particularly relevant given the association between ADHD symptoms and poor subjective health status. ADHD is a behavioral syndrome that is treatable, with medical intervention having a potential impact. By recognizing this interictal phenomenon, we have the opportunity to intervene with proper treatment and effect positive change in the overall HRQOL in these children.

▶ MEASURING TOOLS TO SCREEN FOR PSYCHOPATHOLOGY IN CHILDREN WITH EPILEPSY

Over the past recent years, the use of self-report rating scales has been used to screen for depression in patients with epilepsy. Though an in-depth psychiatric interview conducted directly with the patient is of great importance when assessing for psychiatric comorbidity, the rating scales assist in providing valuable information, and can help the clinician determine when referral to a psychiatrist is warranted.

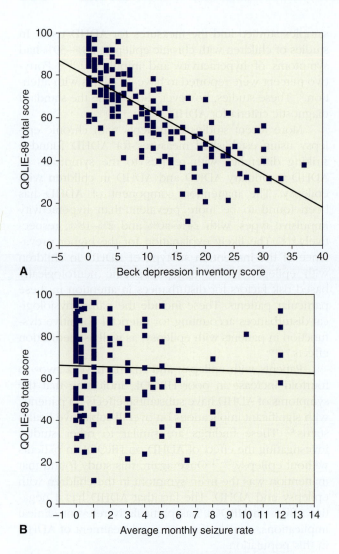

Figure 45–1. (A) Scatterplot of correlation of health-related quality of life (Quality of Life—89 global score) with depression symptoms ($r = -0.49$, $p < 0.001$) ($n = 200$). **(B)** Scatterplot of correlation of average monthly seizure rate with depression symptoms ($r = -0.01$, $p = 0.93$) ($n = 200$). (From Gilliam F, Kanner AM. Treatment of depressive disorders in epilepsy patients. *Epilepsy Behav* 2002;3:2–9.)

Many depression scales have been developed over the years for assessing psychopathology in adults with epilepsy.

- The Beck Depression Inventory (BDI) is the most commonly used self-rating scale. It was designed to detect current (past 2 weeks) depressive symptoms. The BDI contains 21 descriptive statements regarding depressive symptoms frequently reported by individuals diagnosed with depression.[72] The statements can be rated on a 4-point severity-rating scale. The BDI was found to have a high sensitivity and specificity as a screening instrument.[73,74]

- The Structured Clinical Interview for DSM-IV: Research Version (SCID-I) and Mini International Neuropsychiatric Interview (MINI) are two effective instruments used primarily in research to screen for Axis I disorders,[75,76] but administration time is approximately 15–20 minutes and are thus impractical for use in a busy practice setting. The Center for Epidemiological Studies-Depression (CES-D) scale is a 20-item scale developed to screen for depression in primary-care settings.[77] The CES-D items focus on measuring the frequency of depressive symptoms and the scale has been shown to be a valid and a reliable instrument,[78] with significant ability to identify major depression in epilepsy.[74]

- The Neurological Disorders Depression Inventory Index for Epilepsy (NDDI-E) is a relatively new tool used for a rapid screening for major depressive episodes in adults with epilepsy.[79] The 6-item questionnaire was developed for a brief, yet accurate screening technique that can easily be applied in a busy office setting.

Similarly, screening instruments have been used for children and adolescents with epilepsy.

The Child Behavior Checklist (CBCL) evaluates pathological behaviors and social competence in children and is one of the most widely used scales in clinical practice and research.[80]

The Children's Depression Inventory (CDI) is one of the most frequently used questionnaires for monitoring depression in children.[81] It contains 27 descriptive items that includes three statements of increasing severity.

The Child Symptom Inventories-4 (CSI) screens for behavioral, affective, and cognitive symptoms of many DSM-IV disorders and is also widely used in research.

▶ IMPACT OF PSYCHIATRIC COMORBIDITY ON PARENTS OF CHILDREN WITH EPILEPSY

Families of children with epilepsy appear to have more problems with family functioning than families with healthy children.[82,83] Having a child diagnosed with epilepsy, like other chronic illnesses, likely provokes substantial stress in parents. Parental difficulty in handling and accepting their child's diagnosis has been associated with elevated levels of parental stress.[84] This, in turn, predicts dysfunction with child–parent relationships, which becomes directly related to child psychopathology.[85,86] This idea is supported by recent reports showing that parental psychopathology, particularly anxiety and depression, has a negative effect

▶ **TABLE 45-1.** THE NEUROLOGICAL DISORDERS DEPRESSION INVENTORY FOR EPILEPSY (NDDI-E) FOR THE STATEMENTS IN THE TABLE, PATIENTS ARE ASKED TO CIRCLE THE NUMBER THAT BEST DESCRIBES THEM OVER THE PAST 2 WEEKS, INCLUDING THE DAY OF THE ASSESSMENT

	Always or Often	Sometimes	Rarely	Never
Everything is a struggle	4	3	2	1
Nothing I do is right	4	3	2	1
Feel guilty	4	3	2	1
I'd be better off dead	4	3	2	1
Frustrated	4	3	2	1
Difficulty finding pleasure	4	3	2	1

Source: From Gilliam FG, et al. Rapid detection of major depression in epilepsy: a multicentre study. *Lancet Neurol* 2006;5:399–405.

on patients' HRQOL,[87–90] with some authors concluding that the influence of parental emotion was stronger than the burden of the epilepsy itself.[90] Indeed, parents of children with epilepsy have their own unique set of psychiatric disorders different from their children's. Parental anxiety may lead to them becoming overprotective, promoting a transmission of anxieties to their children. Prevalence of maternal depression was reported to be anywhere between 32% and 37% in mothers of children with epilepsy.[91–93]

Identifying parental psychological symptoms may be beneficial not only to the parent but also to the child, as parental psychopathology may directly impose a negative effect on patients' overall quality of life. Increased awareness of these disorders may help clinicians to develop preventive and interventional measures for the mental health of parents. Ultimately, this should lead to a positive effect on patients' overall HRQOL.

▶ IMPACT OF COGNITIVE COMORBIDITY DUE TO MEDICATION EFFECT IN CHILDREN WITH EPILEPSY

In children, interictal impairment of cognitive functioning and learning disabilities are also associated with poor outcome, independent of seizure frequency.[94,95]

Though much of the cognitive dysfunction experienced by children with epilepsy are secondary to the underlying brain dysfunction related to the disease, it is known that antiepileptic drug (AED) effects contribute to cognitive problems.[96] Several studies have demonstrated the importance of medication-induced problems effecting subjective health status in adults.[87,97–100] The negative effect of AEDs on cognition and overall well-being has become better known recently, and has led to the development of measures to assist clinicians in identifying medication problems. The Adverse Effects Profile (AEP) was designed to enable patients to determine the most important AED side effects from their perspective.[101] The clinical utility of the AEP was recently demonstrated in a single-center study, where AED effects were strongly correlated with poor HRQOL.[102]

Children with epilepsy are at risk for cognitive impairment and subsequent poor academic achievements, with at least some component being attributed to AED effects. AED effects can manifest in overt neurotoxicity, or, over time, in a more subtle fashion, affecting attention and memory. Indeed, phenobarbital has been associated with having a negative impact on IQ.[103] There is a dearth of literature studying the magnitude of the long-term effects AEDs have in children's neurocognitive functioning and school performance.[104]

Toxic effects of medication are also implicated in poor overall HRQOL in children. Symptoms of neurotoxicity were associated with low subjective health status when measured by the QOLIE-AD-48, an epilepsy-specific instrument used to assess HRQOL in children and adolescents.[18] In a survey of elementary and junior high school children with epilepsy, both seizures and medication effects were primary concerns.[105] Total number of medications was associated with a negative influence on HRQOL when parents rated their children's quality of life.[10,89] Concerns about the adverse effects of AEDs were among the main distresses experienced by children in a study using a qualitative focus group methodology.[16] A combination of executive dysfunction and high medication load were among the factors associated with an adverse effect on psychosocial well-being in a recent study investigating pediatric epilepsy and HRQOL.[106]

The effects of AEDs, both acute and chronic, can have clinically relevant implications, particularly affecting neurocognitive functioning. This, in turn, may have a profound effect on subjective health status. Attention should be given to reduce the toxic effects of AEDs in an effort to improve HRQOL in children with epilepsy. Instruments such as the AEP are ideally designed and should be employed routinely.

▶ **TABLE 45–2.** COMPARISON OF MEAN (SD) BASELINE AND FOLLOW-UP SCORES FOR SEIZURE-FREE AND PERSISTENT SEIZURE GROUPS IN CHILDREN UNDERGOING EPILEPSY SURGERY

| | Seizure Free | | Persistent Seizures | | |
| | Baseline | Follow-up | Baseline | Follow-up | Interaction |
Scale	Mean (SD)	Mean (SD)	Mean (SD)	Mean (SD)	P value
Physical restrictions	44.79 (23.66)	70.26 (26.33)	33.78 (18.73)	38.96 (26.63)	0.024
Attention/concentration	46.25 (24.97)	64.31 (30.47)	44.75 (20.38)	42.50 (29.01)	0.046
Anxiety	53.56 (18.78)	72.92 (24.53)	63.67 (18.97)	67.86 (22.76)	0.040
Control/helplessness	51.56 (23.55)	74.06 (20.00)	48.66 (20.24)	50.45 (16.55)	0.035
Self-esteem	62.06 (17.32)	74.50 (21.27)	70.08 (24.44)	59.89 (23.98)	0.009
Social interactions	48.83 (33.53)	72.56 (28.50)	58.22 (25.15)	52.44 (23.20)	0.001
Social activities	42.08 (33.28)	80.21 (26.66)	34.44 (23.12)	40.00 (26.76)	0.013
General health item	42.50 (32.55)	83.75 (26.00)	26.67 (27.49)	35.00 (29.58)	0.010
Quality of life item	42.50 (33.54)	82.50 (29.36)	30.56 (24.37)	33.93 (23.22)	0.003
Overall QOL	51.35 (18.62)	72.66 (20.17)	48.50 (12.17)	49.91 (15.82)	0.008

Source: From Sabaz M, et al. The impact of epilepsy surgery on quality of life in children. *Neurology* 2006;66:557–561.

▶ **IMPACT OF SURGERY ON HEALTH-RELATED QUALITY OF LIFE (HRQOL)**

More than 30% of patients with epilepsy do not achieve complete control of seizures through AED treatment.[107] In children with temporal lobe epilepsy, 35% are resistant to medications, with incomplete response to first AED trial representing a predictor for becoming refractory.[108] Surgery has been used to treat medically intractable epilepsy in childhood for several decades. Surgery was revealed to be far superior to medical therapy in terms of rendering patients seizure-free (58% vs. 8%) in the only randomized controlled trial studying epilepsy surgery.[109] Published studies on surgical outcomes in pediatric epilepsy are reliable but difficult to compare, given the diverse pathological conditions, variety of surgical techniques, and differing definitions of postoperative outcome. Children with hippocampal sclerosis have similar outcomes after temporal lobectomy as adults.[110] Other forms of pathology, particularly low-grade tumors, have been associated with better postoperative outcome when compared to cortical dysplasia (82% vs. 52%).[111]

Epilepsy surgery is effective in improving HRQOL in children, notably having positive effects on cognitive, social, emotional, behavioral, and physical domains of life with improvement in subjective health status being associated with seizure freedom.[112] Epilepsy surgery allows for freedom of seizures, for a substantial reduction in number of AEDs taken postoperatively, and for more independence. Studies investigating patient-oriented outcomes following temporal lobectomy for pharmacoresistant epilepsy in adults showed improvement in HRQOL following surgery, with multivariate regression analysis in the postoperative group demonstrating that factors associated with improved HRQOL included mood status, employment, driving, and AED cessation, but did not include seizure freedom.[99]

The improved subjective health status following successful epilepsy surgery in children is more likely associated with seizure freedom as driving and employment are not applicable in childhood. In addition, many of the quality of life measures used in children with epilepsy are scored by the parents. Freedom of seizures, their accompanying unpredictability, and risk for injury are especially important for families of children with epilepsy. In fact, in surveys assessing concerns of parents with epilepsy, safety and risk for injury were rated as either the first[14] or fourth[113] most common fear among families.

Surgery for medication-resistant epilepsy is a proven treatment modality that can often lead to seizure freedom. Seizure freedom is in turn the strongest predictor of improvement in HRQOL in children with epilepsy. Identifying patients that are pharmacoresistant and possible surgical candidates early may be invaluable in improving their comprehensive care.

▶ **INSTRUMENTS USED TO MEASURE HRQOL IN CHILDREN**

The relatively recent interest in outcomes research in children sparked the development of several scales for measuring HRQOL and associated risk factors in children and adolescents with epilepsy. The scales are either scored by the parent or patient, and are either disease-specific or generic. Generic scales, designed for general use across a multitude of medical conditions, can be used for children with epilepsy. Also, scales differ in the measurement of particular domains of HRQOL. Limitations in the existing research exist, given that many of the instruments are relatively new. Many of the older studies used specifically designed questionnaires that are not necessarily validated.

- The Impact of Childhood Illness (ICI) scale is a measure of HRQOL in children that is not disease-specific. It measures the physical, emotional, and familial aspects of HRQOL. It is a 30-item parent-rated questionnaire that is divided into four sections: impact of the disorder and its treatment, impact on the child's development and adjustment, impact on parents, and impact on the family. Parents rate each item in terms of perceived frequency and degree of concern. This instrument has been validated[114] and has been used in patients with epilepsy.[14,106]

- The Quality of Life in Childhood Epilepsy (QOLCE) questionnaire is a validated parent-rating questionnaire specifically designed for use with children with epilepsy.[20] It consists of 77 items that are ranked on a 5-point scale that are then linearly changed to a 0–100-point scale when scored. Five domains of function are assessed, and include cognitive function, physical function, emotional well-being, social function, and behavior. The subscale scores are averaged into a composite score. The QOLCE has been used in studies of impact of epilepsy surgery,[112] sleep disturbance,[115] and memory[116] in children with epilepsy.

- The Impact of Child Neurologic Handicap (ICNH) scale is a measure of HRQOL in children that is disease-specific to epilepsy. It affords subscale scores in four domains, as well as an overall score of HRQOL. The ICNH was shown to be a valid instrument,[114] but has not been used in any published studies.

- The Hague Restrictions in Epilepsy Scale (HARCES) is a 10-item parent-rated scale that measures the amount of disability resulting from seizure-imposed restrictions. The items used in the instrument reflect everyday activities common to children, such as riding a bicycle, staying elsewhere overnight, and swimming. Eight of the items pertain to activities of daily living, and two items reflect degree of restriction on the child. The HARCES is a tool measuring both the psychosocial and physical domains. It has been shown to be reliable and valid[114,117] and used in studies regarding epilepsy surgery[118] and executive functioning[106] in children with epilepsy.

- The QOLIE-AD-48 is a disease-specific instrument assessing 48 items in eight domains of HRQOL, including health perception, epilepsy impact, cognition, physical functioning, social support, stigma, school behavior, and attitudes toward epilepsy.[17] It is scored by adolescent patients, and consists of 5-point scales, with total and domain scores being translated into scores on a 0–100-response scale, with higher scores indicating better HRQOL.

- The Child Health Questionnaire (CHQ) is a 50-item scale developed to compare children's health status and changes over time across general and specific populations. It is not disease-specific and is parent-rated. The reliability and validity of the CHQ have been confirmed by extensive testing in children. Twelve health concepts are measured, and converted linearly to a 0–100 scale, with higher scores indicating better functioning. The CHQ was used to study the impact of epilepsy surgery outcome in children.[119]

- The Impact of Pediatric Epilepsy Scale (IPES) is a relatively brief instrument that specifically measures the psychosocial impact of pediatric epilepsy on the family.[10] It consists of a parent-rated 11-item scale, assessing the impact on academic achievement, participation in activities, health, family and peer relationships, social activities, self-esteem, and hopes for the child's future. The IPES has been used in the literature to assess HRQOL.[120,121]

▶ CONCLUSIONS

Interictal comorbidities have a substantial effect on HRQOL in children with epilepsy. Traditionally, the management of epilepsy had been focused on the ictal manifestations of the disorder, with seizures considered of paramount importance. In treating patients with epilepsy, attempting to reduce or eliminate seizures is a worthy goal. However, the last decades of research in epilepsy, particularly research relating to comorbidity and HRQOL, have begun to shift the focus of management from the ictal to the interictal period. Recognition of the extensive and persistent interictal factors, negative effects of subjective health status, such as psychiatric comorbidity and cognitive-altering effects of medications, allows us to conclude that the cessation of seizures alone may not suffice in causing a positive impact on HRQOL. Advances in the research in this field have yielded instruments available for use in this population, such as the IPES, AEP, and CDI. Tools such as these can be easily used in clinical practice and are of great value in optimizing the overall health of children with epilepsy.

REFERENCES

1. Preamble to the Constitution of the World Health Organization as adopted by the International Health conference, New York, 19–22 June 1946; Signed on July 1946 by the representatives of 61 states (Official Records of the World Health Organization, No. 2, p. 100) and entered into force on 7 April 1948.

2. Clancy CM, Eisenberg JM. Outcomes research: measuring the end results of health care. *Science* 1998;282:245–246.

3. Baker GA, et al. Commission on Outcome Measurement in Epilepsy, 1994–1997: final report. *Epilespia* 1998;39:213–231.

4. Wiebe S, et al. Burden of epilepsy: the Ontario Health Survey. *Can J Neurol Sci* 1999;26:263–270.

5. Batzel LW, et al. An objective method for the assessment of psychosocial problems in adolescents with epilepsy. *Epilepsia* 1991;32:202–211.

6. Hoare P, Kerley S. Psychosocial adjustment of children with chronic epilepsy and their families. *Dev Med Child Neurol* 1991;33:210–215.

7. Westbrook LE, Bauman LJ, Shinnar S. Applying stigma theory to epilepsy: a test of a conceptual model. *J Pediatr Psychol* 1992;17:633–649.

8. Levin R, Banks S. Stress in parents of children with epilepsy. *Can J Rehabil* 1991;4:229–238.

9. Camfield CS, Breau LM, Camfield PR. The impact of Pediatric Epilepsy Scale: A pilot study. *Can Psych* 1999;40:53.

10. Camfield C, Breau L, Camfield P. Impact of pediatric epilepsy on the family: a new scale for clinical and research use. *Epilepsia* 2001;42:104–112.

11. Carr A. *The Handbook of Child and Adolescent Clinical Psychology: A Contextual Approach.* London and New York: Routledge, 1999.

12. Austin JK, et al. Childhood epilepsy and asthma: comparison of quality of life. *Epilepsia* 1994;35:608–615.

13. Austin JK, et al. Adolescents with active and inactive epilepsy or asthma: a comparison of quality of life. *Epilepsia* 1996;37:1228–1238.

14. Hoare P, Russell M. The quality of life of children with chronic epilepsy and their families: preliminary findings with a new assessment measure. *Dev Med Child Neurol* 1995;37:689–696.

15. Wildrick D, Parker-Fisher S, Morales A. Quality of life in children with well-controlled epilepsy. *J Neurosci Nurs* 1996;28:192–198.

16. Ronen GM, et al. Health-related quality of life in childhood epilepsy: the results of children's participation in identifying the components. *Dev Med Child Neurol* 1999;41:554–559.

17. Cramer JA, et al. Development of quality of life in epilepsy inventory for adolescents: the QOLIE-AD-48. *Epilepsia* 1999;40:1114–1121.

18. Devinsky O, et al. Risk factors for poor health related quality of life in adolescents with epilepsy. *Epilepsia* 1999;40:1725–1720.

19. Norrby U, et al. Self-assessment of well being in a group of children with epilepsy. *Seizure* 1999;8:228–234.

20. Sabaz M, et al. Validation of a new quality of life measure for children with epilepsy. *Epilepsia* 2000;41:765–774.

21. Miller V, Palermo TM, Grewe SD. Quality of life in pediatric epilepsy: demographic and disease-related predictors and comparison with healthy controls. *Epilepsy Behav* 2003;4:36–42.

22. Elliott IM, Lach L, Smith ML. I just want to be normal: a qualitative study exploring how children and adolescents view the impact of intractable epilepsy on their quality of life. *Epilepsy Behav* 2005;7:664–678.

23. Mcewan MJ, Espie CA, Metcalfe J. A systematic review of the contribution of qualitative research to the study of quality of life in children and adolescents with epilepsy. *Seizure* 2004;13:3–14.

24. Kanner AM. Depression in epilepsy: prevalence, clinical semiology, pathogenic mechanisms, and treatment. *Biol Psychiatry* 2003;54:388–398.

25. Gilliam F, Kanner AM. Treatment of depressive disorders in epilepsy patients. *Epilepsy Behav* 2002;3:2–9.

26. Harden CL, Goldstein MA. Mood disorders in patients with epilepsy: epidemiology and management. *CNS Drugs* 2002;16:291–302.

27. Jones JE, et al. Clinical assessment of Axis I psychiatric morbidity in chronic epilepsy: a multicenter investigation. *J Neuropsychiatry Clin Neurosci* 2005;17:172–179.

28. Ettinger AB, et al. Symptoms of anxiety and depression in pediatric epilepsy patients. *Epilepsia* 1998;39:595–599.

29. Ott D, et al. Behavioral disorders in pediatric epilepsy: unmet psychiatric needs. *Epilepsia* 2003;44:591–597.

30. Taylor DC. Psychosocial components of childhood epilepsy In: Hermann BP, Seidenberg M (eds), *Childhood Epilepsies: Neuropsychological, Psychosocial and Intervention Aspects.* Chichester: John Wiley & Sons, 1989.

31. Hermann BP, Whitman S. Psychopathology in epilepsy: the role of psychology in altering paradigms of research, treatment, and prevention. *Am Psychol* 1992;47:1134–1138.

32. Dunn DW, Austin JK, Huster GA. Behavioral problems in children with new-onset epilepsy. *Seizure* 1997;6:283–287.

33. Austin J, et al. Behavior problems in children before first recognized seizures. *Pediatrics* 2001;107:115–122.

34. Gilliam FG, et al. Depression in epilepsy: ignoring clinical expression of neuronal network dysfunction? *Epilepsia* 2004;45:28–33.

35. Bromfield EB, et al. Cerebral metabolism and depression in patients with complex partial seizures. *Arch Neurol* 1992;49:617–623.

36. Quiske A, et al. Depression in patients with temporal lobe epilepsy is related to mesial temporal sclerosis. *Epilepsy Res* 2000;39:121–129.

37. Savic I, et al. Limbic reductions of 5-HT1A receptor binding in human temporal lobe epilepsy. *Neurology* 2004;62:1343–1351.

38. Giovacchini G, et al. 5-HT1A receptors are reduced in temporal lobe epilepsy after partial volume correction. *J Nucl Med* 2005;46:1128–1135.

39. Dam M. Children with epilepsy: the effect of seizures, syndromes, and etiological factors on cognitive functioning. *Epilepsia* 1990;31(Suppl 4):S26–S29.

40. Besag FM. Behavioral aspects of pediatric epilepsy syndromes. *Epilepsy Behav* 2004;5(Suppl 1):S3–S13.

41. Caplan R, Guthrie D, Shields WD. Formal thought disorder in pediatric complex partial seizure disorder. *J Child Psychiatry Psychol* 1992;33:1399–1412.

42. Trinka E, et al. Psychiatric comorbidity in juvenile myoclonic epilepsy. *Epilepsia* 2006;47:1086–2091.

43. Kanner AM, Weisbrodt DM. Psychiatric evaluation of the adult and pediatric patient with epilepsy, a practical approach for the "nonpsychiatrist." In: Ettinger AB, Kanner AM (eds), *Psychiatric Issues in Epilepsy: A Practical Guide to Diagnosis and Treatment.* Philadelphia: Lippincott Williams & Wilkins, 2007; p. 121.

44. Weil A. Ictal emotions occurring in temporal lobe dysfunction. *Arch Neurol* 1959;1:87–97.

45. Kanner AM, Soto A, Gross-Kanner H. Prevalence and clinical characteristics of postictal psychiatric symptoms in partial epilepsy. *Neurology* 2004;62:708–713.

46. Perrine K, Congett S. Neurobehavioral problems in epilepsy. *Neurol Clin North Am* 1994;12:129–152.

47. Mendez MF, Cummings JL, Benson DF. Depression in epilepsy. Significance and phenomenology. *Arch Neurol* 1996;43:766–770.

48. Hermann BP, Seidenberg M, Bell B. Psychiatric comorbidity in chronic epilepsy: identification, consequences, and treatment of major depression. *Epilepsia* 2000;41(Suppl 2): S31–S41.

49. Gilliam FG. Diagnosis and treatment of mood disorders in persons with epilepsy. *Curr Opin Neurol* 2005;18: 129–133.

50. Dunn DW, Austin JK. Symptoms of depression in adolescents with epilepsy. *J Am Acad Child Adolesc Psychiatry* 1999;38:1132–1138.

51. Weisbrodt DM, Ettinger AB. Psychiatric aspects of pediatric epilepsy. In: Ettinger AB, Kanner AM (eds), *Psychiatric Issues in Epilepsy: A Practical Guide to Diagnosis and Treatment.* Philadelphia: Lippincott Williams & Wilkins, 2007; p. 137.

52. Boylan LS, et al. Depression but not seizure frequency predicts quality of life in treatment-resistant epilepsy. *Neurology* 2004;45:28–33.

53. Loring DW, Meador KJ, Lee GP. Determinants of quality of life in epilepsy. *Epilepsy Behav* 2004;5:976–980.

54. Hoare P, Mann H. Self-esteem and behavioral adjustment in children with epilepsy and children with diabetes. *J Psychosom Res* 1994;38:859–869.

55. Rappley MD. Attention deficit-hyperactivity disorder. *New Engl J Med* 2005;352:165–173.

56. Polanczyk G, et al. The worldwide prevalence of ADHD: a systematic review and metaregression analysis. *Am J Psychiatry* 2007;164:942–948.

57. Wilens TE, Biederman J, Spencer TJ. Attention deficit/ hyperactivity disorder across the lifespan. *Annu Rev Med* 2002;53:113–131.

58. Spencer TJ, Biederman J, Mick E. Attention-deficit/ hyperactivity disorder: diagnosis, lifespan, comorbidities, and neurobiology. *Ambul Pediatr* 2007;7:73–81.

59. Pelham WE, Foster EM, Robb JA. The economic impact of attention deficit/hyperactivity disorder in children and adolescents. *Ambul Pediatr* 2007;7:121–131.

60. Ounstead C. The hyperkinetic syndrome in epileptic children. *Lancet* 1955;13:301–311.

61. McDermott S, Mani S, Krishnaswami S. A population-based analysis of specific behavior problems associated with childhood seizure disorders. *J Epilepsy* 1995;8: 110–118.

62. Carlton-Ford S, et al. Epilepsy and children's social and psychological adjustment. *J Health Soc Behav* 1995; 36:285–301.

63. Holdsworth L, Whitmore K. A study of children with epilepsy attending ordinary schools I: their seizure patterns, progress, and behavior in school. *Dev Med Child Neurol* 1991;33:201–215.

64. Dunn DW, et al. ADHD and epilepsy in childhood. *Dev Med Child Neurol* 2003;45:50–54.

65. Sherman EM, Slick DJ, Connolly MB. ADHD, neurological correlates and health-related quality of life in severe pediatric epilepsy. *Epilepsia* 2007;48:1083–1091.

66. Espie CA, et al. Cognitive functioning in people with epilepsy plus severe learning disabilities: a systematic analysis of predictors of daytime arousal and attention. *Seizure* 1999;8:73–80.

67. Meador KJ. Cognitive outcomes and predictive factors in epilepsy. *Neurology* 2002;58(Suppl 5):S21–S26.

68. Helmstaeder C, et al. Chronic epilepsy and cognition: a longitudinal study in temporal lobe epilepsy. *Ann Neurol* 2003;54:425–432.

69. Matza LS, et al. The link between health-related quality of life and clinical symptoms among children with attention deficit hyperactivity disorder. *Dev Behav Pediatr* 2004;25:166–174.

70. Topolski TD, et al. Quality of life of adolescent males with attention deficit hyperactivity disorder. *J Atten Disord* 2004;7:163–173.

71. Escobar R, et al. Worse quality of life for children with newly diagnosed attention deficit/hyperactivity disorder, compared with asthmatic and healthy children. *Pediatrics* 2005;116:364–369.

72. Beck AT, Steer RA, Brown GK. *Beck Depression Inventory Manual.* San Antonio: The Psychological Corporation, 1996; 2nd edn.

73. Beck AT, et al. An inventory for measuring depression. *Arch Gen Psychiatry* 1961;4:561–571.

74. Jones JE, et al. Screening for major depression in epilepsy with common self-report depression inventories. *Epilepsia* 2005;46:731–735.

75. First MB, et al. *Structured Clinical Interview for DSM-IV-TR Axis I Disorders: Non-Patient Edition (SCI-I/NP-2/2001 Revision).* New York: Biometrics Research Department, 2001.

76. Sheehan DV, et al. The Mini-International Neuropsychiatric Interview (M.I.N.I.): the development and validation of a structured diagnostic psychiatric interview for DSM-IV and ICD-10. *J Clin Psychiatry* 1998;59(Suppl 20):22–33.

77. Radloff LS. The CES-D Scale: a self-report depression scale for research in the general population. *J Appl Psychol Measur* 1977;1:385–401.

78. Weissman MM, et al. Assessing depressive symptoms in five psychiatric populations: a validation study. *Am J Epidemiol* 1977;106:203–214.

79. Gilliam FG, et al. Rapid detection of major depression in epilepsy: a multicentre study. *Lancet Neurol* 2006;5:399–405.

80. Achenbach TM, Elderbrock CS. *Child Behavior Checklist.* Burlington: TM Achenbach, 1986.

81. Kovaks M. The Children's Depression Inventory (CDI). *Psychopharmacol Bull* 1985;21:605–620.

82. Matthews WS, Barabas G, Ferrari M. Emotional concomitants of childhood epilepsy. *Epilepsia* 1982; 23:671–681.

83. Ferrari M, Matthews WS, Barabas G. The family and the child with epilepsy. *Fam Process* 1983;22:53–59.

84. Sheeran T, Marvin RS, Pianta RC. Mothers' resolution of their child's diagnosis and self-reported measures of parenting stress, marital relations, and social support. *J Pediatr Psychol* 1997;22:197–212.

85. Marvin RS, Pianta RC. Mothers' reaction to their child's diagnosis: relations with security of attachment. *J Clin Child Psychol* 1996;25:436–445.

86. Dekovic M. Risk and protective factors in the development of problem behavior during adolescence. *J Youth Adolesc* 1999;28:667–685.

87. Raty L, Hamrin E, Soderfeldt B. Quality of life in newly debuted epilepsy. An empirical study. *Acta Neurol Scand* 1999;100:221–226.

88. Williams J, et al. Parental anxiety and quality of life in children with epilepsy. *Epilepsy Behav* 2003;4:483–486.

89. Yong L, Chengye J, Jiong Q. Factors affecting the quality of life in childhood epilepsy in China. *Acta Neurol Scand* 2006;113:167–173.

90. Cramer JA, et al. The influence of comorbid depression on quality of life for people with epilepsy. *Epilepsy Behav* 2003;4:515–521.

91. Hodes M, et al. Maternal expressed emotion and adjustment in children with epilepsy. *J Child Psychol Psychiatry* 1999;40:1083–1093.

92. Dunn DW, et al. Symptoms of depression in adolescents with epilepsy. *J Am Acad Child Adolesc Psychiatry* 1999;38:1133–1138.

93. Shore CP, et al. Identifying risk factors for maternal depression in families of adolescents with epilepsy. *J Specialists Pediatr Nurs* 2002;7:71–80.

94. Kokkonen J, et al. Psychosocial outcome of young adults with epilepsy in childhood. *J Neurol Neurosurg Psychiatry* 1997;62:265–268.

95. Caplan R, et al. Psychopathology and pediatric complex partial seizures: seizure-related, cognitive, and linguistic variables. *Epilepsia* 2004;45:1273–1281.

96. Meador KJ. Cognitive side effects of epilepsy and of antiepileptic medications. In: Wyllie E (ed), *The Treatment of Epilepsy: Principles and Practices.* Philadelphia: Lippincott Williams & Wilkins, 2005; 4th edn: pp. 1215–1226.

97. Matsuura M. Patient satisfaction with polypharmacy reduction in chronic epileptics. *Psychiatry Clin Neurosci* 2000;54:249–253.

98. Gilliam F, et al. Patient-validated content of epilepsy-specific quality-of-life measurements. *Epilepsia* 1997; 38:233–236.

99. Gilliam F, et al. Patient-oriented outcome assessment after temporal lobectomy for refractory epilepsy. *Neurology* 1999;53:687–694.

100. Fisher RS, et al. The impact of epilepsy from the patient's perspective II: views about therapy and health care. *Epilepsy Res* 2000;41:53–61.

101. Baker GA, Frances P, Middleton E. Initial development, reliability, and validity of a patient-based adverse events scale. *Epilepsia* 1994;35(Suppl 7):80.

102. Gilliam FG, et al. Systematic screening allows reduction of adverse antiepileptic drug effects. A randomized trial. *Neurology* 2004;62:23–27.

103. Farwell JR, et al. Phenobarbital for febrile seizures-effects on intelligence and on seizure recurrence. *N Engl J Med* 1990;322:364–369.

104. Loring DW, Meador KJ. Cognitive side effects of antiepileptic drugs in children. *Neurology* 2004;62:872–877.

105. Hanai T. Quality of life in children with epilepsy. *Epilepsia* 1996;37:28–32.

106. Sherman EM, Slick DJ, Eyrl KL. Executive dysfunction is a significant predictor of poor quality of life in children with epilepsy. *Epilepsia* 2006;47:1936–1942.

107. Kwan P, Brodie MJ. Early identification of refractory epilepsy. *N Engl J Med* 2000;342:314–319.

108. Dlugos DJ, et al. Response to first drug trial predicts outcome in childhood temporal lobe epilepsy. *Neurology* 2001;57:2259–2264.

109. Wiebe S, et al. A randomized, controlled trial of surgery for temporal lobe-epilepsy. *N Engl J Med* 2001;345:311–318.

110. Mohamed A, et al. Temporal lobe epilepsy due to hippocampal sclerosis in pediatric candidates for epilepsy surgery. *Neurology* 2001;56:1643–1649.

111. Wyllie E, et al. Seizure outcome alter epilepsy surgery in children and adolescents. *Ann Neurol* 1998;44:740–748.

112. Sabaz M, et al. The impact of epilepsy surgery on quality of life in children. *Neurology* 2006;66:557–561.

113. Arunkumar G, et al. Parent- and patient-validated content for pediatric epilepsy quality-of-life assessment. *Epilepsia* 2000;41:1474–1484.

114. Sherman EM, et al. Validity of three measures of health-related quality of life in children with intractable epilepsy. *Epilepsia* 2002;43:1230–1238.

115. Wirrell E, et al. Sleep disturbances in children with epilepsy compared to their nearest-aged siblings. *Dev Med Child Neurol* 2005;47:754–759.

116. Northcott E, et al. Memory and phonological awareness in children with Benign Rolandic Epilepsy compared to a matched control group. *Epilepsy Res* 2007;75:57–62.

117. Carpay H, et al. Disability due to restrictions in childhood epilepsy. *Dev Med Child Neurol* 1997;39:521–526.

118. van Empelen R, et al. Functional consequences of hemispherectomy. *Brain* 2004;127:2071–2079.

119. Gilliam F, et al. Epilepsy surgery outcome: comprehensive assessment in children. *Neurology* 1997;48:1368–1374.

120. Datta SS, et al. Impact of pediatric epilepsy on Indian families: influence of psychopathology and seizure-related variables. *Epilepsy Behav* 2006;9:145–151.

121. Turky A, et al. Psychopathology of children and adolescents with epilepsy: an investigation of predictive variables. *Epilepsy Behav* 2008;12:136–144.

SECTION IX

Medical, Dietary, and Nursing Treatment

CHAPTER 46

Medical and Surgical Treatment of Pediatric Epilepsy

Willem F. Arts

▶ OVERVIEW

Antiepileptic drugs (AEDs) are a treatment modality for the suppression of seizures. Medical therapy is usually the first option once it is established that seizures should be prevented. This is a worthwhile goal not only with a confirmed diagnosis of epilepsy but also when there is a clear indication to prevent further (acute symptomatic) seizures. Several possible indications for initiating AEDs will be discussed in this chapter.

The decision to start long-term AED treatment should never be undertaken by the treating physician alone as it requires exhaustive information and discussion with the parents, and—if the age and intelligence are appropriate—with the child. This discussion should consider the expected efficacy as well as the tolerability of treatment. The balance between possible benefit and risks will ultimately determine whether the child will be treated.

In established epilepsy, the benefit of the first AED will be seizure-freedom in about 50%, while the risks of (serious) adverse events or side effects is approximately 15%. The frequency and severity of the seizures as well as the prognosis of the particular epilepsy type should be taken into account. Therefore, the approach to AED therapy must be individualized as the patient's individual reaction to an AED is difficult to predict, both as regards seizure reduction as well as side effects. In this chapter, we will consider the possible indications to start an AED for the prevention of seizures.

▶ THE DECISION TO START AED TREATMENT

The clearest indication for initiating AED maintenance therapy is the proven recurrence of epileptic seizures. The diagnosis of epilepsy should be firmly established through clinical signs while the characteristic EEG features help confirm the type of epilepsy.

However, there are other situations where AEDs are advocated when the diagnosis of epilepsy is questionable or where seizures have been provoked acutely. Figures 46–1 to 46–4 review the various situations that invite consideration of the use of AED therapy to prevent (further) seizures. Each is briefly discussed.

STARTING AEDS FOR CONFIRMED SEIZURES OR EPILEPSY

The current belief is that AEDs suppress seizures, but do not heal the epilepsy. Gower's paradigm ("Seizures beget seizures") was formerly popular, and AEDs were thought to prevent intractable epilepsy.[1,2] It is now understood that medical intractability is not based on the number or severity of seizures but on the nature of the underlying neurological disorder.[3] Others[4] could not confirm that a decreasing interval between seizures facilitates further seizures.

From a clinical standpoint, the course of the epilepsy is favorable if it remits spontaneously and unfavorable if severe underlying disease or conventional medical suppression of seizures are insufficient to prevent intractability.[3,5] In the latter situation, epilepsy can be considered a "progressive" disorder. However, this situation is highly variable as the course of epilepsy may change during long-term follow-up.[6]

Currently, the decision to start AED therapy is based on the goal of suppressing seizures because their number, severity, etiology, and other variables unfavorably influence long-term prognosis.[6,7] In children, the influence of seizures and accompanying epileptic discharges on cognitive development is also an important consideration.

AEDs FOR SEIZURE PROPHYLAXIS

AED Prophylaxis for Febrile Seizures

The morbidity and mortality of febrile seizures is generally low, and the risk of future epilepsy is only slightly increased as compared to the general population. A history of complex febrile seizures will significantly increase the risk of future epilepsy. Complex febrile seizures are defined by prolonged duration, focal onset, or one or more recurrences during the same febrile period. Antipyretic drugs administered during the fever do not prevent febrile seizure recurrence.[8]

Current consensus holds that it is not useful to start maintenance therapy with AEDs after multiple simple febrile seizures, because medication does not reduce the risk of subsequent epilepsy.[9] Phenobarbital and sodium valproate reduce febrile seizure recurrence, but are associated with considerable side effects. Febrile seizure recurrence is preferably prevented with intermittent diazepam or clobazam prophylaxis during the period of fever (Fig. 46–1).

Oral benzodiazepines have been shown to significantly lower the risk of febrile seizure recurrence.[10–13]

Acute Neurological Disorders or Neurosurgical Procedures

Certain acute or subacute neurologic disorders promote the development of acute symptomatic seizures. Examples include brain trauma, meningitis or encephalitis, stroke, intracerebral and subarachnoid hemorrhage, and intracranial neurosurgical procedures. AEDs are employed to prevent seizures or status epilepticus (Fig. 46–2). However, careful studies and meta-analyses reveal that prophylactic long-term AED treatment does not prevent late symptomatic epilepsy.[14,15] Current guidelines state that AED prophylaxis is only indicated for a period of 1 week after onset of the disease, trauma, or neurosurgical procedure. The routine use of AEDs after 1 week is not recommended to prevent late symptomatic seizures (epilepsy).[16]

Most neonatal seizures are also acutely symptomatic. Treatment starts with phenobarbital, followed by other drugs if initial treatment is unsuccessful. AED treatment is indicated in the acute stage only.

Prophylaxis After a Single Unprovoked Paroxysmal Event

Prescribing an AED after a single epileptic seizure is of limited benefit. The AAN Practice Parameter[17] states that AED treatment is not indicated to prevent epilepsy, and that treatment to reduce the risk of further seizures is indicated only when the expected benefits outweigh potential side effects. Studies in adults demonstrate that the end results of the treated and untreated groups are similar for terminal remission.[18] Even if status epilepticus occurs as a solitary seizure, the prognosis for terminal remission is unaltered at long-term follow-up, and should not influence the decision to wait and see rather than initiate AED treatment.

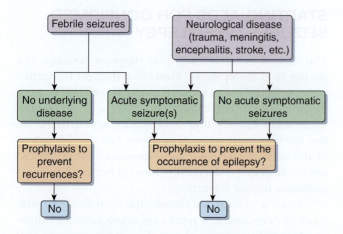

Figure 46–1. Prophylaxis after acute symptomatic seizures or acute neurological insult?

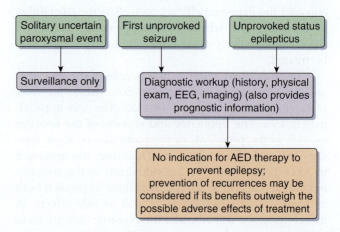

Figure 46–2. Prophylaxis after a single unprovoked paroxysmal event?

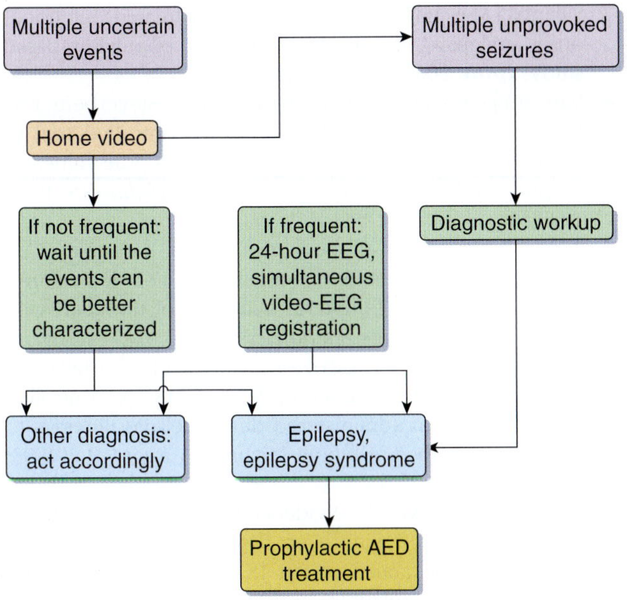

Figure 46–3. Prophylaxis after multiple paroxysmal events?

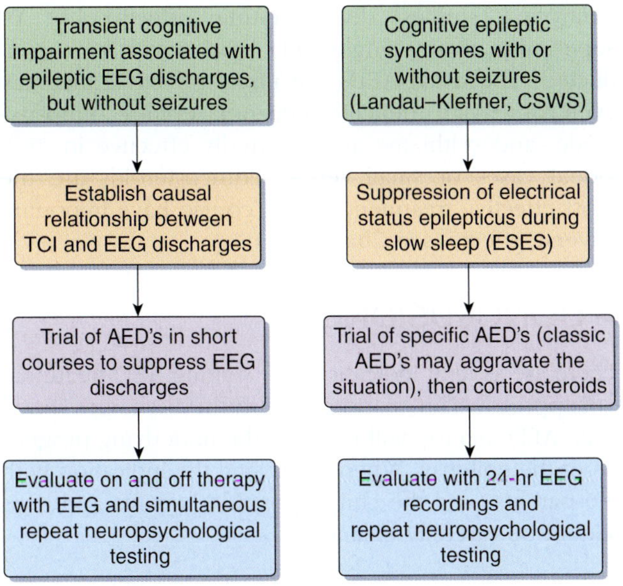

Figure 46–4. AED treatment in epileptic conditions with mainly cognitive effects.

Multiple Paroxysmal Events

After a proven diagnosis of epileptic seizures, prophylactic AED therapy is warranted in most cases. As outlined earlier, AED treatment is directed toward preventing further seizures or status epilepticus, and cannot alleviate the underlying epilepsy or prevent intractability.[5] However, seizures in many benign epilepsy syndromes are rarely harmful, occur only rarely or both. In these cases, maintenance therapy may not be necessary (Fig. 46–3). In cases of benign partial epilepsy with rolandic spikes (BPERS) and children with rare generalized tonic–clonic seizures consideration may be given to withholding therapy. Other benign syndromes including benign myoclonic epilepsy of infancy or the most benign variant of childhood absence seizures usually need only a short course of treatment to induce remission, or initially may be indistinguishable from more serious variants, and must be treated for that reason.

Multiple events, whose epileptic nature cannot be proven with certainty, should be approached independently. If their frequency is too low, they cannot be captured on long-term EEG or video-EEG monitoring. One may ask the parents for a home video, and otherwise, it is best to withhold treatment. If events occur more frequently, it is best to record them to prove or disprove the diagnosis of epilepsy. AEDs should never be used as a means to confirm a diagnosis. Neither the sensitivity nor the specificity of such a diagnostic trial is sufficient to establish the nature of paroxysmal events.

AEDs TO PREVENT COGNITIVE IMPAIRMENT WITH CONCOMITANT EPILEPTIC EEG DISCHARGES

As illustrated in Figure 46–4, two distinctly different cognitive issues must be differentiated—Transient Cognitive Impairment (TCI) associated with interictal epileptic EEG discharges in the absence of seizures and the occurrence of Continuous Spike-Waves during slow Sleep (CSWS) associated with language, cognitive, or even behavioral deterioration. Language deterioration in this context is termed Acquired Epileptic Aphasia or Landau–Kleffner syndrome (see Chapter 18).

It may be hard to prove a definite relation between TCI and cognitive problems and EEG abnormalities. A careful approach is in order beginning with an initial period of monitoring the course of the child's cognitive abilities. If stagnation or regression is clearly evident after a few weeks to months of observation, a carefully conducted therapeutic trial should be conducted. Evaluation by EEG and standardized neuropsychological test procedures before and during therapy is required. Various drugs can be tried in short periods successively as there are no studies proving the benefit of one AED over another or the clear superiority of a single agent. If a relation between the clinical signs and the EEG abnormalities cannot be established, and the child has no seizures, AED therapy should not be started.

AED therapy is definitely indicated in Landau–Kleffner or CSWS syndrome even without clinically manifest seizures. The goal is to suppress the electrical status epilepticus during slow sleep (ESES). However, controlled studies demonstrating effectiveness or superiority of any single AED have never been conducted. The usual AEDs are rarely effective and may even aggravate deficits; benzodiazepines, ethosuximide, and sulthiame are reportedly effective in individual cases or small series. Corticosteroids are the most effective treatment, but of course have important adverse effects (see Chapter 18).

► CONCLUSIONS

There are several indications for starting AED treatment to suppress seizures and epileptiform discharges; however, AED therapy will not alter the underlying prognosis of the epilepsy. When discussing the indication with the parents (and the child), possible benefits and risks should be carefully balanced.

REFERENCES

1. Reynolds EH, Elwes RDC, Shorvon SD. Why does epilepsy become intractable? *Lancet* 1983;II:952–954.
2. Elwes RDC, Johnson AL, Reynolds EH. The course of untreated epilepsy. *BMJ* 1988;297:948–950.
3. Berg AT, Shinnar S. Do seizures beget seizures? An assessment of the clinical evidence in humans. *J Clin Neurophysiol* 1997;14:102–110.
4. Van Donselaar CA, Brouwer OF, Geerts AT, Arts WFM, Stroink H, Peters ACB. Clinical course of untreated tonic-clonic seizures in childhood: prospective, longitudinal study. *BMJ* 1997;314:401–404.
5. Shinnar S, Berg AT. Does antiepileptic drug therapy alter the prognosis of childhood seizures and prevent the development of chronic epilepsy? *Semin Pediatr Neurol* 1994;1:111–117.
6. Arts WF, Brouwer OF, Peters AC, Stroink H, Peeters EA, Schmitz PI, Van Donselaar CA, Geerts AT. Course and prognosis of childhood epilepsy: 5-year follow-up of the Dutch study of epilepsy in childhood. *Brain* 2004;127:1774–1784.
7. Sillanpää M, Schmidt D. Natural history of treated childhood-onset epilepsy: prospective, long-term population-based study. *Brain* 2006;129:617–624.
8. Van Stuijvenberg M, Derksen-Lubsen A, Steyerberg EW, Habbema JD, Moll HA. Randomized, controlled trial of ibuprofen syrup administered during febrile illnesses to prevent febrile seizure recurrences. *Pediatrics* 1998; 102:E51.
9. American Academy of Pediatrics (AAP). Committee on Quality Improvement, Subcommittee on Febrile Seizures. Practice Parameter: long-term treatment of the child with simple febrile seizures. *Pediatrics* 1999;103:1307–1309.
10. Rosman NP, Colton T, Labazzo J, Gilbert PL, Gardella NB, Kaye EM, Van Bennekom C, Winter MR. A controlled trial of diazepam administered during febrile illnesses to prevent recurrence of febrile seizures. *N Engl J Med* 1993; 329:79–84.
11. Offringa M, Moyer V. Evidence-based management of seizures associated with fever. *BMJ* 2001;323:1111–1114.
12. Rose W, Kirubakaran C, Scott JX. Intermittent clobazam therapy in febrile seizures. *Indian J Pediatr* 2005;72:31–33.
13. Pavlidou E, Tzitiridou M, Panteliadis C. Effectiveness of intermittent diazepam prophylaxis in febrile seizures: long-term prospective controlled study. *J Child Neurol* 2006;21:1036–1040.
14. Temkin NR. Anti-epileptogenesis and seizure prevention trials with antiepileptic drugs: meta-analysis of controlled trials. *Epilepsia* 2001;42:515–524.
15. Temkin NR. Prophylactic anticonvulsants after neurosurgery. *Epilepsy Curr* 2002;2:105–107.
16. Glantz MJ, Cole BF, Forsyth PA, Recht LD, Wen PY, Chamberlain MC, Grossman SA, Cairncross JG. Practice parameter: anticonvulsant prophylaxis in patients with newly diagnosed brain tumors. *Neurology* 2000;54:1886–1893.
17. Hirtz D, Berg A, Bettis D, Camfield C, Camfield P, Crumrine P, Gaillard WD, Schneider S, Shinnar S. Practice parameter: treatment of the child with a first unprovoked seizure. *Neurology* 2003;60:166–175.
18. Musicco M, Beghi E, Solari A, Viani F. Treatment of first tonic-clonic seizure does not improve the prognosis of epilepsy. First Seizure Trial Group (FIRST Group). *Neurology* 1997;49:991–998.

CHAPTER 47

Antiepileptic Drugs: How to Choose

John M. Pellock

Following the diagnosis of epilepsy and making the decision to start a treatment, as discussed in the prior chapter, the clinician must choose the most appropriate initial medication. This decision requires knowledge of the clinical pharmacology of medications used for the treatment of epilepsy and an ability to individualize treatment to the child in question.[1] The ultimate goal is complete control of seizures without producing adverse effects. Although the perfect drug does not exist, the current therapeutic armamentarium offers a broader range of choices than available ever before with each drug having some advantages and disadvantages. A single drug should be chosen so that the child is treated with monotherapy, which has the likelihood of producing the fewest number of side effects.[2,3] The first issue in deciding upon initial therapy depends on seizure type. An appreciation of epilepsy syndrome is also extremely important, as it may select for or against an agent and may exacerbate seizure types, which have not been yet appreciated in the child.

Besides the expected efficacy of the medication for the seizure type(s), other important aspects that must be considered in children with epilepsy include the spectrum of toxicity, side effects, likelihood of compliance, ease of administration, and the potential for additional side effects following long-term therapy, if prolonged treatment is thought to be probable. Besides possible immediate age-specific organ toxicities, potential side effects affecting cognition and behavior must be considered. Effects upon daily activity such as sleeping, eating, and behavior are of most concern to caregivers, but the potential for developing rare but life-threatening adverse effects must be carefully reviewed and appropriately discussed.

▶ FINDING THE DRUG OF CHOICE

Following the establishment of the need to treat and having a clear description of seizure type, the clinician and caregiver should together decide upon initial therapy. The clinician advising the family regarding antiepileptic drug (AED) use will frequently recommend an agent that is comfortable.

This comfort comes from prior experience in prescribing the medication, recommendations of experts and peers derived from multiple types of studies. For some, randomized clinical trials (RCTs) offer the strongest evidence concerning which AEDs should be selected as first line.

THE ROLE OF CLINICAL TRIALS IN CHOOSING A DRUG

RCTs of AEDs applicable to treatment of children with epilepsy are performed only following studies in adults with refractory partial seizures. Pediatric partial seizure trials are initiated and then recommendations follow. Specialized studies in children with the Lennox–Gastaut syndrome and childhood absence epilepsy have only recently generated specific recommendations for the use of AEDs in these disorders.[1] Thus, the timing of the performance and reporting of the most rigorous type of studies applicable to the treatment of children with epilepsy may be substantially delayed following the approval and introduction of a newer AED. A discussion of clinical trials versus antedoctal reports is presented in subsequent chapters. Nevertheless, many AEDs are never formally studied in specific childhood epilepsy syndromes because of significant procedural difficulties in conducting these studies, particularly in infants and young children with relatively uncommon syndromes.

The clinician must therefore balance the importance of RCTs, comparative studies, and expert opinion with their own experience when individualizing to selecting the drug of choice for a specific child. Thus, effectiveness rather than pure efficacy is a guiding principle of AED treatment.

Classic studies demonstrated a near equipoise in the treatment of convulsive pediatric epilepsy with phenobarbital, carbamazepine, phenytoin, and valproate; however, the intolerability of barbiturates was quickly identified as other agents became available; phenobarbital became a second-line medication because of its lack of tolerability, rather than its efficacy.[4]

▶ THE ROLE OF RECOMMENDATIONS AND GUIDELINES IN CHOOSING A DRUG

Various authoritative agencies recommended approval for the use of newer AEDs, such as lamotrigine,

▶ **TABLE 47-1. COMPARISON OF RECOMMENDATIONS FOR THE TREATMENT OF PEDIATRIC EPILEPSY**

Seizure Type or Epilepsy Syndrome	Pediatric Expert Consensus Survey	ILAE	SIGN	NICE	French Study	FDA Approved
Partial onset	OXC, CBZ	A: OXC B: None C: CBZ, PB, PHT, TPM, VPA	PHT, VPA, CBZ, LTG, TPM, OXC, VGB, CLB	CBZ, VPA, LTG, OXC, TPM	OXC, CBZ, LTG (adult males)	PB. PHT, CBZ, OXC, TPM
Benign epilepsy of childhood with centrotemporal spikes	OXC, CBZ	A, B: None C: CBZ, VPA	Not specifically mentioned	CBZ, OXC, LTG, VPA	Not surveyed	None
Childhood absence epilepsy	ESM	A, B: None C: ESM, CBZ, VPA	VPA, ESM, LTG	VPA, ESM, LTG	VPA, LTG	ESM, VPA, LTG[a]
Juvenile myoclonic epilepsy	VPA, LTG	A, B, C: None	VPA, LTG, TPM	VPA, LTG	VAP, LTG	TPM, LEV[a]
Lennox–Gastaut syndrome	VPA, TPM, LTG	Not reviewed	Not specifically mentioned	LTG, VPA, TPM	Not surveyed	FLB, TPM, LTG, RFM, CLB

Source: Modified from Wheless JW, Clarke DF, Carpenter D. Treatment of pediatric epilepsy: expert opinion, 2005. *J Child Neurol* 2005;20:S1–S56.
CBZ, carbamazepine; CLB, clobazam; ESM, ethosuximide; FLB, felbamate; LTG, lamotrigine; OXC, oxcarbazepine; PB, phenobarbital; PHT, phenytoin; RFM, rufinamide; TPM, topiramate; VPA, valproate; VGB, vigabatrin; LEV, levetiracetam.
[a]Recently approved after publication cited.

oxcarbazepine, topiramate, and levetiracetam for partial onset seizures and lamotrigine has been added to prior approvals of ethosuximide and valproate for absence epilepsy.[1] Topiramate and levetiracetam have recently been approved to treat primary generalized epilepsy, primarily based on trials involving patients with juvenile myoclonic epilepsy. Felbamate, topiramate, and lamotrigine have proven efficacious for seizures associated with Lennox–Gastaut syndrome in well-controlled RCTs.[1]

The case of infantile spasms demonstrates the difficulties in doing large trials in a relatively rare disorder. Following extensive review, the American Academy of Neurology has published a guideline establishing ACTH as probably effective and vigabatrin as possibly effective for the treatment of this encephalopathic epilepsy despite significant side effects of both agents. Although other AEDs including valproate, topiramate, and zonisamide may be efficacious in some children with infantile spasms, the published studies are frequently too small to allow establishing definitive guidelines.[5]

Recommendations from the National Institutes of Clinical Excellence[6] state that the newer AEDs including gabapentin, lamotrigine, oxcarbazepine, tiagabine, topiramate, and vigabatrin are recommended for epilepsy management in children when used within their licensed indications and in children who have not benefited from treatment with older agents such as

carbamazepine or valproate, or in those for whom the more established AEDs were inappropriate. Within the NICE Guidelines, vigabatrin is recommended as first-line therapy for infantile spasms. Other recommendations are given in Table 47–1. Expert opinion surveys performed using similar methodology have recently been published.[7–9] Through these clinically based expert surveys, it becomes obvious that certain AEDs such as carbamazepine, oxcarbazepine, and valproate are well-established agents and are utilized widely despite their potential adverse effects. These consensus surveys also demonstrate that the newer agents such as lamotrigine, topiramate, and levetiracetam have become somewhat more popular over time.

Valproate remains the treatment of choice for Lennox–Gastaut syndrome with topiramate and lamotrigine also first line. For the acute treatment of prolonged seizures (with or without fever) and clusters of seizures rectal diazepam was most preferred. For benign childhood epilepsy with centrotemporal spikes (BECTS), oxcarbazepine and carbamazepine were treatments of choice with gabapentin, lamotrigine, and levetiracetam also first line. Ethosuximide was rated as the first choice for childhood absence epilepsy, with valproate and lamotrigine also first line. For juvenile absence epilepsy, valproate and lamotrigine were treatments of choice. For juvenile myoclonic epilepsy in adolescent males, valproate and lamotrigine were preferred with topiramate also being first line, whereas in adolescent females lamotrigine was favored with topiramate and valproate other first-line options. First-line treatment for neonatal status epilepticus was intravenous phenobarbital, with lorazepam, and fosphenytoin also first line. Valproate was more commonly recommended by experts internationally as first-line therapy than in the United States.[10]

Levetiracetam use has recently grown in popularity in the United States. It is also apparent from the expert consensus surveys that gender dictates a significant difference in the choice of antiepileptic drug; valproate is less frequently acceptable to clinicians for the treatment of girls nearing puberty or women of childbearing age because of its potential for teratogenic effects. Although differences exist, expert opinion surveys and guidelines significantly overlap (Table 47–1). Pediatric epileptologists while awaiting formal controlled studies, extrapolate results from studies of adult refractory epilepsy and seemingly add to this foundation from various sources.[4] Many licensing authorities require pediatric pharmacokinetic data as part of submission, allowing some data concerning dosing, even before definitive childhood epilepsy studies are complete.[4]

NEGOTIATED CHOICE

Thus, the physician treating epilepsy must frequently go beyond guidelines and expert opinion when recommending which AED to begin. Clinical experience, expertise, depth of knowledge, and discussing all possibilities with caregivers will guide the decision regarding the choice of the initial and subsequent preferred AED. Existing comorbidities and considerations of potential adverse effects frequently lead to the decision for or against particular agents. These comorbidities exist in over 50% of children in epilepsy, either as etiologic factors for the epilepsy itself or as part of the total medical history, age, gender, and life situation of the child. Possible comorbidities are listed in Table 47–2.

It is important to determine all coexisting medical and behavioral characteristics of the patient prior to the administration of an AED. A careful history recording past adverse reactions to previously prescribed medications must be established, be they AEDs or others, especially for idiosyncratic reactions such as rash and hypersensitivity reactions, as some are genetically predisposed. More frequently, a worsening of the symptom over time is interpreted to be the result of AED therapy versus part of the natural course of the disorder.

SPECIAL CONSIDERATIONS IN CHOOSING A DRUG

As noted previously, women, infants, elderly, and all those with associated medical/psychiatric illness require special considerations when treating their epilepsy.

▶ **TABLE 47–2. COMORBIDITIES OF EPILEPSY**

• Renal	• Stroke
• Hepatic	• Anoxic ischemic encephalopathy
• Connective tissue	• Endocrine/reproductive
• Cardiac/cerebrovascular	• Infection/immunizations
• Immunodeficiency (HIV)	• Degenerative/dementia
• ETOH and drugs	• Trauma
• Pulmonary	• Migraine
• Metabolic abnormalities	• Behavioral/psychiatric
• Glucose, Na Ca	• Mental retardation
	• Depression
• Bone	• ADHD
• Cerebral palsy	

Source: From Pellock JM. Bridging the gap between clinical guidelines and individualized patient treatment. In: Ryvlin P, Beghi E, Camfield P, Hesdorffer D (eds), *Progress in Epileptic Disorders. From First Unprovoked Seizure to Newly Diagnosed Epilepsy, Volume 3.* France: John Libbey Eurotext, 2007.

Even in young girls, many physicians will not prescribe medication which may potentiate adverse effects during puberty or thereafter. Teratogenic and hormonal considerations play a large part in the choice of anticonvulsant medications. Birth control hormonal preparations may be affected by enzyme inducing AEDs and only recently has the interaction between hormonal therapy and lamotrigine clearance been appreciated.[11] Teratogenesis and effects upon the unborn require using medications with less risk. The potential for *in-utero* exposure to valproate and other AEDs leading to possible negative cognitive consequences in children in women with epilepsy add to this dilemma.[12] In children, adolescents, and young adults, bone health may be significantly affected by AEDs, especially enzyme inducers such as carbamazepine, phenytoin, and phenobarbital. In young children where these drugs are most often prescribed, the potential for affecting primary bone development may be the highest.[13,14]

Although it is sometimes difficult to separate the cognitive and behavioral effects of epilepsy itself from those of prescribed AEDs, both positive and negative changes are frequently reported.[15] The prior development of adverse psychiatric events may well define a higher risk population.[15] Furthermore, investigational studies suggest that classic AEDs used to treat neonatal seizures might actually promote apoptosis,[16] but alternatives are not currently accepted. As noted previously, young infants may undergo an evolution of their epilepsy such that the initial medication may actually aggravate other seizure types[17] as a child evolves to other syndromes (Table 47–3). Frequent reevaluation may be necessary to ascertain that the seizure manifestations remain constant and that other activity does not represent seizures. Children with comorbid

▶ **TABLE 47–3.** AGGRAVATION OF SEIZURES OR EPILEPSY SYNDROMES

Seizures/Syndrome	CBZ	PHT	LTG	GBP	VGB	TGB	BDZ
Absence seizures	X	X		X	X	X	
Myoclonic seizures	X	X	X	X	X		
JME	X	X	X				
LGS/MAE	X	X	X	X	X		X
BECTS	X		X				
SMEI	X		X		X		
LKS/ESES	X	X					
Unverricht–Lundborg disease	X						

Source: From Sazgar M, Bourgeois BF. Aggravation of epilepsy by antiepileptic drugs. *Pediatr Neurol* 2005;33(4):227–234.
CBZ, carbamazepine; PHT, phenytoin; LTG, lamotrigine; GBP, gabapentin; VGB, vigabatrin; TGB, tiagabine; BDZ, benzodiazepine; JME, Juvenile myoclonic epilepsy; LGS, Lennox–Gastaut syndrome; MAE, myoclonic astatic epilepsy; BECTS, Benign epilepsy of childhood with centrotemporal spikes; SMEI, severe myoclonic epilepsy of infancy; LKS, Landau–Kleffner syndrome; ESES, electrical status epilepticus of sleep.

cerebral palsy, intellectual disability, and psychiatric diagnosis may require multiple medications, which may significantly affect the pharmacokinetics and pharmacodynamics of prescribed AEDs. In children receiving chemotherapy for neoplastic disease, nonenzyme inducing AED should be prescribed whenever possible.

▶ MONITORING AFTER FIRST CHOICE DRUG GIVEN

During initiation of medication, the physician will frequently need to titrate medication to a specified chronic dose. With some medications, titration is slow because of the potential for systemic complication, such as lamotrigine-associated rash. With other AEDs, a slower titration leads to better tolerability with a decrease of gastrointestinal effects or neurotoxicity. Extended release formulations may offer specific advantage for some children in reducing both gastrointestinal and neurotoxicity. During the titration phase, physicians should carefully discuss a plan for seizure emergencies or recurrence when medications are not yet established at the appropriate dosing. Even after an appropriate dose of medication is established, seizure emergencies should be discussed with caregivers of children with epilepsy. Appropriate and rapid treatment for prolonged seizure clusters occurring out of hospital is now the standard.[18] Patients with brief seizures or nonconvulsive events are at lower risk, whereas those who present with initial clusters or prolonged seizures are at greater risk for recurrences requiring emergency intervention.

▶ APPROACH TO TREATMENT

Once the decision has been made to treat a child with epilepsy, the physician and caregivers must weigh the risks and benefits of using a medication and choose the agent most likely to render the patient seizure free while producing little or the least toxicity. Counseling and discussion with patient and caregivers should determine the preferred agent, which is presumed to hold the best promise for tolerability and effectiveness. Seizure type, epilepsy syndrome, and comorbidities are all weighed and establish not only the AEDs most appropriate but also those least likely to exacerbate associated comorbidities or seizure types as yet unappreciated. The general approach for appropriate medications for partial and generalized seizures is shown in Figure 47–1.

Initially, the first medication is chosen because of its presumptive efficacy against a particular identified seizure type, partial or generalized at onset.[1,4] The identification of the entire epilepsy syndrome as early on as possible may aid in outlining the treatment plan in regard to likelihood of prolonged versus a briefer period of treatment, as discussed in other chapters. It is of utmost importance to involve the patient and family in discussion of which drug is to be initiated and for how long. They must clearly understand risk versus benefit. This understanding will allow the medical team to establish a meaningful rapport and devise plans for potential adverse effects, both life threatening and less serious. Identifying symptoms associated with potentially life-threatening adverse reactions is extremely important as there is rarely only one drug of choice for the treatment of each patient.

Discussion of available information regarding efficacy and its application to the child's diagnosis is usually followed by delineation of the AED's potential for side effects. Behavior, cognition, sleep, and weight issues are usually of primary concern. As noted earlier, patients on multiple medications with comorbid diagnoses must have careful consideration given to drug interactions and potential to lead to further difficulties as non-AEDs are added or deleted from the therapeutic mix. Lastly, those with suspected refractory epilepsy must have a careful review of all previously administered medications. For patients taking multiple medications, reduction of agents and simplifying dosing may

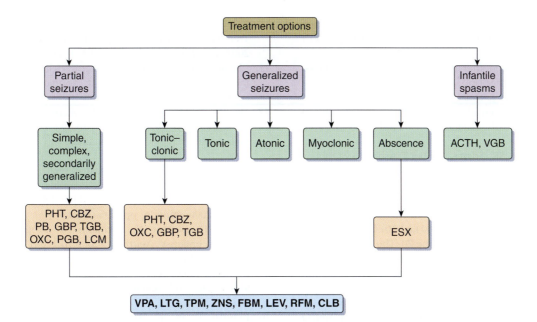

Figure 47–1. Clinical utility of established and newer AEDs. (Modified from Pellock JM. *Epilepsy in patients with multiple handicaps.* In: Wylie E (ed), *The Treatment of Epilepsy: Principles and Practice.* Philadelphia: Wolters Kluwer/LWW, 2011; 5th edn: pp. 451–457.)

best lead to success while moving toward a potentially more appropriate regimen. An important question for the family is if any previous AED worked better than others. The response may determine the choice of the next medication or even reinstitution of a previously used AED. Although it may be said that a drug has failed, careful questioning may uncover an inappropriate dose, too rapid titration, or even administration while other drugs were being changed, so that a clear picture of its efficacy and side-effect profile is not possible. Reevaluation with imaging and surgical consideration may yield important information. AED polytherapy is of limited utility over monotherapy in most patients. Moreover, rescue medication must be given judiciously and not become chronic. The removal of sedating medications or those producing aberrant behavior will lead to an overall improvement in the child with epilepsy.

▶ CONCLUSION

The choice of the best AED for each patient requires the balance of knowledge of AED pharmacology and the art of the practice of medicine. One takes all available information concerning medications and the epilepsy in the patient. A discussion or risk and benefit of treatment follows with the family and caregiver, so that a unified decision is established. Furthermore, this discussion leads to a practical plan for medication administration, usually dosing no more than twice daily whenever possible. Adversity encountered as side effect or lack of complete efficacy is not uncommon. Thus, outlining the steps for the plan and alternative adjustments or a true change in therapy is best performed at the initiation of therapy. In some, this plan will be reviewed frequently, whereas in others it is rarely discussed, usually regarding medication discontinuation. The patient should be given or referred to information to help guide the decisions and further care. This information should be in regards to epilepsy itself and the various treatments for the child's seizures. As noted earlier, a plan for seizure emergencies and lifestyle should also be discussed. Depending upon the child's age and ability to take part in the discussion regarding choice of medication, the family and physician may truly be surprised at their first choice medication. This discussion with the patient and caregivers is the single most important aspect in determining ongoing compliance and is the most helpful step in aiding the clinician in choosing the proper first choice of therapy. Individualization of epilepsy treatment occurs when careful consideration is given to the entirety of the child's needs and wishes and a meaningful agreement is reached. No AED is perfect for every patient, but preferred therapy can be established and followed. The goal of the treater and the child is the same: no seizures, no side effects.

REFERENCES

1. Pellock JM. Bridging the gap between clinical guidelines and individualized patient treatment. In: Ryvlin P, Beghi E, Camfield P, Hesdorffer D (eds), *Progress in Epileptic Disorders. From First Unprovoked Seizure to Newly Diagnosed Epilepsy.* France: John Libbey Eurotext, 2007.

2. Sachdeo MD. The evidence-based rationale for monotherapy in appropriate patients with epilepsy. *Neurology* 2007; 69(Suppl 3):S1–S2.

3. Wilfong MD. Monotherapy in children and infants. *Neurology* 2007;69(Suppl 3):S17–S22.

4. Pellock JM, Nordli J, Dulac O. Drug treatment in children with epilepsy. In: Engel J, Pedley TA (eds), *Epilepsy: A Comprehensive Textbook*. Philadelphia: LWW, 2008; 2nd edn: pp. 1249–1258.

5. Mckay MT, Weiss SK, Adams-Webber T, Ashwal S, Stephens D, Ballaban-Gill K, Baram TZ, Duchowny M, Hirtz D, Pellock JM, Shields WD, Shinnar S, Wyllie E, Snead III OC. Practice parameter: medical treatment of infantile spasms. Report of the American Academy of Neurology and Child Neurology Society. *Neurology* 2004;62(10):1668–1681.

6. NICE Guidelines. Clinical guideline 20. The epilepsies: the diagnosis and management of the epilepsies in adults and children in primary and secondary care. www.nice.org. uk/CGO20NICEguideline, 2004.

7. Wheless JW, Clarke DF, Carpenter D. Treatment of pediatric epilepsy: expert opinion, 2005. *J Child Neurol* 2005;20:S1–S56.

8. Karceski S, Morrell M, Carpenter D. The expert consensus guideline series: treatment of epilepsy. *Epilepsy Behav* 2001;2(Suppl):A1–A50.

9. Karceski S, Morrell MJ, Carpenter D. Treatment of epilepsy in adults: expert opinion, 2005. *Epilepsy Behav* 2005;7(Suppl 1):S1–S64.

10. Wheless JW, Clarke DF, Arzimaniglou A, Carpenter D. Treatment of pediatric epilepsy: European expert opinion, 2007. *Epileptic Disorders* 2007;9:353–412.

11. Christensen J, et al. Oral contraceptives induce lamotrigine metabolism: evidence from a double-blind, placebo-controlled trial. *Epilepsia* 2007;48:484–489.

12. Meador KJ. Cognitive effects of epilepsy and antiepileptic medications. In: Wyllie E (ed), *The Treatment of Epilepsy*. Philadelphia: Lippincott-Raven, 2006; 4th edn: pp. 1185–1196.

13. Morrell MJ. Hormones, catamenial epilepsy and reproductive and bone health in epilepsy. In: Wyllie E (ed), *The Treatment of Epilepsy*. Philadelphia: Lippincott-Raven, 2006; 4th edn: pp. 695–704.

14. Sheth RD, Binkley N, Hermann BP. Progressive bone deficit in epilepsy. *Neurology* 2008;70:170–176.

15. Mula M, Trimble MR, Sander JW. Are psychiatric adverse events of antiepileptic drugs a unique entity? A study on topiramate and levetiracetam. *Epilepsia* 2007;48:2322–2326.

16. Bittigau P, et al. Antiepileptic drugs and apoptotic neurodegeneration in the developing brain. *Proc Natl Acad Sci USA* 2002;99:15089–15094.

17. Sazgar M, Bourgeois BF. Aggravation of epilepsy by antiepileptic drugs. *Pediatr Neurol* 2005;33:227–234.

18. Pellock JM, Shinnar S. Conclusion: having a plan to manage seizure emergencies. *J Child Neurol* 2007;22(Suppl 5):S71–S73.

CHAPTER 48

Antiepileptic Drug Follow-up and Withdrawal

James W. Wheless

▶ OVERVIEW

The aim of epilepsy treatment is cessation of seizures without side effects. In the course of treating the child, the family should be informed, based on their level of medical sophistication, about choices of treatment and options for dealing with the condition and its consequences. Both seizures and therapies carry risks and optimal patient care requires thoughtful balancing of these risks and benefits. To provide the best care, the physician must be aware of the available options and individualize them to the needs of the specific child (see Chapter 2).

The goals of treatment will differ considerably depending upon the severity of the epilepsy syndrome. Many childhood epilepsies are easily controlled with modest doses of medication (i.e., childhood absence epilepsy, benign epilepsy with centrotemporal spikes, and idiopathic generalized epilepsies). For these children, selecting a treatment that has no major adverse effects, yet produces seizure control in a convenient manner is a reasonable goal. Contrasted to this are children with severe forms of epilepsy, often with multiple seizure types and pharmacoresistant seizures (i.e., infantile spasms, Lennox–Gastaut syndrome and symptomatic partial onset epilepsies). For these disorders, selecting a treatment with an elevated risk–benefit ratio may be acceptable to gain improvement in seizure control. Additionally, in this group considerations of all therapeutic options should be undertaken. Finally, realistic goals for seizure control should be balanced with chronic medication side effects (especially sedation). The management of epilepsy should be conceived as a global therapeutic strategy applied to an individual child. This chapter will provide general recommendations for antiepileptic drug (AED) follow-up and withdrawal, which the physician must individualize for each child by forming a therapeutic alliance with the family.

▶ AED FOLLOW-UP

ENSURING THAT A CHOSEN DRUG IS EFFECTIVE

Treatment should always be initiated with a single antiepileptic drug and the dose slowly increased until the seizures are controlled or until clinical toxicity occurs.

Antiepileptic drugs should never be stopped abruptly unless a serious adverse event occurs (i.e., rash).

Only one in five children with epilepsy will have "smooth sailing epilepsy" (i.e., they start on an antiepileptic drug, become instantly seizure-free, and eventually come off medication and remain in remission). However, an additional 40% of children will become seizure-free with the first antiepileptic drug, after some dose adjustment to deal with subsequent seizures.[1] In general, the first antiepileptic drug will eventually be successful in controlling the seizures in 50%–70% of children. Antiepileptic drug therapy should be assessed in light of the epilepsy syndrome and a risk-to-benefit profile established when considering the various antiepileptic drugs. Initiation of antiepileptic therapy should be done with a realization that about half of the time the initial antiepileptic drug will be changed. As a result, compatibility of the initial antiepileptic drug with future antiepileptic drugs should be considered when initial therapy is begun. If monotherapy fails, and a combination of antiepileptic drugs is used, then drugs effective for the particular seizure type with low risk of pharmacokinetic interaction and differing mechanisms of actions are preferred.

FREQUENCY OF FOLLOW-UP

There are no studies that address the optimal approach to outpatient care for children being treated with antiepileptic drug. Physician or epilepsy nurse contacts need to be frequent enough to maximize drug efficacy, monitor side effects, and screen for psychosocial or other health issues. How frequently this occurs will vary from child to child. It is realistic to evaluate children who are doing well 4–6 weeks after beginning treatment, at 3 months, and then every 6 months thereafter. The initial visit is particularly important to assess behavioral and cognitive side effects of antiepileptic drugs.

Medication Adherence

Medication adherence should be assessed at each visit. Using a 7-day pill dispenser, strategies for dealing with missed doses, and physician interest in the number of misses doses helps improve adherence with an antiepileptic drug treatment plan. The family should have a detailed plan for what to do if a medication dose is missed and for a seizure emergency.

► CHANGING OR ADDING MEDICATIONS

When seizures continue at the maximally tolerated dosage, the most common strategy is to substitute a second drug for the first, given as monotherapy.[2,3] In practice, to minimize the risk of withdrawal seizures, it is preferable to avoid abrupt discontinuation of the preexisting antiepileptic drug when switching to an alternative medication. A therapeutic strategy that is an intermediate step between alternative monotherapy and combination therapy involves adding a second drug, stabilizing the patient for a period sufficient to access the response to combination therapy, and then proceeding with the gradual removal of the initial drug, if a good response has been achieved. This transition phase allows the effect of the combination of the two drugs to be tested. If the child needs the drug combination to remain seizure-free, this will become apparent and the withdrawal procedure can be rapidly reversed. Historically, this procedure had the major drawback of possibly exposing the patient to adverse drug interactions and to side effects of polytherapy. However, the newer antiepileptic drugs have fewer interactions and are better tolerated, potentially making this option more attractive.

Choosing an alternative monotherapy or adding a second drug is a matter of personal preference, as no sound evidence is available to indicate that one choice is superior to the other.[4,5] The inability to document improved efficacy with two drugs, combined with the potential for increased adverse events and cost, is probably why surveyed experts suggest a second trial of monotherapy prior to polytherapy.[2] Combination therapy should be reserved for patients who are refractory to two or more sequential monotherapy trials.

Clinical evidence only indicates a few drug combinations that are more advantageous than others. The best examples of useful antiepileptic drug combinations are valproate and ethosuximide in the management of refractory absence seizures and valproate–lamotrigine in refractory partial onset seizures.

► ASSESSING THERAPEUTIC RESPONSE

Under usual circumstances, the assessment of therapeutic response is based on observation of seizures. Parents should carefully record all seizures in a diary, utilizing simple codes that allow differentiation by seizure type. In addition to recording seizure type and the date on which it occurs, the length of the seizure, time of day when it occurred, and days when medication doses were missed should also be recorded.

Baseline seizure frequency needs to be considered: if at baseline the child is having one seizure every 2 or 3 weeks, it may take up to 2 months, three to four times the baseline interval, to determine with confidence whether a change in drug therapy led to seizure freedom.

Antiepileptic drug therapy is typically aimed at suppressing the clinical manifestation of seizures whereas normalization of the EEG is typically not a primary or attainable goal. However, in some epilepsy syndromes, suppression of epileptiform EEG abnormalities is a justifiable therapeutic goal. This occurs when there is a close correlation between clinical seizures and EEG paroxysms, and seizures are not easily quantifiable clinically as in childhood absence epilepsy and photosensitive epilepsies. In infants and children with severe epileptiform abnormalities coexisting with encephalopathy, the extent of the EEG-related dysfunction should be determined and vigorous treatment may abate its effect. Examples include infantile spasms and Landau–Kleffner syndrome or CSWS (continuous spikes in slow-wave sleep). Monitoring EEG responsiveness in these patients can be useful in optimizing therapy.

► MAKING THE DECISION TO WITHDRAW AN AED

A CONCEPTUAL FRAMEWORK

Rarely do clinical trials address some of the critical decisions that are essential to patient management: when to stop using a particular antiepileptic drug or when to switch to another medication. However, a basic conceptual framework that is evidence-based can help in deciding when to stop and when to switch antiepileptic drugs for an individual child. This conceptual framework has changed in the last two decades because of an increased number of available treatment options and a better understanding of epilepsy response to antiepileptic drug therapy.

Historically, clinicians would titrate a single drug to seizure control or toxicity. Evidence from recent studies can be used to support a new conceptual framework for pursuing antiepileptic drug polytherapy (Fig. 48–1). The first principle is that most children who are responders to a given antiepileptic drug respond to treatment early. Second, most responders do so at low to moderate doses. Data for antiepileptic drugs suggest a steep response curve, so that very high doses only account for another 5%–10% of responders. Keeping these two principles in mind, it is probably unnecessary to push a drug to maximum doses before deciding if the patient will likely respond. However, if the child shows a partial response to a low to moderate does, this identifies a drug that should be increased to either seizure control or toxicity. Finally, initiate therapy with an antiepileptic drug that has few pharmacokinetic or pharmacodynamic interactions and add a second antiepileptic drug if it shares the same properties. Keeping these principles in

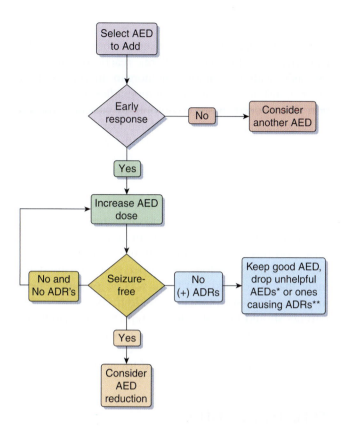

Figure 48–1. Antiepileptic drug polytherapy: decision-making. *AED, antiepileptic drug; **ADRs, adverse drug reactions.

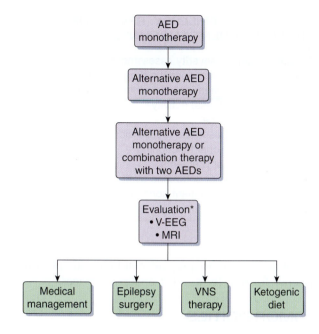

Figure 48–2. Overall therapeutic sequence for uncontrolled seizures.*Minimal evaluation. AED, antiepileptic drug; V-EEG, video-electroencephalogram scalp monitoring; MRI, magnetic resonance image of the brain using an epilepsy protocol.

mind allows the clinician to establish a rational methodologic approach to antiepileptic drug management.

First, select an appropriate antiepileptic drug based on the epilepsy syndrome and individual patient characteristics, targeting a midrange dose. Next, critically reevaluate the antiepileptic drug response soon after each change, typically in 4–6 weeks. If the child has shown a greater than 50% reduction in seizure frequency, but is not seizure-free, increase the drug dose until side effects occur or there is seizure freedom. However, if there is no significant response, select a new antiepileptic drug and stop the prior one. This strategy allows the most efficacious and best-tolerated medication selection and an efficient use of time to determine the best combination drug therapy. This strategy is employed after critical evaluation in a specialized pediatric epilepsy monitoring unit, with consideration of all nonpharmacologic and pharmacologic treatment options for the given epilepsy syndrome and etiology (Fig. 48–2).[2,6] Using this conceptual framework will allow a rational approach to polytherapy for the child with seizures that are difficult to control.

WHEN SEIZURE CONTROL IS INCOMPLETE AT MAXIMUM DOSE

In patients whose seizures cannot be controlled completely by anticonvulsant medication at maximally tolerated dosage, it is a secondary aim to suppress or reduce the frequency of those seizures that have the worst impact on the patient's quality of life. For example, control of drop attacks in patients with Lennox–Gastaut syndrome may produce far greater benefits than suppression of associated atypical absence seizures. Treatment that prevents secondary generalization of seizures would be expected to have a major impact on the quality of life of a patient with simple partial seizures.

Although achieving seizure control is usually the most important objective of medical management, seizures are not the only cause for concern in patients with epilepsy. Associated neurologic, intellectual, psychological, and social handicaps must also be addressed (Table 48–1). Whenever complete seizure freedom proves to be a nonrealistic goal, optimal treatment results from a compromise between the desire to minimize seizure frequency and the need to maintain side effects within acceptable limits.

ADOLESCENCE

Specific issues unique to adolescents must be addressed to allow the teenager to pass successfully from childhood to adulthood. The concerns, which need to be addressed, as voiced by teenagers, include choices of further education and career, the possibility and risk of withdrawing from anticonvulsants, driving regulations, the inheritance of epilepsy, leisure activities, alcohol use, pregnancy, and contraception.[7] The pediatric

▶ **TABLE 48–1. EPILEPSY: REVIEW OF THE OUTPATIENT ENCOUNTER**

Seizure frequency, severity assessment
Screen for adverse antiepileptic drug effects
Review all drugs, vitamins, and other treatments
Assess physical fitness, activity
Review sleep hygiene
Screen for mood disorders (depression, anxiety)
Screen for educational functioning
Screen for behavior problems
Review symptoms of endocrine dysfunction
Assess other family, patient concerns
Admonitions

neurologist needs to prepare children with persistent epilepsy for transfer to adult epilepsy services.

COMORBIDITIES

The majority of children with epilepsy have other neurologic comorbidities at the time of diagnosis. These comorbidities may have a greater impact on a child's life than do seizures.[8] The initial and follow-up assessments for epilepsy should include thorough questioning about cognitive and behavioral problems and sleep difficulties.[9] Screening questionnaires can be very revealing.

ADVERSE DRUG REACTIONS

Prescription of antiepileptic medication entails a significant risk of side effects. Choice of drug and dosage needs to be tailored to individual needs. In many patients with newly diagnosed epilepsy, it is realistic to expect seizure control at dosages that produce no toxicity. For a given seizure type or epilepsy syndrome, there are often two or more antiepileptic drugs with relatively similar efficacy; thus the choice of drug may be largely determined by the side effect profile.

It is critical that the child being treated for epilepsy be monitored carefully, not only for seizure activity but also for potential adverse events. It is important to inform the family about side effects that may be anticipated and any action that may need to be taken, particularly with respect to early signs of serious toxicity. While laboratory safety monitoring may be recommended for certain drugs (felbamate, most notably) for detection of serious adverse effects, it is much more important to alert the patient about the need to recognize immediately any warning symptoms.[10] For example, bleeding, bruising, and infections may be manifestations of a blood dyscrasia, whereas vomiting, anorexia, sedation, and increased seizure frequency in a patient treated with valproate should raise the possibility of liver toxicity. It is especially important to appreciate age-specific organ toxicities.

Acute idiosyncratic reactions are rare, unpredictable, and necessitate immediate withdrawal of the causative drug. In children, allergic reactions manifested by rash, with or without multiorgan involvement or fever, constitute the most common idiosyncratic reaction. These occur more commonly in patients exposed to carbamazepine, phenytoin, phenobarbital, or lamotrigine. Patients should be counseled with regard to the timing of occurrence (typically the first 4 weeks) of this reaction and have a plan for contacting the prescribing physician.

Two studies address the lack of value of routine blood work for assessment of toxicity in asymptomatic children with epilepsy taking an antiepileptic drug. Based on this evidence, in 1989, the Canadian Associates for Child Neurology developed a consensus statement that concluded that there was no proven benefit in screening asymptomatic children, but rather that parents should be instructed to report early symptoms or signs of a possible drug reaction, which should then be investigated.[11] Chronic toxicity can affect any organ system and should be monitored for at regular follow-up visits.

TERATOGENICITY

Teratogenicity is a special issue that must be reviewed in all adolescents of childbearing age. Different antiepileptic drugs carry differing risks of teratogenicity,[12] and increased drug burden appears to elevate this risk. Review of the antiepileptic drug, its risk of teratogenicity, and the need for ongoing antiepileptic drug therapy should be discussed with every adolescent female with epilepsy, and changes made in their drug therapy, if appropriate.

ANTIEPILEPTIC DRUG-RELATED SEIZURE EXACERBATION

Once a diagnosis of epilepsy is ascertained, the physician must guide the family and arrive at the best-tolerated and most efficacious medication for treatment of the child's epilepsy syndrome or seizure type. Besides establishing a medication that would be appropriate based on seizure type, the physician must use medications that will not exacerbate seizures.[5,13] (Tables 48–2 and 48–3 summarize these data.) In general, antiepileptic drugs with a broad spectrum of activity rarely lead to seizure exacerbation, unless patients are rendered toxic with a high dose. The exacerbation or new onset of myoclonic seizures by lamotrigine is a prominent exception. The antiepileptic drugs that are primarily used for the treatment of partial onset seizures have been more commonly identified as those leading to exacerbation with the appearance of generalized seizures, notably myoclonic or absence events.

▶ **TABLE 48–2. ANTIEPILEPTIC DRUGS (AEDs) ASSOCIATED WITH SEIZURE EXACERBATION**

AED	Seizure Type Exacerbated
Carbamazepine	Absence, atonic, myoclonic
Oxcarbazepine	Atonic, myoclonic
Phenytoin	Absence, atonic, myoclonic
Phenobarbital	Absence, atonic
Tiagabine	Absence, myoclonic
Vigabatrin	Absence, myoclonic
Gabapentin	Myoclonic
Lamotrigine	Myoclonic

▶ MONITORING

One of the major advances in the treatment of epilepsy is the recognition that dose requirements vary greatly between patients and throughout the pediatric age range. This variability results primarily from pharmacokinetic differences, but pharmacodynamic variation may be equally important. If therapeutic success is to be achieved, tailoring dosage to meet individual needs is important. Optimizing the antiepileptic drug dosage is a complex process. Unfortunately, for most antiepileptic drugs starting doses and guidelines for dose escalation are poorly defined. The physician typically aims for an initial target maintenance dose defined as the lowest daily dose expected to produce seizure control in that individual child.

Pharmacokinetic principles tell us that about five half-lives are required to reach steady state plasma concentrations after stabilizing the child on given medication dosages. Response to the antiepileptic drug treatment cannot be fully evaluated before this time, and it should be considered the minimal interval that should elapse before assessing the need for dosage adjustments.

PLASMA CONCENTRATIONS

Monitoring the plasma concentrations can be helpful in deciding the need for and extent of dose adjustments. While dose adjustments should be based primarily on clinical response, the serum level may help gauge the appropriate range.

The pharmacokinetics of most antiepileptic drugs exhibit remarkable interindividual variation, resulting in wide differences in plasma drug concentrations at steady state among patients receiving the same dose. Since the concentration of the antiepileptic drug in plasma is in equilibrium with brain concentrations, this variability will affect the degree of pharmacologic response achieved at any given dosage, and therapeutic and toxic effects correlate better with the drug concentration in plasma than the prescribed daily dose.[14] Based on these considerations, therapeutic drug monitoring has been found to provide a useful guide to adjusting the dose of many antiepileptic drugs. The physician should always have a specific question in mind when antiepileptic drug serum levels are obtained (Table 48–4). The therapeutic decision should be based on the direct evaluation of clinical response. However, the information obtained from assessing the serum antiepileptic drug level may assist the clinical decision-making in some scenarios. Ranges of drug concentrations have been described for many antiepileptic drugs (Table 48–5). These ranges are representative of the plasma concentrations at which most patients respond. Patients with easily manageable forms of epilepsy tend to be controlled at the lower end of the range, whereas

▶ **TABLE 48–3.** AEDs ASSOCIATED WITH SEIZURE AGGRAVATION

Drug	Epilepsy Syndrome	Possible Worsening
Carbamazepine	Absence epilepsy	Absence, myoclonus
	Juvenile myoclonic epilepsy	Myoclonus
	Progressive myoclonic epilepsies	Myoclonus
	BECTs	Negative myoclonus, ESES
Phenytoin	Absence epilepsy	Absence
	PMEs (Unverricht–Lundborg disease)	Worsening of ataxia
Phenobarbital	Absence epilepsy	Absence (high doses)
Benzodiazepines	LGS	Tonic seizures
Vigabatrin	Absence epilepsy	Absence
	Epilepsies with myoclonus	Myoclonus
Gabapentin	Absence epilepsy	Absence
	Epilepsies with myoclonus	Myoclonus
Lamotrigine	Dravet syndrome	Myoclonic, clonic, tonic–clonic
	JME	Myoclonic
Tiagabine	IGEs	Absence

AEDs, antiepileptic drugs; BECTS, benign epilepsy with centro-temporal spikes; ESES, electrical status epilepticus in slow-wave sleep; PMEs, progressive myoclonic epilepsies; LGS, Lennox–Gastaut syndrome; JME, juvenile myoclonic epilepsy; IGE, idiopathic generalized epilepsies.

▶ **TABLE 48–4.** USE OF ANTIEPILEPTIC DRUG LEVEL MONITORING

Establish "baseline" effective concentrations.
Evaluate potential causes for lack of efficacy:
- "Fast metabolizers"
- Partial adherence

Evaluate potential causes for toxicity:
- Altered drug utilization as a consequence of physiological conditions (puberty)
- "Slow metabolizers"
- Altered drug utilization as a consequence of pathological conditions (renal failure, liver failure)
- Drug–drug interactions

Evaluate potential causes for loss of efficacy:
- Altered drug utilization as a consequence of physiological conditions (e.g., neonates, infants, young children, or pregnancy)
- Altered drug utilization as a consequence of pathological conditions
- Drug–drug interactions

Judge "room to move" or when to change AEDs.
Minimize predictable problems (e.g., interaction between phenytoin and valproate)

patients with more difficult to control epilepsies tend to require higher levels. It is far more important for the physician to listen to and examine the patient after initiating antiepileptic drug therapy than to guide therapy strictly by the serum concentration. Surveillance for drug toxicity and side effects is critical.

▶ **TABLE 48–5.** THERAPEUTIC DRUG MANAGEMENT: SERUM AED LEVELS

AED	Therapeutic Range (mcg/mL)
Carbamazepine	3–12
Ethosuximide	40–100
Felbamate	30–100
Gabapentin	4–20
Lacosamide	3–12
Lamotrigine	2–20
Levetiracetam	20–60
Oxcarbazepine (MHD)	10–45
Phenobarbital	10–40
Phenytoin	10–20
Pregabalin	2–16
Primidone	4–12
Rufinamide	5–50
Tiagabine	5–70
Topiramate	2–20
Valproate	50–100
Zonisamide	10–40

AED, antiepileptic drug.

SERUM CONCENTRATIONS

Serum drug concentrations are useful guidelines in assessing therapy. Each patient has his or her own therapeutic range: the key to successful epilepsy management is to keep the patient within that range. Once the patient achieves a serum antiepileptic drug concentration that controls seizures without producing adverse effects, it is important to maintain it. Fluctuation of this concentration resulting from either partial adherence or drug interactions places a patient at risk for recurrent seizures or adverse effects.

More recently, there has been increasing interest in genetic factors that are associated with treatment outcomes. Most of the positive findings are polymorphisms that predict serious adverse events,[15] with much less success in finding genetic polymorphisms associated with treatment success (seizure control). In the future, genetic analysis for polymorphisms important in drug metabolism may be performed prior to initiating therapy to allow selection of an initial medication that is least likely to cause side effects in a given patient.

▶ WITHDRAWAL

For most children, seizure disorders are not life-long. When children have experienced a period of seizure freedom, this raises an important question: are the seizures under control because of continued antiepileptic drug therapy, or has the tendency for seizures passed and the antiepileptic drugs are unnecessary (seizure remission)? Antiepileptic drug discontinuation should be considered a therapeutic trial, just as starting a new antiepileptic drug is exploratory. Consider antiepileptic drug reduction as a first step and compromise, especially in the developmentally disabled child. Listen to what the family wants. Some are not ready for antiepileptic drug discontinuation the first time the topic is proposed.

SPONTANEOUS REMISSION

Many types of epilepsy are prone to undergo spontaneous remission, so the possibility of discontinuing antiepileptic drugs after an adequate period of seizure freedom should be considered. This is especially important in children who have a higher prevalence of self-remitting epilepsy syndromes and in whom the psychosocial consequences of seizure relapse are less severe than in adults. The option of discontinuing treatment should be discussed with the child and the family, taking into account the probability of relapse, side effects of treatment, and consequences of seizure recurrence. The consequences of seizure recurrence are usually more important in adults, whereas potential medication side effects are more important in children.

Antiepileptic drugs that are used to prevent seizures may have long-term adverse effects. The potential adverse effects of medication must be balanced against the risk of further seizures. Seizure recurrence is the risk associated with discontinuing antiepileptic drug therapy. The seizure is usually brief and any injuries are usually related to the resultant fall. When discussing antiepileptic drug discontinuation, the parents should be given a plan about how to manage further seizures if they occur. This should include consideration as to when is a good time for the child and family to pursue antiepileptic drug withdrawal (i.e., not while traveling on vacation). In females, especially in the teenage years, the risk of continuing on antiepileptic drug treatment must include consideration of the potential for teratogenicity of medications. For this reason, medication may be withdrawn in adolescent females who have been seizure-free for 2 years. If the female adolescent or family is hesitant, consideration should be given to switching to another antiepileptic drug for their seizure type if they are taking an antiepileptic drug with a Category D rating (currently this applies to phenytoin, phenobarbital, carbamazepine, and valproate). This approach allows the adolescent female to either be off antiepileptic drug therapy or on a less teratogenic therapy and seizure-free prior to pregnancy.

ADOLESCENCE

A major event for adolescents is obtaining a driver's license. It is usually easier to attempt withdrawal of an antiepileptic drug therapy before a driver's license has been obtained. For this reason, it is prudent to withdraw antiepileptic drug therapy in adolescents who have been seizure-free for 2 years, before they obtain their driver's license. An exception to this policy is the adolescent with juvenile myoclonic epilepsy.

MAKING THE DECISION

The decision regarding antiepileptic drug withdrawal should be a joint one made by the physician, the patient, and the family after careful discussion of the risks and benefits of treatment, and a review of the measures to be taken if the seizures recur. When epilepsy is in remission, it may be in the child's best interest to discontinue medication. However, the timing of withdrawal is a difficult issue. Two important questions are: (1) how long should a child be seizure-free before discontinuing antiepileptic drugs and (2) how quickly (or slowly) can antiepileptic drugs be withdrawn in a child whose epilepsy is in remission?

Approximately 50% of patients with childhood onset epilepsy will have remission of their seizures and another 20% will have remission after a relapse.[16] The success rate of discontinuation of antiepileptic drug treatment is approximately the same once a child has spent 1, 2, 4, or 5 years seizure-free.[17]

While there are risk factors that predict the likelihood of successful discontinuation, there is no way to predict accurately that any given child will be successful in discontinuing medication. The child who is seizure-free on treatment must weigh the risk of possible seizure recurrence if medications are withdrawn against the risk of continuing long-term antiepileptic drug therapy. The child and family should decide if taking antiepileptic drugs is more or less concerning than the risk of another seizure. If another seizure does occur, the family can be reassured that the vast majority of seizures come back under good control with the previous medication.[18] Additionally, studies show that if there is failure of an initial discontinuation attempt, another 60% will again become seizure-free, and 60%–70% of these children will be successful with the second attempt to stop medication.[19]

About 50% of childhood epilepsy does not resolve prior to adulthood. These children and families must be prepared and anticipate an adult life with continuation of the epilepsy. Many will have a primary generalized epilepsy.

How long should a child be seizure-free before attempting to withdraw medication? This decision must be individualized and is influenced by several factors: the epilepsy syndrome, the probability of remaining seizure-free after withdrawal, the potential risk of injury from seizure recurrence, and the potential risk of continuing antiepileptic drug therapy.

The majority of children who are seizure-free on medication for at least 2 years remain seizure-free when medication is withdrawn. Over 10 studies, performed over the last four decades and involving hundreds of children, provide consistent information with which to counsel families.[17,20,21] When medication is withdrawn in children who have been seizure-free for more than 2 years, between 60% and 75% remain seizure-free. The majority of recurrences occur shortly after medication withdrawal; about half of the relapses occur within the first 6 months after medication withdrawal, and 60%–80% occur within 1 year.[20,21] Knowing the duration of highest risk of seizure recurrence after medication withdrawal assists a clinician when counseling the family about the need for ongoing lifestyle restrictions in a child who has been seizure-free and is now having medication withdrawn.

A recent Cochrane review representing 924 children revealed a higher relapse rate after antiepileptic drug withdrawal for children who were seizure-free for less than 2 years versus those who were seizure-free for more than 2 years.[22] The earlier discontinuation was associated with the greatest relapse rates in children with partial seizures or an abnormal EEG.

There seems to be a consensus that a child should be seizure-free for 2 years before considering stopping antiepileptic drug therapy. The available data indicate children who are seizure-free for 2 years or more have a very high likelihood of remaining in remission off the medication. In selected children, medication withdrawal after an even shorter seizure-free interval may be possible.[23]

Ranganathan et al reviewed the effect of seizure recurrence after rapid taper (3 months or less) or slow taper (more than 3 months) of medication in children whose epilepsy was in remission.[24] Only one study found no difference in seizure-free rates during follow-up as long as 5 years. Methodological deficiencies and the small sample size in the single study do not allow reliable conclusions regarding the optimal rate of tapering of antiepileptic drugs. Most pediatric neurologists taper medication over 6 weeks (typically by reducing the dose by 25% every 2 weeks), with longer time periods for some medications (i.e., barbiturates, benzodiazepines), to minimize possible withdrawal seizures.

Risk Factors

Several potential risk factors have been investigated in an attempt to allow clinicians to identify subgroups of children with better prognoses and subgroups with much less favorable prognoses for remaining in remission off medications (Tables 48–6 and 48–7). The most important prognostic factor is the epilepsy syndrome, with the relapse rate being very rare in childhood epilepsy with centrotemporal spikes, relatively rare in childhood absence epilepsy, intermediate in cryptogenic or symptomatic partial epilepsies, and high in juvenile myoclonic epilepsy. In childhood epilepsy, age of onset above 12 years of age is an important risk factor for recurrence.[21] Onset at a young age (under 2 years) was associated with a less favorable prognosis only in those with remote symptomatic seizures. An EEG at time of medication withdrawal may indicate recurrence risk; however, the EEG at the time of diagnosis may also have predictive value. Characteristic EEG patterns associated with specific epilepsy syndromes,

► **TABLE 48–6. POTENTIAL RISK FACTORS FOR SEIZURE RECURRENCE AFTER ANTIEPILEPTIC DRUG WITHDRAWAL**

Remote symptomatic etiology
Age of onset >12 years of age
Age of onset <2 years of age
Number of seizures (>30 GTC seizures)
Multiple seizure types
Abnormal EEG before medicine withdrawal (primarily if cryptogenic or idiopathic epilepsy)
Epilepsy syndrome
Juvenile myoclonic epilepsy
Lennox–Gastaut syndrome

► **TABLE 48–7. GUIDELINE FOR DISCONTINUING ANTIEPILEPTIC DRUGS (AEDs) IN SEIZURE-FREE PATIENTS (AMERICAN ACADEMY OF NEUROLOGY)**

Practice parameter conclusion: Consider AED withdrawal if patient meets the following profile:
- Seizure-free 2–5 years on AEDs
- Single type of partial or generalized seizures
- Normal IQ/neurologic exam
- EEG normalized with treatment

Discontinuance of AEDs may also be appropriate in patients not meeting this profile

Source: From American Academy of Neurology. Practice parameter: a guideline for discontinuing antiepileptic drugs in seizure-free patients—summary statement. *Neurol* 1996;47(2):600–602.

such as benign rolandic epilepsy or juvenile myoclonic epilepsy, provide prognostic information. Children with benign rolandic epilepsy have a very favorable prognosis even with an abnormal EEG.

SEIZURE RECURRANCE AFTER WITHDRAWAL

If seizures recur after antiepileptic drug withdrawal, the majority of patients attain seizure control after medication is restarted.[25] The Medical Research Council (MRC) study found that the prognosis for seizure control after recurrence was no different in those who were withdrawn from antiepileptic drug therapy and relapsed as compared to those who relapsed while on antiepileptic drug therapy.[25]

Rarely, there may be late recurrences of seizures; however, the rate of late recurrence does not appear to differ in those who continue antiepileptic drug therapy or in those in whom antiepileptic drugs were discontinued.[20]

One important issue for management in a child whose seizures relapse after at least a 2-year seizure-free period is how often reinstitution of therapy promptly controls epilepsy. Recent studies provide reassurance to the clinician as a vast majority of children who relapse either require no further treatment or have seizures that are readily controlled with reinitiation of therapy. Patients only rarely develop intractable epilepsy (1%–2%).[18] Additionally, all three studies identified remote symptomatic etiology, mental impairment, and localization-related epilepsy as risk factors for difficult-to-control epilepsy in children who relapse after a seizure-free period, although predictions of individual outcome before withdrawal remain uncertain.

► CONCLUSIONS

The effective follow-up of a child with epilepsy relies on critical communication between the child, the family, and physician. Follow-up must not only include assessment of seizure response to antiepileptic drug therapy but also evaluation for medication side effects, behavioral, psychosocial, or school difficulties. The physician and family must come to a mutual agreement on a plan for treatment of seizures and comorbid conditions. Both seizures and therapies carry risks and optimal patient care requires careful balancing of these risks and benefits, which may change as new information becomes available. This risk-to-benefit approach is useful in consideration of antiepileptic drug therapy and other treatment decisions. This must be done with an understanding that individual patients and doctors place different values on different outcomes and the acceptability of certain risks.

In children and adolescents who are seizure-free on antiepileptic drugs for at least 2 years, at least one attempt should be made to withdraw medication, even if risk factors for recurrence are present.

REFERENCES

1. Camfield PR, Camfield CS. Childhood epilepsy: What is the evidence for what we think and what we do? *J Child Neurol* 2003;18:272–287.

2. Wheless JW, Clarke DF, Carpenter D. Treatment of pediatric epilepsy: expert opinion, 2005. *J Child Neurol* 2005;20:S1–S60.

3. Karceski S, Morrell MJ, Carpenter D. Treatment of epilepsy in adults: expert opinion, 2005. *Epilepsy Behav* 2005;7:S1–S64.

4. Beghi E, et al. Adjunctive therapy versus alternative monotherapy in patients with partial epilepsy failing on a single drug: a multicentre, randomized, pragmatic controlled trial. *Epilepsy Res* 2003;57(1):1–13.

5. Guerrini R, Parmeggiani L. Practitioner Review: use of antiepileptic drugs in children. *J Child Psychol Psychiatry* 2006;47(2):115–126.

6. Cross JH, et al. Proposed criteria for referral and evaluation of children for epilepsy surgery: recommendations of the subcommission for pediatric epilepsy surgery. *Epilepsia* 2006;47(6):952–959.

7. Appleton RE, Chadwick D, Sweeney A. Managing the teenager with epilepsy: pediatric to adult care. *Seizure* 1997;6:27–30.

8. Austin JK, et al. Recurrent seizures and behavior problems in children with first recognized seizures: a prospective study. *Epilepsia* 2002;43:1564–1573.

9. Gilliam FG, Mendiratta A, Pack AM, Bazil CW. Epilepsy and common comorbidities: improving the outpatient epilepsy encounter. *Epileptic Disord* 2005;7(Suppl 1):S27–S33.

10. Pellock JM, Willmore LJ. A rational guide to routine blood monitoring in patients receiving antiepileptic drugs. *Neurol* 1991;41(7):961–964.

11. Camfield PR, et al. Routine screening of blood and urine for severe reactions to anti-convulsant drugs in asymptomatic patients is of doubtful value. *Can Med Assoc J* 1989;140:1303–1305.

12. Ornov A. Neuroteratogens in man: an overview with special emphasis on the teratogenicity of antiepileptic drugs in pregnancy. *Reprod Toxicol* 2006;22(2):214–226.

13. Gayatri NA, Livingston JH. Aggravation of epilepsy by anti-epileptic drugs. *Dev Med Child Neurol* 2006;48(5):394–398.

14. Glauser TA, Pippenger CE. Controversies in blood-level monitoring. Re-examining its role in the treatment of epilepsy. *Epilepsia* 2000;41(Suppl 8):S6–S15.

15. Pirmohamed M. Genetic factors in the predisposition to drug-induced hypersensitivity reactions. *AAPS J* 2006; 8(1):E20–E26.

16. Sillanpaa M, Schmidt D. Natural history of treated childhood-onset epilepsy. Prospective, long-term population-based study. *Brain* 2006;129:617–624.

17. Berg AT, Shinnar S. Relapse following discontinuation of anti-epileptic drugs: meta-analysis. *Neurol* 1994;44:601–608.

18. Camfield PR, Camfield CS. The frequency of intractable seizures after stopping AEDs in seizure-free children with epilepsy. *Neurol* 2005;64:973–975.

19. Berg AT, et al. Two-year remission and subsequent relapse in children with newly diagnosed epilepsy. *Epilepsia* 2001;42:1553–1562.

20. Medical Research Council (MRC). Antiepileptic Drug Withdrawal Study Group. Randomized study of antiepileptic drug withdrawal in patient with remission. *Lancet* 1991;337:1175–1180.

21. Shinnar S, et al. Discontinuing antiepileptic drugs in children with epilepsy: a prospective study. *Ann Neurol* 1994;35:534–545.

22. Sirven JI, Sperling M, Wingerchuk DM. Early versus late antiepileptic drug withdrawal for people with epilepsy in remission. *Cochrane Database Syst Rev* 2001; (3):CD0019202.

23. Dooley JM, et al. Discontinuation of anticonvulsant therapy in children free of seizures for one year: a prospective study. *Neurol* 1996;456:969–974.

24. Ranganathan LN, Ramaratnam S. Rapid versus slow withdrawal of antiepileptic drugs. *Cochrane Database Syst Rev* 2006;(2):CD 005003.

25. Chadwick D, Taylor J, Johnson T. Outcomes after seizure recurrence in people with well-controlled epilepsy and the factors that influence it. The MRC Antiepileptic Drug Withdrawal Group. *Epilepsia* 1996;37:1043–1050.

26. American Academy of Neurology. Practice parameter: a guideline for discontinuing antiepileptic drugs in seizure-free patients—summary statement. *Neurol* 1996;47(2):600–602.

SUGGESTED READINGS

Adab N. Birth defects and epilepsy medication. *Expert Rev Neurother* 2006;6(6):833–845.

Arts WFM. The Dutch study of epilepsy in childhood: early discontinuation. *Epilepsia* 1995;36(Suppl 3):S29.

Arts WFM, et al. Follow-up of 146 children with epilepsy after withdrawal of antiepileptic therapy. *Epilepsia* 1988;29:244–250.

Austin JK, et al. Behavioral issues involving children and adolescents with epilepsy and the impact of their families: recent research data. *Epilepsy Behavior* 2004;5:S33–S41.

Bouma PAD, et al. Discontinuation of antiepileptic therapy: a prospective trial in children. *J Neurol Neurosurg Psychiatry* 1987;50:1579–1583.

Bouma PAD, Peters ACB, Brouwer OF. Long-term course of childhood epilepsy following relapse after antiepileptic drug withdrawal. *J Neurol Neurosurg Psychiatry* 2002;72:507–510.

Braathen G, Melander H. Early discontinuation of treatment in children with uncomplicated epilepsy: a prospective study with a model for prediction of outcome. *Epilepsia* 1997;38:561–569.

Brodie MJ, Yuen AWC 105 Study Group. Lamotrigine substitution study. Evidence for synergism with sodium valproate. *Epilepsy Res* 1997;26:423–432.

Callaghan N, Garrett A, Goggin T. Withdrawal of anticonvulsant drugs in patients free of seizures for two years. *N Engl J Med* 1988;318:942–946.

Camfield CS, et al. Predicting the outcome of childhood epilepsy—A population-based study yielding a simple scoring system. *J Pediatr* 1993;122:861–868.

Camfield CS, et al. Asymptomatic children with epilepsy: little benefit from screening for anti-convulsant-induced liver, blood or renal damage. *Neurol* 1986;36:838–841.

Camfield P, Camfield C. The frequency of intractable seizures after stopping AEDs in seizure-free children with epilepsy. *Neurol* 2005;64:973–975.

Camfield P, Camfield C. The office management of epilepsy. *Semin Pediatr Neurol* 2006;13(4):201–207.

Camfield PR, Camfield CS. Treatment of children with "ordinary" epilepsy. *Epileptic Disorders* 2000;2(1):45–51.

Camfield PR, et al. If a first antiepileptic drug fails to control a child's epilepsy, what are the chances of success with the next drug? *J Pediatr* 1997;131:821–824.

Cerminara C, et al. Lamogrigine-induced seizure aggravation and negative myoclonus in idiopathic rolandic epilepsy. *Neurol* 2004;63(2):373–375.

Chadwick D representing the MRC Antiepileptic Drug Withdrawal Study Group. Does withdrawal of different antiepileptic drugs have different effects on seizure recurrence? Further results from the MRC Antiepileptic Drug Withdrawal Study. *Brain* 1999;122:441–448.

Chadwick D. Starting and stopping treatment for seizures and epilepsy. *Epilepsia* 2006;47(Suppl 1):58–61.

Chaves J, Sander JW. Seizure aggravation in idiopathic generalized epilepsies. *Epilepsia* 2005; 46(Suppl 9):133–139.

Emerson R, et al. Stopping medication in children with epilepsy: predictors of outcome. *N Engl J Med* 1981;304:1125–1129.

Gilliam F. Optimizing health outcomes in active epilepsy. *Neurol* 2002;58(Suppl 5):S9–S19.

Holmes GL. Critical issues in the treatment of epilepsy. *Am J Hosp Pharm* 1993;50(12, Suppl 5):S5–S16.

Holowach J, Thurston DL, O'Leary J. Prognosis in childhood epilepsy: follow-up study of 148 cases in which therapy had been suspended after prolonged anticonvulsant control. *N Engl J Med* 1972;286:169–174.

Jalava M, et al. Social adjustment and competence 35 years after onset of childhood epilepsy: A prospective controlled study. *Epilepsia* 1997;38:708–715.

Kadir ZA, Chadwick DW. Principles of treatment of epilepsy. *Drugs Today (Barc)* 1999;35(1):35–41.

Marson A, et al. Medical Research Council MESS Study Group: immediate versus deferred antiepileptic drug treatment for early epilepsy and single seizures: A randomized controlled trial. *Lancet* 2005;365:2007–2013.

Mattson RH, Cramer JA, Collins JF the Department of Veteran Affairs Epilepsy Co-operative Study Group. Connective tissue changes, hypersensitivity rash, and blood laboratory test changes associated with antiepileptic drug therapy. *Ann Neurol* 1986;20:119.

Oostrom KJ, et al. Three to four years after diagnosis: cognition and behavior in children with "epilepsy only." A prospective, controlled study. *Brain* 2005;128:1546–1555.

Panayiotopoulos CP, et al. Interaction of lamotrigine with sodium valproate. *Lancet* 1993;341:445.

Perucca E, et al. Antiepileptic drugs as a cause of worsening seizures. *Epilepsia* 1998;39(1):5–17.

Peters ACB, et al. Randomized prospective study of early discontinuation of antiepileptic drugs in children with epilepsy. *Neurol* 1998;50(3):724–730.

Pisani F, et al. The efficacy of valproate-lamotrigine comedication in refractory complex partial seizures. Evidence for a pharmacodynamic interaction. *Epilepsia* 1999;40:1141–1146.

Rowan AJ, et al. Valproate ethosuximide combination therapy for refractory absence seizures. *Arch Neurol* 1983;40:797–802.

Sazgar M, Bourgeois BFD. Aggravation of epilepsy by antiepileptic drugs, *Pediatr Neurol* 2005;33(4):227–234.

Shinnar S, et al. What happens to children with epilepsy who experience a seizure recurrence after withdrawl of antiepileptic drugs. *Ann Neurol* 1996;40:301–302.

Shinnar S, et al. Discontinuing antiepileptic medication in children with epilepsy after two years without seizures: a prospective study. *N Engl J Med* 1985;313:976–980.

Sillanpaa M. Children with epilepsy as adults. Outcome after 30 years of follow-up. *Acta Paediatr Scand* 1990; 368(Suppl):1–78.

Sillanpaa M, Jalava M, Shinnar S. Epilepsy syndromes in patients with childhood-onset epilepsy. *Pediatr Neurol* 1999; 21:533–537.

Sillanpaa M, Schmidt D. Prognosis of seizure recurrence after stopping antiepileptic drugs in seizure-free patients: A long-term population-based study of childhood-onset epilepsy. *Epilepsy Behavior* 2006;8:713–719.

Smith D, Chadwick D. The management of epilepsy. *J Neurol Neurosurg Psychiatry* 2001;70(Suppl 11):II15–II21.

Somerville ER. Aggravation of partial seizures by antiepileptic drugs: is there evidence from clinical trials? *Neurol* 2002; 59(1):79–83.

Tatum WO. Use of antiepileptic drugs in pregnancy. *Expert Rev Neurother* 2006;6(7):1077–1086.

Tennison M, et al. Discontinuing antiepileptic drugs in children with epilepsy. A comparison of a six-week and a nine-month taper period. *N Engl J Med* 1994;330(20):1407–1410.

Todt H. The late prognosis of epilepsy in childhood: results of a prospective follow-up study. *Epilepsia* 1984;25:137–144.

CHAPTER 49

Clinical Trials Versus Anecdotal Reports

Mona Nabulsi and Mohamad A. Mikati

▶ OVERVIEW

The choice of antiepileptic drugs (AEDs) entails a number of considerations detailed later. All these considerations cannot be fully or adequately addressed by controlled studies alone, and are thus grounds for individualization of therapy. Although evidence-based data from randomized controlled trials (RCTs) on drug efficacy are a critical part of the choice, as they provide an objective method to compare efficacy, they often do not address many other aspects that are important in such choices such as comparative efficacy, comorbidity, and ease of use.

▶ FACTORS AFFECTING AED INITIATION

During the process of patient evaluation and medication decision, several considerations affect treatment choices. These include:

1. *Comparative efficacy:* This refers to the ability of medication to control seizures and is usually best determined by RCTs. However, efficacy of drugs in specific epilepsy syndromes and long-term efficacy over years, even for common seizure types, are difficult to determine using RCTs, and data are limited. Furthermore, the phenomenon of seizure aggravation from AEDs has not been studied adequately but will affect the choice of an AED.

2. *Relative tolerability:* This refers to the medication adverse effect profile, which varies for each patient. A prominent example is the increased risk of liver toxicity for valproate (VPA) therapy in children under the age of 2 years with metabolic disorders. Relative tolerability also applies to lifestyle side effects including weight gain, gingival hyperplasia, alopecia, hyperactivity, and others. Children with behavior problems and/or with attention deficit disorder are particularly hyperactive with GABA-ergic drugs such as benzodiazepines barbiturates or VPA.

3. *Cost and availability:* The cost of the newer AEDs may prevent their use, particularly in developing countries. Furthermore, many drugs are available only in some countries either because they are too expensive or because, paradoxically, they are too inexpensive (with little financial incentive for their importation), or for regulatory reasons.

4. *Ease of initiation of the antiepileptic drug:* Medications that are titrated gradually such as lamotrigine (LTG) and topiramate (TPM) may not be chosen if rapid therapeutic levels are required. In these situations, medications with intravenous preparations or rapid oral titration schedules such as VPA, phenytoin (PHT), or levetiracetam (LEV) are alternative choices.

5. *Preexisiting medications and the potential for pharmacokinetic drug interactions:* An example is the reciprocal ability of VPA to increase the epoxide level of carbamazepine (CBZ) and CBZ lowering the level of VPA.

6. *Availability of syndrome-specific and age-specific efficacy and tolerability data:* Many AEDs are only proven to be effective in adult symptomatic and cryptogenic partial epilepsy, but have not been fully studied in children. In addition, some unique epilepsy syndromes and seizure types in childhood including neonatal seizures, West syndrome, early myoclonic encephalopathy, Ohtahara syndrome, and several other syndromes do not occur in adults. Furthermore, many of these disorders are relatively uncommon or rare and controlled studies are not available. This is also the case in more common pediatric epilepsy syndromes such as benign occipital epilepsy of childhood.

7. *The presence of comorbid conditions:* For example, the presence of migraine in a patient with epilepsy may suggest a medication effective against both disorders such as VPA or TPM. Obesity may dictate against medications such as VPA. Other comorbid conditions include malignancies like leukemia where enzyme inducers reduce the efficacy of chemotherapy or increase the risk of relapse. Thus, enzyme inducers should be avoided in patients with cancer. In adolescent females of childbearing potential,

enzyme-inducing AEDs may interfere with birth control pills or increase the risk of fetal malformation.

8. *Coexisting seizures:* The presence of multiple seizure types also influences AED choice. Some medications have a broad spectrum of antiseizure effects whereas others exhibit a more limited spectrum. The presence of both absence and generalized tonic–clonic seizures may favor LTG and VPA rather than ethosuximide (ESM) or CBZ alone or their combination.

9. *History of prior response to specific antiepileptic drugs:* For example, if a patient had previously responded to a GABA-ergic drug, then introduction of another GABA-ergic drug may be beneficial.

10. *Mechanism of drug actions:* At present, the understanding of the pathophysiology of epilepsy does not allow for specific choice of AEDs based on the assumed pathophysiology of the epilepsy, and the presumed AED mechanism of action. However, it is preferable to not combine medications with similar mechanisms of action such as PHT and CBZ whose major effects are on sodium channels. In contrast, several combinations including LTG and VPA and TPM and LTG are anecdotally reported to have synergistic effects, possibly through different mechanisms of action. When combining AEDs, the choice of the second may depend on the background drug (i.e., the first drug preceding the second) and on the combined mechanisms of action. Thus, pharmacodynamic interactions and not just pharmacokinetic interactions may be important.

11. *Ease of use:* This is particularly important in children. Medications administered once or twice daily are easier to use than medications given three or four times daily. In addition, a pediatric liquid preparation rather than tablets or capsules is an important consideration in children under age 6 years.

12. *Ability to monitor the medication and adjust the dose:* It is difficult to maintain stable plasma concentrations of some AEDs and frequent AED blood levels may be required. The prototype is PHT, but many of the older medications also require blood level monitoring.

13. *Patient and family preferences:* All things being equal, the choice between two or more acceptable alternative AEDs also depends on patient or family preferences. For example, patients or their parents may want to avoid gingival hyperplasia and hirsutism but may tolerate weight loss, or vice versa.

► **EXPERT OPINION SURVEYS**

Some, but not necessarily all of the previous considerations have been addressed through "expert opinion" surveys[1] or guidelines developed by professional societies such as the International League Against Epilepsy (ILAE),[2] National Institute for Clinical Excellence (NICE),[3] Scottish Intercollegiate Guidelines Network (SIGN),[4] or the American Academy of Neurology (AAN).[5,6] Some guidelines are evidence-based (AAN), while others (NICE, SIGN) incorporate other considerations. However, no guidelines incorporate all considerations relevant to each patient. Thus, the process of choosing an AED involves incorporating evidence from RCTs, guidelines, expert opinion surveys, and all the previous considerations for individualizing therapy.

► **INDIVIDUALIZING THE APPROACH**

Individualization is time-consuming and requires expertise that may not be present in all treating physicians outside tertiary referral centers. Physicians can rely on algorithms based on guidelines or expert opinion, as well as on RCTs. These algorithms are not designed to replace sound clinical judgment or subspecialty referral. In complex patients, decisions are typically made by the treating neurologist or epileptologist.

► **MAKING EVIDENCE-BASED DECISIONS**

INITIATING THERAPY

The decision to initiate antiepileptic therapy following a first seizure is based on several considerations. These include patient age, gender, vocation, driving status, epilepsy or seizure type, EEG findings, physical examination, neuroimaging findings, as well as relevant data from randomized clinical trials.[7–11] Only one study (performed on adults after a single seizure) was placebo-controlled.[8] In general, all studies reveal a reduced risk of seizure recurrence in patients randomized to treatment, but a corresponding increase in adverse drug effects. The decision to treat is therefore complex when considering the risk of a new seizure, an abnormal EEG, radiologic, or neurologic abnormalities. Social and personal patient preferences also influence the decision-making process. Three studies examining long-term remission found that earlier treatment did not affect its incidence.[7,9,11] Two studies[9,11] included both adults and children and one included only children.[7]

Choosing an Initial Drug

Choosing an AED for the initial treatment of a new-onset seizure disorder is challenging due to a lack of randomized, double-blind, placebo-controlled trial data. The SANAD study,[12,13] which was open label and included adults and children older than 4 years, attempted to address this issue. Newly diagnosed patients whose physicians thought CBZ was the appropriate initial drug were randomized to carbamazepine, oxcarbazepine (OXC), LTG, gabapentin (GBP), or TPM,[12] and those whose physicians thought VPA was the appropriate drug to VPA, LTG, or TPM.[13] In the first group, LTG was more acceptable than CBZ due to differences in adverse effects, and both were more successful than GBP due to its decreased efficacy, or TPM-induced adverse effects. In the second group, VPA was more successful than LTG because of greater efficacy, and both were superior to TPM due to its side effects. This study has been criticized because AED doses and titration schedules could have substantially biased the results.

Currently, the choices of initial monotherapy for old and new AEDs exist in guidelines from the ILAE,[2] SIGN,[4] NICE,[3] and the AAN[5] (Table 49–1).

Adding an AED

There are no RCTs that address the choice of a second AED when the first has failed. Furthermore, no trials address the choice of a first drug in febrile seizures or specific pediatric epilepsy syndromes with the exception of refractory partial seizures or resistant Lennox–Gastaut syndrome (LGS). Several studies of partial seizures patients achieved seizure control leading to approval for monotherapy use. Whereas the choice of AEDs is often influenced by the results of these studies, in the final decision is often individualized. Guidelines from NICE,[3] SIGN,[4] and AAN[6] (Table 49–1) currently exist for add-on therapy in different seizure and epilepsy types.

EFFICACY AND TOLERABILITY

In 2004, the Quality Standards Subcommittee (QSS) and the Therapeutics and Technology Assessment (TTA) Subcommittee of the American Academy of Neurology and the American Epilepsy Society published two reports assessing the evidence on efficacy and tolerability of the new AEDs for new onset[5] and refractory epilepsy.[6] Studies were evaluated for their class of

► TABLE 49–1. COMPARISON OF RECOMMENDATIONS FOR THE TREATMENT OF PEDIATRIC EPILEPSY

Seizure Type or Epilepsy Syndrome	Pediatric Expert Consensus Survey[1]	ILAE[2]	NICE[3]	SIGN[4]	AAN[5,6]	FDA Approved
Partial-onset	OXC, CBZ	A: OXC; B: none; C: CBZ, PB, PHT TPM, VPA	CBZ, VPA, LTG, OXC, TPM	PHT, VPA, CBZ, LTG, TPM, OXC, VGB, CLB	OXC, CBZ, LTG (adult males)	PB, PHT, CBZ, OXC, TPM, LTG, LEV
BECT	OXC, CBZ	A, B: none; C: CBZ, VPA	CBZ, OXC, LTG, VPA	Not specifically mentioned	Not surveyed	None
Childhood absence epilepsy	ESM	A, B: none; C: ESM, LTG, VPA	VPA, ESM, LTG	VPA, ESM, LTG	VPA, LTG	ESM, VPA
Juvenile myoclonic epilepsy	VPA, LTG	A, B, C: none	VPA, LTG	VPA, LTG, TPM	VPA, LTG	TPM, LEV, LTG
Lennox–Gastaut syndrome	VPA, TPM, LTG	Not reviewed	LTG, VPA, TPM	Not specifically mentioned	Not surveyed	FLB, TPM, LTG
Infantile spasms	VGB, ACTH	Not reviewed	VGB, corticosteroids	Not specifically mentioned	Not surveyed	None

Source: Adapted from Wheless JW, Clarke DF, Carpenter D. Treatment of pediatric epilepsy: expert opinion. *J Child Neurol* 2005;20(Suppl 1):S1–S56.
ACTH, adrenocorticotropic hormone; BECT, benign childhood epilepsy with centrotemporal spikes; CBZ, carbamazepine; CLB, clobazam; ESM, ethosuximide; FLB, felbamate; LTG, lamotrigine; OXC, oxcarbazepine; PB, phenobarbital; PHT, phenytoin; TPM, topiramate; VPA, valproate; VGB, vigabatrin.

[2]Recommendations listed according to levels of evidence supporting the efficacy of the options. Level A: ≥1 class I RCT or ≥2 class II RCTs; level B: 1 class II RCT; level C: ≥2 class III RCTs.

evidence based on study design and methodology into four classes (I–IV). Evidence was translated into recommendations, rating in strength from Level A to Level U.

In 2006, the ILAE published evidence-based treatment guidelines on antiepileptic drug efficacy and effectiveness as initial monotherapy for epileptic seizures and syndromes.[2] The criteria used to evaluate the studies for their class of evidence, as well as level-of-evidence of the recommendations were adapted from the US Agency for Health and Policy Research[14] and the American Academy of Neurology[15] scoring systems. The criteria used to rate the studies in the ILAE treatment guidelines share many similarities to those of the TAA and QSS subcommittees' reports but include more stringent criteria, such as longer study duration and absence of forced-exit criteria. For instance, some studies that met a class I rating by the TAA and QSS criteria would be classified as class III by ILAE criteria. In reviewing the literature for this chapter, we adopted the ILAE study classification and rating of evidence for the sake of consistency with the guidelines.[2] In addition, and since the focus of this chapter is on pediatric and adolescent epilepsy, studies that did not include children below 16 years of age were excluded.

First Generation AEDs

First generation AEDs include drugs used broadly for the treatment of both partial-onset and primary generalized tonic–clonic seizures such as VPA, or predominantly partial seizures such as CBZ, PHT, and phenobarbital (PB). Other drugs like ESM) and adrenocorticotropic hormone (ACTH) are primarily used to treat very specific seizure types such as absence seizures or infantile spasms (IS).

With the advent of the second and third generation AEDs, antiepileptic treatment recommendations are changing in favor of newer agents, with some older agents like acetazolamide (ACZ) or bromides (Br) becoming obsolete. The use of older AEDs for pediatric epilepsy was mostly based on uncontrolled trials, extrapolation from studies done on adults and anecdotal reports. Most have not been rigorously tested in clinical trials for efficacy or tolerability. Table 49–2 summarizes the available evidence on the efficacy/effectiveness of the older AEDs for the treatment of pediatric epilepsies. The rating of evidence is based on the highest level available in the literature, consistent with ILAE classification of studies and rating of evidence.[2]

Acetazolamide

ACZ is used as adjunctive treatment for catamenial epilepsy based on class IV retrospective studies. Similarly, several class IV studies report the use of ACZ as add-on treatment for refractory absence, partial-onset, or myoclonic seizures with significant decrease in seizure frequency.[16–20]

▶ **TABLE 49–2.** FIRST GENERATION AED'S IN PEDIATRIC EPILEPSY AND TREATMENT RECOMMENDATIONS LISTED ACCORDING TO LEVELS OF EVIDENCE SUPPORTING DRUG EFFICACY (CONSISTENT WITH ILAE[2] SYSTEM OF CLASSIFICATION)

	Partial	PGCS	Myoclonic	Absence	IS	Neonatal	BECCTS	LGS
ACZ	Adjunctive (E)	Adjunctive (E)	Adjunctive (E)	Adjunctive (E)	—	—		
ACTH	—	—	MonoRx (E)	—	MonoRx (C)	—	—	MonoRx (E)
Br	Adjunctive (E)	MonoRx/ adjunctive (E)	Adjunctive (E)	—	—	—	—	—
CBZ	MonoRx (C)	MonoRx (C)	—	—	—	—	MonoRx (C)	—
ESM	—	—	Adjunctive (E)	MonoRx (C)	—	—	—	—
MSX	Adjunctive (D)	—	MonoRx (D)	MonoRx (D)	—	—	—	—
PB	MonoRx (C)	MonoRx (C)	—	—	—	MonoRx (C)	—	—
PHT	MonoRx (C)	MonoRx (C)	—	—	—	MonoRx (C)	—	—
VPA	MonoRx (C)	MonoRx (C)	MonoRx (D)	MonoRx (D)	MonoRx (D)	—	—	MonoRx (D)

ACZ, acetazolamide; ACTH, adrenocorticotropic hormone; Br, bromides; CBZ, carbamazepine; ESM, ethosuximide; MSX, methsuximide; PB, phenobarbital; PHT, phenytoin; VPA, valproate; MonoRx, monotherapy.
Recommendation level: Level C: ≥2 class III RCTs; level D: 1 class III RCT; level E: ≥1 class IV studies or expert opinion.

ACTH and Oral Corticosteroids

ACTH and oral corticosteroids (prednisone) are indicated for the treatment of IS. However, there are no clinical trials that compared the effectiveness of ACTH or oral corticosteroids versus placebo in controlling IS. Two class III RCTs revealed that ACTH was superior to prednisone in spasm cessation.[21,22] When compared to vigabatrin (VGB), ACTH results in a higher and faster response rate in spasm control, with similar cognitive development after 9–44 months of treatment[23] (class III). In another class III open-label RCT, ACTH had similar short-term efficacy and tolerability to nitrazepam for the treatment of cryptogenic IS.[24] ACTH may therefore be considered for initial monotherapy of IS, while oral corticosteroids may be considered as alternative first-line monotherapy. In addition, few class IV studies have reported the use of ACTH for the treatment of myoclonic seizures[25] and LGS[26,27] with variable response rates.

Clobazam. Evidence from one class III double-blind and one class III open-label trials suggest that clobazam is possibly equally effective to PHT or CBZ as initial monotherapy for partial or generalized-onset epilepsy.[28,29] Based on several class III double-blind, single-blind, and open-label trials, clobazam is possibly efficacious as adjunctive treatment or monotherapy for refractory epilepsy of mixed types, and for catamenial epilepsy. However, all studies suffered from small sample sizes.[30] A recent class III double-blind, placebo-controlled crossover study in 24 women with refractory catamenial epilepsy reported effectiveness in 78% of subjects.[31]

Clonazepam. Evidence from one class IV study found clonazepam to be effective for treatment of myoclonic, atonic and tonic seizures in patients with mental retardation.[32] A class III double-blind RCT compared clonazepam to CBZ as initial monotherapy of psychomotor seizures and found similar efficacy and tolerability.[33] A class IV comparative study of 40 children with benign epilepsy of childhood with centrotemporal spikes (BECTS), aged 3–11 years, revealed that *clonzazepam* resulted in disappearance of rolandic discharges in 75% patients as compared to 10% of children receiving VPA and 0% of children treated with CBZ. However, seizure incidence, type, and clonazepam blood levels were similar between patients whose discharges disappeared and those who did not.[34] In a class III double-blind, placebo-controlled RCT, administration of a single adjunctive low dose of intramuscular clonazepam to 15 children with focal or generalized epilepsy reduced epileptiform discharges on long-term EEG monitoring as compared to placebo with a concomitant reduction of seizures.[35]

Clorazepate. One class IV study reported excellent results with clorazepate when used in 59 patients (ages 7 months to 45 years) with intractable seizures of different types.[36]

Midazolam. A class III open-label RCT compared *intranasal midazolam* to *intravenous diazepam* in 47 children (6 months to 5 years in age) with febrile seizures lasting more than 10 minutes. Intranasal midazolam was as safe and effective as intravenous diazepam. Seizures were controlled faster with diazepam but overall time to cessation of seizures after arrival to hospital was faster with midazolam,[37] due to the easy and fast intranasal drug administration.

Nitrazepam. A case series (class IV study) of 35 children (ages 7 months to 19 years) with different seizure types (petit mal, IS, myoclonic, psychomotor) reported the use of nitrazepam as add-on treatment with no placebo control. There was very good response in atonic seizures and IS, whereas there were poor and variable responses in myoclonic seizures, petit mal, "myoclonic type of absence, and complex partial seizures.[38] In IS, two case series (class IV) reported cessation of spasms in 30%–54% of patients with resolution of hypsarrythmia in 46%.[39]

Another class III unblinded RCT compared the efficacy and safety of nitrazepam versus ACTH in 52 patients below 2 years of age with cryptogenic IS over 4 weeks. Both treatments were similarly effective in reducing spasms. Adverse events were similar in frequency for both drugs but more severe in the ACTH group.[24]

Oxazepam. Oxazepam was introduced in 12 patients, ages 2–58 years, with complex partial seizures as monotherapy or as adjunctive treatment in a class IV nonrandomized, placebo-controlled, blind crossover study for 4 months followed by an open-label, 3–6-month phase. There was an excellent response in 10 patients; transient drowsiness or ataxia were observed.[40]

Bromide (Br)

First used as an antiepileptic about 150 years ago, Br is currently restricted to the treatment of severely refractory seizures of different types.[41–45] The use of Br is based on anecdotal reports as there are no RCTs that assessed efficacy as initial or adjunctive therapy for refractory seizures.

Carbamazepine

CBZ is an initial monotherapy for the treatment of partial-onset and generalized-onset seizures. However, CBZ has not been tested against placebo in double-blind RCTs. In several comparative RCTs, CBZ was tested against VPA, PB, GBP, LMG, TPM, and OXC. One systematic review of class III studies found that in patients 2–68 years of age with either partial or generalized tonic–clonic seizure, CBZ was equally effective to PB and better tolerated as monotherapy for either type of seizures.[46] In a meta-analysis of class III studies, CBZ was more effective than VPA as first-line monotherapy for partial-onset seizures and equally effective to VPA as first-line monotherapy for generalized-onset seizures.[47] Several class I and II studies found CBZ equally effective to GBP,[48] LTG,[49] TPM,[50] and OXC[51] as monotherapy for new-onset epilepsy (partial or primary generalized). Based on the available evidence, CBZ is possibly effective as first-line drug for the treatment of partial-onset and primary generalized seizures.

Ethosuximide/Methsuximide

Available evidence from limited class III clinical trials suggest that ESM is equally effective to VPA in controlling absence seizures.[52] However, the studies are of poor quality, and there are no placebo-controlled double-blind RCTs assessing efficacy of ESM in absence-seizures. Anecdotal reports (class IV studies) suggest that combining ESM with VPA may reduce seizures in epilepsy with myoclonic absence, eyelid myoclonia with absence and juvenile myoclonic epilepsy (JME).[53]

Methsuximide (MSX) use in pediatric epilepsy is based on small retrospective studies and case series (class IV studies). These studies suggest that MSX is potentially efficacious as adjunctive therapy in refractory epilepsy.[54–56] MSX use for absence seizures is based on anecdotal reports. A single small series reported excellent control of JME with MSX monotherapy.[57] Currently, there is insufficient evidence to recommend MSX for absence seizures or JME.

Phenobarbital

PB is commonly used as initial monotherapy for partial-onset, primary generalized, febrile and neonatal seizures.[58] One meta-analysis of two pediatric and two adult studies included a heterogeneous group of patients. Both pediatric studies were open-label, class III randomized studies that compared PB and PHT in partial and primary generalized tonic–clonic seizures. Efficacy of both drugs was found to be similar, with higher discontinuation rates with PB. However, studies may have lacked power.[59] In two class III open-label studies, PB was compared to CBZ and there were no differences in terms of time to discontinuation or time to 12-month remission of partial and primary generalized seizures.[60,61] PB is thus possibly efficacious as initial monotherapy for partial or primary generalized seizures.

A meta-analysis of nine RCTs in febrile seizures including four with PB found that continuous PB therapy effectively reduced recurrences with an estimated number needed to treat of eight.[62] In neonatal seizures, available class III and class IV studies suggest that PB is efficacious in about half of the patients, a rate that is similar to the response rate with PHT.[63–65] Based on the available evidence, PB is probably efficacious in reducing febrile seizure recurrences and is possibly efficacious in controlling neonatal seizures.

Phenytoin

In partial epilepsy, PHT may be used as a first-line treatment for children with partial seizures. However, this is based primarily on adult studies supplemented by open-label controlled and uncontrolled pediatric studies and clinical experience (class III and class IV).[66] PHT was shown to have equal efficacy to PB as initial monotherapy for partial or primary generalized epilepsy.[59] Based on available evidence, PHT is possibly efficacious as first-line treatment of partial or primary generalized epilepsy.

In neonatal seizures, a Cochrane review reported equal efficacy of PB and PHT with about 50% response rates based on one single-blind comparative short-term class III RCT. There are no studies comparing PHT to placebo.[67] PHT is thus possibly efficacious as initial monotherapy for neonatal seizures.

For the prevention of early posttraumatic seizures, a Cochrane review found that the early use of PHT decreased the risk of early seizures (RR = 0.34; 95% CI: 0.21–0.54). However, these studies included both pediatric and adult patients.[68]

There is no conclusive evidence that PHT is efficacious in preventing late posttraumatic seizures, since all studies are limited by loss of follow-up exceeding 20%. PHT is thus possibly efficacious in preventing early posttraumatic seizures.

Valproate

VPA is a broad spectrum AED used in generalized, partial-onset and absence seizures, febrile seizure prophylaxis, and myoclonic jerks. In partial and primary generalized seizures, a meta-analysis of five class III studies (including children and adults) revealed equal effectiveness of VPA and CBZ as initial monotherapy for the outcomes "time to treatment discontinuation" and "time to 12-month remission." However, the outcome "time to first seizure" was longer with CBZ. No subgroup analysis by age was done.[47]

Two other class III RCTs revealed equal efficacy to CBZ and TPM in monotherapy of newly diagnosed epilepsy.[50,69] In absence seizures, available class III trials suggest that VPA is effective in absence seizures both as monotherapy and as add-on treatment. It is slightly more effective than ESM and equally effective to LTG.[52] A recent class III study in children (3–13 years) suggests equal efficacy to LTG as monotherapy but a faster action.[70]

In febrile seizures, one class III and two class IV studies suggest that VPA is more effective than placebo and PB in preventing recurrences.[71] Class IV studies suggest that VPA may potentially be efficacious in the treatment of myoclonic epilepsies,[72] IS,[39] West syndrome, and LGS.[73] Based on the available evidence, VPA is possibly efficacious for the treatment of partial, primary generalized or febrile seizures, and is potentially efficacious for the treatment of myoclonic seizures, IS, West syndrome, and LGS.

SECOND GENERATION AEDs (TABLE 49–3)

Felbamate

Due to its hepatic and hematologic toxicities, felbamate (FLB) is often used as a last resort when other less toxic AEDs fail to control seizures. Two double-blind RCTs reported the use of FLB as monotherapy in partial epilepsy. The first was a placebo-controlled class III trial in 40 subjects, ages 14–55 years. FLB was effective in reducing seizures; however, the study was underpowered due to withdrawals.[74] The second trial was a class III study that compared FLB monotherapy to VPA in 111 subjects, ages 16–67 years. FLB was more effective and better tolerated than VPA.[75]

FLB was also used as adjunctive treatment for LGS. A class III double-blind, placebo-controlled crossover trial reported the use of FLB as add-on to VPA therapy in 14 children, ages 4.2–15.7 years with LGS. FLB was efficacious in controlling drop attacks, apparently due to synergism between the two drugs.[76] Another class III double-blind, placebo-controlled trial reported that FLB was effective in controlling drop attacks and generalized tonic–clonic seizures in 73 patients (ages 4–36 years) with LGS when used as add-on therapy. These effects were maintained in the 12-month open-label follow-up study.[77,78] FLB is thus possibly efficacious as initial monotherapy for adolescents with partial epilepsy, and as adjunctive therapy for children and adolescents with LGS.

▶ **TABLE 49–3.** SECOND GENERATION AEDs IN PEDIATRIC EPILEPSIES AND LEVEL OF EVIDENCE OF TREATMENT RECOMMENDATION

	Partial	PGCS	Myoclonic	Absence	IS	LGS	BECTS
FLB	MonoRx (C)	—	—	—	—	Adjunctive (C)	—
GBP	Adjunctive (B)	—	—	—	—	—	—
LTG	MonoRx adjunctive (C)	MonoRx (C) adjunctive (B)	Adjunctive (E)	MonoRx (C)	MonoRx (D)	Adjunctive (A)	—
LEV	Adjunctive (C)	—	—	—	—	—	—
OXC	MonoRx adjunctive (A)	—	—	—	—	—	—
PGB	Adjunctive (D)	Adjunctive (D)	—	—	—	—	—
STP	—	—	Adjunctive (C)	—	—	—	—
STM	—	—	—	—	Adjunctive (C)	—	MonoRx (C)
TGB	Adjunctive (D)	—	—	—	—	—	—
TPM	MonoRx; adjunctive (A)	MonoRx; adjunctive (A)	MonoRx (U)	—	—	Adjunctive (A)	—
VGB	MonoRx (D)	—	—	—	MonoRx (C)	—	—
ZNS	Adjunctive (A)	—	—	—	—	—	—

Source: Adapted from Glauser T, et al. ILAE treatment guidelines: evidence-based analysis of antiepileptic drug efficacy and effectiveness as initial monotherapy for epileptic seizures and syndromes. *Epilepsia* 2006;47:1094–1120.
FLB, felbamate; GBP, gabapentin; LTG, lamotrigine; LEV, levetiracetam; OXC, oxcarbamazepine; PGB, progabide; STP, stiripentol; STM, sulthiame; TGB, tiagabine; TPM, topiramate; VGB, vigabatrin; ZNS, zonisamide; MonoRx, monotherapy.
Recommendation level: Level A: ≥1 class I RCT or ≥2 class II RCTs; level B: 1 class II RCT; level C: ≥2 class III RCTs; level D: 1 class III RCT; level E: ≥1 class IV studies or expert opinion.

Gabapentin

There is evidence from two class III double-blind, placebo-controlled trials[79,80] and one open-label RCT[81] that GBP is possibly effective and tolerable in refractory partial epilepsy. GBP is FDA approved as adjunctive treatment in partial epilepsy for children 3 years of age and older.

Lamotrigine

In newly diagnosed partial or generalized-onset seizures, evidence from one systematic review,[49] two double-blind,[82,83] and one open-label[84] RCTs (all are class III) reveal that LTG is possibly efficacious as monotherapy in controlling seizures and is equivalent to CBZ,[49,83,84] VPA,[83,84] PHA,[84] or GBP.[82] One class III study revealed that LTG is equally effective as adjunctive treatment for refractory partial epilepsy.[85] Another class II study suggests that LTG is probably effective as adjunctive treatment for refractory primary generalized seizures.[86] A Cochrane review compared LTG to VPA for treatment of absence seizures. Class III studies included in the review suggested that LTG was equally effective to VPA. LTG is thus possibly effective as monotherapy for absence seizures.[52]

A recent open-label class III study in children (ages 3–13 years) suggests equal efficacy to VPA as monotherapy but a slower action.[71] In LGS syndrome, one class I and one class II studies suggest that LTG is probably effective as add-on treatment for secondarily generalized seizures.[6] A review of case series and anecdotal reports suggests that LTG may be efficacious as adjunctive treatment for myoclonic seizures, but it may also cause worsening of seizures.[53]

Levetiracetam

One class III double-blind[87] and one open-label[88] clinical trials (ages >4 years) suggest that LEV is possibly efficacious and tolerable as add-on treatment for resistant partial seizures.

Oxcarbazepine

One class I evidence RCT,[89] one Cochrane review,[90] and several recent class III clinical trials suggest that OXC is effective, safe, and well tolerated both as monotherapy and as add-on treatment for partial-onset epilepsy in children.[91–93] OXC is FDA approved as monotherapy for partial-onset epilepsy in children ≥4 years and as adjunctive therapy for resistant partial-onset epilepsy in children ≥2 years.

Progabide

One class III double-blind, placebo-controlled, crossover RCT reported the use of progabide (PGB) in 20 patients (ages 7–47 years) as add-on treatment for refractory partial or generalized seizures and found it to be effective and well tolerated.[94]

Stiripentol

Two class III studies suggest that stiripentol (STP) is possibly efficacious as add-on treatment for severe myoclonic epilepsy in infants. An open-label study reported that STP reduced seizure frequency by more than 50% in half of the patients.[95] A double-blind, placebo-controlled trial found STP to be efficacious in 71% of the patients.[96]

Sulthiame

Sulthiame (STM) is potentially efficacious in West syndrome. One class III double-blind, placebo-controlled trial found STM to be effective in newly diagnosed infants with West syndrome, including tuberous sclerosis.[97] STM is also potentially effective in benign epilepsy with centrotemporal spikes (BECTS) based on results from one class III double-blind, placebo-controlled trial.[98]

Tiagabine

One class III open-label study in 243 patients (age ≥12 years) with refractory partial epilepsy found tiagabine (TGB) to be effective and tolerable treatment.[99]

Topiramate

Several class III double-blind trials suggest that TPM is possibly efficacious as monotherapy for newly diagnosed partial or generalized-onset seizures and as add-on treatment for refractory partial or generalized-onset epilepsy.[69,100,101–104] In LGS, evidence from one class I double-blind and two class III open-label studies suggest that add-on treatment with TPM is effective in reducing drop attacks.[105–107] One pilot study found TPM to have similar efficacy to VPA in JME.[108]

Vigabatrin

Evidence from several class III studies suggests that VGB is possibly efficacious as initial monotherapy for IS or West syndrome, especially in patients with tuberous sclerosis. An open-label RCT compared VGB to prednisolone or tetracosactide in 107 infants with IS (excluding tuberous sclerosis). More patients (76%) in the hormonal therapy group had cessation of spasms after 2 weeks, as compared to 54% in the VGB group. Follow-up at 12–14 months revealed similar rates of spasm control in both groups. However, in the subgroup of patients with cryptogenic IS, subjects who received hormonal therapy had a better neurodevelopmental outcome than those who received VGB.[109,110]

Another double-blind, placebo-controlled trial on 40 infants with West syndrome reported seizure control in 35% of patients receiving VGB as compared to 10% in the placebo arm.[111] One open-label RCT compared VGB to hydrocortisone in 22 patients with IS and tuberous sclerosis for 1 month. All patients receiving VGB responded as compared to 45% in the hydrocortisone group.[112]

In an open-label, crossover RCT, ACTH treatment resulted in a higher and quicker response compared to VGB. There was no difference in cognitive development between the two groups after 9–44 months of follow-up.[23] VGB has been tried as monotherapy for newly diagnosed partial seizures in a class III open-label RCT versus CBZ and was found to be equally safe and effective.[113]

Zonisamide

Evidence from one class III study in adults and children (ages >12 years) suggested that zonisamide (ZNS) was effective and well tolerated as adjunctive therapy in refractory partial seizures. No subgroup analysis by age was performed.[114]

ANTIEPILEPTICS IN STATUS EPILEPTICUS

Benzodiazepines

In general, benzodiazepines are first-line drugs for treatment of acute seizures and status epilepticus (SE).

Lorazepam. In SE, evidence from one class III open-label RCT[115] and one class IV comparative study[116] suggest that *intravenous lorazepam* is probably as efficacious as *intravenous diazepam* in controlling seizures in emergency room settings. *Intravenous lorazepam* controlled seizures within 5 minutes in 65%–75% of patients. Another class III open-label RCT compared *intranasal lorazepam* to *intramuscular paraldehyde* in 2 months to 12-year-old children with protracted convulsions. Intranasal lorazepam was equally effective in stopping convulsions within 10 minutes from administration. No clinically significant adverse effects were seen in either group.[117]

Midazolam. In refractory status epilepticus (RSE), several class III and IV studies suggest that intravenous, intramuscular, intranasal, or buccal midazolam is efficacious in terminating RSE. One class IV study reported case series of *intravenous midazolam* (as bolus or continuous) infusions in patients (35 weeks to 12 years of age) with SE. Intravenous midazolam was effective in terminating refractory seizures and was well tolerated.[118] *Continuous infusion of midazolam*

was also compared to *continuous infusion of diazepam* in a class III open-label study involving 40 patients (ages 2 months to 12 years) with RSE. Both drugs were equally effective in seizure control, but midazolam was associated with more recurrences.[119]

Two class III RCTs in children of different ages compared *intramuscular midazolam* to *intravenous diazepam*. Midazolam resulted in a faster cessation of seizures with minimal side effects.[120,121]

Intranasal midazolam was found to be equally effective and safe when compared to *intravenous diazepam* in 70 children (ages 2 months to 15 years) with acute seizures (class III).[122] *Intranasal midazolam* was also compared to *rectal diazepam* in two class III and class IV trials. Midazolam was more effective than diazepam in seizure cessation with no serious adverse events.[123,124]

Two class III RCTs compared *buccal midazolam* to *rectal diazepam* in children with prolonged acute seizures. Both drugs were equally effective and safe but buccal midazolam was more "socially" acceptable.[125,126]

Diazepam. A review of 76 case reports indicated that diazepam was extremely effective in a wide range of SE, in agreement with expert opinion that considered intravenous diazepam as the drug of choice in this condition (class IV).[127]

Several case series and retrospective studies reported the use of rectal diazepam in SE or prolonged febrile and nonfebrile seizures. Rectal diazepam was found to be rapidly absorbed and equally effective to intravenous diazepam (class IV studies).[128]

A class III double-blind, placebo-controlled RCT reported that home treatment of repetitive seizures with rectal diazepam (Diastat) in 114 patients ≥2 years of age was efficacious in reducing seizures.[129]

Phenobarbital

Very high-dose PB (80 mg/kg) was found to be effective in controlling seizures in three children with RSE with mild adverse events reported in comparison to thiopental (class IV).[130]

Pentobarbital

Pentobarbital coma is the most universally accepted treatment of RSE, defined as persistent seizures lasting 60 minutes or more despite appropriate AED treatment. However, the duration of drug treatment and optimal drug dosage is still uncertain. Currently, limited data exists in the pediatric literature since the use of pentobarbital coma is based primarily on case series. One series in 23 patients (ages 0–13 years) reported 52% response rate. Nonresponders had a high mortality rate (91%) as opposed to 0% in responders. Survival rate

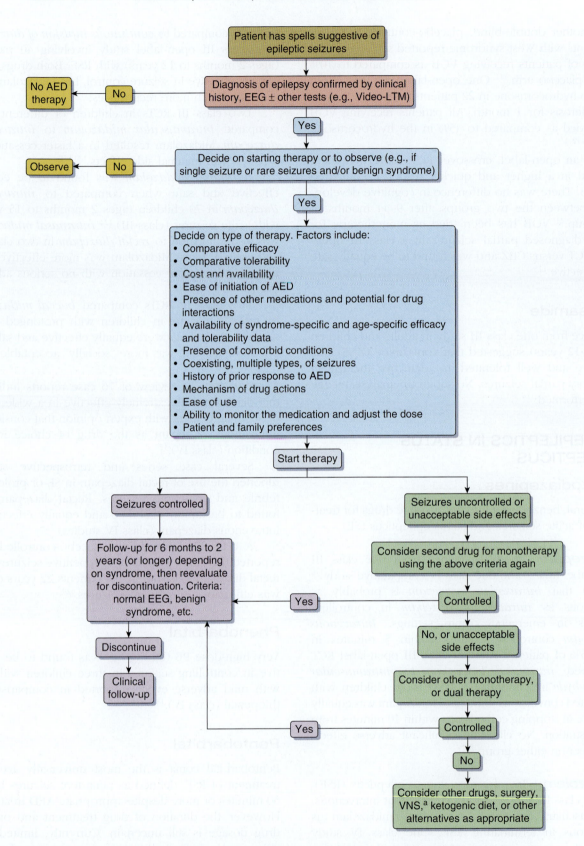

Figure 49–1. Flow chart illustrating general approach to the therapy of epilepsy.

was greater among toddlers as compared to neonates (class IV). Pentobarbital coma has serious complications such as hypotension, and bradycardia, especially in neonates, necessitating continuous monitoring.[131]

Propofol

Propofol has a rapid onset of action and quick recovery time. Its use in RSE is primarily based on case reports and small case series (class IV evidence). A retrospective study reported the experience with propofol versus thiopental in the treatment of 34 episodes of RSE. RSE could be controlled in 14 of 22 episodes (64%) treated with propofol as compared to 11 of 20 (55%) episodes treated with thiopental. Adverse events include rhabdomyolysis, hypertriglyceridemia, elevation in creatine kinase, metabolic acidosis, and cardiovascular collapse. Dosages above 5 mg/kg per hour and/or prolonged use (propofol infusion syndrome) have been associated with high mortality.[132]

Thiopental

Thiopental was compared to propofol in RSE in the retrospective study summarized previously.[132] Thiopental can result in serious adverse events associated with fatalities such as acute hepatic failure, pulmonary damage, multiple organ dysfunction, increased risk of infections especially pulmonary infections or sepsis.

Topiramate

One class IV study reported the use of TPM in three children (ages 4.5 months to 11 years) who had RSE. TPM stopped seizures in all three children.[133]

Valproate

One class IV study in children ≥1 year of age with SE found VPA to be more effective in seizure control than PHT, both as monotherapy and as a second-line treatment. Intravenous VPA is potentially effective as second-line therapy after benzodiazepines in myoclonic, absence or generalized tonic–clonic status.[134]

► CONCLUSIONS

Therapy of epilepsy is usually based on multiple considerations including controlled and uncontrolled data (Fig. 49–1). It is not based on correcting the primary underlying etiology but reducing neuronal excitability that is the final common pathway in epileptic seizures.

After a first seizure, treatment may be withheld in favor of further observation. However, if therapy has to be initiated, several factors should be considered: comparative efficacy and relative tolerability, cost and availability, ease of initiation of AED, presence of background medications with potential for drug interactions, availability of syndrome-specific and age-specific efficacy and tolerability data, presence of comorbid conditions, coexisting seizures, history of prior response to AEDs, mechanisms of drug actions, ease of use, ability to monitor the medication and adjust the dose, as well as patient and family preferences. In addition, guidelines by concerned organizations and evidence-based resources are useful in the decision-making process including the Cochrane database, ILAE, AAN, NICE, and SIGN guidelines.

Once seizures are controlled, follow-up should be performed for 2 years or longer depending on the syndrome. Reevaluation for AED discontinuation depends on certain criteria such as type of epilepsy syndrome and normalization of the EEG. If the seizures are uncontrolled, then other medications (whether mono- or dual therapy) should be considered. Finally, if all treatments do not provide adequate seizure control, surgery, or vagal nerve stimulation (VNS) should be considered.

REFERENCES

1. Wheless JW, Clarke DF, Carpenter D. Treatment of pediatric epilepsy: expert opinion, 2005. *J Child Neurol* 2005;20(Suppl 1):S1–S56.
2. Glauser T, et al. ILAE treatment guidelines: evidence-based analysis of antiepileptic drug efficacy and effectiveness as initial monotherapy for epileptic seizures and syndromes. *Epilepsia* 2006;47:1094–1120.
3. National Institute for Clinical Excellence (NICE). *Technology Appraisal Guidance 79, Newer Drugs for Epilepsy in Children* (Available at http://guidance.nice.org.uk/TA79/guidance/pdf/English) and *Clinical Guideline 20, The Epilepsies: The Diagnosis and Management of the Epilepsies in Adults and Children in Primary and Secondary Care*, (Available at http://guidance.nice.org.uk/CG20/niceguidance/pdf/English), 2004.
4. Scottish Intercollegiate Guidelines Network. *Diagnosis and Management of Epilepsies in Children and Young People: A National Clinical Guideline*. Edinburgh: Scottish Intercollegiate Guidelines Network, 2005. Available at http://www.sign.ac.uk/pdf/sign81.pdf.
5. French JA, et al. Efficacy and tolerability of the new antiepileptic drugs I: treatment of new onset epilepsy. Report of the Therapeutics and Technology Assessment Subcommittee and Quality Standards Subcommittee of the American Academy of Neurology and the American Epilepsy Society. *Neurology* 2004;62:1252–1260.
6. French JA, et al. Efficacy and tolerability of the new antiepileptic drugs II: treatment of refractory epilepsy. Report of the TTA and QSS Subcommittees of the American Academy of Neurology and the American Epilepsy Society. *Epilepsia* 2004;45:410–423.
7. Camfield P, Camfield C, Dooley J, Smith E, Garner B. A randomized study of carbamazepine versus no medication after a first unprovoked seizure in childhood. *Neurology* 1989;39:851–852.

8. Chandra B. First seizure in adults: to treat or not to treat. *Clin Neurol Neurosurg* 1992;94(Suppl):S61–S63.

9. Musicco M, Beghi E, Solari A, Viani F, First Seizure Trial Group (FIRST Group). Treatment of first tonic–clonic seizure does not improve the prognosis of epilepsy. *Neurology* 1997;49:991–998.

10. Gilad R, Lampl Y, Gabbay U, Eshel Y, Sarova-Pinhas I. Early treatment of a single generalized tonic–clonic seizure to prevent recurrence. *Arch Neurol* 1996;53:1149–1152.

11. Marson A, Jacoby A, Johnson A, Kim L, Gamble C, Chadwick D. Immediate versus deferred antiepileptic drug treatment for early epilepsy and single seizures: a randomised controlled trial. *Lancet* 2005;365:2007–2013.

12. Marson AG, et al. The SANAD study of effectiveness of carbamazepine, gabapentin, lamotrigine, oxcarbazepine, or topiramate for treatment of partial epilepsy: an unblinded randomized controlled trial. *Lancet* 2007;369:1000–1015.

13. Marson AG, et al. The SANAD study of effectiveness of valproate, lamotrigine, or topiramate for generalized and unclassifiable epilepsy: an unblinded randomized controlled trial. *Lancet* 2007;369:1016–1026.

14. US Department of Health and Human Services. *Acute Pain Management: Operative or Medical Procedures and Trauma, in Clinical Practice Guideline No. 1.* Rockville: Agency for Healthcare Policy and Research, 1993; p. 107.

15. Edlund W, Gronseth G, So Y, Franklin G. *American Academy of Neurology Clinical Practice Guideline Process Manual.* St. Paul: American Academy of Neurology, 2004.

16. Reiss WG, Oles KS. Acetazolamide in the treatment of seizures. *Ann Pharmacother* 1996;30:514–519.

17. Katayama F, Miura H, Takanashi S. Long-term effectiveness and side effects of acetazolamide as an adjunct to other anticonvulsants in the treatment of refractory epilepsies. *Brain Dev* 2002;24:150–154.

18. Forsythe WI, Owens JR, Toothill C. Effectiveness of acetazolamide in the treatment of carbamazepine-resistant epilepsy in children. *Develop Med Child Neurol* 1981;23:761–769.

19. Oles KS, Penry JK, Cole DLW, Howard G. Use of acetazolamide as an adjunct to carbamazepine in refractory partial seizures. *Epilepsia* 1989;30:74–78.

20. Resor SR, Resor LD. Chronic acetazolamide monotherapy in the treatment of juvenile myoclonic epilepsy. *Neurology* 1990;40:1677–1681.

21. Baram TZ, Mitchell WG, Tournay A, Snead OC, Hanson RA, Horton EJ. High-dose corticotrophin (ACTH) versus prednisone for infantile spasms: a prospective, randomized, blinded study. *Pediatrics* 1996;97:375–379.

22. Hrachovy RA, Frost JD, Kellaway P, Zion TE. Double blind study of ACTH vs. prednisone in infantile spasms. *J Pediatr* 1983;103:641–645.

23. Vigevano F, Cilio MR. Vigabatrin versus ACTH as the first line treatment of infantile spasms. *Epilepsia* 1997;38:1270–1274.

24. Dreifuss F, et al. Infantile spasms. Comparative trial of nitrazepam and corticotrophin. *Arch Neurol* 1986;43:1107–1110.

25. Snead OC 3rd, Benton JW, Myers GJ. ACTH and prednisone in childhood seizure disorders. *Neurology* 1983;33:966–970.

26. Yamatogi Y, et al. Treatment of the Lennox–Gastaut syndrome with ACTH: a clinical and electroencephalographic study. *Brain Dev* 1979;1:267–276.

27. O'Reagan ME, Brown JK. ACTH in the treatment of epilepsy. *Dev Med Child Neurol* 1998;40:82–89.

28. Canadian Study Group for Childhood Epilepsy. Clobazam has equivalent efficacy to carbamazepine and phenytoin as monotherapy for childhood epilepsy. *Epilepsia* 1998;39:952–959.

29. Kaushal S, Rani A, Chopra SC, Singh G. Safety and efficacy of clobazam versus phenytoin-sodium in the antiepileptic drug treatment of solitary cysticercus granulomas. *Neurol India* 2006;54:157–160.

30. Robertson MM. Current status of the 1,4- and 1,5-benzodiazepines in the treatment of epilepsy: the place of clobazam. *Epilepsia* 1986;27(Suppl 1):S27–S41.

31. Foldvary-Schaefer N, Falcone T. Catamenial epilepsy: pathophysiology, diagnosis, and management. *Neurology* 2003;61(Suppl 2):S2–S15.

32. Eeg-Olofsson O. Experiences with Rivotril® in the treatment of epilepsy—particularly minor motor epilepsy—in mentally retarded children. *Acta Neurol Scandinav* 1973;49(Suppl 53):29–31.

33. Mikkelsen B, Berggreen P, Joensen P, Kristensen O, Køhler O, Mikkelsen BO. Clonazepam (Rivotril®) and carbamazepine (Tegretol®) in psychomotor epilepsy: a randomized multicenter trial. *Epilepsia* 1981;22:415–420.

34. Mitsudome A, et al. The effectiveness of clonazepam on the Rolandic discharges. *Brain Dev* 1997;19:274–278.

35. Dahlin M, Knutsson E, Åmark P, Nergårdh A. Reduction of epileptiform activity in response to low-dose clonazepam in children with epilepsy: a randomized double-blind study. *Epilepsia* 2000;41:308–315.

36. Booker HE. Clorazepate dipotassium in the treatment of intractable epilepsy. *JAMA* 1974;229:552–555.

37. Lahat E, Goldman M, Barr J, Bistritzer T, Berkovitch M. Comparison of intranasal midazolam with intravenous diazepam for treating febrile seizures in children: prospective randomised study. *BMJ* 2000;321:83–86.

38. Hagberg B. The chlordiazepoxide HCl (Librium) analogue nitrazepam (Mogadon) in the treatment of epilepsy in children. *Develop Med Child Neurol* 1968;10:302–308.

39. Mackay MT, et al. Practice parameter: medical treatment of infantile spasms. Report of the American Academy of Neurology and the Child Neurology Society. *Neurology* 2004;62:1668–1681.

40. Lou HOC. Oxazepam in the treatment of psychomotor epilepsy. *Neurology* 1968;18:986–990.

41. Kagitani-Shimono K, et al. Epilepsy in Wolf–Hirschhorn syndrome (4p-). *Epilepsia* 2005;46:150–155.

42. Takayanagi M, et al. Two successful cases of bromide therapy for refractory symptomatic localization-related epilepsy. *Brain Dev* 2002;24:194–196.

43. Oguni H, et al. Treatment of severe myoclonic epilepsy in infants with bromide and its borderline variant. *Epilepsia* 1994;35:1140–1145.

44. Steinhoff B, Kruse R. Bromide treatment of pharmaco-resistant epilepsies with generalized tonic–clonic seizures: a clinical study. *Brain Dev* 1992;14:144–149.

45. Ernst JP, Doose H, Baier WK. Bromides were effective in intractable epilepsy with generalized tonic–clonic seizures and onset in early childhood. *Brain Dev* 1988;10:385–388.

46. Tudur Smith C, Marson AG, Williamson PR. Carbamazepine versus phenobarbitone monotherapy for epilepsy. *Cochrane Database Syst Rev* 2003;CD001904.

47. Marson AG, Williamson PR, Clough H, Hutton JL, Chadwick DW, Epilepsy Monotherapy Trial Group. Carbamazepine versus valproate monotherapy for epilepsy: a meta-analysis. *Epilepsia* 2002;43:505–513.

48. Chadwick DW, et al. A double-blind trial of gabapentin monotherapy for newly diagnosed partial seizures. International Gabapentin Monotherapy Study Group 945–77. *Neurology* 1998;51:1282–1288.

49. Gamble CL, Williamson PR, Marson AG. Lamotrigine versus carbamazepine monotherapy for epilepsy. *Cochrane Database Syst Rev* 2006;CD001031.

50. Wheless JW, Neto W, Wang S, EPMN-105 Study Group. Topiramate, carbamazepine, and valproate monotherapy: double-blind comparison in children with newly diagnosed epilepsy. *J Child Neurol* 2004;19:135–141.

51. Dam M, Ekberg R, Loyning Y, Waltimo O, Jakobsen K. A double-blind study comparing oxcarbazepine and carbamazepine in patients with newly diagnosed, previously untreated epilepsy. *Epilepsy Res* 1989;3:70–76.

52. Posner EB, Mohamed K, Marson AG. Ethosuximide, sodium valproate or lamotrigine for absence seizures in children and adolescents. *Cochrane Database Syst Rev* 2005;4:CD003032.

53. Wallace SJ. Myoclonus and epilepsy in childhood: a review of treatment with valproate, ethosuximide, lamotrigine and zonisamide. *Epilepsy Res* 1998;29:147–154.

54. Tennison MB, Greenwood RS, Miles MV. Methsuximide for intractable childhood seizures. *Pediatrics* 1991;87:186–189.

55. Sigler M, Strassburg HM, Boenigk HE. Effective and safe but forgotten: methsuximide in intractable epilepsies in childhood. *Seizure* 2001;10:120–124.

56. Wilder BJ, Buchanan RA. Methsuximide for refractory complex seizures. *Neurology* 1981;31:741–744.

57. Hurst DL. Methsuximide therapy of juvenile myoclonic epilepsy. *Seizure* 1996;5:47–50.

58. Kwan P, Brodie MJ. Phenobarbital for the treatment of epilepsy in the 21st century: a critical review. *Epilepsia* 2004;45:1141–1149.

59. Taylor S, Tudur Smith C, Williamson PR, Marson AG. Phenobarbitone versus phenytoin monotherapy for partial onset seizures and generalized onset tonic–clonic seizures. *Cochrane Database Syst Rev* 2003;2: CD002217.

60. De Silva M, et al. Randomised comparative monotherapy trial of phenobarbitone, phenytoin, carbamazepine, or sodium valproate for newly diagnosed childhood epilepsy. *Lancet* 1996;347:709–713.

61. Pal DK, Das T, Chaudhury G, Johnson AL, Neville BG. Randomised controlled trial to assess acceptability of phenobarbital for childhood epilepsy in rural India. *Lancet* 1998;351:19–23.

62. Rantala H, Tarkka R, Ubari M. A meta-analytic review of the preventive treatment of recurrences of febrile seizures. *J Pediatr* 1997;131:922–925.

63. Boylan GB, Rennie JM, Pressler RM, Wilson G, Morton M, Binnie CD. Phenobarbitone, neonatal seizures, and video-EEG. *Arch Dis Child Fetal Neonatal Ed* 2002; 86(3):F165–F170.

64. Painter MJ, et al. Phenobarbital compared with phenytoin for the treatment of neonatal seizures. *N Engl J Med* 1999; 341:485–489.

65. Castro Conde JR, Hernandez Borges AA, Domenech Martinez E, Gonzales Campo C, Perera Soler R. Midazolam in neonatal seizures with no response to phenobarbital. *Neurology* 2005;64:876–879.

66. Dodson WE, Bourgeois BFD. Pharmacology and therapeutic aspects of antiepileptic drugs in pediatrics. *J Child Neurol* 1994;9:281–287.

67. Booth D, Evans DJ. Anticonvulsants for neonates with seizures. *Cochrane Database Syst Rev* 2004;3:CD004218.

68. Schierhout G, Roberts I. Anti-epileptic drugs for preventing seizures following acute traumatic brain injury. *Cochrane Database Syst Rev* 2001;(4):CD000173.

69. Privitera MD, Brodie MJ, Mattson RH, Chadwick DW, Neto W, Wang S, EPMN 105 Study Group. Topiramate, carbamazepine and valproate monotherapy: double-blind comparison in newly diagnosed epilepsy. *Acta Neurol Scand* 2003;107:165–175.

70. Coppola G, Auricchio G, Federico R, Carotenuto M, Pascotto A. Lamotrigine versus valproic acid as first-line monotherapy in newly diagnosed typical absence seizures: an open-label, randomized, parallel-group study. *Epilepsia* 2004;45:1049–1053.

71. Baumann RJ. Technical report: treatment of the child with simple febrile seizures. *Pediatrics* 1999;103:e86.

72. Aldenkamp A, Vigevano F, Arzimanoglou A, Covanis A. Role of valproate across the ages: treatment of epilepsy in children. *Acta Neurol Scand* 2006;114(Suppl 184): 1–13.

73. Guerrini R. Valproate as a mainstay of therapy for pediatric epilepsy. *Pediatr Drugs* 2006;8:113–129.

74. Theodore WH, et al. Felbamate monotherapy: implications for antiepileptic drug development. *Epilepsia* 1995;36:1105–1110.

75. Faught E, et al. Felbamate monotherapy for partial-onset seizures: an active-control trial. *Neurology* 1993;43:688–692.

76. Siegel H, et al. The efficacy of felbamate as add-on therapy to valproic acid in the Lennox–Gastaut syndrome. *Epilepsy Res* 1999;34:91–97.

77. The felbamate Study group in Lennox–Gastaut Syndrome. Efficacy of felbamate in childhood epileptic encephalopathy (Lennox–Gastaut syndrome). *N Engl J Med* 1993;328:29–33.

78. Dodson WE. Felbamate in the treatment of Lennox–Gastaut Syndrome: results of a 12-month open-label study following a randomized clinical trial. *Epilepsia* 1993;34(Suppl 7):S18–S24.

79. Appleton R, et al. Gabapentin as add-on therapy in children with refractory partial seizures: a 12-week, multicentre, double-blind, placebo-controlled study. Gabapentin Paediatric Study Group. *Epilepsia* 1999;40:1147–1154.

80. Yamauchi T, Kaneko S, Yagi K, Sase S. Treatment of partial seizures with gabapentin: double-blind, placebo-controlled, parallel-group study. *Psychiatry Clin Neurosci* 2006;60:507–515.

81. Korn-Merker E, Borusiak P, Boenigk HE. Gabapentin in childhood epilepsy: a prospective evaluation of efficacy and safety. *Epilepsy Res* 2000;38:27–32.

82. Brodie MJ, et al. Gabapentin versus lamotrigine monotherapy: a double-blind comparison in newly diagnosed epilepsy. *Epilepsia* 2002;43:993–1000.

83. Steinhoff BJ, Ueberall MA, Siemes H, Kurlemann G, Schmitz B, Bergmann L. The LAM-SAFE Study: lamotrigine versus carbamazepine or valproic acid in newly diagnosed focal and generalised epilepsies in adolescents and adults. *Seizure* 2005;14:597–605.

84. Kaminow L, Schimschock JR, Hammer AE, Vuong A. Lamotrigine monotherapy compared with carbamazepine, phenytoin, or valproate monotherapy in patients with epilepsy. *Epilepsy Behavior* 2003;4:659–666.

85. Duchowny M, et al. A placebo-controlled trial of lamotrigine add-on therapy for partial seizures in children: Lamictal Pediatric Partial Seizure Study Group. *Neurology* 1999;53:1724–1731.

86. Trevathan E, Kerls SP, Hammer AE, Vuong A, Messenheimer JA. Lamotrigine adjunctive therapy among children and adolescents with primary generalized tonic–clonic seizures. *Pediatrics* 2006;118:e371–e378.

87. Glauser TA, et al. Double-blind placebo-controlled trial of adjunctive levetiracetam in pediatric partial seizures. *Neurology* 2006;66:1654–1660.

88. Glauser TA, et al. Efficacy and safety of levetiracetam in children with partial seizures: an open-label trial. *Epilepsia* 2002;43:518–524.

89. Guerreiro MM, et al. A double-blind controlled clinical trial of oxcarbazepine versus phenytoin in children and adolescents with epilepsy. *Epilepsy Res* 1997;27:205–213.

90. Castillo S, Schmidt DB, White S. Oxcarbazepine add-on for drug-resistant partial epilepsy. *Cochrane Database of Sys Rev* 2000; (3):CD002028.

91. Beydoun A, Sachdeo RC, Kutluay E, McCague K, D'Souza J. Sustained efficacy and long-term safety of oxcarbazepine: one-year open-label extension of study in refractory partial epilepsy. *Epilepsia* 2003;44:1160–1165.

92. Piña-Garza JE, et al. Oxcarbazepine adjunctive therapy in infants and young children with partial seizures. *Neurology* 2005;65:1370–1375.

93. Donati F, et al. Effects of oxcarbazepine on cognitive function in children and adolescents with partial seizures. *Neurology* 2006;67:679–682.

94. Loiseau P, Bossi L, Guyot M, Orofiamma B, Morselli PL. Double-blind crossover trial of progabide versus placebo in severe epilepsies. *Epilepsia* 1983;24:703–715.

95. Perez J, et al. Stiripentol: efficacy and tolerability in epileptic children. *Epilepsia* 1999;40:1618–1626.

96. Chiron C, et al. Stiripentol in severe myoclonic epilepsy in infancy: a randomized placebo-controlled syndrome-dedicated trial. *Lancet* 2000;356:1638–1642.

97. Debus OM, Kurlemann G, for the Sulthiame Study Group. Sulthiame in the primary therapy of West Syndrome: a randomized double-blind placebo-controlled add-on trial on baseline pyridoxine medication. *Epilepsia* 2004;45:103–108.

98. Rating D, Wolf C, Bast T, Sulthiame Study Group. Sulthiame as monotherapy in children with benign childhood epilepsy with centrotemporal spikes: a 6-month randomized, double-blind, placebo-controlled study. *Epilepsia* 2000;41:1284–1288.

99. Arroyo S, et al. A randomised open-label study of tiagabine given two or three times daily in refractory epilepsy. *Seizure* 2005;14:81–84.

100. Gilliam FG, et al. A dose-comparison trial of topiramate as monotherapy in recently diagnosed partial epilepsy. *Neurology* 2003;60:196–202.

101. Arroyo S, et al. Randomized dose-controlled study of topiramate as first-line therapy in epilepsy. *Acta Neurol Scand* 2005;112:214–222.

102. Reife R, Pledger G, Wu SC. Topiramate as add-on therapy: pooled analysis of randomized controlled trials in adults. *Epilepsia* 2000;41(Suppl 1):S66–S71.

103. Elterman RD, Glauser TA, Wyllie E, Reife R, Wu SC, Pedger G. A double-blind, randomized trial of topiramate as adjunctive therapy for partial-onset seizures in children: Topiramate YP Study Group. *Neurology* 1999;52:1338–1344.

104. Biton V, et al. A randomized, placebo-controlled study of topiramate in primary generalized tonic–clonic seizures: Topiramate YTC Study Group. *Neurology* 1999;52:1330–1337.

105. Sachdeo RC, Glauser TA, Ritter F, Reife R, Lim P, Pledger G. A double-blind, randomized trial of topiramate in Lennox–Gastaut syndrome: Topiramate YL Study Group. *Neurology* 1999;52:1882–1887.

106. Glauser TA, Levisohn PM, Ritter F, Sachdeo RC. Topiramate in Lennox–Gastaut syndrome: open-label treatment of patients completing a randomized controlled trial: Topirmate YL Study Group. *Epilepsia* 2000;41:S86–S90.

107. Coppola G, et al. Topiramate as add-on drug in children, adolescents and young adults with Lennox–Gastaut syndrome: an Italian multicentric study. *Epilepsy Res* 2002;51:147–153.

108. Levisohn PM, Hulihan JF, Fisher AC. Topiramate versus valproate in patients with juvenile myoclonic epilepsy. *Epilepsia* 2003;44(Suppl 9):267.

109. Lux AL, et al. The United Kingdom Infantile Spasms Study (UKISS) comparing vigabatrin with prednisolone or tetracosactide at 14 days: a multicentre, randomised controlled trial. *Lancet* 2004;364:1773–1778.

110. Lux AL, et al. The United Kingdom Infantile Spasms Study (UKISS) comparing hormone treatment with vigabatrin on developmental and epilepsy outcomes to age 14 months: a multicentre randomized trial. *Lancet* 2005;4:712–717.

111. Appleton RE, Peters ACB, Mumford JP, Shaw DE. Randomised, placebo-controlled study of vigabatrin as first-line treatment of infantile spasms. *Epilepsia* 1991; 40:1627–1633.

112. Chiron C, Dumas C, Jambaque I, Mumford J, Dulac O. Randomised trial comparing vigabatrin and hydrocortisone in infantile spasms due to tuberous sclerosis. *Epilepsy Res* 1997;26:389–395.

113. Sobaniec W, Kutac W, Strzelecka J, Śmigielska-Kuzia J, Boćkowski L. A comparative study of vigabatrin versus carbamazepine in monotherapy of newly diagnosed partial seizures in children. *Pharmacol Rep* 2005;57:646–653.

114. Brodie MJ, Duncan R, Vespignani H, Solyom A, Bitensky V, Lucas C. Dose-dependent safety and efficacy of zonisamide: a randomized, double-blind, placebo-controlled study in patients with refractory partial seizures. *Epilepsia* 2005;46:31–41.

115. Appleton RE, Sweeney A, Choonara I, Robson J, Molyneux E. Lorazepam versus diazepam in the acute treatment of epileptic seizures and status epilepticus. *Dev Med Child Neurol* 1995;37:682–688.

116. Qureshi A, Wassmer E, Davies P, Berry K, Whitehouse WP. Comparative audit of intravenous lorazepam and diazepam in the emergency treatment of convulsive status epilepticus in children. *Seizure* 2002;11:141–144.

117. Ahmad S, Ellis JC, Kamwendo H, Molyneux E. Efficacy and safety of intranasal lorazepam versus intramuscular paraldehyde for protracted convulsions in children: an open randomized trial. *Lancet* 2006;367:1591–1597.

118. Holmes GL, Riviello JJ Jr. Midazolam and pentobarbital for refractory status epilepticus. *Pediatr Neurol* 1999; 20:259–264.

119. Singhi S, Murthy A, Singhi P, Jayashree M. Continuous midazolam versus diazepam infusion for refractory convulsive status epilepticus. *J Child Neurol* 2002;17:106–110.

120. Chamberlain JM, Altieri MA, Futterman C, Young GM, Ochsenschlager DW, Waisman Y. A prospective, randomized study comparing intramuscular midazolam with intravenous diazepam for the treatment of seizures in children. *Pediatr Emerg Care* 1997;13:92–94.

121. Shah I, Deshmukh CT. Intramuscular midazolam vs. intravenous diazepam for acute seizures. *Indian J Pediatr* 2005;72:667–670.

122. Mahmoudian T, Mohammadi Zadeh M. Comparison of intranasal midazolam with intravenous diazepam for treating acute seizures in children. *Epilep Behaviour* 2004;5:253–255.

123. Fişgin T, et al. Effects of intranasal midazolam and rectal diazepam on acute convulsions in children: prospective randomized study. *J Child Neurol* 2002;17:123–126.

124. Bhattacharyya M, Karla V, Gulati S. Intranasal midazolam vs. rectal diazepam in acute childhood seizures. *Pediatr Neurol* 2006;34:355–359.

125. Scott RC, Besag FM, Neville BGR. Buccal midazolam and rectal diazepam for treatment of prolonged seizures in childhood and adolescence: a randomised trial. *Lancet* 1999;353:623–626.

126. McIntyre J, et al. Safety and efficacy of buccal midazolam versus rectal diazepam for emergency treatment of seizures in children: a randomized controlled trial. *Lancet* 2005;366:205–210.

127. Browne TR, Penry JK. Benzodiazepines in the treatment of epilepsy. A review. *Epilepsia (Amst.)* 1973;14:277–310.

128. Sieger RS. The administration of rectal diazepam for acute management of seizures. *J Emerg Med* 1990;8:155–159.

129. Cereghinon JJ, et al. Treating repetitive seizures with a rectal diazepam formulation. A randomized study. *Neurology* 1998;51:1274–1282.

130. Lee WK, Liu KT, Young BWY. Very-high-dose phenobarbital for childhood refractory status epilepticus. *Pediatr Neurol* 2006;34:63–65.

131. Kim SJ, Lee DY, Kim JS. Neurologic outcomes of pediatric epileptic patients with pentobarbital coma. *Pediatr Neurol* 2001;25:217–220.

132. van Gestel JPJ, van Oud-Alblas B, Malingre M, Ververs FFT, Braun KPJ, van Nieuwenhuizen O. Propofol and thiopental for refractory status epilepticus in children. *Neurology* 2005;65:591–592.

133. Kahriman M, Minecan D, Kutluay E, Selwa L, Beydoun A. Efficacy of topiramate in children with refractory status epilepticus. *Epilepsia* 2003;44:1353–1356.

134. Wheless JW. Acute management of seizures in the syndromes of idiopathic generalized epilepsies. *Epilepsia* 2003;44(Suppl 2):2–26.

CHAPTER 50

A Practical Guide to AED Pharmacology

Jamie T. Gilman and Kim West

Almost half of the patients who initially present with epilepsy will become seizure free on their first antiepileptic drug (AED). The prognosis for the remaining half who fail initial treatment is less optimistic with response rates plummeting lower with each successive treatment failure.[1] This data underscore the importance of selecting an agent with a high probability of success early in treatment. In children, agent selection is often the foundation for successful therapy.

Pediatric therapy is confounded by the need to choose an appropriate dosage regimen and formulation that are compatible with a higher metabolic rate, heightened sensitivity to adverse drug effects, and drug–drug/drug–food compatibility issues in childhood. Achieving therapy goals is fraught with challenges as many product formulations are not pediatric-friendly. Furthermore, organogenesis complicates medication dosing by a continuum of pharmacokinetic changes that necessitate frequent monitoring and possible custom drug formulations.[2,3] Inadequate dosage regimens easily lead to treatment failure and an undeserved label of intractable epilepsy.[4] Thus, pharmacoresistance in childhood can have complex etiologies.

▶ EFFICACY ISSUES

Hepatic Phase I biotransformation reactions are diminished in infants during the first 6 months of life but subsequently attain and supersede adult values resulting in rapid drug elimination. This can cause ineffective drug exposure and an inadequate therapeutic response. While serum AED concentration monitoring is not typically encouraged, it remains useful to gain insight into dosing pitfalls in unresponsive children. *Routine* monitoring has not provided value for patient care for the second generation AEDs. Unlike the older AEDs, the newer agents lack convincing and consistent evidence of a therapeutic correlation with serum drug concentrations.[5,6]

The value of *routine* monitoring for older AEDs has also been questioned, particularly for asymptomatic patients.[7] Serum concentration determinations may yield useful information regarding developmental pharmacokinetic changes in childhood.[8] Children who fail treatment despite higher than recommended doses warrant serum concentration assessments even with the second generation AEDs. In situations where serum concentrations are only slightly low, a minor dosage, dosing interval, or dosage form alteration may significantly improve response. Extremely low values, however, are suggestive of a more complicated problem.

The differential diagnoses for exceedingly low drug concentrations include: rapid drug clearance, impaired oral absorption, generic substitution problems, drug interactions (producing changes in protein binding, volume of distribution, or metabolism), dispensing errors, or medication noncompliance. Differentiating between these causative factors enables regimen changes that may improve therapeutic response.[2] The possibility of a diagnostic reassessment (e.g., seizure reclassification, consideration oft pseudoseizures, etc.) in unresponsive children with adequate serum AED concentrations should not be overlooked.

The distinction between poor oral absorption, rapid drug elimination, and medication noncompliance can be determined by basic drug clearance determinations. This method requires at least three serial serum AED concentrations within the same dosage interval (i.e., no drug administered between blood draws).[9] The time interval between the first and third specimen should be equivalent or longer than the half-life of the AED. It is frequently necessary to delay the next scheduled dose to allow an appropriate time lapse between specimens.

A bolus dose may be necessary if baseline serum concentrations are extremely low. This boost facilitates a sufficiently high serum concentration to demonstrate a suitable decline between specimens with a measurable value on the last sample. It is also important that the first specimen be obtained after the drug absorption phase, so that all specimens are drawn only on the elimination side of the serum concentration time curve. The first blood draw can usually be obtained 2 hours after drug administration as this is typically sufficient for completion of the absorption phase of most immediate release formulations.

For extended release (ER) formulations, the absorption phase may be as long as 6–8 hours after the dose. Serial testing with these products requires the elimination of a dose to allow both completion of the absorption phase and an acceptable time (one half-life) between the first and last specimen. The procedure and formulas for drug elimination calculations are reviewed elsewhere.[9]

Rapid AED clearance is likely when serum drug concentrations drop rapidly (>50%) between serial blood specimens. There are three primary methods to overcome hypermetabolism and maintain an effective drug exposure: (1) increasing dosing frequency and drug dose (e.g., from bid to tid dosing) to accommodate the high elimination rate, (2) use a sustained release formulation, (3) change to an AED with a longer drug half-life or renal excretion.

ER formulations retard drug release and are popular to maintain stable serum concentrations. Sustained release products release drug continuously into the system protecting the total dose from immediate metabolism. Even ER products require more frequent dosing in children compared to adults (e.g., every 8 hours vs. every 12 hours). However, they maintain more consistent serum concentrations and avoid large peak-to-trough variation.

Suspensions or liquid formulations are not recommended in children due to rapid drug clearance. They are also absorbed rapidly and would require very frequent dosing (e.g., every 3–4 hours).[2,9]

Children also may exhibit erratic and unpredictable drug absorption. Predisposing factors include: delayed gastric emptying time in infants, diminished intestinal transit times (limits absorption of ER formulations), reduced absorptive surface area, intestinal disorders (e.g., acute diarrhea), and drug interactions with milk and infant formulas.[2,3] Absorption problems lead to low or erratic serum concentrations and a poor therapeutic response. Impaired oral absorption should be suspected if peak concentrations are much lower than expected and either decline normally between specimens or fail to show expected peak and trough variations.

Coadministered medications, food and liquids should be reviewed for interactions producing malabsorption.[2,9] Some solid dosage forms are poorly absorbed in children due to shorter transit time through the gastrointestinal tract. Solid formulations recovered from the stool contain significant amounts of drug and are particularly problematic with some AEDs.[10,11] Inconsistent generic substitution or generic brand switching is another cause of erratic serum concentration in generic products.[12]

Lastly, medication noncompliance is prevalent in children with chronic illnesses. Compliance issues are a primary cause of low or widely fluctuating serum concentrations and inadequate drug exposure. Noncompliance rates may reach 30%–40% in pediatric patients and increase proportionately to the number of medications.[13] Serial drug concentrations may appear normal when taken after an observed dose. However, the clinical assessment does not correlate with levels obtained at home.

Compliance can also be evaluated with serial trough serum concentrations at the same time of the day—several days to a week apart. The values should not vary by more than 10% with full compliance and the same testing laboratory. Pill counts and prescription refill records can also be used to check compliance. Counseling is sometimes effective but a change to a less frequently administered medication may be necessary.[2]

Determining the cause of incomplete treatment response in children can be frustrating and time consuming. Figure 50–1 represents a cognitive algorithm for inadequate treatment response that may prove useful in sorting out drug therapy issues.

▶ ADVERSE DRUG EFFECTS

In pediatric epilepsy, drug safety and tolerability are equally if not more important than efficacy. Efficacy of the approved AEDs is fairly equal for epilepsy types and syndromes but the adverse effect (AE) profile often determines AED selection.[14] An individualized treatment approach will take into account the patient's seizure type or syndrome, family history, and AED safety and efficacy profile. It is important to carefully balance AED morbidity with efficacy profile and potential consequences of recurrent seizures.

Approximately 33%–61% of patients on AED therapy will experience at least one AE during the course of their treatment.[15,16] For the purpose of prescription drug labeling, the FDA defines adverse reaction as an undesirable effect, reasonably associated with use of a drug, that may occur as part of the pharmacological action of the drug or may be unpredictable in its occurrence. This definition does not include all adverse events during drug usage, only those for which there is some basis to ascribe a causal relationship between the drug and adverse event occurrence.[17] These effects are further characterized by body system, reaction severity, incidence of occurrence, or by a combination. Updated safety requirements further separate adverse reactions from clinical trials and postmarketing spontaneous reports.

AEs associated with AEDs are generally classified as acute (including idiosyncratic) or chronic and can vary considerably between the adult and pediatric population.[7,15,18] AEs that are mild in young adults may be more pronounced in children, especially behavioral and neurological effects.[15] Some AEs in children are more difficult to identify particularly cognitive and behavioral effects. It is therefore important to determine whether an observed effect is related to the neurological disorder or its treatment.[19] AEs associated with specific AEDs are listed in Table 50–1.

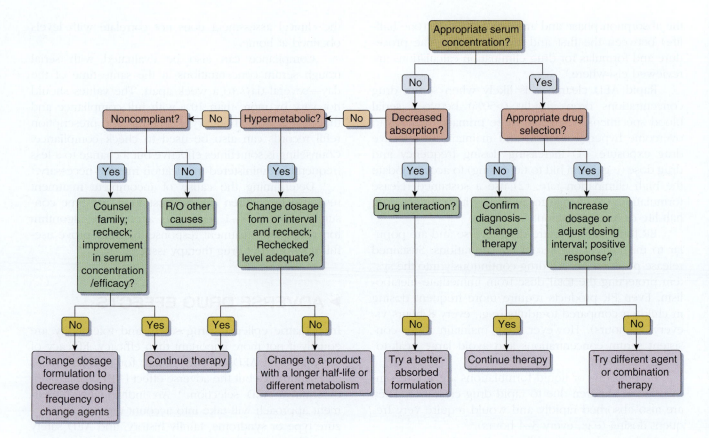

Figure 50–1. Algorithm for inadequate response.

Acute AEs generally occur within the first 6 months of treatment and range from bothersome to life threatening. Common acute reactions are usually reversible, related to the known primary or ancillary AED mechanism, and are usually dose- or concentration-dependent. Included with acute effects are a number of neurologic or cognitive effects including sedation, dizziness, fatigue, visual disturbances, difficulty with concentration, and ataxia.[15,21] These are almost always diminished or alleviated by dosage reduction.

Idiosyncratic reactions are unrelated to the primary mechanisms of drug action. They are considered to result from individual susceptibility due to genetic or acquired mechanisms. Idiosyncratic reactions occur mostly during the first few weeks or months of therapy and are related to starting dose and/or rate of titration. Some idiosyncratic reactions, however, may not be recognized or associated with an AED until years after drug approval and marketing. Hypersensitivity reactions are included in this category and are usually mild, but carry a risk of becoming more serious when one or more organ systems become involved.[20]

Other types of idiosyncratic reactions include hepatitis, blood dyscrasias, aplastic anemia, glaucoma, hepatotoxicity, and other immune-mediated reactions. Life-threatening idiosyncratic reactions include Stevens

Johnson Syndrome, fulminant liver toxicity, and aplastic anemia. (other examples include pancreatitis from VPA).

Chronic AEs generally involve "biological" dysfunction or behavioral and cognitive problems and fully manifest after a prolonged period of exposure, usually several months to years. The mechanisms are poorly understood or may result from known alterations of biochemical or metabolic pathways. They can appear despite serum concentrations within the accepted therapeutic or even subtherapeutic range. Chronic effects generally develop more slowly and may be overlooked without a proper level of vigilance. Examples of chronic AEs associated with AEDs include connective tissue and endocrine disorders, vitamin D and folate deficiency, weight gain or loss, gingival hyperplasia, hirsutism, visual field loss, cognitive and behavioral effects.[15]

It is not uncommon to observe cognitive or behavioral dysfunction in medically treated children with epilepsy.[21–23] While it is well recognized that AEDs have the potential to impair cognition and impact behavior, it is important to discern whether the dysfunction is AED related or part of an underlying disorder.[24] An attempt should be made to exclude other causes.[19,24] Baseline deficits can be documented with neuropsychological testing prior to AED introduction. Testing not only

▶ **TABLE 50–1.** RELEVENT ADVERSE REACTIONS OF AEDs

AED	CNS	Blood	Rash	Liver	BW	Miscellaneous	Serious and Life-Threatening
Phenobarbital	Sedation, irritability, hyper-activity, ↓ cognition, and concentration	+	+	+		Exacerbation of por-phyria, ↓ vitamin A, D, and folic acid	SJS, AHS
Phenytoin	Nystagmus, ataxia, drowsiness, lethargy, sedation	+	+	+		Gingivinal hypertrophy, hirsutism, osteoporo-sis, SLE	SJS, AHS, renal and hepatic failure
Benzodiazepine	Sedation, ataxia, drowsi-ness, hyperactivity, ↓ cognition, depression	+	+	+	↑	Exacerbation of sei-zures, tolerance and withdrawal syndrome	No
Ethosuximide	Sedation, dizziness, head-aches, photophobia movement disorders	+	+		↓	Gastric upset, ano-rexia, vomiting, SLE	SJS, AHS, renal and hepatic failure
Carbamazepine	Sedation, ataxia, head-ache, nystagmus, diplopia, tremor, movement disorders	+	+	+	↑	Hyponatremia, osteo-malacia, atrioven-tricular blockade, arrhythmias, SLE	SJS, AHS, and hepatic failure
Valproate	Tremor, sedation, fatigue, ataxia, behavioral changes	+	+	++	↑↑	GI irritation, PCOS, alopecia	Hepatic and pan-creatic failure
Vigabatrin	Fatigue, sedation, change mood, psychosis				↑		Irreversible visual field defects
Felbamate	Headache, dizziness, tremor, diplopia	++	+		↓	Urolithiasis, hyponatremia	Aplastic anemia, hepatic failure
Lamotrigine	Headache, asthenia, dizziness, insomnia, mild hand tremor, tics		++	+		Gastrointestinal distur-bances, pseudolym-phoma	SJS, DIC, multior-gan or hepatic failure
Gabapentin	Somnolence, dizziness, nystagmus diplopia, tremor, memory difficul-ties, fatigue, behavioral changes, exacerbation of psychosis				↑	Aggravation of absences and cause myoclonus, move-ment disorders GI effects	No
Topiramate	Somnolence, dizziness, ataxia, diplopia, dif-ficulty in memory and concentration, speech problems				↓↓	Kidney stones; oligo-hidrosis, none with ketogenic diet	Hepatic failure
Oxcarbazepine	Dizziness, nausea, headache, drowsiness, ataxia, diplopia, fatigue		+			Hyponatremia	AHS, hematologic
Zonisamide	Somnolence, ataxia, diz-ziness, fatigue, difficulty in concentration and language, psychosis	+			↓	Kidney stones, oligo-hidrosis, and hyper-thermia	SJS, AHS, aplas-tic, anemia
Levetiracetam	Irritability, behavioral changes, dizziness, insomnia					Increase seizure frequency	No

Source: From Kothare SV, Kaleyias J. The adverse effects of antiepileptic drugs in children. *Expert Opin Drug Saf* 2007;6(3):251–265.
AED, antiepileptic drug; AHS, anticonvulsant hypersensitivity syndrome; BW, body weight; DIC, disseminated intravascular coagulation; GI, gastrointestinal; PCOS, polycystic ovary syndrome; SJS, Stevens-Johnson syndrome; SLE, systemic lupus erythematosus.

avoids attributing deficits to drug therapy but also may influence AED selection.[21]

While permanent, progressive cognitive deficits do not occur in most pediatric patients with uncomplicated epilepsy, cognitive decline has been documented in subgroups of patients.[22] Predictors of cognitive impairment include overmedication, poor seizure control, early onset of epilepsy, and symptomatic epilepsy. Medications are rarely the sole cause of cognitive deficits. When AEDs have been identified as the source of the problem, their cognitive effects can be minimized or eliminated by discontinuing the AED, decreasing the dose, or switching to another medication.[22]

Older AEDs are more often associated with cognitive dysfunction when compared with the second generation AEDs, placebo, or nondrug options. While there are few notable differences between individual agents, phenobarbital consistently performs more poorly in this regard.[22] Although there is less data on second generation AEDs, they generally have a more favorable cognitive profile with the possible exception of topiramate.[22]

It is helpful to consider the mechanisms of action of the available AEDs when assessing behavioral and psychiatric AEs in pediatric patients. There is evidence suggesting a relationship between the type and frequency of AEs and AED mechanism of action.[25] AEDs with GABA-ergic mechanisms are associated with the most troublesome behavioral and psychiatric profiles; hyperactivity and major depressive disorder are most commonly reported (particularly with phenobarbital).[25,26]

AEDs that modulate voltage-gated cationic channels produce fewer behavioral AEs overall but higher rates of sedation (somnolence, drowsiness); these are most consistently reported with phenytoin (PHT), carbamazepine (CBZ), and oxcarbazepine (OXC).[25] Multiple AEDs, preexisting behavioral difficulties, developmental delay, and family history of psychiatric illness are considered risk factors for AED-related behavioral and psychiatric AEs in this population.[25]

AEs may result from an AED's pharmacokinetic properties. Protein-binding displacement may occur when a highly protein-bound AED is added to the regimen of a child taking other medications. This produces a potentially significant increase in the compound's free fraction (pharmacologically relevant).[21] AEDs that are enzyme inducers may increase the metabolism of inducible compounds, lowering their serum concentration, and compromising efficacy. Conversely, AEDs known to be enzyme inhibitors may slow the metabolism of concomitant agents competing for the same cytochrome P450 pathway, increasing their serum concentration, and exposing them to the risk of toxicity.

Pharmacokinetic differences may contribute to age-related differences in the incidence of AEs.[18] Likewise, factors affecting an AED's pharmacokinetic properties may vary among children and fluctuate with age,

necessitating dose adjustments over time. There is some evidence that renally excreted AEDs are less likely to be problematic.[27,28] Basic pharmacokinetic properties and drug–drug interactions must be considered when optimizing AED therapy, especially when AEDs are used concomitantly.[21]

In addition to their pharmacokinetic effects, concomitant drug therapy can affect the emergence of AEs through pharmacodynamic alterations. Pharmacodynamics is the study of the relationship between the concentration of a drug and the response obtained in a patient.[29] Pharmacodynamic drug interactions impact the sensitivity or responsiveness of the target site to one or both drugs involved, with combined effects that may be synergistic, additive, or antagonistic. As most of our knowledge of pharmacodynamic interactions is derived from animal studies, they are more difficult to predict in man than pharmacokinetic interactions.[30]

Whether drug–drug interactions (DDIs) are pharmacokinetic or pharmacodynamic, the possibility of a concomitantly administered drug (AED or other drug) altering the effects or effectiveness of an AED must always be considered. These interactions may result in enhanced or diminished effects of either drug or may result in an unanticipated effect seen with neither drug alone. The consequences of DDIs are especially important for AEDs with a low therapeutic index and/or known serious toxicities. Indeed, at least one study has demonstrated that multidrug use is strongly associated with an increased probability of AEs, showing a significant correlation between the number of reported AEs and the number of medications used concurrently.[16]

While it is not possible to accurately predict their occurrence, a goal of treatment to identify, minimize, and monitor for AEs. The association of some AEDs with acute, severe reactions has prompted manufacturers to recommend routine regular blood and urine screening in asymptomatic patients, a practice which rarely proves useful.[7] This recommendation is based on two assumptions: (1) there are biological markers present in asymptomatic patients that can predict an impending AE and (2) altering therapy in the asymptomatic phase will alter the outcome.

While pharmacogenomic research is being conducted to identify predictive markers, the previous assumptions have not been evaluated systematically.[7] The most commonly reported chronic AEs due to AEDs—reduction in bone mineral density, obesity, and polycystic ovary disease—can be monitored although there are currently no published algorithms. Some clinicians choose to monitor AED serum concentrations in an attempt to improve seizure control, reduce AEs, and verify compliance.

It is often assumed that seizures are more likely to be controlled and AEs minimized if an AED concentration is within the proposed "therapeutic range."[7] Limitations with this approach include: lack of standardization for determining AED therapeutic range, and difficulty interpreting AED concentrations. In three randomized trials, AED concentrations were found to be of no clinical value. Assessment of serum concentrations may prove useful for patients taking several AEDs with neurotoxic symptoms and/or uncontrolled seizures.[7] Serum concentrations may also help sort out pharmacokinetic dosing issues.

▶ DRUG SAFETY

New drugs for epilepsy are increasingly administered to children despite a lack of evidence for their long-term safety. Collection of safety data in children is critically important since common AEs as well as long-term safety frequently differs between adults and children.[27,31] Efficacy trials are generally too short and may

not include all suitable patient populations to accurately assess effects on growth, development, behavior, and cognitive function. Long-term studies are needed within clinical development programs to accurately collect and assess this data.[31]

Attention to a few basic principles may aid in avoiding or minimizing the emergence of AED-related AEs. Careful diagnosis and selection of the appropriate AED for the identified epilepsy syndrome will prevent increased seizure frequency, severity, and the emergence of new seizure types. Baseline laboratory studies should be performed when indicated prior to initiation of therapy. AEDs should be introduced at a low dose and titrated according to published recommendations. Patients and families should receive counseling regarding appropriate medication administration and AE monitoring. An algorithm on the general approach to AEs is presented in Figure 50–2.

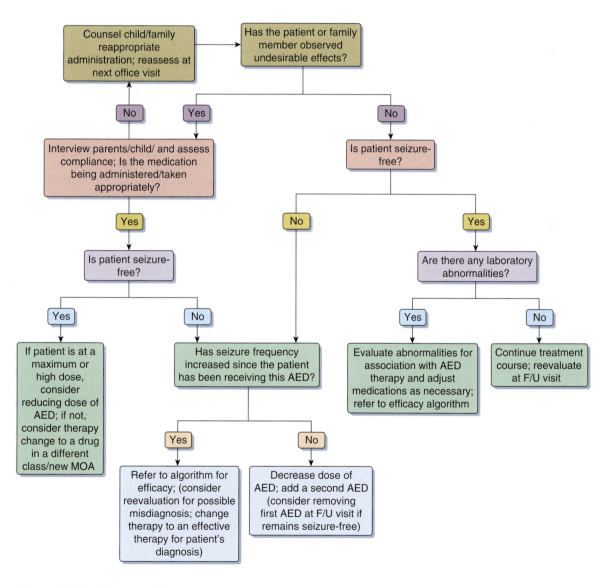

Figure 50–2. Adverse effects.

▶ SUMMARY

The treatment of childhood epilepsy can be confounding in children with pharmacokinetic, pharmacodynamic, and/or sensitivities to the AEs of AEDs. A multidisciplinary approach with pediatric epileptologists, pharmacologists for clinical pharmacokinetics/pharmacodynamics, and neuropsychologists often improves the chances of successful treatment in difficult patients.

REFERENCES

1. Kwan P, Brodie MJ. Early identification of refractory epilepsy. *N Engl J Med* 2000;342:314–319.
2. Gilman JT, Duchowny M, Campo AE. Pharmacokinetic considerations in the treatment of childhood epilepsy. *Pediatr Drugs* 2003;5(4):267–277.
3. Bartelink I, et al. Guidelines on paediatric dosing on the basis of developmental physiology and pharmacokinetic considerations. *Clin Pharmacokinet* 2006;45(11):1077–1097.
4. Gilman JT, et al. Medical intractability in children evaluated for epilepsy surgery. *Neurology* 1994;44:1341–1343.
5. Johannessen SI, Thomson T. Pharmacokinetic variability of new antiepileptic drugs: When is monitoring needed? *Clin Pharmacokinet* 2006;45(11):1061–1075.
6. Perucca E. Is there a role for therapeutic drug monitoring of new anticonvulsants? *Clin Pharmacokinet* 2000;38(3):191–204.
7. Camfield P, Camfield C. Monitoring for adverse effects of antiepileptic drugs. *Epilepsia* 2006;47(Suppl 1):31–34.
8. Johannessen SI. Can pharmacokinetic variability be controlled for the patient's benefit? *Ther Drug Monit* 2005;27(6):710–713.
9. Gilman JT. Intractable childhood epilepsy: issues in pharmacotherapy. *J Epilepsy* 1990;3(Suppl):21–34.
10. Gilman JT, Duchowny MS, Hershorin ER. Carbamazepine malabsorption: a case report. *Pediatrics* 1988;82(3):518–519.
11. Gilman JT. Carbamazepine dosing for pediatric seizure disorders: the highs and lows. *DICP* 1991;25:1109–1112.
12. Gilman JT, Alvarez LA, Duchowny M. Carbamazepine toxicity resulting from generic substitution. *Neurology* 1993;43:2696–2697.
13. Cramer JA. Optimizing long-term patient compliance. *Neurology* 1995;45(Suppl 1):S25–S28.
14. Greenwood RS. Adverse effects of antiepileptic drugs. *Epilepsia* 2000;41(Suppl 2):S42–S52.
15. Perucca E, Meador KJ. Adverse effects of antiepileptic drugs. *Acta Neurol Scand* 2005;112(Suppl 181):30–35.
16. Beghi E, Mascio R-c D, Sasanelli F. Adverse reactions to antiepileptic drugs: a multicenter survey of clinical practice.. *Epilepsia* 1986;27(4):323–330.
17. US Food and Drug Administration. Code of Federal Regulations, Title 21, Volume 4, Part 201—Labeling. http://www.accessdata.fda.gov/scripts/cdrh/cfdocs/cfcfr/CFRSearch.cfm?fr=201.57, 2007.
18. Kothare SV, Kaleyias J. The adverse effects of antiepileptic drugs in children. *Expert Opin Drug Saf* 2007;6(3):251–265.
19. Shinnar S, Gross-Tsur V. Discontinuing antiepileptic drug therapy. In: Wyllie E (ed), *The Treatment of Epilepsy: Principles & Practice*. 2001; pp. 811–819.
20. Gidal DE, Garnett WR, Graves N. Epilepsy. In: DiPiro JT (ed), *Pharmacotherapy: A Pathophysiologic Approach*. 2002; pp. 1031–1059.
21. Hadjiloizou SM, Bourgeois BFD. Antiepileptic drug treatment in children. *Expert Rev Neurother* 2007;7(2):179–193.
22. Bourgeois BFD. Determining the effects of antiepileptic drugs on cognitive function in pediatric patients with epilepsy. *J Child Neurol* 2004;19(Suppl 1):S15–S24.
23. Wolf SM, McGoldrick PE. Recognition and management of pediatric seizures. *Pediatr Ann* 2006;35(5):332–344.
24. Aldenkamp AP, Bodde N. Behavior, cognition and epilepsy. *Acta Neurol Scand* 2005;112(Suppl 182):19–25.
25. Glauser TA. Behavioral and psychiatric adverse events associated with antiepileptic drugs commonly used in pediatric patients. *J Child Neurol* 2004;19(Suppl 1):S25–S38.
26. Crumrine PK. Antiepileptic drug selection in pediatric epilepsy. *J Child Neurol* 2002;17:2S2–2S8.
27. Dulac O. Issues in paediatric epilepsy. *Acta Neurol Scand* 2005;112(Suppl 182):9–11.
28. Perucca E. Pharmacological problems in the management of epilepsy in children. *Seizure* 1995;4:139–143.
29. Bauer LA. Clinical pharmacokinetics and pharmacodynamics. In: DiPiro JT (ed), *Pharmacotherapy: A Pathophysiologic Approach*. 2002; pp. 33–54.
30. Bourgeois BFD. Pharmacokinetics and pharmacodynamics of antiepileptic drugs. In Wyllie E (ed), *The Treatment of Epilepsy: Principles & Practice*. 2001; pp. 729–739 .
31. Garofalo E. Clinical development of antiepileptic drugs for children. *Neurotherapeutics* 2007;4(1):70–74.

CHAPTER 51

Teratogenicity of Antiepileptic Drugs

Eija Gaily and Dick Lindhout

▶ INTRODUCTION

In most women with epilepsy, it is necessary to continue antiepileptic drug (AED) treatment during pregnancy to reduce the risks caused by epileptic seizures for both mother and child.[1–3] The risk of maternal death during pregnancy has been estimated to be ten times higher in women with epilepsy compared to the general population,[4] possibly due to poor compliance with AED treatment and seizure occurrence. Seizure-related accidents and convulsive status epilepticus during pregnancy are associated with an increased risk of fetal death.[5] Even brief generalized tonic–clonic seizures during pregnancy may have an unfavorable effect on cognitive outcome based on retrospective data,[4] although this has not been confirmed prospectively.[6,7]

Foetal exposure to AEDs occurs in 0.3%–0.5% of all pregnancies; of them, 17%–47% are exposed to two or more drugs.[8,9] Since both seizures during pregnancy and the medication needed to prevent seizures may have adverse foetal effects, the treatment of maternal epilepsy is a matter of balance by weighing advantages and disadvantages.

AEDs are freely transported across the placenta, and the foetal serum levels for most drugs are roughly the same as the maternal levels; valproate and possibly gabapentin seem to accumulate in the fetus.[10,11] There is some evidence that infants born to women with epilepsy have low birth weight more commonly than infants of women with no chronic diseases.[12,13] One minute Apgar scores may also be lower and the need for care in the neonatal ward is increased in the infants of mothers with epilepsy.[9] These effects do not seem to be very strong and are not readily explained by pregnancy complications, exposure to specific AEDs, or seizures during pregnancy.[9,12,14]

STRUCTURAL AND FUNCTIONAL TERATOGENESIS

Structural teratogenesis resulting in malformations occurs during the first trimester of pregnancy. The vulnerable period for functional teratogenesis producing cognitive and behavioral disturbances covers the whole pregnancy as neuronal migration and organization are teratogen-sensitive processes continuing also in the second and third trimesters.[15] Animal studies have demonstrated that AEDs have dose-dependent teratogenic effects. The doses required for functional deficits are generally lower than those producing structural anomalies.[16]

The prevalence of major malformations in the general population is approximately 2.2%–2.8% according to population-based studies.[8,17] It is well established that prenatal exposure to AEDs increases the prevalence of major malformations in humans (Fig. 51–1).[18] The magnitude of the risk is approximately two- to threefold for most monotherapies compared to the baseline rate. The most common malformations are the same that are common in the general population (e.g., heart defects and facial clefts). The highest relative risk in children of mothers with epilepsy has been observed in spina bifida and congenital anomalies of genital organs.[17] Comparisons between different studies and pooling of data are not always straightforward because of differences in definitions of major malformations, of sampling, observational periods, and in whether terminated pregnancies are included in the analysis.[19] Recently, the EURAP study contributed new data on major malformations showing dose-dependency of the risk for four monotherapies in a prospective series of near 5000 pregnancies with follow-up until the first year of postnatal life (Table 51–1).[20]

The risk of major malformations does not appear to be significantly increased by epilepsy *per se*.[21]

Maternal epilepsy is associated with mildly but significantly reduced intelligence in the offspring, based on a large population-based cohort study.[13] IQ scores of 1207 young men whose mothers had epilepsy during pregnancy were compared with a control group of 316,554 males of similar age. No individual AED exposure data were available from that study. Differential effects of individual AEDs on cognitive development are difficult to estimate as there are many confounding factors and long follow-up periods carry the risk of selective loss to follow-up. Moderate to severe mental deficiency may be diagnosed in the first years of life, but milder cognitive deficits cannot be reliably studied before preschool or early school age and standardized neuropsychological testing are always needed. Good-quality studies on the effects of AEDs on cognitive development are scarce.[22]

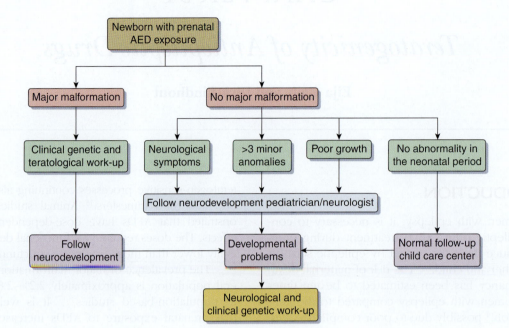

Figure 51–1. Algorithm.

CONFOUNDING FACTORS

Epilepsy type and severity are associated with AED choice, dosage and whether monotherapy is sufficient or if polytherapy is indicated, leading to a risk of confounding by indication especially in studies investigating cognitive outcome. There are some data suggesting that genetic epilepsy-related factors could sometimes contribute to cognitive outcome in children of mothers with epilepsy. For example, centrotemporal EEG spikes may be genetically determined[23] and may also

be associated with increased cognitive[24] or attentional dysfunction[25] even in the absence of epilepsy. Idiopathic epilepsies which may have familial predisposition are associated with mild cognitive and behavioral dysfunction which is not totally explained by epileptiform discharges[26] and which may be present before seizure onset.[27] The effects of epilepsy on male and female reproductive fitness may differ[28] which implies that comparing offspring of fathers and mothers with similar types of epilepsy does not solve the problem of confounding by indication.

▶ **TABLE 51–1.** COMPARISON OF MALFORMATION RATES AT 1 YEAR AFTER BIRTH WITH FOUR AEDs IN MONOTHERAPY AND DOSE DEPENDENCY (EURAP STUDY)[20]

		Malformations up to 12 Months		
Drug, Daily Dose (mg)	Number	N	(%)	95% CI
Carbamazepine				
<400	148	5	3.4	1.11–7.71
≥700 to <1000	1047	56	5.3	4.07–6.89
≥1000	207	18	8.7	5.24–13.39
Lamotrigine				
<300	836	17	2.0	1.19–3.24
≥300	444	20	4.5	2.77–6.87
Phenobarbital				
<150	166	9	5.4	2.51–10.04
≥150	51	7	13.7	5.70–26.26
Valproate				
<700	431	24	5.6	3.60–8.17
≥700 to <1500	480	50	10.4	7.83–13.50
≥1500	99	24	24.2	16.19–33.89

Epilepsy is associated with psychosocial and socio-economic difficulties, especially in patients who are not seizure-free.[29] In addition to possible environmental effects to the offspring, it is conceivable that epilepsy may cause a disadvantage in partner choice,[30] expressed in one study by smaller head circumferences in fathers of children whose mothers had epilepsy.[31]

GENETIC VARIABILITY IN SUSCEPTIBILITY TO TERATOGENIC EFFECTS

Pharmacogenetic factors may influence vulnerability for teratogenic effects.[32] Low epoxide hydrolase activity is associated with an increased risk of developmental defects after prenatal phenytoin exposure.[33] Dizygotic or heteropaternal twins or triplets from phenytoin-exposed multiple pregnancies have shown different outcomes, some infants being healthy while others with identical exposure have congenital defects.[34,35] Repeated occurrence of developmental defects in siblings after prenatal valproate[36–38] or phenytoin[39] exposure has been described. These observations suggest that AEDs exert their teratogenic effects in interaction with a specific genetic susceptibility.

The nature of genetic susceptibility factors is not well studied in human maternal epilepsy but probably subject to extensive polygenetic heterogeneity, both at the level of metabolism and pharmacodynamics. In addition, one has to take into account that genetic factors related to the maternal phenotype as well as independently segregating genetic factors may play a role in the occurrence of abnormalities in the offspring.

PHENYTOIN

Recent prospective cohort and registry studies have reported 2.4%–3.7% prevalence of major malformations after prenatal exposure to phenytoin monotherapy.[14,40] A meta-analysis of five prospective European studies found malformations in 9 of 141 monotherapy exposed pregnancies (6%),[19] not significantly different from non-exposed controls.

The foetal hydantoin syndrome was first described in 1975.[41] Five unrelated children of mothers with epilepsy had been prenatally exposed to either 100–400 mg of phenytoin (four children, only one monotherapy) or 300 mg of another hydantoin, mephenytoin. The characteristic pattern of minor anomalies included a short nose with low nasal bridge, hypertelorism, and hypoplasia of nails and distal phalanges. Other syndrome features were postnatal growth deficiency and motor or mental deficiency. The frequency of the foetal hydantoin syndrome among phenytoin-exposed children is unknown. The first estimation was as high as 11%,[42] but

this has not been confirmed in prospective population-based studies.[6,43]

The facial features of the foetal hydantoin syndrome have been observed in controlled prospective and retrospective studies in exposed and nonexposed children of mothers with epilepsy and also as part of normal variation.[43,44] Distal digital hypoplasia, however, seems to be consistently associated with prenatal phenytoin exposure. This has been shown in prospective-controlled studies blinded to exposure using clinical[43,45] or anthropometric methods.[46,47] Prospective studies found no association between digital hypoplasia or deficient growth, and abnormal cognitive development.[6,47]

Developmental data obtained with standardized methods in preschool or school-aged children with prenatal phenytoin exposure and maternal epilepsy are available from three studies—prospective, controlled, population-based—with evaluation blinded for prenatal exposure.[6,48,49] Two studies[6,48] controlled for socioeconomic class or maternal educational level. A total of 364 children of women with epilepsy were included, and approximately 50%–60% of the population were covered in each study. Out of the total, 222 children were exposed to phenytoin, 96 of them to monotherapy. IQ was assessed at age 4 (Stanford–Binet)[48] or 5.5 years (age-appropriate Wechsler scale),[6] or a developmental quotient was obtained in six domains by the Griffiths test at age 2–8 years.[49] The results were compared with 40 nonexposed children of women with epilepsy and over 27,000 control children of mothers without epilepsy. The mean phenytoin dose was reported in only one study (253 mg/day).[49] Maternal phenytoin levels during pregnancy were reported in another study;[6] most were within the reference range. Two studies[6,48] reported lower IQ values in children of women with epilepsy compared to control children of mothers without epilepsy, but no significant associations were observed to phenytoin or other drug exposure. The 15 children exposed to phenytoin monotherapy assessed by the Griffiths test had significantly lower scores in locomotor function; no difference was found in the other domains.[49]

Prospective IQ data at 7 years were also reported by Hanson et al[42] from the same database as Shapiro et al.[48] The results were controlled for socioeconomic status. The mean IQ of 83 children exposed to phenytoin (number with monotherapy not stated, but 25% at most) was five points lower than control children of mothers without epilepsy. All children of women with epilepsy were exposed to phenytoin; thus the independent drug effect cannot be estimated.

The prevalence of mental deficiency (IQ below 70) can be estimated from a prospective population-based study comprising 103 phenytoin-exposed children (54 monotherapy).[6] One child exposed to phenytoin, carbamazepine, and alcohol had mental deficiency (IQ below 70). Of the children exposed to phenytoin monotherapy, one had borderline IQ (below 85). For comparison, the prevalence of mental deficiency was found to be 1.4% among 8–9-year-old children in a population-based study from the same country.[50]

PHENOBARBITAL AND PRIMIDONE

A prospective registry study[51] observed an increased risk of major malformations (5/77 or 6.5%) in pregnancies exposed to phenobarbitone monotherapy (1.6%, RR 4.2, 95% CI 1.5–9.4). Based on another prospective registry study, the risk is dose-dependent (Table 51–1).[20] A large retrospective study comprising 172 monotherapy exposed pregnancies[52] observed five malformed infants (3%), which was not increased compared to nonepileptic controls. However, the study revealed the unexpected finding that the combination of phenobarbitone with caffeine was associated with a significantly elevated malformation risk.

Prospective-controlled data on cognitive outcome at 4 years of age after prenatal exposure to phenobarbital monotherapy have been reported in 35 exposed children of women with epilepsy and 4705 children of mothers without epilepsy but with phenobarbital exposure.[48] There was no IQ difference compared to unexposed control children.

Another study of male subjects whose mothers did not have epilepsy but were treated with phenobarbital for at least 10 days during pregnancy for variable obstetric indications[53] showed different results. The data was acquired from the Danish Perinatal Cohort, comprising the offspring of 9006 deliveries that took place at one hospital in Copenhagen from 1959 to 1961. An attempt was made to match for maternal phenobarbital indication among other potential confounders. Drugs used during pregnancy were recorded prospectively. Total phenobarbital dosages during pregnancy ranged from 225 mg to 22,500 mg. On standardized IQ testing at a mean age around 20 years, men exposed to phenobarbital showed significantly lower IQ scores (approximately 0.5 SD) than controls. The IQ impairment was greatest after exposure in the third trimester, especially in subjects of low socioeconomic background who were offspring of unwanted pregnancy.

Data on primidone-exposed pregnancies are scarce. A pattern of minor anomalies similar to phenytoin combined with developmental delay has been described in association with prenatal primidone exposure[54] but not confirmed as a separate syndrome. The only prospective results on cognitive outcome after prenatal exposure to primidone monotherapy are based on nine children who were tested at age 11–18 years.[55] There were no differences compared to 49 control children of mothers without epilepsy.

CARBAMAZEPINE

A meta-analysis of prospective studies included 795 exposures to carbamazepine monotherapy;[56] major malformations were observed in 5.3% that was significantly increased compared to controls without epilepsy (2.3%, OR 2.4, 95% CI 1.6–3.4). A recent UK registry study[40] found major malformations in 20/900 pregnancies exposed to carbamazepine monotherapy (2.2%, 95% CI 1.4–3.4) that was not significantly increased compared to unexposed pregnancies of women with epilepsy. Like valproate, maternal carbamazepine use is also associated with an increased risk of neural tube defects, although the risk is lower (0.5%–1.0%).[57] The risk of malformations is dose-dependent (Table 51–1).[20]

A pattern of minor anomalies together with developmental delay has been described in a case series of children with prenatal carbamazepine exposure.[58] Many of the typical features overlap with dysmorphic features described after other exposures or with no exposure,[43,44] and the existence of a specific carbamazepine syndrome has not been confirmed.

Two recent population-based prospective controlled evaluator-blinded studies have reported cognitive outcome measured by standardized methods at preschool to school age in children with prenatal exposure to carbamazepine monotherapy. One study[49] found no difference in the results of the Griffiths test at 2–8 years between 35 carbamazepine-exposed children and 66 control children of mothers without epilepsy. The other study[7] included 86 children exposed to carbamazepine, 45 nonexposed children, and 141 control children of mothers without epilepsy; there were no differences between these groups in the IQ scores obtained by the age-appropriate Wechsler scale at 5–11 years.

Data on the prevalence of mental deficiency in children exposed to carbamazepine monotherapy *in utero* are available from two prospective population-based studies.[6,7] Two of 105 exposed children had an IQ under 70 (1.9%). One of the two children had intractable West syndrome.

The prevalence of autistic spectrum disorder in AED-exposed children of mothers with epilepsy has been investigated in only one study, a retrospective population-based survey including 80 children exposed to carbamazepine monotherapy.[59] The participants were estimated to represent 42% of the population. The risk was 2.5% (95% CI 0–6) among carbamazepine-exposed children compared to 0.25% (95% CI 0.17–0.33) in the general population.

VALPROATE

Recent prospective registry studies[40,60] and a population-based retrospective registry study[61] have observed 6.2%–10.7% malformation rates in pregnancies exposed to monotherapy; this is significantly increased compared to carbamazepine monotherapy or nonexposed children. In the population-based study,[61] the risk was about four times as high as in nonexposed pregnancies (OR 4.2, 95% CI 2.3–7.0). A significant dose-response effect has been observed in a number of studies.[19,20,61,62] Compared to lamotrigine doses below 300 mg, valproate exposure at all doses is associated with higher malformation rates (Table 51–1).[20]

A causal association between maternal valproate use and spina bifida aperta was first suggested by an unexpectedly large number of cases of spina bifida reported from the birth defects registry in the Rhônes-Alpes region in France.[63] This has been confirmed by a retrospective case study,[64] a multicenter prospective cohort study,[65] a prospective cohort study showing a dose-response effect of valproate,[62] and a registry study.[60] On average, the risk of spina bifida aperta has been estimated at 1%–2%, which has made maternal valproate use an indication for offering prenatal diagnosis. Another specific but rare malformation associated with valproate is bilateral radial aplasia.[57]

The foetal valproate syndrome was first described in 1984 and is now well documented.[66] The characteristic craniofacial features include metopic ridge, trigonocephaly, bifrontal narrowing with indentation of the outer orbital ridge, medial deficiency of eyebrows, long shallow philtrum with long and thin upper vermillion, broad or flat nasal bridge and low-set poorly developed ear shelves. The typical facial features may also occur in association with major malformations. Developmental delay is observed in most children with the syndrome features. Pre- and postnatal growth is usually normal. The prevalence of the valproate syndrome is unknown as no population-based data are available.

Prospective population-based data on cognitive outcome at 5 years of age or later after foetal valproate exposure are available from two studies,[7,67] which included a total of 26 children exposed to valproate monotherapy. Both studies found a 11–13 points lower verbal IQ in the valproate group than in children with no AED exposure or exposed to carbamazepine monotherapy (not statistically significant in either study). Reduced verbal IQ was associated with impaired auditory working memory in valproate-exposed children.[68] Both studies were confounded by lower educational level or IQ of valproate using mothers. Pooled data from the same studies show mental deficiency in 3 of 34 (8.8%) children exposed to valproate monotherapy compared to 1 of 94 (1.1%) children whose mothers had used other AED monotherapy.

Data on early (at 2–3 years) cognitive development of children exposed to valproate monotherapy are available from a prospective blinded registry study conducted in the United States and United Kingdom.[69] Other exposure groups included phenytoin,

carbamazepine, and lamotrigine monotherapy. Maternal IQ was measured and women with IQ less than 70 were excluded. Cognitive assessments were conducted in 83.5% of the 309 children who had been enrolled prenatally and were born alive, including 53 children exposed to valproate. The mean IQ (95% CI) of valproate-exposed children was 92 (88–97), which was significantly lower than in the other exposure subgroups, and was not explained by confounding factors such as maternal IQ.

A retrospective clinic-based study[4] reported cognitive outcome in 41 children exposed to valproate monotherapy *in utero*. Verbal IQ was approximately 10 points lower in the valproate group than unexposed and other monotherapy groups. The finding was statistically significant and not explained by maternal IQ scores that in this study were not lower in valproate users compared to other mothers with epilepsy.

A retrospective population-based study[59] including 56 children with prenatal exposure to valproate monotherapy reported an autistic spectrum disorder in 5 or 8.9% (95% CI 1.3–16.5), which was significantly increased compared to the general population.

LAMOTRIGINE

Three prospective registries have reported data on altogether 1061 pregnancies exposed to lamotrigine monotherapy in the first trimester.[20,70,40] Major malformations were observed in 2.9%–3.2%. Two studies observed a dose-response effect with higher rates after exposure to more than 200 mg or 300 mg per day.[20,40] Exposure to lamotrigine doses less than 300 mg per day was associated with significantly lower rates of major malformations than valproate or phenobarbitone at all doses, or carbamazepine more than 400 mg per day (Table 51–1).[20]

Preliminary data from the North American Antiepileptic Drug (NAAED) pregnancy registry[71,72] suggested an unexpectedly high prevalence of isolated, nonsyndromic, cleft palate and/or cleft lip in infants exposed to lamotrigine monotherapy during the first trimester of pregnancy. Five oral cleft cases (two isolated cleft lip, three isolated cleft palate) occurred in 564 pregnant women treated with lamotrigine monotherapy resulting in a total prevalence of 8.9 per 1000, whereas the prevalence of prevalence of nonsyndromic oral clefts among infants of nonepileptic mothers not taking lamotrigine in other studies from the United States, Australia, and Europe ranged from 0.50 to 2.16 per 1000. These observations need further confirmation by independent studies from other registries.

With regard to cognitive outcome, the prospective blinded registry study described earlier in connection to valproate[69] also included 84 children exposed to lamotrigine monotherapy. Their mean IQ (95% CI) at age 2–3 years was 101 (98–104) that was significantly higher than in the valproate group and did not differ from phenytoin or carbamazepine.

LEVETIRACETAM

A prospective registry study[73] included 39 pregnancies exposed to 500–4000 mg of levetiracetam in monotherapy. There were 35 live births, three abortions (one induced), and one stillbirth. No malformations were observed. A preliminary study of a retrospective and prospective case series of pregnancies with levetiracetam including monotherapies as well as polytherapies in the Netherlands showed an overrepresentation of cases with low birth weight (corrected for pregnancy duration) of less than the fifth centile.[74,75]

Data on early cognitive development of children with prenatal exposure to levetiracetam monotherapy are available from only one prospective registry study.[76] Children born to women with epilepsy were enrolled during pregnancy, and consent for the developmental assessment was obtained postnatally. Included were 51 children exposed to levetiracetam monotherapy and 44 children exposed to valproate monotherapy. Of those invited to participate, more valproate (57%) than levetiracetam users (37%) declined. Valproate was the prevalent drug in women with generalized epilepsy and levetiracetam in those with focal epilepsy. The comparison group comprised 97 children born to women without epilepsy. The Griffiths Mental Development Scale was administered at a mean age of 14 months (range 3–24 months). Developmental scores of children exposed to levetiracetam did not differ from control children and were significantly higher than of valproate-exposed children, even when maternal IQ was controlled for. No data for more long-term cognitive outcome after levetiracetam exposure are available.

OTHER AEDS IN MONOTHERAPY

Topiramate. A prospective registry study[40] included 28 monotherapy exposures, two of which showed a major malformation (one cleft lip and palate, one hypospadias).

Gabapentin. A retrospective study included 17 fetuses exposed to gabapentin monotherapy in the first trimester; one had a major malformation at birth (single kidney).[77] A prospective registry study enrolled 31 exposed pregnancies and observed one major malformation (ventricular septal defect) (3.2%, 95% CI 0.6–16.2).[40]

Oxcarbazepine. A multicenter registry study in Argentina[78] reported 35 monotherapy exposed pregnancies none of which resulted in a malformation. One major malformation (urogenital) was observed among 99 pregnancies exposed to monotherapy in a population-based retrospective registry study.[61]

Benzodiazepines. A retrospective registry study included 33 infants who had been exposed to clonazepam monotherapy in the first trimester.[79] One infant (3%) had a major malformation (Fallot tetralogy).

There are no human data on functional teratogenesis of these AEDs.

POLYTHERAPY

The risk of major malformations in mothers taking multiple AEDs is increased compared to monotherapy exposures,[18] especially for combinations including valproate.[61,40]

Prospective population-based data on IQ scores after AED polytherapy exposure are available from two controlled evaluator-blinded studies. The first study[48] included 107 children exposed to a combination of phenytoin and phenobarbital. They did not differ from other children of mothers with epilepsy. The second study[7] compared the mean IQ of 30 children exposed to AED polytherapy to 107 monotherapy-exposed children. Seventeen AED combinations included valproate and 13 were combinations of valproate with carbamazepine. The mean verbal IQ in the polytherapy group was significantly decreased, even when controlled for maternal education.

A prospective long-term clinic-based study[55] also compared cognitive outcome in 23 children exposed to AED polytherapy exposure with 31 children exposed to monotherapy. Polytherapy was associated with impaired verbal and nonverbal IQ. The most common drugs were phenytoin and primidone.

Prospective population-based data on mental deficiency in AED polytherapy-exposed children are available from only two studies.[6,7] The observed prevalence of mental deficiency in the pooled data was 1/84 or 1.2%. The affected child had been exposed phenytoin, carbamazepine, and alcohol.

CLINICAL EVALUATION OF ABNORMALITIES IN THE OFFSPRING

Not every abnormality in the offspring of mothers on AEDs is due to maternal medication. Each child with congenital abnormalities deserves a full clinical evaluation of all relevant potential causes of the defects observed. This is important for genetic and teratogenic counseling with respect to future offspring. Identification of a major genetic cause that by its nature excludes a teratogenic causation implies that the recurrence risk cannot be changed by change of treatment regimen like dose reduction, change of drug or reduction of polytherapy. On the other hand, assuming a genetic cause may lead to recurrence of teratogenic abnormality due to unaltered medication in a subsequent pregnancy and in larger series to wrong or less precise outcome of human teratological studies.

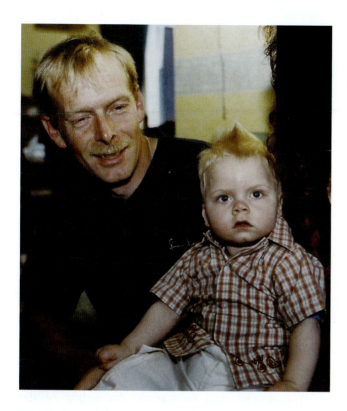

Figure 51–2. A boy with prenatal exposure to valproate and lamotrigine together with his father. The boy shows several typical features of the foetal valproate syndrome (see Table 51–1).

The comprehensive approach needed is best illustrated by the history of a boy depicted with his father in Figure 51–2. This case has been briefly described previously in an abstract.[80] The mother had epileptic seizures, which were predominantly nocturnal and difficult to classify. The etiology of her epilepsy was unknown. The boy was prenatally exposed to a combination of valproate and lamotrigine. The valproate dose was 1500 mg/day divided in three daily doses. The lamotrigine dose was initiated at 50 mg/day and increased to 150 mg/day later during pregnancy. One record noted that lamotrigine had been increased up to a dose of 1000 mg/day but that could not be verified. The mother had an unknown number of nocturnal seizures during pregnancy. Severe maternal pneumonia requiring artificial ventilation occurred at the tenth gestational week and was treated with erythromycin and cefuroxime. Birth was at term and birth weight was 2665 grams. After birth the boy showed dysmorphic features. He also developed epilepsy and neurodevelopmental deficits.

Table 51–2 presents the minor anomalies observed in a physical examination of the boy and his parents. The father's philtrum was difficult to assess in adulthood because of his moustache but a photograph taken of him at elementary school age (Fig. 51–3) shows that he had a similar smooth philtrum and thin upper vermillion as his son. The paternal grandmother did not have epilepsy and did not use antiepileptic medication. The boy shows a combination of features most of which are typical of the fetal valproate syndrome. However, a number of his features can also be found in his parents and can be equally well explained by paternal and maternal inheritance. This leaves only three features that with more certainty may be attributed to prenatal valproate exposure now that we have common knowledge about the existence of this syndrome. Even more

▶ **TABLE 51–2. MINOR ANOMALIES AND FUNCTIONAL ABNORMALITIES IN A CHILD PRENATALLY EXPOSED TO VALPROATE AND LAMOTRIGINE**

Minor Anomalies and Functional Abnormalities Present in the Child	Present in Mother or Father	Typical of Foetal Valproate Syndrome	Possible Effects of Lamotrigine or the Drug Combination	Possible Effects of Maternal Epilepsy	Possible Effects of Maternal Critical Illness[a]
Abnormal ear shelves	–	+	?	–	–
Metopic ridge	–	+	?	–	–
Trigonocephaly	–	+	?	–	–
Overlapping toes	–	+	?	–	–
Neonatal hirsutism	?	+	?	–	–
Midfacial hypoplasia (as child)	?	+	?	–	–
High arched palate	+ (mother)	+	?	–	–
Thin upper vermillion	+ (father)	+	?	–	–
Long, smooth philtrum	+ (father)	+	?	–	–
Dimple on chin	+ (father)	–	?	–	–
"Mohican haircut"	–	–	?	–	–
Epilepsy	+ (mother)	–	?	+	?
Neurodevelopmental deficits	–	+	?	+/–	?

[a]Severe pneumonia at tenth gestational weeks treated with erythromycin and cefuroxime.

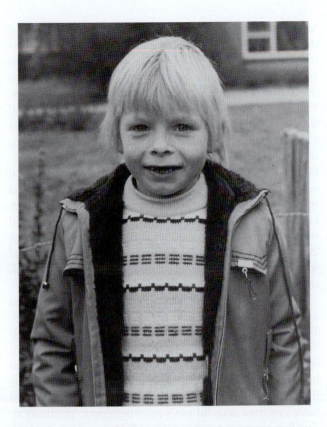

Figure 51–3. The father of the child shown in Figure 51–2 at elementary school age. The nonexposed father has a long, smooth philtrum, which is typical of the foetal valproate syndrome.

carefulness is needed with evaluation of the pregnancy outcome after new drugs, when such prior knowledge about potential teratogenic risks is not yet available.

▶ SUMMARY

Exposure to AEDs during pregnancy increases the risk of major malformations. For phenytoin, phenobarbitone, carbamazepine, and lamotrigine in monotherapy, the prevalence seems to be at most 2–3 times higher than in the general population. A significantly higher risk is associated with fetal exposure to valproate and to polytherapy, especially combinations including valproate. Dose-dependency has been shown for lamotrigine, valproate, carbamazepine, and phenobarbitone. The most common malformations are similar to those observed in the general population, except that there are specific associations of valproate and carbamazepine exposures to spina bifida. Insufficient data are available on other AEDs.

Fetal exposure to phenytoin or valproate may result in syndromes consisting of typical craniofacial features and developmental delay. The prevalence of

these syndromes are not known for lack of sufficiently large population-based studies but they are probably rare. Syndromes specific to other AED exposures have not been established.

Population-based studies suggest that the risk of cognitive impairment after fetal exposure to phenytoin or carbamazepine monotherapy below toxic levels is low. Data on developmental effects of fetal valproate exposure are much more limited but raise a serious concern that valproate monotherapy may be harmful for cognitive and possibly also for social development in the prenatally exposed offspring of mothers with epilepsy. The data on phenobarbital are incongruent. Reports on early cognitive development after lamotrigine or levetiracetam monotherapy exposure have been reassuring, but more studies are needed before conclusions can be drawn. There are no data on cognitive effects of other newer generation AEDs.

Polytherapy exposure during pregnancy appears to increase the risk of cognitive impairment. The little data available on the effects of different combinations suggest that polytherapy including valproate may be especially harmful.

For genetic and teratogenic counseling of the families, it is important to give every child with abnormalities after prenatal drug exposure a full clinical evaluation with an effort to separate the effects of AEDs from other relevant potential causes.

REFERENCES

1. Hiilesmaa VK, Bardy A, Teramo K. Obstetric outcome in women with epilepsy. *Am J Obstet Gynecol* 1985; 152(5):499–504.
2. Spitz MC. Injuries and death as a consequence of seizures in people with epilepsy. *Epilepsia* 1998;39(8):904–907.
3. Tomson T, Walczak T, Sillanpaa M, Sander JW. Sudden unexpected death in epilepsy: a review of incidence and risk factors. *Epilepsia* 2005;46(Suppl 11):54–61.
4. Adab N, et al. The longer term outcome of children born to mothers with epilepsy. *J Neurol Neurosurg Psychiatry* 2004;75:1575–1583.
5. EURAP Study Group. Seizure control and treatment in pregnancy: observations from the EURAP epilepsy pregnancy registry. *Neurology* 2006;66(3):354–360.
6. Gaily E, Kantola-Sorsa E, Granstrom ML. Intelligence of children of epileptic mothers. *J Pediatr* 1988;113(4):677–684.
7. Gaily E, Kantola-Sorsa E, Hiilesmaa V, Isoaho M, Matila R, Kotila M, Nylund T, Bardy A, Kaaja E, Granstrom ML. Normal intelligence in children with prenatal exposure to carbamazepine. *Neurology* 2004;62(1):28–32.
8. Olafsson E, Hallgrimsson JT, Hauser WA, Ludvigsson P, Gudmundsson G. Pregnancies of women with epilepsy: a population-based study in Iceland. *Epilepsia* 1998;39:887–892.

9. Viinikainen K, Heinonen S, Eriksson K, Kalviainen R. Community-based, prospective, controlled study of obstetric and neonatal outcome of 179 pregnancies in women with epilepsy. *Epilepsia* 2006;47(1):186–192.

10. Pennell PB. Antiepileptic drug pharmacokinetics during pregnancy and lactation. *Neurology* 2003;61(6 Suppl 2):S35–S42.

11. Ohman I, Vitols S, Tomson T. Pharmacokinetics of gabapentin during delivery, in the neonatal period, and lactation: does a fetal accumulation occur during pregnancy? *Epilepsia* 2005;46(10):1621–1624.

12. Hvas CL, Henriksen TB, Ostergaard JR. Birth weight in offspring of women with epilepsy. *Epidemiol Rev* 2000;22(2):275–282.

13. Oyen N, Vollset SE, Eide MG, Bjerkedal T, Skjaerven R. Maternal epilepsy and offsprings' adult intelligence: a population-based study from Norway. *Epilepsia* 2007;48(9):1731–1738.

14. Kaaja E, Kaaja R, Hiilesmaa V. Major malformations in offspring of women with epilepsy. *Neurology* 2003;60(4):575–579.

15. Schaefer GB, Sheth RD, Bodensteiner JB. Cerebral dysgenesis. An overview. *Neurol Clin* 1994;12:773–788.

16. Adams J, Vorhees CV, Middaugh LD. Developmental neurotoxicity of anticonvulsants: human and animal evidence on phenytoin. *Neurotoxicol Teratol* 1990;12:203–214.

17. Artama M, Ritvanen A, Gissler M, Isojarvi J, Auvinen A. Congenital structural anomalies in offspring of women with epilepsy—a population-based cohort study in Finland. *Int J Epidemiol* 2006;35:280–287.

18. Perucca E. Birth defects after prenatal exposure to antiepileptic drugs. *Lancet Neurol* 2005;4(11):781–786.

19. Samrén EB, van Duijn CM, Koch S, Hiilesmaa VK, Klepel H, Bardy AH, Beck MG, Deichl AW, Gaily E, Granstrom ML, Meinardi H, Grobbee DE, Hofman A, Janz D, Lindhout D. Maternal use of anti-epileptic drugs and the risk of major congenital malformations: a joint European prospective study of human teratogenesis associated with maternal epilepsy. *Epilepsia* 1997;38:981–990.

20. Tomson T, Battino D, Bonizzoni E, Craig J, Lindhout D, Sabers A, Perucca E, Vajda F. Dose-dependent risk of malformations with antiepileptic drugs: an analysis of data from the EURAP epilepsy and pregnancy registry. *Lancet Neurol* 2011;10:609–617.

21. Fried S, Kozer E, Nulman I, Einarson TR. Koren G. Malformation rates in children of women with untreated epilepsy: a meta-analysis. *Drug Safety* 2004;27(3):197–202.

22. Adab N, Tudur Smith C, Vinten J, Williamson PR, Winterbottom JJ. Common antiepileptic drugs in pregnancy in women with epilepsy. *Cochrane Database Syst Rev* 2004b;(Issue 3):CD004848. DOI: 10.1002/14651858.CD004848.

23. Neubauer BA, Fiedler B, Himmelein B, Kampfer F, Lassker U, Schwabe G, Spanier I, Tams D, Bretscher C, Moldenhauer K, Kurlemann G, Weise S, Tedroff K, Eeg-Olofsson O, Wadelius C, Stephani U. Centrotemporal spikes in families with Rolandic epilepsy: linkage to chromosome 15q14. *Neurology* 1998;51(6):1608–1612.

24. Weglage J, Demsky A, Pietsch M, Kurlemann G. Neuropsychological, intellectual, and behavioral findings in patients with centrotemporal spikes with and without seizures. *Dev Med Child Neurol* 1997;39(10):646–651.

25. Carlsson G, Igelbrink-Schulze N, Neubauer BA, Stephani U. Neuropsychological long-term outcome of Rolandic EEG traits. *Epileptic Disorders* 2000;2(Suppl 1):S63–S66.

26. Hommet C, Sauerwein HC, de Toffol B, Lassonde M. Idiopathic epileptic syndromes and cognition. *Neurosci Behav Rev* 2006;30:85–96.

27. Hermann B, Jones J, Sheth R, Dow C, Koehn M, Seidenberg M. Children with new-onset epilepsy: neuropsychological status and brain structure. *Brain* 2006;129(Pt 10):2609–2619.

28. Schupf N, Ottman R. Reproduction among individuals with idiopathic/cryptogenic epilepsy: risk factors for spontaneous abortion. *Epilepsia* 1997;38(7):824–829.

29. Baker GA. The psychosocial burden of epilepsy. *Epilepsia* 2002;43(Suppl 6):26–30.

30. Jalava M, Sillanpaa M. Reproductive activity and offspring health of young adults with childhood-onset epilepsy: a controlled study. *Epilepsia* 1997;38(5):532–540.

31. Gaily EK, Granstrom ML, Hiilesmaa VK, Bardy AH. Head circumference in children of epileptic mothers: contributions of drug exposure and genetic background. *Epilepsy Res* 1990;5(3):217–222.

32. Lindhout D. Pharmacogenetics and drug interactions: role in antiepileptic-drug-induced teratogenesis. *Neurology* 1992;42(4 Suppl 5):43–47.

33. Buehler BA, Delimont D, van Waes M, Finnell RH. Prenatal prediction of risk of the fetal hydantoin syndrome. *N Engl J Med* 1990;322:1567–1572.

34. Phelan MC, Pellock JM, Nance WE. Discordant expression of fetal hydantoin syndrome in heteropaternal dizygotic twins. *N Engl J Med* 1982;307(2):99–101.

35. Bustamante SA, Stumpff LC. Fetal hydantoin syndrome in triplets. A unique experiment of nature. *Am J Dis Child* 1978;132:978–979.

36. Duncan S, Mercho S, Lopes-Cendes I, Seni MH, Benjamin A. Dubeau F, Andermann F, Andermann E. Repeated neural tube defects and valproate monotherapy suggest a pharmacogenetic abnormality. *Epilepsia* 2001;42(6):750–753.

37. Kozma C. Valproic acid embryopathy. Report of two siblings with further expansion of the phenotypic abnormalities and review of the literature. *Am J Med Genet* 2001;98:168–175.

38. Malm H, Kajantie E, Kivirikko S, Kaariainen H, Peippo M, Somer M. Valproate embryopathy in three sets of siblings: further proof of hereditary susceptibility. *Neurology* 2002;59(4):630–633.

39. Van Dyke DC, Hodge SE, Heide F, Hill LR. Family studies in fetal phenytoin exposure. *J Pediatr* 1988;113(2):301–306.

40. Morrow J, Russell A, Guthrie E, Parsons L, Robertson I, Waddell R, Irwin B, McGivern RC, Morrison PJ, Craig J. Malformation risks of antiepileptic drugs in pregnancy: a prospective study from the UK Epilepsy and Pregnancy Register. *J Neurol Neurosurg Psychiatry* 2006;77(2):193–198.

41. Hanson JW, Smith DW. The fetal hydantoin syndrome. *J Pediatr* 1975;87(2):285–290.

42. Hanson JW, Myrianthopoulos NC, Harvey MA, Smith DW. Risks to the offspring of women treated with hydantoin anticonvulsants, with emphasis on the fetal hydantoin syndrome. *J Pediatr* 1976;89(4):662–668.

43. Gaily E, Granstrom ML, Hiilesmaa V, Bardy A. Minor anomalies in offspring of epileptic mothers. *J Pediatr* 1988;112(4):520–529.

44. Kini U, Adab N, Vinten J, Fryer A, Clayton-Smith J. Liverpool and Manchester Neurodevelopmental Study Group. Dysmorphic features: an important clue to the diagnosis and severity of fetal anticonvulsant syndromes. *Arch Dis Child Fetal Neonatal Ed* 2006;91(2):F90–F95.

45. Kelly TE, Edwards P, Rein M, Miller FQ, Dreifuss FE. Teratogenicity of anticonvulsant drugs II: a prospective study. *Am J Med Genet* 1984;19:435–443.

46. Kelly TE. Teratogenicity of anticonvulsant drugs. III: Radiographic hand analysis of children exposed in utero to diphenyl hydantoin. *Am J Med Genet* 1984;19:445–450.

47. Gaily E. Distal phalangeal hypoplasia in children with prenatal phenytoin exposure: results of a controlled anthropometric study. *Am J Med Genet* 1990;35(4):574–578.

48. Shapiro S, Hartz SC, Siskind V, Mitchell AA, Slone D, Rosenberg L, Monson RR, Heinonen OP. Anticonvulsants and parental epilepsy in the development of birth defects. *Lancet* 1976;1(7954):272–275.

49. Wide K, Hening E, Tomson T, Winbladh B. Psychomotor development in preschool children exposed to antiepileptic drugs in utero. *Acta Paediatr* 2002;91:409–414.

50. Airaksinen EM, et al. A population-based study on epilepsy in mentally retarded children. *Epilepsia* 2000;41:1214–1220.

51. Holmes LB, Wyszynski DF, Lieberman E. The AED (antiepileptic drug) pregnancy registry: a 6-year experience. *Arch Neurol* 2004;61(5):673–678.

52. Samrén EB, van Duijn CM, Christiaens GCML, Hofman A, Lindhout D. Antiepileptic drug regimens associated with major congenital abnormalities in the offspring. *Ann Neurol* 1999;46:739–746.

53. Reinisch JM, Sanders SA, Mortensen EL, Rubin DB. In utero exposure to phenobarbital and intelligence deficits in adult men. *JAMA* 1995;274(19):1518–1525.

54. Myhre SA, Williams R. Teratogenic effects associated with maternal primidone therapy. *J Pediatr* 1981;99(1):160–162.

55. Koch S, Titze K, Zimmermann RB, Schroder M, Lehmkuhl U, Rauh H. Long-term neuropsychological consequences of maternal epilepsy and anticonvulsant treatment during pregnancy for school-age children and adolescents. *Epilepsia* 1999;40(9):1237–1243.

56. Matalon S, Schechtman S, Goldzweig G, Ornoy A. The teratogenic effect of carbamazepine: a meta-analysis of 1255 exposures. *Reprod Toxicol* 2002;16(1):9–17.

57. Lindhout D, Omtzigt JG. Pregnancy and the risk of teratogenicity. *Epilepsia* 1992;33(Suppl 4):S41–S48.

58. Jones KL, Lacro RV, Johnson KA, Adams J. Pattern of malformations in the children of women treated with carbamazepine during pregnancy. *N Engl J Med* 1989;320(25):1661–1666.

59. Rasalam AD, Hailey H, Williams LHG, Moore SJ, Turnpenny PD, Lloyd DJ, Dean JCS. Characteristics of fetal anticonvulsant syndrome associated autistic disorder. *Dev Med Child Neurol* 2005;47:551–555.

60. Wyszynski DF, Nambisan M, Surve T, Alsdorf RM, Smith CR, Holmes LB. Antiepileptic Drug Pregnancy Registry. Increased rate of major malformations in offspring exposed to valproate during pregnancy. *Neurology* 2005;64(6):961–965.

61. Artama M, Auvinen A, Raudaskoski T, Isojarvi I, Isojarvi J. Antiepileptic drug use of women with epilepsy and congenital malformations in offspring. *Neurology* 2005;64:1874–1878.

62. Omtzigt JGC, Nau H, Los FJ, Pijpers L, Lindhout D. The disposition of valproate and its metabolites in the late first trimester and early second trimester of pregnancy in maternal serum, urine, and amniotic fluid: effect of dose, co-medication, and the presence of spina bifida. *Eur J Clin Pharmacol* 1992;43:381–388.

63. Robert E, Guibaud P. Maternal valproic acid and congenital neural tube defects. *Lancet* 1982;2(8304):937.

64. Lindhout D, Meinardi H. Spina bifida and in-utero exposure to valproate. *Lancet* 1984;2(8399):396.

65. Lindhout D, Schmidt D. In-utero exposure to valproate and neural tube defects. *Lancet* 1986;1(8494):1392–1393.

66. Clayton-Smith J, Donnai D. Fetal valproate syndrome. *J Med Genet* 1995;32:724–727.

67. Eriksson K, Viinikainen K, Mönkkönen A, Äikiä M, Nieminen P, Heinonen S, Kälviäinen R. Children exposed to valproate in utero—Population-based evaluation of risks and confounding factors for long-term neurocognitive development. *Epilepsy Res* 2005;65:189–200.

68. Kantola-Sorsa E, Gaily E, Isoaho M, Korkman M. Neuropsychological outcomes in children of mothers with epilepsy. *J Int Neuropsychol Soc* 2007;13:642–652.

69. Meador K, Baker GA, Browning N, Clayton-Smith J, Combs-Cantrell DT, Cohen M, Kalayjian LA, Kanner A, Liporace JD, Pennell PB, Privitera M, Loring DW. Cognitive function at three years of age after fetal exposure to antiepileptic drugs. *New Engl J Med* 2009;360:1597–1605.

70. Cunnington M, Tennis P. International Lamotrigine Pregnancy Registry Scientific Advisory Committee. Lamotrigine and the risk of malformations in pregnancy. *Neurology* 2005;64(6):955–960.

71. Holmes LB, Wyszynski DF, Baldwin EJ, Habecker E, Glassman LH, Smith CR. Increased risk for non-syndromic cleft palate among infants exposed to lamotrigine during pregnancy (abstract). *Birth Defects Res A Clin Mol Teratol* 2006;76(5):318.

72. FDA. Alert for Health Care Providers. http://www.fda.gov/CDER/Drug/InfoSheets/HCP/lamotrigineHCP.htm, 2006.

73. Hunt S, Craig J, Russell A, Guthrie E, Parsons L, Robertson I, Waddell R, Irwin B, Morrison PJ, Morrow J. Levetiracetam in pregnancy: preliminary experience from the UK Epilepsy and Pregnancy Register. *Neurology* 2006;67(10):1876–1879.

74. ten Berg K, Samrén EB, van Oppen AC, Engelsman M, Lindhout D. Levetiracetam use and pregnancy outcome. *Reprod Toxicol* 2005;20:175–178.

75. ten Berg K, Van Oppen AC, Van Donselaar CA, Wentges-Van Holthe JM, Koppe WM, Tamminga P, Lindhout D. Outcomes of human pregnancies with levetiracetam exposure (abstract). *Birth Defects Res A Clin Mol Teratol* 2006;76(5):318.

76. Shallcross R, Bromley RL, Irwin B, Bonnett LJ, Morrow J, Baker GA. Child development following in utero exposure. Levetiracetam vs. sodium valproate. *Neurology* 2011;76:383–389.

77. Montouris G. Gabapentin exposure in human pregnancy: results from the Gabapentin Pregnancy Registry. *Epilepsy Behav* 2003;4(3):310–317.

78. Meischenguiser R, D'Giano CH, Ferraro SM. Oxcarbazepine in pregnancy: clinical experience in Argentina. *Epilepsy Behav* 2004;5(2):163–167.

79. Lin AE, Peller AJ, Westgate MN, Houde K, Franz A, Holmes LB. Clonazepam use in pregnancy and the risk of malformations. *Birth Defects Res* 2004;70(8):534–536.

80. ten Berg K, Veenstra-Knol HE, van Pinxteren-Nagler E, Engstrom LJ, Lindhout D. Congenital abnormalities in maternal epilepsy treated with lamotrigine–valproate combination: clinical assessment of phenotype (abstract). *Reprod Toxicol* 2004;18:721–722.

CHAPTER 52

Comorbidities of Treatment with Antiepileptic Drugs

Dominique M. IJff and Albert P. Aldenkamp

► SUMMARY

All commonly used antiepileptic drugs (AEDs) have some effect on cognitive function, and the effect may be substantial when crucial functions are involved, such as learning in children, driving ability in adults, or already vulnerable functions such as memory in elderly patients. For the commonly used AEDs the effect of phenobarbitone on memory and long-term treatment with phenytoin on mental speed are well established. There is no serious impact on cognition for carbamazepine and valproate and the evidence for ethosuximide is inconclusive.

The available evidence is insufficient to support definite conclusions about the cognitive effects of five of the newer AEDs vigabatrin, zonisamide, tiagabine, gabapentin, and levetiracetam. Better evidence is available for lamotrigine, topiramate, and, to a lesser degree, oxcarbazepine. Oxcarbazepine appears not to affect cognitive function. A relatively large number of studies are available for lamotrigine, which has demonstrated a favorable cognitive profile overall, both in volunteers and in patients with epilepsy. Although dose and titration speed may be confounding factors in some of the studies of topiramate, there is clear evidence that this agent does affect cognitive function, with specific effects on attention and verbal function. For lamotrigine, attempts have been made to correlate cognitive effects with what is known of the drug's mechanism of action. This is an area of research that deserves further exploration with regard to other AEDs.

► INTRODUCTION

Cognitive impairment is the most common comorbid disorder in epilepsy.[1,2] Memory impairments, mental slowing, and attentional deficits are the most frequently reported cognitive disorders.[3,4] These consequences may be even more debilitating than the seizures; thus, it is worthwhile to explore factors leading to cognitive impairment. Although many factors may induce such cognitive impairment, we will here concentrate on the unwanted effects of antiepileptic medication on cognitive function.[5]

In clinical practice, most cognitive problems are multifactorial in origin and the three aforementioned factors are responsible for most cognitive problems. Moreover, the factors are related leading to therapeutic dilemmas when seizure control can only be achieved with treatment-induced cognitive side effects.

Interest in the cognitive effects of antiepileptic drug (AED) treatment is of recent origin. The possibility that cognitive impairment is a consequence or aftermath of epilepsy was raised as early as 1885 when Gowers described "epileptic dementia" as an effect of the pathological sequela of seizures. Nonetheless, the topic was not coupled to AED treatment until the 1970s,[6,7] probably stimulated by the widening range of possibilities associated with the introduction of carbamazepine and valproate. A plethora of subsequent studies have been published focussing on the commonly used AEDs: valproate (VPA), carbamazepine (CBZ), and phenytoin (PHT).

Several new AEDs have been introduced in the last decade. Despite claims that newer AEDs have different efficacy profiles and are particularly efficacious in specific syndromes, head-to-head comparisons between the new AEDs and classical AEDs (such as CBZ and VPA) are rare. Nonetheless, meta-analyses[8,9] do not show significant differences in efficacy between the newer or classical AEDs.

Studies analyzing long-term retention also do not show significant differences.[10,11] Several studies reveal that retention rate is the best predictor of long-term clinical usefulness.[12] Retention rate is a composite of drug efficacy and drug safety and assesses the willingness of patients to continue drug treatment and is the best standard for evaluating the clinical relevance of side effects. The 1-year retention rate is reported to be less than 55% for topiramate (TPM),[13] 60% for lamotrigine (LTG), 58% for VGB, and 45% for gabapentin (GBP).[14] Long-term (mostly 3-year) retention is about 35% for all newer AEDs.[15]

Side effects appear to be the major factor affecting long-term retention for most drugs.[16,17] In clinical practice, tolerability is therefore a major issue and the choice of AED is at least partially based on comparison of tolerability profiles.[18] The tolerability profiles of the newer drugs are also an important issue in drug development, stimulated by the interest of regulatory agencies.[17] Cognitive side effects are one of the most important tolerability problems in chronic AED treatment.

▶ METHOD

An evidence-based approach[5,19,20] is useful to evaluate studies of the cognitive effects of AEDs. Two types of data are evaluated:

a. Absolute drug effects, i.e., the effects of drug treatment against no-treatment (nondrugs) in the same subjects or in a control condition yield the most valuable information.
b. Relative drug effects, i.e., the comparison of the cognitive side effects of a drug with the effects of another drug. Although this clinical information is relevant, this type of comparison does not exclude the possibility that two drugs do not differ if they both impair cognitive function to the same extent.

Data concerning the cognitive side effects of AEDs in pediatric studies are of critical importance when prescribing these drugs in children who are at greater risk for learning disabilities. Children are potentially more susceptible to the adverse effects of AEDs because of the effect of AEDs on neurodevelopment. Even a modest cognitive effect may have significant consequences for neurodevelopment. Therefore, cognitive side effects of the AEDs have emerged as an important consideration when an AED is being selected for the treatment of childhood epilepsy.[21]

▶ RESULTS

PHENOBARBITAL (PB)

The main anticonvulsant mechanism of action is the increase of the duration (not the frequency) of the GABA activated chloride ion channel opening,[22] hence potentiating GABA mediated inhibitory neurotransmission. PB also activates the $GABA_A$ receptor in the absence of GABA, which is a putative mechanism for its sedative properties. PB has been used to treat epilepsy since the discovery of its antiepileptic effect by Hauptman in 1912.

For (PB) one study[23] evaluating the cognitive effects of PB relative to a nondrug condition revealed significant memory impairment (short-term memory recall) in 19 patients with epilepsy.

Comparisons with other AEDs are available from five studies,[24–27] all with patients with epilepsy. One revealed greater impairment for PB than phenytoin (PHT) or carbamazepine (CBZ) on visuomotor and memory tests[27] while two others had convincing and

clinically highly relevant impairments of intelligence scores after long-term PB treatment in comparison with valproate (VPA).[24,25] Only the study by Meador et al (1990) does not show differences between PB and PHT or CBZ.[26]

When the cognitive and behavior effects of PB were assessed in toddlers in a randomized, placebo-controlled study of patients who had febrile seizures, no differences were found in IQ scores between placebo and phenobarbital groups after eight to twelve months of therapy,[28] a finding debated in other studies.[29,30] Effects of PB in children are generally found on memory and comprehension. Schubert reports evidence that PB produces a clinically significant impairment in attention in children[31] and long-term adverse effects on reading skills.[32] There were differences for PB in children when compared to VPA and CBZ.[33]

PHENYTOIN (PHT)

The main anticonvulsant mechanism of action is use-dependent (voltage- and frequency-dependent) sodium channel blocking.[34] PHT binds to the fast inactivated state of the channel, reducing high frequency neuronal firing. PHT has a stronger effect on the sodium channel than CBZ, delaying recovery stronger than CBZ. PHT may also have mild effects on the excitatory glutamate system and on the inhibitory GABA system.

Which mechanism of action is responsible for DPH-induced side effects is unknown. PHT has been used as an AED since 1938 by Merritt and Putnam, and for 20 years PHT was (together with PB) the universal treatment of epilepsy. PHT has excellent anticonvulsant properties and is used as a broad spectrum AED.

Five studies of cognitive comorbidity[35–39] compare PHT with drug-naïve patients. All reveal PHT-induced cognitive impairment in attention, memory and especially mental speed. The magnitude of the reported effects is moderate to large but studies were carried out in normal volunteers, which opens the possibility that these effects represent short-term drug outcomes.

The results of head-to-head comparisons with other AEDs are unclear. Using an ingenious long-term treatment and withdrawal design, Gallassi and coworkers[27] found more cognitive impairment than CBZ. This finding was confirmed in a study with children.[40] However, no differences were reported in comparison to CBZ, VPA, and PB.[26,38–42]

ETHOSUXIMIDE (ESX)

ESX modifies the properties of voltage-dependent calcium channels, reducing the T-type currents and thereby preventing synchronized firing. The reduction is most prominent at negative membrane potentials and less prominent at more positive membrane potentials. Most of the effect is assumed to take place in thalamocortical relay neurons. ESX was introduced in 1960 and is mainly used to treat generalized absence seizures.

A recent study by Mandelbaum et al (2009) shows mild and temporary attentional problems in children with idiopathic epilepsy (mostly absence seizures) in comparison to a nontreatment baseline.[21] However, more recently, a double-blind, randomized, controlled clinical trial with children with newly diagnosed childhood absence epilepsy showed that ethosuximide was associated with fewer adverse attentional effects than valproic acid or lamotrigine.[43]

CARBAMAZEPINE (CBZ)

The main anticonvulsant mechanism of action is similar to PHT with a smaller "slowing" effect in the recovery state compared to PHT. The mechanism of action is also voltage- and frequency-dependent. CBZ was first synthesized in the early 1950s[44,45] and introduced in Europe by Bonduelle in 1964. CBZ is used to treat partial complex seizures with or without secondary generalization. Approval by the FDA for use in the United States followed much later (1978) because of concerns about serious hematological toxicity (e.g., aplastic anemia).

Three studies, one in normal volunteers,[36] one in patients with epilepsy,[40] and one in children with symptomatic partial epilepsy[46] report "no cognitive impairment" for CBZ compared to a nondrug condition. However, Meador and coworkers[38,39] reported impairments in memory, attention and mental speed, similar to the adverse effect profile for phenytoin. In children, poorer performance than controls was seen early in treatment with carbamazepine in the pegboard measure of visuomotor coordination.[47] Moreover, they were faster on a visual search task and better on recalled stories compared to a nondrug condition.[48] Mandelbaum et al (2009) reported persistence of attentional problem compared to a nondrug baseline when newly diagnosed children with localization-related epilepsy were treated over a period of 1 year.[21]

In comparisons of CBZ with other AEDs, Gallassi and coworkers demonstrated a more favorable profile compared with PHT and PB[27] whereas Meador and coworkers[26,38,39] found no differences in similar comparisons. Chen and coworkers found no differences between CBZ and PB and VPA in children.[33] However, Forsythe and coworkers[41] reported that CBZ in moderate dosage adversely affected memory in children, whereas VPA and PHT did not.

VALPROATE (VPA)

VPA is one of the most effective drugs against generalized absence seizures. It is a fatty acid and is believed to possess multiple mechanisms of action. Several studies have demonstrated an effect on sodium channels that is different from PHT and CBZ. An effect on T-type calcium channels has also been reported. Recent studies have demonstrated a predominant effect in its interaction with the GABA-ergic neurotransmitter system by elevating brain GABA levels and potentiating GABA responses, possibly by enhancing GABA synthesis and inhibiting degradation. Theoretically, such mechanisms of action may cause cognitive side effects. Furthermore, VPA may also augment GABA release and block the reuptake of GABA into glial cells.

Three studies[49–51] of VPAs have absolute effects reveal mild to moderate impairments of psychomotor and mental speed. Comparison to other AEDs reveal reduced memory and visuomotor function compared to CBZ[27] and a favorable profile compared to PHB on tests of intelligence.[24,25] One study revealed no difference from PHT,[41] and another withdrawal design study of children in remission reported "no cognitive impairment" compared to a nondrug condition.[40] Hyperammonemia is an indirect effect of valproate that may result in mental slowing.[52]

OXCARBAZEPINE (OXC)

OXC is a keto homologue prodrug of CBZ. It is structurally similar to CBZ, but has a different metabolic profile. In humans, the keto group is rapidly and quantitatively reduced to a monohydroxy derivative that is the main active anticonvulsant agent. Metabolism of OXC does not result in the formation of 10,11-epoxy carbamazepine that is considered the main metabolite causing side effects. The mechanism of action is similar to CBZ, but OXC also reduces presynaptic glutamate release, possibly by reduction of high-threshold calcium currents.

OXC was approved in the European Union in 1999 and is indicated for use as a monotherapy or adjunctive therapy for partial seizures with or without secondarily generalized tonic–clonic seizures in patients ≥6 years of age.

The effects of OXC on cognitive function were evaluated in one study of healthy volunteers and five studies of patients with epilepsy. A double-blind, placebo-controlled, crossover study conducted in 12 healthy volunteers[53] compared the effects of two doses of OXC (300 mg per day and 600 mg per day) and placebo on cognitive function and psychomotor performance. Treatment duration for each condition was 2 weeks. Cognitive function was assessed before treatment initiation and 4 hours after the morning doses on days 1, 8, and 15. OXC improved performance on a focused attention task, increased manual writing speed, and had no effect on long-term memory processes.

In patients with epilepsy, four monotherapy comparative studies are available to evaluate the effects of OXC on cognitive functions in adult patients with newly diagnosed epilepsy. The first study[54] was a double-blind, active-control study evaluating the effects of CBZ and OXC on memory and attention in 41 patients with newly diagnosed epilepsy. Treatment duration was 1 year. Cognitive function and intelligence was assessed before treatment initiation and after 1 year of treatment. The results indicated no deterioration of memory or attention with either CBZ or OXC.

The second study was an active-control study that evaluated the effects of CBZ, VPA, and OXC on intelligence, learning and memory, attention, psychomotor speed, verbal span, and visuospatial construction in 32 patients with newly diagnosed epilepsy.[55] The treatment duration was 4 months. Cognitive function and intelligence were evaluated before treatment initiation and after 4 months of treatment. There was no deterioration of cognitive function in any treatment group. Significant improvements in learning and memory tests were found for the CBZ- and OXC-treated patients. Improvements also occurred in attention and psychomotor speed tests for the VPA-treated patients and partly for the CBZ-treated patients.

The third study was a double-blind, randomized, active-control study that evaluated the effects of PHT and OXC on memory, attention, and psychomotor speed in 29 patients with newly diagnosed epilepsy[56] treated for 1 year. Cognitive function tests were administered before treatment initiation and after 6 and 12 months of treatment. There were no significant differential cognitive effects between PHT and OXC during the first year of treatment in patients with newly diagnosed epilepsy who achieved adequate seizure control.

In the fourth study,[57] three groups of 12 patients taking either CBZ, VPA, or PHT received a single 600-mg dose of OXC followed 7 days later by 3 weeks of treatment with OXC 300 mg thrice daily and matched placebo in random order. Seven untreated patients, acting as controls, were prescribed the single OXC dose and 3 weeks of active treatment only. There were no significant changes in cognitive function during administration of OXC compared with placebo.

The effects in children have been studied in only one study, comparing OXC with CBZ and VPA.[58,59] The study was an open-label, randomized, active-control, three-arm, parallel-group, 6-month study comparing 55 newly diagnosed patients on OXC monotherapy versus 57 patients taking CBZ or VPA. There were no statistically significant differences between the two arms for seven cognitive tests. As in adults some mild improvements were reported on the attentional tests.

TOPIRAMATE (TPM)

TPM is a sulfamate-substituted monosaccharide that has multiple mechanisms of action.[60] TPM blocks neuronal sodium channels in a voltage- and frequency-dependent manner, inhibits CA, promotes the action of GABA at the $GABA_A$ receptor complex, and GABA brain concentrations by about 60% at 3 and 6 hours after a single dose—an increase that is maintained with 4 weeks of TPM administration.[61] TPM is a carbonic anhydrase inhibiting agent that is effective in refractory chronic partial epilepsy.[62,63]

During the initial add-on clinical trials, central nervous system-related "cognitive" subjective complaints were frequently reported, including mental slowing, attentional deficits, speech problems and memory difficulties.[63] However, higher target doses and faster titration schedules were used than are now common in clinical practice (see Faught et al, 1996 for a discussion of dose and titration speed). Recent studies with TPM-treated patients confirm high levels of adverse cognitive effects based on subjective complaints.[64,65] A follow-up study[66] showed long-term retention of 30% at 4-year follow-up. For about half of the 70% of patients who discontinued treatment, side effects were the major reason, with cognitive side effects being mentioned most frequently.

A study of six normal volunteers[67] used an acute dose of 2.8 mg/kg (~200 mg per day) followed by a titration to 5.7 mg/kg (~400 mg per day) in 4 weeks, resulting in weekly dose escalations of about 100 mg. The rate at which TPM was escalated in this study was very similar to the dose escalation used in the initial TPM adjunctive-therapy trials[62] escalating the TPM dose to 200 or 400 mg per day over 2–3 weeks, and was associated with somnolence, psychomotor slowing, speech disorders, and concentration and memory difficulties.[61] The neuropsychometric changes were commensurate with the CNS effects. The cognitive effects of an acute starting dose of 200 mg per day were impairments of verbal function (word finding and verbal fluency) of approximately two standard deviations (a very serious impairment) and sustained attention. Titration to 400 mg per day in 4 weeks resulted in impairments of verbal memory and mental speed of more than two standard deviations.

Five studies involving patients with epilepsy are available. In a study by Meador (1997) of 155 patients with epilepsy, the effects of the gradual introduction of TPM as add-on (a 50-mg starting dose, followed by increments of 50 mg per week over 8 weeks) were compared with a more rapid dose escalation (initial dose of 100 mg, followed by two consecutive weekly increments of 100 and 200 mg). In a test battery of 23 variables representing selective attention, word fluency, and visuomotor speed, subjects on a slow-titration schedule treated with one background AED displayed TPM-associated abnormalities of more than one third but less than one standard deviation.[68]

A study by Aldenkamp et al (2000) was specifically designed to compare cognitive effects of TPM and VPA added to therapeutic dosages of CBZ in 59 patients with epilepsy. A slow titration speed was used with a starting dose of 25 mg per day TPM and weekly increments of 25 mg.[69] Moreover, the average achieved dose (approximately 250 mg) was relatively low. Neuropsychometric testing was conducted 8 weeks after the last dosage increase (20 weeks after the start of TPM therapy). The study used optimal conditions (i.e., slow titration, relatively low dose, and a longer treatment period), allowing for patient habituation to the effects of TPM therapy. Nonetheless, cognitive impairment was found for verbal memory function both during the titration and at end point.

Burton and Harden (1997) assessed attention weekly in ten subjects receiving TPM over a 3-month period.[70] Four of nine subjects showed significant correlations between TPM dosage and forward digit span. In a study by Thompson et al (2000), the neuropsychological test scores of 18 patients obtained before and after the introduction of treatment with TPM (median dose 300 mg) and controls were retrospectively evaluated. Patients taking TPM showed significant deterioration in many domains including verbal IQ, verbal fluency, and verbal learning.[71] In an open, prospective study, 41 patients with intractable epilepsy initially received either TPM or Tiagabine (TGB) as add-on treatment.[72] Of these 21 patients were assessed at baseline; after a three month titration phase and after a 3-month maintenance phase. The patients were assessed on various aspects of cognitive functioning such as attention, memory, language and self-report mood and quality of life. The TPM group performed worse on measures of verbal fluency and working memory and reported more depression than the TGB group. They also felt that they were suffering from more adverse effects due to the TPM medication. However, TPM patients did report an increase in mental flexibility between titration and maintenance phase. In another study, patients treated with TPM worsened in the cognitive domains of cognitive speed and verbal fluency, as well as verbal and visual short-term memory compared to patients treated with LEV.[73]

Few studies have psychometrically measured cognitive changes in children on TPM. In a randomized, double-blind, placebo-controlled study comparing topiramate in different dosages (50 mg per day and 100 mg per day) and placebo, the topiramate 100 mg per day dose was associated with slowing in psychomotor reaction times.[74] Learning, memory and executive function were unchanged. In another study, the digit symbol test and verbal learning memory test were administered at baseline and study endpoint in children treated with topiramate started either in monotherapy or add-on therapy. Cognitive testing revealed no significant changes during TPM therapy. Comparing pre–post differences, TPM monotherapy was associated with better cognitive outcomes than add-on therapy.[75] However, the results of this 12-week open-label study must be interpreted with caution given the short study duration and heterogeneity of the study population.

When cognitive effects of TPM were compared with CBZ in children (5–15 years) with benign rolandic epilepsy after 28 weeks of treatment, patients who received carbamazepine showed an improvement on the subtest maze from the WISC-R and children with TPM had a poorer performance on the subtest arithmetic.[76] However, when the patients who had maintained the minimum target dose were compared, the TPM group improved on the subtest object assembly compared to the carbamazepine treatment group. This study and the study of Coppola et al (2008) corroborate the finding in adults. A high percentage of children (>20%) suffer from a broad range of cognitive side effects that persist even at assessments for more than 1 year.[77]

LAMOTRIGINE (LTG)

LTG is a phenyltriazine with weak antifolate activity. It was introduced in Europe in 1991 and in the United States in 1994. The main anticonvulsant mechanism of action is to block voltage-dependent sodium channels that result in voltage- and frequency-dependent inhibition of the channel. This suggests that the mechanism of action is similar to PHT and CBZ. However in LTG treatment this mechanism prevents presynaptic excitatory neurotransmitter release and the extent to which the mechanisms of action differ from CBZ is debatable.[78] Clinical evidence indicates that LTG is effective against partial and secondarily generalized tonic–clonic seizures, as well as idiopathic (primary) generalized epilepsy.

A large number of cognitive studies are available for LTG (see Aldenkamp & Baker[79] for an overview). Six volunteer studies have been conducted with LTG. Doses of 120 mg and 240 mg did not produce a significant change in cognitive function compared with baseline when administered to 12 normal volunteers in an acute 1-day study.[80] Similarly, five volunteers who received LTG (acute dose 3.5 mg/kg titrated to a maximum of 7.1 mg/kg) in a single-blind manner were assessed for change in cognitive function after 2 and 4 weeks.[67] There was no significant change in any of the neurocognitive measures relative to baseline performance.

LTG and CBZ were compared in 12 healthy male volunteers and associations were made between the observed cognitive effects and plasma concentrations.[81] AED effects were studied utilizing adaptive tracking which assesses eye–hand coordination and effects of attention, and eye movement. LTG treatment did not significantly differ from placebo, but increased CBZ saliva concentrations were significantly associated with impaired adaptive tracking and smooth and saccadic eye movements.

The long-term effects of LTG and CBZ were compared in 23 volunteers in a 10-week crossover study.[82] A neuropsychological battery included 19 instruments yielding 40 variables, including both subjective and objective measures. LTG was significantly associated with better performance or fewer side effects in 19 (48%) of the variables. The cognitive and behavioral effects of LTG and TPM were compared in 47 healthy adults using a double-blind, randomized crossover design with two 12-week treatment periods.[83] Neuropsychological evaluation included 17 measures yielding 41 variables of cognitive function and subjective behavioral effects. Better performance on 33 (80%) variables was observed for LTG, but none for TPM. Even after adjustment for blood levels, performance was better on 19 (46%) variables for LTG, but none for TPM. Differences concerned both objective cognitive and subjective behavioral measures.

Finally, a study by Aldenkamp et al (2002) in 30 volunteers (12 days of treatment, using a daily dose of 50 mg of LTG) showed evidence for a selective positive effect of LTG on cognitive activation, relative to both placebo and VPA. Although the results of these volunteer studies provide a preliminary insight into the impact of LTG on cognition, the generalizability of the results from these studies to patients with epilepsy receiving long-term AED treatment is limited.[84]

The effects of LTG on cognitive function were compared with CBZ in patients with newly diagnosed epilepsy. Patients completed tests of verbal learning, memory, attention, and mental flexibility at baseline and were reassessed for up to 48 weeks. Significant differences favoring LTG over CBZ were observed for semantic processing, verbal learning, and attention.[85] The authors concluded that LTG may have a favorable long-term effect on cognitive function when compared with CBZ.

Other studies have reported positive cognitive effects of LTG used as adjunctive therapy. Three independent double-blind, randomized, crossover studies examined the cognitive effects of LTG as add-on therapy.[86–88] Two included patients with a history of partial seizures (at least once weekly during the preceding 3 months) who had received no more than two other AEDs or VPA monotherapy. Both studies also used two treatment periods (12 and 18 weeks), which were separated by a washout period (4 and 6 weeks). Despite the similarity in trial design and patients, there

is some inconsistency between the findings of these three studies.

One study revealed a marginal reduction in "cerebral efficiency" (an indirect measure of cognitive function) following LTG treatment.[87] Conversely, significant improvements were reported in the second study[86] and in the third study when compared with TPM.[88] In an uncontrolled add-on study[89] using CBZ as a baseline drug, no deterioration on any of the cognitive tests was found after introducing LTG (200 mg). LTG therapy in seven patients with epilepsy and mental retardation caused both positive and negative psychotropic effects.[90] These findings were based on the observations of parents and supervising staff. Positive effects included reduced irritability and increased compliance with simple instructions, while negative effects included behavioral deterioration with temper tantrums, restlessness, and hyperactivity. Similarly, a second study in 67 patients with mental retardation showed that following adjunctive treatment with LTG, social functioning was stable or improved in 90% of patients.[91]

In addition to clinical studies of the impact of LTG on cognitive function, LTG may impact electroencephalographic (EEG) parameters. Subclinical epileptiform discharges may be associated with transient deterioration in cognitive function.[92–94] Data from several studies indicate that LTG may reduce spontaneous epileptiform discharges, which may partially explain the favorable cognitive profile of LTG. In five patients with interictal EEG discharges, a single dose of LTG (120 mg or 240 mg in addition to existing medication) resulted in a substantial reduction of discharges within a 24-hour period.[95]

The long-term effects of LTG on paroxysmal abnormalities have also been monitored with a computer-based analysis system.[96] Twenty-one patients with intractable epilepsy (twenty of whom were receiving multiple AED therapy) were evaluated for EEG ictal events and number of spikes in a 10-minute period before and after LTG treatment. At baseline, patients typically showed diffuse spike–wave complexes. At 4 months, ictal discharges were replaced by diffuse slow wave activity with no adverse effect on background activity. Nineteen of the 21 patients also evidenced reduced seizure frequency.

The effect of LTG add-on therapy in 11 patients with refractory partial seizures with or without secondary generalization has also been reported.[97] LTG was added to existing therapy consisting of CBZ with at least one additional AED. EEG recordings were made at rest with eyes closed, during an attentive task (blocking reaction induced by several episodes of eyes open lasting 8–9 seconds), during cognitive tasks, and while performing mental arithmetic. In addition, a battery of neuropsychological tests was performed. Before LTG treatment, the EEG revealed decreased fast activity at rest and a reduction in alpha and beta bands during attentive and cognitive tasks. LTG treatment resulted in a selective increase in alpha reactivity and beta power during the attentive tasks with no other detectable changes. During cortical activation, subtle changes were observed that were taken as indicative of a slight improvement in attention. Neuropsychological evaluation revealed no deterioration in cognitive function after 3 months of LTG therapy.

LTG also shows a promising cognitive profile in elderly patients suffering from age-associated memory impairment.[98] A neuropsychological test battery in combination with auditory event-related potentials (ERPs) was used to measure the impact of LTG on cognitive function. LTG treatment caused a reduction in amplitude of the P_{300} component of the ERP and a corresponding improvement in immediate and delayed visual memory and delayed logical memory. LTG may therefore improve simple memory functions in a memory-impaired elderly population.

In the first placebo-controlled, double-blind, crossover study on the cognitive effects of lamotrigine in children with epilepsy, children with well-controlled or mild epilepsy were randomly assigned to add-on therapy with either lamotrigine followed by placebo or placebo followed by lamotrigine.[99] For children on sodium valproate, lamotrigine was titrated to 2 mg/kg per day (≤12 years old) or 150 mg per day (>12 years old). For children not on sodium valproate, lamotrigine was titrated to 10 mg/kg per day (≤12 years old) or 300 mg per day (>12 years old). Each treatment phase lasted 9 weeks, with a crossover period of 5 weeks. A neuropsychological test battery was performed during EEG monitoring at baseline and at the end of placebo and drug phases. There were no cognitive effects for LTG in adjunctive therapy in children with epilepsy. A favorable cognitive profile was also reported after long-term treatment based on physicians' and parents' experience.[100] More positive changes in concentration and vigilance were reported.

LEVETIRACETAM (LEV)

LEV is structurally and mechanistically dissimilar to other AEDs. It is believed to bind to a specific, as yet undetermined, site on the synaptic plasma membrane. Moreover, LEV reduces GABA turnover in the striatum by reducing GABA synthesis and increasing GABA metabolism. It is effective in reducing partial seizures in patients with epilepsy, both as adjunctive treatment and as monotherapy.

LEV has many therapeutic advantages for patients with epilepsy. It has favorable pharmacokinetic characteristics (good bioavailability, linear pharmacokinetics, insignificant protein binding, lack of hepatic metabolism, and rapid achievement of steady-state concentrations) and a low potential for drug interactions. It is licensed for use as adjunctive treatment for partial seizures, with or without secondary generalization, in people aged over 16 years.

Only limited data are available from a small pilot study on cognitive function.[101] A prospective, multicenter, open-label study showed that adjunctive therapy or monotherapy with LEV in adults with epilepsy improved cognitive and neuropsychological functions such as recall and language.[102] Recently, Bootsma et al (2009) showed favorable effects.[103] An international (UK/The Netherlands) cognitive study is presently being carried out. This study employs a first-line add-on design to, compare the cognitive effects of LEV with CBZ and VPA. In comparison to CBZ, LEV has a positive stimulating effect on cognition.[104]

The effects of adjunctive LEV on memory and attention in children have been investigated in a randomized, double-blind, placebo-controlled study. The behavioral and emotional effects of adjunctive LEV treatment in children and adolescents (4–16 years old) with uncontrolled partial-onset seizures were also evaluated in a randomized, double-blind, placebo-controlled study.[106] Patients received adjunctive LEV 20–60 mg/kg per day or placebo for 12 weeks. Selective aspects of behavioral and emotional functioning, specifically aggressive behavior, were affected by adjunctive LEV treatment. The Aggressive Behavior score of the Achenbach Child Behavior Checklist (CBCL) worsened in the LEV group, which led to treatment group differences on the composite scores of Externalizing Syndromes and Total Problems. Patterns of spontaneous treatment-emergent adverse events were consistent with these outcomes. However, no patient discontinued the trial because of aggressive behavior-related events.

VIGABATRIN (VGB)

A small sample showed no change from baseline after patients with partial epilepsy were treated with 2 g of VGB for 6 months.[107] This finding was supported by Thomas and Trimble (1996) in a healthy volunteer study.[108] No serious cognitive impairment was found in a retrospective chart review of 84 children. In fact, a shorter period from onset of infantile spasms to treatment with VGB was associated with superior cognitive outcome.[109] In contrast, Gaily et al (1999) reported cognitive impairments during treatment with VGB in a minority of their sample with uncontrolled epilepsy.[110]

TIAGABINE (TGB)

Tiagabine (TGB) is a γ-aminobutyric acid (GABA) uptake inhibitor that is structurally related to the prototypic GABA uptake blocker nipecotic acid, but has an improved ability to cross the blood–brain barrier.

TGB temporarily prolongs the presence of GABA in the synaptic cleft by delayed clearance. Clinical trials have shown that TGB is effective as add-on therapy in the management of patients with refractory partial epilepsy. As TGB was recently marketed certain aspects of its development are unfinished.

Three cognitive studies are available. Dodrill et al[111] included 162 patients who received the following treatments: placebo (n = 57), 16 mg per day TGB (n = 34), 32 mg per day TGB (n = 45), or 56 mg per day TGB (n = 26) at a fixed dose for 12 weeks after a 4-week dose titration period. Eight cognitive tests and three measures of mood and adjustment were administered during the baseline period and again during the double-blind period near the end of treatment (or at the time of dropout). The results showed no cognitive effects of monotherapy with TGB at a low or high dose, but there was some evidence for mood effects of add-on treatment with TGB at higher dosing, possibly related to titration speed.[111]

Thirty seven patients with partial epilepsy were studied in the add-on polytherapy study by Kälviäinen et al (1996). The study protocol consisted of a randomized, double-blind, placebo-controlled, parallel-group add-on study with open-label extension.[112] During the 3-month double-blind low-dose phase (30 mg per day), TGB treatment did not produce cognitive changes compared to placebo. TGB treatment also did not cause deterioration in cognitive performance during longer follow-up with successful treatment on higher doses after 6 to 12 months (mean 65.7 mg per day, range 30–80 mg per day) and after 18–24 months (mean dose 67.6 mg per day, range 24–80 mg per day).

Finally, Sveinbjornsdottir et al (1994) conducted an open trial of 22 adult patients with refractory partial epilepsy followed by a double-blind, placebo-controlled, crossover trial in 12 subjects. Nineteen patients completed the initial open titration and fixed-dose phase of the study and 11 patients completed the double-blind phase. The median daily TGB dose was 32 mg during the open fixed-dose and 24 mg during the double-blind period. Neuropsychological evaluation did not show any significant effect on cognitive function in the open or double-blind phase.[113]

GABAPENTIN (GBP)

GBP (1-(aminomethyl) cyclohexane-acetic acid) is a novel AED utilized primarily as add-on therapy in patients with partial and generalized tonic–clonic seizures. GBP is a cyclic GABA analogue, originally designed as a GABA agonist.[114] Further research has clearly shown a specific effect of GBP on GABA-ergic neurotransmitter systems, especially influencing GABA turnover. Investigations using nuclear magnetic resonance imaging spectroscopy have confirmed that GBP elevates GABA concentrations, specifically in the occipital cortex of patients with epilepsy.[61]

Two volunteer studies and one clinical study are available to interpret the cognitive effects.

Martin et al (1999) used an acute dose and rapid titration in six volunteers and did not find cognitive effects of GBP.[67] Meador et al (1999) compared the cognitive effects of GBP and CBZ in 35 healthy subjects by using a double-blind, randomized, crossover design with two 5-week treatment periods. During each treatment condition, subjects received either GBP 2400 mg per day or CBZ (mean 731 mg per day). Subjects were tested at the end of each AED treatment period and in four drug-free conditions (two pretreatment baselines and two posttreatment washout periods [1 month after each AED]). A neuropsychological test battery included 17 measures yielding 31 total variables. Significantly better performance on eight variables was found for GBP, but on no variables for CBZ. Comparison of CBZ and GBP with the nondrug average revealed significant statistical differences for 15 (48%) of 31 variables.[115] Leach et al (1997) studied GBP in 21 patients in an add-on polytherapy study after 4 weeks of adjunctive therapy and found no change in psychomotor and memory tests.[116] Drowsiness was more often found in higher dosing (2400 mg). Mortimore et al (1998) did not find a difference between continued polytherapy and an add-on with GBP in measures of quality of life.[117]

No studies are available for children.

ZONISAMIDE (ZNS)

The anticonvulsant properties of ZNS were discovered through extensive testing of a variety of sulfonamide compounds. Like TPM it has multiple mechanisms of action: blockade of voltage-gated sodium channels, reducing sustained repetitive firing, blocking T-type calcium channels, and inhibiting ligand binding tot the GABA$_A$ receptor. Like TPM, ZNS is a carbonic anhydrase inhibiting drug. Although there is longer experience with ZNS in Japan (where it was developed), it was recently introduced in the United States and in Europe for partial onset seizures in refractory epilepsy.

Anecdotal clinical experience reveals a cognitive side-effect profile very similar to TPM but no controlled studies are available. Two studies are currently in preparation. No studies are available for children.

RUFINAMIDE (RUF)

Rufinamide (RUF 331; 1-(2,6-difluoro-phenyl)methyl-1H-1,2,3-triazole-4-carboxamide) is a structurally novel compound which limits the frequency of sodium-dependent neuronal action potentials. One study is available to assess the cognitive effects.[118] The study used a multicenter, multinational double-blind, randomized, placebo-controlled parallel study design with four different doses of RUF (based on prior studies): 200 mg per day, 400 mg per day, 800 mg per day and 1600 mg per day as add-on to the existing medication. Cognitive assessment was performed at baseline (before the start with RUF treatment) and at endpoint (after 3 months of treatment). The most significant finding is the absence of any statistically significant worsening on cognitive measures at any dose of RUF after 12 weeks of treatment. There were also no statistically significant differences between RUF and placebo. No data are available for children.

▶ CONCLUSION

Although cognitive side effects are generally considered to be mild to moderate for most AEDs,[19] all of the commonly used AEDs have some impact on cognitive function. A mild impact may be amplified in specific conditions and become substantial when crucial functions, such as learning in children[4] or driving capacities in adults (often requiring millisecond precision) are involved. This also holds true for functions that are already vulnerable, such as memory function in the elderly.[119] Moreover, the cognitive side are present long term and may increase with prolonged AED therapy, impacting on quality of life in refractory epilepsies.[120] The current evidence is summarized in Table 52–1 and Fig. 52–1.

Definite evidence for drug-induced cognitive impairment is now established for PB (especially memory impairment), PHT (mental slowing) and TPM (mental slowing and verbal impairments/dysphasia). Mild effects (mostly psychomotor slowing) were found for CBZ and VPA. No cognitive effects were found for VGB, RUF, TGB, and GBP, although the evidence requires confirmation. No cognitive side effects and even some mild cognitive activating effects were observed for LTG and OXC. The cognitive effects for ESX, LEV, and ZNS are inconclusive.

▶ **TABLE 52–1. COGNITIVE EFFECTS OF AEDs**

	Absolute Effects (Comparison with a Nondrug Condition)	Relative Effects (Impairment When Compared with Other Antiepileptic Drugs)
Phenobarbital (PB)	1 study reporting impairment • Memory impairment	4 studies, 3 reporting impairment • Memory and visuomotor impairment when compared with PHT and CBZ • Impairment of intelligence after long-term treatment when compared to VPA
Phenytoin (PHT)	5 studies, all reporting impairment • Attentional deficits, memory impairment, and mental slowing (mental slowing most frequently reported)	6 studies, 2 reporting impairment • Global cognitive impairment and mental slowing
Ethosuximide (ESX)	No studies	No studies
Carbamazepine (CBZ)	3 studies, 1 reporting impairment • Attentional deficits and mental slowing	2 studies, none reporting impairment
Valproate (VPA)	4 studies, all reporting mild impairment • Psychomotor and mental slowing	1 study, reporting no impairment
Oxcarbazepine (OXC)	1 study, reporting no impairment	5 studies, none reporting impairment
Topiramate (TPM)	1 study, reporting impairment • Attentional deficits, verbal impairments	5 studies, all reporting impairment • Verbal impairments (especially word finding problems/dysphasia), memory impairment, and mental slowing
Lamotrigine (LTG)	5 studies, none reporting impairment and 4 reporting activating effects	8 studies, none reporting impairment; the majority reporting psychotropic effects (activation)
Levetiracetam (LEV)	No studies	1 study, reporting no impairment
Vigabatrin (VGB)	No studies	No studies
Tiagabine (TGB)	3 studies, none reporting impairment	No studies
Gabapentin (GBP)	1 study, reporting no impairment	2 studies, not reporting impairment
Zonisamide (ZNS)	No studies	No studies
Rufinamide (RUF)	No studies	1 study, reporting no impairment

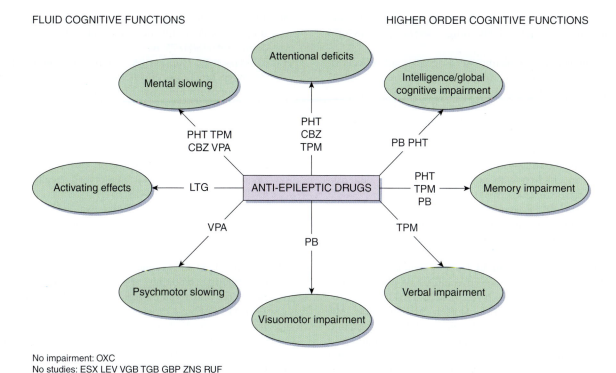

Figure 52-1. Dominant impairment per antiepileptic drug.

REFERENCES

1. Aldenkamp AP, Dodson WE (eds). Epilepsy and education; cognitive factors in learning behavior. *Epilepsia* 1990;31(Suppl 4):S9–S20.

2. Dodson WE, Pellock JM. *Pediatric Epilepsy: Diagnosis and Treatment.* New York: Demos Publications, 1993.

3. Dodson WE, Trimble MR. *Epilepsy and Quality of Life.* New York: Raven Press, 1994.

4. Aldenkamp AP, Dreifuss FE, Renier WO, Suumeijer PBM. Epilepsy in Children and Adolescents. Boca Raton: CRC Press, 1995.

5. Aldenkamp AP. Antiepileptic drug treatment and epileptic seizures—effects on cognitive function. In: Trimble M, Schmitz B (eds), *The Neuropsychiatry of Epilepsy.* New York: Cambridge University Press, 2002; pp. 256–267.

6. Ideström CM, Schalling D, Carlquist U, Sjöqvist F. Behavioral and psychophysiological studies: acute effects of diphenylhydantoin in relation to plasma levels. *Psychol Med* 1972;2:111–120.

7. Dodrill CB, Troupin AS. Psychotropic effects of carbamazepine in epilepsy: a double-blind comparison with phenytoin. *Neurology* 1977;27:1023–1028.

8. Marson AG, Kadir ZA, Hutton JL, Chadwick DW. The new antiepileptic drugs: a systematic review of their efficacy and tolerability. *Epilepsia* 1997;38:859–880.

9. Jette NJ, Marson AG, Hutton JL. Topiramate add-on for drug-resistant partial epilepsy. *Cochrane Database Syst Rev* 2002;3:CD001417.

10. Wong IC. New antiepileptic drugs. Study suggests that under a quarter of patients will still be taking the new drugs after six years. *BMJ* 1997;314:603–604.

11. Stefan H, Krämer G, Mamoli B (eds). *Challenge Epilepsy – New Antiepileptic Drugs.* Berlin: Blackwell Science, 1998.

12. Lhatoo SD, Wong IC, Polizzi G, Sander JW. Long-term retention rates of lamotrigine, gabapentin, and topiramate in chronic epilepsy. *Epilepsia* 2000;41:592–596.

13. Kellett MW, Smith DF, Stockton PA, Chadwick DW. Topiramate in clinical practice: first year's postlicensing experience in a specialist epilepsy clinic. *J Neurol Neurosurg Psychiatry* 1999;66:759–763.

14. Marson AG, Kadir ZA, Hutton JL, Chadwick DW. Gabapentin for drug-resistant partial epilepsy. *Cochrane Database Syst Rev* 2000;2:CD001415.

15. Marson AG, Hutton JL, Leach JP, Castillo S, Schmidt D, White S, Chaisewikul R, Privitera M, Chadwick DW. Levetiracetam, oxcarbazepine, remacemide and zonisamide for drug resistant localization-related epilepsy: a systematic review. *Epilepsy Res* 2001;46:259–270.

16. Chadwick DW, Marson T, Kadir Z. Clinical administration of new antiepileptic drugs: an overview of safety and efficacy. *Epilepsia* 1996;37:S17–S22.

17. Aldenkamp AP. Cognitive and behavioural assessment in clinical trials: when should they be done? *Epilepsy Res* 2001;45:155–159.

18. Bootsma HP, Ricker L, Hekster YA, Hulsman J, Lambrechts D, Majoie M, Schellekens A, de Krom M, Aldenkamp

AP. The impact of side effects on long-term retention in three new antiepileptic drugs. *Seizure* 2009;18:327–331.

19. Vermeulen J, Aldenkamp AP. Cognitive side-effects of chronic antiepileptic drug treatment: a review of 25 years of research. *Epilepsy Res* 1995;22:65–95.

20. Aldenkamp AP, De Krom M, Reijs R. Newer antiepileptic drugs and cognitive issues. *Epilepsia* 2003;44(Suppl 4): 21–29.

21. Mandelbaum DE, Burack GD, Bhise VV. Impact of antiepileptic drugs on cognition, behaviour, and motor skills in children with new-onset, idiopathic epilepsy. *Epilepsy Behav* 2009;16:341–344.

22. Twyman RE, Rogers CJ, Macdonald RL. Differential regulation of gamma-aminobutyric acid receptor channels by diazepam and phenobarbital. *Ann Neurol* 1989;25:213–220.

23. MacLeod CM, Dekaban AS, Hunt E. Memory impairment in epileptic patients: selective effects of phenobarbital concentration. *Science* 1978;202:1102–1104.

24. Vining EP, Mellits ED, Dorsen MM, Cataldo MF, Quaskey SA, Spielberg SP, Freeman JM. Psychologic and behavioral effects of antiepileptic drugs in children: a double-blind comparison between phenobarbital and valproic acid. *Pediatrics* 1987;80(2):165–174.

25. Calandre EP, et al. Cognitive effects of long-term treatment with phenobarbital and valproic acid in school children. *Acta Neur Scand* 1990;81:504–506.

26. Meador KJM, Loring DW, Huh K, Gallagher BB, King DW. Comparative cognitive effects of anticonvulsants. *Neurology* 1990;40:391–394.

27. Gallassi R, Morreale A, Di Sarro R, Marra M, Lugaresi E, Baruzzi A. Cognitive effects of antiepileptic drug discontinuation. *Epilepsia* 1992;33(Suppl 6):S41–S44.

28. Camfield CS, Chaplin S, Doyle AB, Shapiro SH, Cummings C, Camfield PR. Side effects of phenobarbital in toddlers; behavioural and cognitive aspects. *J Pediatr* 1979;95:361–365.

29. Wolf SM, Forsythe A, Studen AA, Friedman R, Diamond H. Long-term effect of phenobarbital on cognitive function in children with febrile convulsions. *Pediatrics* 1981;68:820–823.

30. Farwell JR, et al. Phenobarbital for febrile seizures—effects on intelligence and on seizure recurrence. *N Engl J Med* 1990;322:364–369.

31. Schubert R. Attention deficit disorder and epilepsy. *Pediatr Neurol* 2005;32:1–10.

32. Sulzbacher S, Farwell JR, Temkin N, Lu AS, Hirtz DG. Late cognitive effects of early treatment with phenobarbital. *Clin Pediatr* 1999;38:387–394.

33. Chen YJ, Chow JC, Lee IC. Comparison the cognitive effect of anti-epileptic drugs in seizure-free children with epilepsy before and after drug withdrawal. *Epilepsy Res* 2001;44:65–70.

34. Schwarz JR, Grigat G. Phenytoin and carbamazepine: potential- and frequency-dependent black of NA currents in mammalian myelinated nerve fibers. *Epilepsia* 1989;30:286–294.

35. Smith WL, Lowrey JB. Effects of diphenylhydantoin on mental abilities in the elderly. *J Am Geriatr Soc* 1975;23:207–211.

36. Thompson PJ, Huppert F, Trimble MR. Anticonvulsant drugs, cognitive function and memory. *Acta Neurol Scand* 1980;(S80):75–80.

37. Thompson PJ, Huppert FA, Trimble MR. Phenytoin and cognitive functions: effects on normal volunteers and implications for epilepsy. *Br J Clin Psychol* 1981;20:155–162.

38. Meador KJM, et al. Comparative cognitive effects of carbamazepine and phenytoin in healthy adults. *Neurology* 1991;41:1537–1540.

39. Meador KJM, et al. Effects of carbamazepine and phenytoin on EEG and memory in healthy adults. *Epilepsia* 1993;34(1):153–157.

40. Aldenkamp AP, et al. Withdrawal of antiepileptic medication—effects on cognitive function in children: The Multicentre Holmfrid Study. *Neurology* 1993;43:41–50.

41. Forsythe I, et al. Cognitive impairment in new cases of epilepsy randomly assigned to carbamazepine, phenytoin and sodium valproate. *Dev Med Child Neurol* 1991;33:524–534.

42. Jha S, Kumar V, Mishra VN. Effect of common anti-epileptic drugs on cognition in schoolchildren with epilepsy. *Indian J Physiol Pharmacol* 2001;45:507–510.

43. Glauser TA, et al. Ethosuximide, valproic acid and lamotrigine in childhood absence epilepsy. *N Engl J Med* 2010;362:790–799.

44. Parnas J, Flachs H, Gram L. Psychotropic effect of antiepileptic drugs. *Acta Neurol Scand* 1979;60:329–343.

45. Parnas J, Gram L, Flachs H. Psychopharmacological aspects of antiepileptic treatment. *Prog Neurobiol* 1980;15: 119–138.

46. Riva D, Devoti M. Carbamazepine withdrawal in children with previous symptomatic partial epilepsy: effects on neuropsychologic function. *J Child Neuro* 1999;14:357–362.

47. Stores G, Williams PL, Styles E, Zaiwalla Z. Psychological effects of sodium valproate and carbamazepine in epilepsy. *Arch Dis Child* 1992;67:1330–1337.

48. Seidel WT, Mitchel WG. Cognitive and behavioural effects of carbamazepine in children: data from benign Rolandic epilepsy. *J Child Neurol* 1999;14:716–723.

49. Thompson PJ, Trimble MR. Sodium valproate and cognitive functioning in normal volunteers. *Br J Clin Pharmacol* 1981;12:819–824.

50. Craig I, Tallis R. Impact of valproate and phenytoin on cognitive function in elderly patients: results of a single-blind randomized comparative study. *Epilepsia* 1994;35:381–390.

51. Prevey ML, Delaney RC, Cramer JA, Cattanach L, Collins JF, Mattson RH. The Department of Veterans Affairs Epilepsy Cooperative Study 264 Group. Effect of valproate on cognitive function. Comparison with carbamazepine. *Arch Neuro* 1996;53:1008–1016.

52. Nicolai J, et al. Cognitive side-effects of valproate-acid-induced hyperammonemia in children with epilepsy. *J Clin Psychopharmacol* 2007;27:221–224.

53. Curran HV, Java R. Memory and psychomotor effects of oxcarbazepine in healthy human volunteers. *Eur J Clin Pharmacol* 1993;44:529–533.

54. Laaksonen R, Kaimola K, Grahn-Teräväinen E, Waltimo O. A controlled clinical trial of the effects of carbamazepine and oxcarbazepine on memory and attention. *16th International Epilepsy Congress*, Hamburg, 1985 (abstract).

55. Sabers A, et al. Cognitive function and anticonvulsant therapy: effect of monotherapy in epilepsy. *Acta Neurol Scand* 1995;92:19–27.

56. Äikiä M, Kälviäinen R, Sivenius J, Halonen T, Riekkinen RJ. Cognitive effects of oxcarbazepine and phenytoin monotherapy in newly diagnosed epilepsy: one year follow-up. *Epilepsy Res* 1992;11:199–203.

57. McKee PJ, et al. A double-blind, placebo-controlled interaction study between oxcarbazepine and carbamazepine, sodium valproate and phenytoin in epileptic patients. *Br J Clin Pharmacol* 1994;37:27–32.

58. Donati F, Gobbi G, Campistol J, Rapatz G, Daehler M, Sturm Y, Aldenkamp AP. Effects of oxcarbazepine on cognitive function in children and adolescents with partial seizures. *Neurology* 2006;67:679–682.

59. Donati F, et al. Oxcarbazepine Cognitive Study Group. The cognitive effects of oxcarbazepine versus carbamazepine or valproate in newly diagnosed children with partial seizures. *Seizure* 2007;16:670–679.

60. White HS. Clinical significance of animal seizure models and mechanism of action studies of potential antiepileptic drugs. *Epilepsia* 1997;38(Suppl 1):S9–S17.

61. Petroff OAC, et al. The effect of gabapentin on brain gamma-aminobutyric acid in patients with epilepsy. *Ann Neurol* 1996;39:95–99.

62. Privitera M, et al. Topiramate placebo-controlled dose-ranging trial in refractory partial epilepsy using 600-, 800-, and 1000-mg daily dosages. *Neurology* 1996;46:1678–1683.

63. Faught E, et al. Topiramate placebo-controlled dose-ranging trial in refractory partial epilepsy using 200-, 400, and 600-mg daily dosages. *Neurology* 1996;46:1684–1690.

64. Ketter TA, Post RM, Theodore WH. Positive and negative psychiatric effects of antiepileptic drugs in patients with seizure disorders. *Neurology* 1999;53(5 suppl 2):53–67.

65. Tatum WO, et al. Postmarketing experience with topiramate and cognition. *Epilepsia* 2001;42:1134–1140.

66. Bootsma HP, Coolen F, Aldenkamp AP, Arends J, Diepman L, Hulsman J, Lambrechts D, Leenen L, Majoie M, Schellekens A, de Krom M. Topiramate in clinical practice: long-term experience in patients with refractory epilepsy referred to a tertiary epilepsy center. *Epilepsy Behav* 2004;5:380–387.

67. Martin R, et al. Cognitive effects of topiramate, gabapentin, and lamotrigine in healthy young adults. *Neurology* 1999;52:321–327.

68. Meador KJ. Assessing cognitive effects of a new AED without the bias of practice effects [abstract]. *Epilepsia* 1997;38(Suppl 3):60.

69. Aldenkamp AP, et al. A multicentre randomized clinical study to evaluate the effect on cognitive function of topiramate compared with valproate as add-on therapy to carbamazepine in patients with partial-onset seizures. *Epilepsia* 2000;41:1167–1178.

70. Burton LA, Harden C. Effect of topiramate on attention. *Epilepsy Res* 1997;27:29–32.

71. Thompson PJ, Baxendale SA, Duncan JS, Sander JW. Effects of topiramate on cognitive function. *J Neurol Neurosurg Psychiatry* 2000;69:636–641.

72. Fritz N, Glogau S, Hoffmann J, Rademacher M, Elger CE, Helmstaedter C. Efficacy and cognitive side effects of tiagabine and topiramate in patients with epilepsy. *Epilepsy Behav* 2005;6:373–381.

73. Gomer B, et al. The influence of antiepileptic drugs on cognition: a comparison of levetiracetam and topiramate. *Epilepsy Behav* 2007;10:486–494.

74. Pandina GJ, et al. Cognitive effects of topiramate in migraine patients aged 12 through 17 years. *Pediatr Neurol* 2010;42:187–195.

75. Brandl U, Kurlemann G, Neubauer B, Retig K, Schäuble B, Schreiner A. Seizure and cognitive outcomes in children and adolescents with epilepsy treated with topiramate. *Neuropediatrics* 2010;41:113–120.

76. Kang HC, et al. The effects on cognitive function and behavioural problems of topiramate compared to carbamazepine as monotherapy for children with benign rolandic epilepsy. *Epilepsia* 2007;48:1716–1723.

77. Coppola G, et al. Topiramate in children and adolescents with epilepsy and mental retardation: a prospective study on behavior and cognitive effects. *Epilepsy Behav* 2008;12:253–256.

78. Leach MJ, Lees G, Riddall DR. Lamotrigine: mechanisms of action. In: Levy RH, Mattson RH, Meldrum BS (eds), *Antiepileptic Drugs*. New York: Raven Press, 1995; 4th edn: pp. 861–869.

79. Aldenkamp AP, Baker G. A systematic review of the effects of lamotrigine on cognitive function and quality of life. *Epilepsy Behav* 2001;2:85–91.

80. Cohen AF, Ashby L, Crowley D, Land G, Peck AW, Miller AA. Lamotrigine (BW430C), a potential anticonvulsant. Effects on the central nervous system in comparison with phenytoin and diazepam. *Br J Clin Pharmacol* 1985;20:619–629.

81. Hamilton MJ, et al. Carbamazepine and lamotrigine in healthy volunteers: relevance to early tolerance and clinical trial dosage. *Epilepsia* 1993;34:166–173.

82. Meador KJ, Loring DW, Ray PG, Perrine KR, Bazquez BR, Kalbosa T. Differential effects of carbamazepine and lamotrigine. *Neurology* 2001;56:1177–1182.

83. Meador KJ, et al. Cognitive and behavioural effects of lamotrigine and topiramate in healthy volunteers. *Neurology* 2005;64:2108–2114.

84. Aldenkamp AP, et al. Randomized, double-blind parallel-group study comparing cognitive effects of a low-dose lamotrigine with valproate and placebo in healthy volunteers. *Epilepsia* 2002;43:19–26.

85. Gillham R, Kane K, Bryant-Comstock L, Brodie MJ. A double-blind comparison of lamotrigine and carbamazepine in newly diagnosed epilepsy with health-related quality of life as an outcome measure. *Seizure* 2000;9:375–379.

86. Smith D, Baker G, Davies G, Dewey M, Chadwick DW. Outcomes of add-on treatment with lamotrigine in partial epilepsy. *Epilepsia* 1993;34:312–322.

87. Banks GK, Beran RG. Neuropsychological assessment in lamotrigine treated epileptic patients. *Clin Exp Neurol* 1991;28:230–237.

88. Blum D, et al. Cognitive effects of lamotrigine compared with topiramate in patients with epilepsy. *Neurology* 2006;67:400–406.

89. Aldenkamp AP, Mulder OG, Overweg J. Cognitive effects of lamotrigine as first line add-on in patients with localized related (partial) epilepsy. *J Epilepsy* 1997;10:117–121.

90. Ettinger AB, Weisbrot DM, Saracco J, Dhoon A, Kanner A, Devinsky O. Positive and negative psychotropic effects of lamotrigine in patients with epilepsy and mental retardation. *Epilepsia* 1998;39:874–877.

91. Earl N, et al. Lamotrigine adjunctive therapy in patients with refractory epilepsy and mental retardation [abstract]. *Epilepsia* 2000;41(Suppl 1):72.

92. Aarts JH, Binnie CD, Smit AM, Wilkins AJ. Selective cognitive impairment during focal and generalized epileptiform EEG activity. *Brain* 1984;107:293–308.

93. Aldenkamp AP, et al. Acute cognitive effects of nonconvulsive difficult-to-detect epileptic seizures and epileptiform electroencephalographic discharges. *J Child Neurol* 2001;16:119–123.

94. Aldenkamp AP, Arends J. The relative influence of epileptic EEG discharges, short nonconvulsive seizures and type of epilepsy on cognitive function. *Epilepsia* 2004;45:54–63.

95. Binnie CD, et al. Acute effects of lamotrigine (BW430C) in persons with epilepsy. *Epilepsia* 1986;27:248–254.

96. Marciani MG, et al. Effect of lamotrigine on EEG paroxysmal abnormalities and background activity: a computerized analysis. *Br J Clin Pharmacol* 1996;42:621–627.

97. Marciani MG, et al. Lamotrigine add-on therapy in focal epilepsy: electroencephalographic and neuropsychological evaluation. *Clin Neuropharmacol* 1998;21:41–47.

98. Mervaala E, et al. Electrophysiological and neuropsychological profiles of lamotrigine in young and age-associated memory impairment (AAMI) subjects [abstract]. *Neurology* 1995;45(Suppl 4):A259.

99. Pressler RM, Binnie CD, Coleshill SG, Chorley GA, Robinson RO. Effect of lamotrigine on cognition in children with epilepsy. *Neurology* 2006;66:1495–1499.

100. Brodbeck V, et al. Long-term profile of lamotrigine in 119 children with epilepsy. *Eur J Paediatr Neurol* 2006;10:135–141.

101. Neyens LGJ, Alpherts WCJ, Aldenkamp AP. Cognitive effects of a new pyrrolidine derivative (levetiracetam) in patients with epilepsy. *Prog Neuropsychopharmacol Biol Psychiatry* 1995;19:411–419.

102. Wu T, et al. Clinical efficacy and cognitive and neuropsychological effects of levetiracetam in epilepsy: an open-label multicenter study. *Epilepsy Behav* 2009;16:468–474.

103. Bootsma HP, et al. The impact of side effects on long-term retention in three new antiepileptic drugs. *Seizure* 2009;18:327–331.

104. Helmstaedter C, Witt JA. Cognitive outcome of antiepileptic treatment with levetiracetam versus carbamazepine monotherapy: a non-interventional surveillance trial. *Epilepsy Behav* 2010;18:74–80.

105. Levisohn PM, Mintz M, Hunter SJ, Yang H, Jones J. Neurocognitive effects of adjunctive levetiracetam in children with partial-onset seizures: a randomized, double-blind, placebo-controlled, noninferiority trial. *Epilepsia* 2009;50:2377–2389.

106. Loge C, Hunter SJ, Schiemann J, Yang H. Assessment of behavioral and emotional functioning using standardized instruments in children and adolescents with partial-onset seizures treated with adjunctive levetiracetam in a randomized, placebo-controlled trial. *Epilepsy Behav* 2010;18:291–298.

107. Monaco F, et al. Lack of association between vigabatrin and impaired cognition. *J Int Med Res* 1997;25:296–301.

108. Thomas L, Trimble M. The effects of vigabatrin on attention, concentration and mood: an investigation in healthy volunteers. *Seizure* 1996;5:205–208.

109. Camposano SE, et al. Vigabatrin in the treatment of childhood epilepsy: a retrospective chart review of efficacy and safety profile. *Epilepsia* 2008;49:1186–1191.

110. Gaily E, et al. Cognitive deficits after cryptogenic infantile spasms with benign seizure evolution. *Dev Med Child Neurol* 1999;41:660–664.

111. Dodrill CB, Arnett JL, Sommerville KW, Shu V. Cognitive and quality of life effects of differing dosages of tiagabine in epilepsy. *Neurology* 1997;48:1025–1031.

112. Kälviäinen R, Äikiä M, Mervaala E, Saukkonen AM, Pitkanen A, Riekkinen PJ Sr. Long-term cognitive and EEG effects of tiagabine in drug-resistant partial epilepsy. *Epilepsy Res* 1996;25:291–297.

113. Sveinbjornsdottir S, Sander JW, Patsalos PN, Upton D, Thompson PJ, Duncan JS. Neuropsychological effects of tiagabine, a potential new antiepileptic drug. *Seizure* 1994;3:29–35.

114. Macdonald RL, Kelly KM. Antiepileptic drug mechanisms of action. *Epilepsia* 1995;36(S2):2–12.

115. Meador KJ, et al. Differential cognitive effects of carbamazepine and gabapentin. *Epilepsia* 1999;40:1279–1285.

116. Leach JP, Girvan J, Paul A, Brodie MJ. Gabapentin and cognition: a double-blind, dose ranging, placebo controlled study in refractory epilepsy. *J Neurol Neurosurg Psychiatry* 1997;62:372–376.

117. Mortimore C, Trimble M, Emmers E. Effects of gabapentin on cognition and quality of life in patients with epilepsy. *Seizure* 1998;7:359–364.

118. Aldenkamp AP, Alpherts WCJ. The effect of the new antiepileptic drug rufinamide on cognitive functions. *Epilepsia* 2006;47(7):1153–1159.

119. Trimble MR. Anticonvulsant drugs and cognitive function: a review of the literature. *Epilepsia* 1987;28(Suppl 3):37–45.

120. American Academy of Pediatrics. Behavioral and cognitive effects of anticonvulsant therapy. Committee on Drugs. *Pediatrics* 1985;76:644–647.

CHAPTER 53

Ketogenic Diets

Eric H. Kossoff and Douglas R. Nordli, Jr.

▶ OVERVIEW: WHAT IS THE KETOGENIC DIET?

The ketogenic diet is a high-fat, adequate-protein, low-carbohydrate diet that is carefully calculated by a dietitian and menus created for a parent to follow.[1] A ketogenic diet ratio of 4:1 describes the ratio of grams of fat to both carbohydrate and protein combined, and provides 90% of calories from fat (Fig. 53–1). A 3:1 ratio is used primarily for infants and adolescents in whom either higher protein or more carbohydrates are needed for either growth or tolerability.

Foods are carefully weighed and measured based on either dietitian-created meal plans or family-oriented computerized exchange program. In most cases, calories are restricted to 75% of daily requirements, although both increases and decreases from this may be made based on the individual child's daily metabolic demands to achieve an ideal body mass index.[1] Fluids are also restricted to 85% of the daily allowance. Neither calorie nor fluid restriction has ever been demonstrated to be effective in children and many dietitians will target either 100% or the baseline prediet intake of each child.

The diet can be provided as solids, liquids (formula), or as a combination of both. Solid foods eaten not only include 36% heavy whipping cream, mayonnaise, oil, butter, cheese, hot dogs, and other high-fat foods but also protein sources typically totaling 1 g/kg body weight per day. The majority of the small amounts of remaining calories include carbohydrates such as fruits and vegetables, which help alleviate constipation. Many families have been very creative in recipe and meal choices (Fig. 53–2).

The diet can also be easily implemented as a formula, either using a single powdered source such as Nutricia KetoCal®, (Fig. 53–3) available in either a 4:1 or now 3:1 preparation, or "modular" components comprised of Ross Carbohydrate-Free® and Polycose® with Novartis Microlipid®.[2] This liquid method of diet administration is used predominantly in infants and gastrostomy-tube fed children and compliance is assured. A formula-only diet has been demonstrated to be very effective, with approximately double the likelihood of a >90% seizure reduction compared to all children on the diet, possibly due to improved compliance.[2,3]

▶ INDICATIONS FOR ITS USE

The ketogenic diet has been used for nearly 90 years in patients with a wide variety of seizure types and epilepsies. Despite this impressive record, there is a paucity of literature regarding its effectiveness for specific clinical circumstances. Earlier publications were retrospective, and therefore subject to ascertainment bias. Later work studied patients with specific seizure types but not epilepsy syndromes. No studies to date have been both prospective and controlled. For these reasons, systematic reviews of the ketogenic diet that are based upon formal medical evidence cannot support efficacy.[4,5] Still, interest in the diet continues to grow worldwide.[6] While most of these studies do not meet the stringent criteria, one would insist for formal drug approval; they can be used to suggest clinical circumstances where the ketogenic diet might be particularly helpful (Fig. 53–4).

PRIMARY THERAPY

The ketogenic diet is first-line therapy for the treatment of seizures in association with glucose-transporter protein deficiency (GLUT1-DS) and pyruvate dehydrogenase deficiency (PDH).[7-9] In both cases, the diet effectively treats seizures while providing essential fuel for brain metabolic activity. Ketone bodies enter the mitochondria and are used in aerobic metabolism, effectively bypassing the limited supply of brain glucose in GLUT1-DS and the enzymatic block that prohibits incorporation of pyruvate into the tricarboxylic acid (TCA) cycle in PDH. The utilization of ketone bodies is thermodynamically very efficient. In this manner, the diet is not only an anticonvulsant treatment, but it is also treats the other nonepileptic manifestations of these diseases that are due to energy deficiency.

SECONDARY TREATMENT

The ketogenic diet has been used historically as an alternative treatment, usually after the failure of valproate, for childhood myoclonic epilepsies including severe myoclonic epilepsy of infancy (Dravet syndrome) and myoclonic-astatic epilepsy (Doose syndrome).[10,11] Given the effectiveness of the diet in the treatment of myoclonic epilepsies, it could possibly

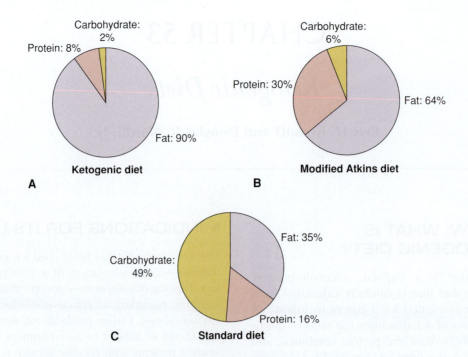

Figure 53–1. Daily calories provided on different diets. (**A**) Ketogenic diet. (**B**) Modified Atkins diet. (**C**) Standard diet.

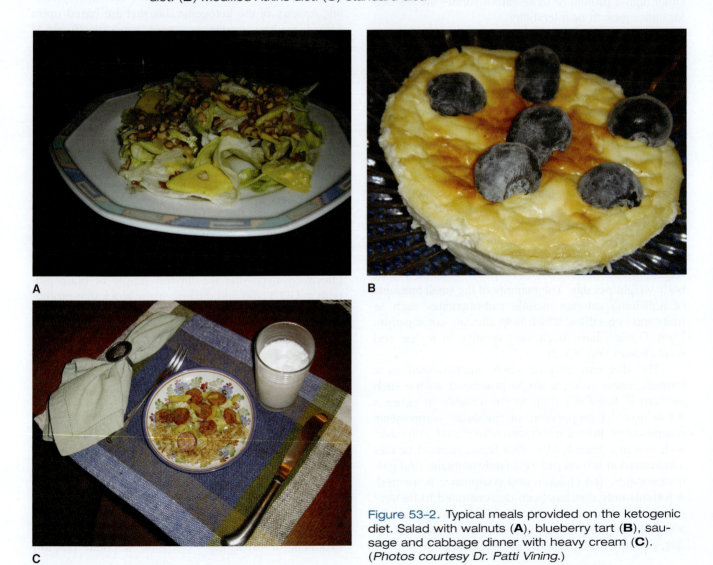

Figure 53–2. Typical meals provided on the ketogenic diet. Salad with walnuts (**A**), blueberry tart (**B**), sausage and cabbage dinner with heavy cream (**C**). (*Photos courtesy Dr. Patti Vining.*)

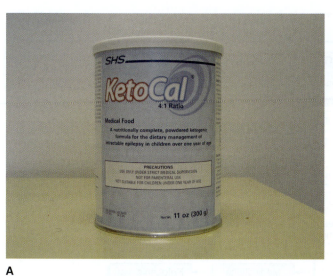

A

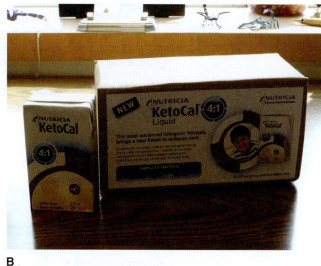

B

Figure 53–3. Nutricia KetoCal®. Powder (**A**), Liquid (**B**).

be considered as first-line treatment for patients with these conditions, but no comparative studies exist. The ketogenic diet can be beneficial in infants with West syndrome who are refractory to corticosteroids and other medications.[12–14]

A prompt response of absence seizures in patients with GLUT1-DS is common. Based upon Keith's data and our own experience, the ketogenic diet may also be useful in the treatment of children with other refractory absence epilepsies, with or without myoclonus.[15] Other forms of dietary treatment may also be useful in absence epilepsies. In one study, a modified Atkins diet was used to treat children with intractable epilepsy. Four out of five children with absence had a greater than 50% seizure reduction and three went at least 1 month without seizures.[16]

EPILEPSIES WITH PROMINENT FOCAL SEIZURES

It is very difficult to precisely determine the efficacy of the diet in the treatment of epilepsies manifesting with predominantly focal seizures. Livingston stated that the diet was not effective for partial seizures. Keith did not classify his patients in a manner that allows one to determine the effectiveness in partial seizures.[15] A recent study of children with a dramatic, seizure-free response to the diet within 2 weeks found that none of these children had solely partial seizures.[17] In kindled animals, a model of focal epilepsy, the diet was shown to have at least transient anticonvulsant properties.[18] To the degree that one can extrapolate from animals to humans, this study bolsters the use of the ketogenic diet in children with refractory partial epilepsy.

Nevertheless, while the diet may be considered in this group, there is no compelling clinical data to favor its use. Therefore, children with refractory focal seizures should be evaluated to determine if they are candidates for focal resective surgery. If they are, then surgery need not be delayed to institute a trial of the ketogenic diet. On the other hand, if drugs have failed and the patient is deemed to be a poor surgical candidate, then the diet should be considered. Based upon our own experience and limited published information infants with migrating partial seizures may not respond favorably to the ketogenic diet.[19]

It would seem inappropriate to treat children with otherwise benign seizure disorders, such as febrile seizures, benign Rolandic epilepsy, benign occipital epilepsy including Panayiotopoulos syndrome, and benign familial neonatal convulsions with the ketogenic diet.

OTHER POSSIBLE INDICATIONS

Preliminary experience showing some beneficial effects of the ketogenic diet have also been reported in the following disorders: seizures in children with tuberous sclerosis complex,[20,21] Rett syndrome,[22] glycogenosis type V,[23] and subacute sclerosing panencephalitis.[24]

PRECAUTIONS

The ketogenic diet could have lethal consequences in certain clinical circumstances where cerebral energy metabolism is deranged. An example of this is pyruvate carboxylase (PC) deficiency. Patients with PC

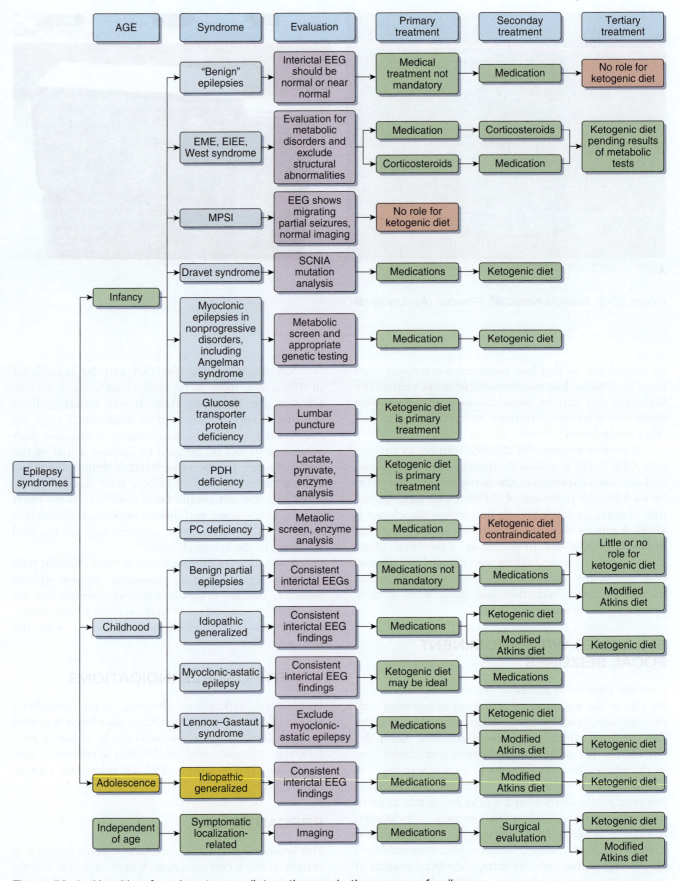

Figure 53–4. Algorithm for when to use dietary therapy in the course of epilepsy.

deficiency may present early in life with refractory myoclonic seizures. PC is the first step in gluconeo-genesis but also controls production of oxaloacetate, the rate-limiting substrate in the Krebs cycle. Patients with PC cannot utilize ketone bodies efficiently so the loss of carbohydrate can have devastating conse-quences.[25] Patients with fatty acid oxidation problems would also be adversely affected by the ketogenic diet, but such patients do not, as a rule, present with seizures. Patients with organic acidurias may worsen with ketogenic diet treatment. Although patients with mitochondrial disorders are not traditionally started on the ketogenic diet, recent evidence suggests safety and efficacy.[26]

▶ INITIATION OF THE KETOGENIC DIET

Perhaps no other aspect of the clinical management of the ketogenic diet has created as much controversy for physicians and anxiety for parents as the initiation pro-tocol. For many decades, the ketogenic diet was started only as an inpatient, with a mandatory fasting period until high levels of urinary ketosis were achieved, fol-lowed by gradually increasing calories over 3 days.[1] Over the past few years, both retrospective and pro-spective studies have analyzed specific aspects of the "Hopkins protocol" (Table 53–1).

Is a fast required? Several retrospective studies have demonstrated that fasting is not necessary when starting the diet.[27–30] The most recent study was a pro-spective, randomized study of a fasting versus gradual initiation approach by the group from Children's Hos-pital of Philadelphia.[27] There was no observed differ-ence in 3-month outcomes and fewer side effects with a gradual approach, although ketosis increased more quickly with a fasting approach.[27] However, fasting is generally well tolerated and may lead to an immediate reduction in seizures even before ketogenic food is provided.[31] Many centers are now individualizing their approach to the start of the diet based on each patient and their families.

The diet has also been reported as effective with-out an inpatient hospitalization. Both the modified Atkins and low-glycemic index diets do not hospitalize children at initiation.[16,32–35] However, hospitalization allows for intensive diet education, monitoring for the potential of acute worsening as ketosis develops, careful examination of medications for carbohydrate contents, and lastly the chance for families to estab-lish support with one another (if admitted in groups). Although an admission is inconvenient for working parents and school-age children, most find the educa-tion immersion helpful for addressing future questions and problems.

▶ TABLE 53–1. JOHNS HOPKINS HOSPITAL PROTOCOL FOR INITIATION OF THE KETOGENIC DIET, 2012

Day prior to admission (Sunday)
- Reduced carbohydrates for 24 h
- Fasting starts the evening before admission with clear no-carbohydrate fluids only

Day 1 (Monday)
- Admitted to the hospital at noon after initial meeting and evaluation by dietitian
- Fasting continues until dinner (24 h total)
- Dinner, given as liquid "eggnog," providing 1/3 of calculated maintenance dinner calorie allowance
- Fluids restricted to 60–75 cc/kg
- Blood glucose monitored every 6 hours, orange juice given for glucose <30 mg/dL
- Change medications to carbohydrate-free versions, solutions generally discontinued
- Parents begin educational program

Day 2 (Tuesday)
- Parents begin to check urine ketones periodically
- Education continues
- Dinner (eggnog), increased to 2/3 of maintenance dinner calorie allowance (ratio kept constant)
- Blood glucose checks typically discontinued after dinner if consistently >50 mg/dL

Day 3 (Wednesday)
- Breakfast and lunch given as eggnog, providing 2/3 of maintenance breakfast and lunch calorie allowance
- Dinner is first full ketogenic meal (solids, not eggnog, if child is able)
- Education continues

Day 4 (Thursday)
- Full ketogenic diet breakfast (100% assigned calories) given
- Education completed
- Prescriptions provided for carbohydrate-free medica-tions, multivitamin, and calcium
- Follow-up appointment arranged (1 month for infants, children at risk; 3 months otherwise)
- Child discharged to home

Source: From Freeman JM, Kossoff EH, Freeman JB, Kelly MT. *The Ketogenic Diet: A Treatment for Epilepsy in Children and Others.* New York: Demos, 2006; 4th edn.

▶ THE MODIFIED ATKINS DIET

Due to the inherent restrictiveness of the ketogenic diet, especially in regards to calorie and protein restric-tion, as well as the weighing and measuring of foods, physicians have long sought alternative, easier dietary methods of providing ketosis. The modified Atkins diet was first reported in 2003 in a case series of six patients, half of whom were actually adults.[32] This diet creates and maintains both ketosis and seizure reduc-tion, but does so with a 1:1 ratio diet with ad lib calories

(Fig. 53–1). In addition, it can be started as an outpatient with minimal education and dietitian involvement. Low-carbohydrate foods and meals can also be ordered in restaurants and groceries, making the diet more accessible and "portable," especially for adolescents and adults. Choosing this diet versus the traditional ketogenic diet depends on each treatment's advantages for the individual patient (Fig. 53–5).

Three prospective, open label studies of this alternative diet have been completed since 2006; two from Johns Hopkins.[16,33,34] The first enrolled 20 children with intractable epilepsy who had never used the traditional ketogenic diet, initially restricting carbohydrates to 10 g per day and following a specific protocol (Table 53–2).[16] Fourteen demonstrated >50% reduction in seizures; of which half had >90% reduction. Although large urinary ketosis was attained rapidly, surprisingly it did not correlate with seizure control. Nine children were able to reduce anticonvulsants. Blood urea nitrogen increased significantly and total cholesterol trended upwards from 192 to 221 mg/dL. Weight loss was infrequent and 80% of the patients completed the 6-month study.

Two additional prospective studies of children found similar results.[32,33] A study from South Korea of 14 children showed 36% with >50% seizure reduction.[32] In a randomized, crossover evaluation of initial carbohydrate limits, a 10 g per day restriction was more likely to lead to >50% seizure reduction at 3 months.[34] However, after that point, increasing to the more palatable 20 g per day limit did not reduce seizure control.

▶ **TABLE 53–2. MODIFIED ATKINS DIET PROTOCOL[16,34]**

- Copy of a carbohydrate counting guide (e.g., The 2012 CalorieKing Calorie, Fat, and carbohydrate counter) provided to family, along with basic recipes and sample meal plans
- Carbohydrates restricted to 10 g per day for the first month (increase afterward if child and family desire)
- Fats (e.g., 36% heavy whipping cream, oils, butter, and mayonnaise) encouraged
- KetoCal® encouraged daily for the initial month
- Clear, carbohydrate-free, fluids not restricted
- Low-carbohydrate multivitamin and calcium supplementation prescribed
- Prescription for Bayer Ketostix™ given, with instructions to check urine ketones semiweekly and weight weekly
- Medications left unchanged for at least the first month, but preparation changed if necessary to tablet or sprinkle (nonliquid)
- Low-carbohydrate, store-bought products (e.g., shakes, candy bars, and baking mixes) discouraged for at least the first month
- Complete blood count, complete metabolic profile (SMA-20), urine calcium and urine creatinine, urinalysis, and fasting lipid profile at baseline, 3 and 6 months with clinic visits

In this study, total and low-density lipoprotein (LDL) cholesterol both significantly increased over time.[34]

Could the modified Atkins diet be effective for adults? A study of the Atkins diet for 30 adults with

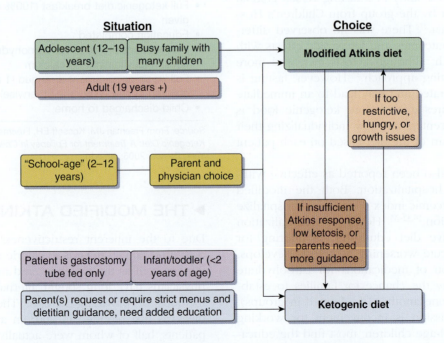

Figure 53–5. Proposed algorithm for choosing between the ketogenic and modified Atkins diets.

epilepsy was presented at the 2006 American Epilepsy Society annual meeting, with 47% of adults aged 18–53 years having at least a 50% reduction in seizures after 3 months. In those with seizure reduction, the median time to improvement was 2 weeks, with a maximum time of 2 months, suggesting that if the modified Atkins diet is not helpful within that time period, it should be discontinued. Considering that 30% of subjects discontinued prior to 3-month-diet duration due to typically restrictiveness, this information is clearly important. The mean weight loss was 6.8 kg, and was a welcome "side effect" for many. Total cholesterol increased, although not significantly.

A low-glycemic index diet has also been studied by the group at Massachusetts General Hospital.[35] Half of the 20 children started on this diet in one retrospective study had >90% seizure reduction. Although the diet ratio is similar to the modified Atkins diet, and children can be started as an outpatient without a fast, there are some differences. First, the actual carbohydrates eaten are specifically low-glycemic (glycemic index less than 50) and daily intake ranges from 40 to 100 g per day. Second, ketosis does not occur, except for minor levels of serum beta-hydroxybutyrate. Lastly, high-fat foods are not encouraged in a manner similar to the modified Atkins diet.

Both "alternative" diets provide welcome choices to the practicing neurologist. These diets may prove to have fewer side effects, especially in terms of growth and dyslipidemia. In addition, they may now offer an option not previously available for adults with epilepsy. Perhaps most exciting, these diets, with their relative ease of use and implementation, may become used in the future as first-line treatments for epilepsy in a motivated family.[36]

► SIDE EFFECTS

Although nearly never life-threatening or requiring diet discontinuation, complications of the ketogenic diet do exist and physicians as well as parents must be observant (Table 53–3). Only a decade ago, side effects of the diet were described only as acidosis, decreased weight gain, constipation, and hypoglycemia during the fasting period.[37,38] Since that time, these side effects have been identified as the "immediate" ones, with dyslipidemia, decreased growth, and kidney stones comprising the long-term effects.[39–41]

The most studied longer term side effects are kidney stones, which occur in approximately 6% of children receiving the ketogenic diet.[39] Both calcium oxalate, calcium carbonate, and uric acid stones may occur, and are associated clinically with hematuria, gritty urine, and pain. In 2000, Furth et al determined

► **TABLE 53–3.** SIDE EFFECTS OF THE KETOGENIC DIET

Common (seen in 80% of patients)
Low-level acidosis
Nausea/vomiting during initiation, especially during the fast
Lack of weight gain
Constipation
Diarrhea and bloating (MCT oil diet)

Less common (5%)
Significant dyslipidemia
Gastrointestinal upset and gastroesophageal reflux
Kidney stones
Inadequate or slowed growth (more problematic in infants)
Inappropriate weight loss
Bone fractures (increased with long-term use)
Rare (case reports)
Prolonged QT interval
Bruising
Selenium and vitamin deficiency (mostly if unsupplemented)
Hypoalbuminemia
Basal ganglia changes
Pancreatitis
Fanconi's renal tubular acidosis

that younger age as well as hypercalciuria were risk factors, and recommended oral alkalinization (Polycitra K®, 2 Meq/kg per day divided twice daily) for the latter.[39] Children with family histories of kidney stones receiving carbonic anhydrase inhibitors (topiramate and zonisamide) are also at higher risk for stones; treatment with Polycitra K® is also recommended.[42] Empiric use of Polycitra K® reduces the risk of kidney stones sevenfold and its routine use may, therefore, be warranted.[43]

Total and LDL cholesterol increase by approximately 30% after 6 months on the diet then plateau over the subsequent 18 months.[40] Long-term effects on atherosclerosis are uncertain, although the majority children do not remain on the diet for more than 2 years. Even so, evidence suggests total cholesterol may decrease after several years, and children with continuous diet durations of 6–22 years had mostly normal values in two studies.[44,45] The modified Atkins diet caused a nonsignificant total cholesterol increase in the first prospective pediatric study, but a significant change in the second.[16,34] Routine lipid profiles are recommended for this diet as well as the ketogenic diet.

Lastly, growth is adversely affected by the diet, especially in young infants and after many years.[41,44] This may be more problematic in high ketosis states.[46] In children on the diet for over 6 years, nearly all were in the tenth percentile for height or lower.[44] Increasing protein and calories may improve this particular side effect if present; the modified Atkins diet may theoretically be advantageous as well.

Rare side effects reported include vitamin and mineral deficiencies (prevented with typical supplementation), selenium deficiency, pancreatitis, cardiomyopathy, bruising, basal ganglia change, and prolonged QT intervals.[38,47] Most of these are limited to single-case series or reports and have not been noted in large series. Increased incidence of bone fractures has been seen in children on the diet for many years, and is the subject of current investigation.[44] This may be due to decreased Vitamin D levels, which even with supplementation decrease on the diet after several months.[48]

▶ DISCONTINUING THE DIET

Discontinuation of the ketogenic diet is handled similarly to anticonvulsant medications, despite the different nature of this therapy.[1] After 2 years of effective use of the diet, most epileptologists will consider discontinuation due to potential long-term health risks as well as a method to "test" if the diet is still effective. However, if there is no improvement after 3–6 months, or seizures worsen, the ketogenic diet can be rapidly discontinued.

It is slightly more complicated in the child receiving the diet for 2 years or longer (Fig. 53–6).[49] If a child has completely responded to the diet and is both seizure and medication free, the diet is typically stopped. Approximately 80% of children will remain seizure free after the diet is discontinued for this reason; with higher risk of recurrence among patients with epileptiform electroencephalograms, focal abnormalities on neuroimaging, and tuberous sclerosis complex.[49] Unfortunately, approximately half of children with recurrence became difficult to control once again, even with resumption of the diet.[49]

Traditionally, the diet is slowly stopped by lowering the ratio (e.g., from 4:1 to 3:1), every month until a 1:1 ratio is achieved, after which calories are rapidly increased to ad lib and sugar-containing foods slowly allowed.[1] However, the diet can also be discontinued more rapidly (over 1–2 months) or even days by switching whole milk then 2%, 1%, and eventually skim milk in the recipes that use 36% heavy whipping cream. This second approach will lead to a rapid loss of ketosis, and is less of a metabolic disruption to the child than introducing high glycemic carbohydrates such as candy, bread, or citrus fruits. Although rarely performed, in situations of significant worsening of seizures by the diet, an

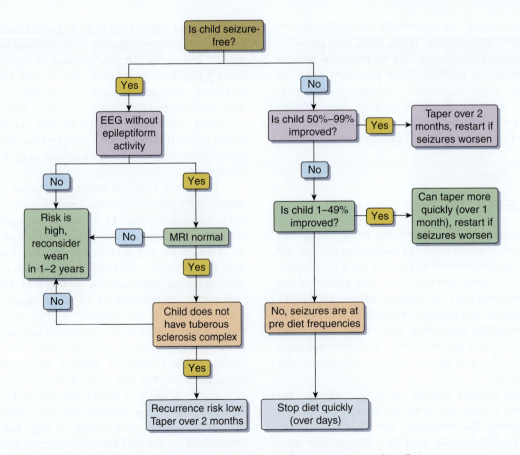

Figure 53–6. Diet discontinuation algorithm, after 2 years on the diet.

abrupt discontinuation of the diet can be made, although we recommend doing this in an inpatient setting (e.g., intensive care unit). Recent data suggests more rapid discontinuations (over weeks not months) are equally safe without a higher risk of seizure worsening.[50]

▶ CONCLUSIONS

The use of diet for epilepsy is one of the most exciting therapies for epilepsy in existence today. Although many anticonvulsants have been introduced in the past decade, the clinical and research interest in the ketogenic diet is at an all-time high. Determining its mechanism(s) of action, which patients are the best candidates, and how to implement it with the least side effects and highest possible tolerability remains area of intense research today.

REFERENCES

1. Freeman JM, Kossoff EH, Freeman JB Kelly MT. *The Ketogenic Diet: A Treatment for Epilepsy in Children and Others.* New York: Demos, 2006; 4th ed.
2. Kossoff EH, McGrogan JR, Freeman JM. Benefits of an all-liquid ketogenic diet. *Epilepsia* 2004;45:1163.
3. Hosain SA, La-Vega-Talbott M, Solomon GE. Ketogenic diet in pediatric epilepsy patients with gastrostomy feeding. *Pediatr Neurol* 2005;32:81–83.
4. Keene DL. A systematic review of the use of the ketogenic diet in childhood epilepsy. *Pediatric Neurol* 2006;35:1–5.
5. Levy R, Cooper P. Ketogenic diet for epilepsy. *Cochrane Database Syst Rev (Online)* 2003;(3):CD001903.
6. Kossoff EH, McGrogan JR. Worldwide use of the ketogenic diet. *Epilepsia* 2005;46:280–289.
7. DeVivo DC, Trifiletti RR, Jacobson RI, Ronen GM, Behmand RA, Harik SI. Defective glucose transport across the blood-brain barrier as a cause of persistent hypoglycorrhachia, seizures, and developmental delay. *New Engl J Med* 1991; 325:713–721.
8. Wexler ID, et al. Outcome of pyruvate dehydrogenase deficiency treated with ketogenic diets: studies in patients with identical mutations. *Neurology* 1997;49:1655–1661.
9. Klepper J. Impaired glucose transport into the brain: the expanding spectrum of glucose transporter type 1 deficiency syndrome. *Current Opin Neurol* 2004;17:193–196.
10. Caraballo RH, Cersosimo RO, Sakr D, Cresta A, Escobal N, Fejerman N. Ketogenic diet in patients with Dravet syndrome. *Epilepsia* 2005;46:1539–1544.
11. Oguni H, et al. Treatment and long-term prognosis of myoclonic-astatic epilepsy of early childhood. *Neuropediatrics* 2002;33:122–132.
12. Nordli DR Jr, et al. Experience with the ketogenic diet in infants. *Pediatrics* 2001;108:129–133.
13. Kossoff EH, Pyzik PL, McGrogan JR, Vining EP, Freeman JM. Efficacy of the ketogenic diet for infantile spasms. *Pediatrics* 2002;109:780–783.
14. Eun SH, Kang HC, Kim DW, Kim HD. Ketogenic diet for treatment of infantile spasms. *Brain Dev* 2006;28:566–571.
15. Groomes LB, et al. Do patients with absence epilepsy respond to ketogenic diets? *J Child Neurol* 2011;26:160–165.
16. Kossoff EH, et.al. A modified Atkins diet is effective for the treatment of intractable pediatric epilepsy. *Epilepsia* 2006;47:421–424.
17. Than KD, Kossoff EH, Rubenstein JE, Pyzik PL, McGrogan JR, Vining EPG. Can you predict an immediate, complete, and sustained response to the ketogenic diet? *Epilepsia* 2005;46:580–582.
18. Hori A, Tandon P, Holmes GL, Stafstrom CE. Ketogenic diet: effects on expression of kindled seizures and behavior in adult rats. *Epilepsia* 1997;38:750–758.
19. Francois LL, Manel V, Rousselle C, David M. Ketogenic regime as anti-epileptic treatment: its use in 29 epileptic children. *Arch Pediatr* 2003;10:300–306.
20. Coppola G, et al. The effects of the ketogenic diet in refractory partial seizures with reference to tuberous sclerosis. *Eur J Paediatr Neurol* 2006;10:148–151.
21. Kossoff EH, Thiele EA, Pfeifer HH, McGrogan JR, Freeman JM. Tuberous sclerosis complex and the ketogenic diet. *Epilepsia* 2005;46:1684–1686.
22. Liebhaber GM, Riemann E, Baumeister FA. Ketogenic diet in Rett syndrome. *J Child Neurol* 2003;18:74–75.
23. Busch V, et al. Treatment of glycogenosis type V with ketogenic diet. *Ann Neurol* 2005;58:341.
24. Bautista RE. The use of the ketogenic diet in a patient with subacute sclerosing panencephalitis. *Seizure* 2003; 12:175–177.
25. DeVivo DC, Haymond MW, Leckie MP, Bussman YL, McDougal DB Jr, Pagliara AS. The clinical and biochemical implications of pyruvate carboxylase deficiency. *J Clin Endocrin Metab* 1977;45:1281–1296.
26. Kang HC, Lee YM, Kim HD, Lee JS, Slama A. Safe and effective use of the ketogenic diet in children with epilepsy and mitochondrial respiratory chain complex defects. *Epilepsia* 2007;48:82–88.
27. Bergqvist AG, et al. Fasting versus gradual initiation of the ketogenic diet: a prospective, randomized clinical trial of efficacy. *Epilepsia* 2005;46:1810–1819.
28. Vaisleib II, Buchhalter JR, Zupanc ML. Ketogenic diet: outpatient initiation, without fluid or caloric restrictions. *Pediatr Neurol* 2004;31:198–202.
29. Wirrell EC, et al. Is a fast necessary when initiating the ketogenic diet? *J Child Neurol* 2002;17:179–182.
30. Kim DW, et al. Benefits of the nonfasting diet compared with the initial fasting ketogenic diet. *Pediatrics* 2004; 114:1627–1630.
31. Freeman JM, Vining EP. Seizures decrease rapidly after fasting: preliminary studies of the ketogenic diet. *Arch Pediatr Adolesc Med* 1999;153:946–949.
32. Kossoff EH, Krauss GL, McGrogan JR, Freeman JM. Efficacy of the Atkins diet as therapy for intractable epilepsy. *Neurology* 2003;61:1789–1791.
33. Kang HC, Lee HS, You SJ, Kang du C, Kim HD. Use of a modified Atkins diet in intractable childhood epilepsy. *Epilepsia* 2007;48:182–186.
34. Kossoff EH, Turner Z, Bluml RM, Pyzik PL, Vining EPG. A randomized, crossover comparison of daily carbohydrate limits using the modified Atkins diet. *Epilepsy Behav* 2007; 10:432–436.

35. Pfeifer HH, Thiele EA. Low-glycemic-index treatment: a liberalized ketogenic diet for treatment of intractable epilepsy. *Neurology* 2005;65:1810–1812.

36. Rubenstein JE, Kossoff EH, Pyzik PL, Vining EPG, McGrogan JR, Freeman JM. Experience in the use of the ketogenic diet as early therapy. *J Child Neurol* 2005; 20:31–34.

37. Wheless JW. The ketogenic diet: An effective medical therapy with side effects. *J Child Neurol* 2001;16:633–635.

38. Kang HC, et al. Early- and late-onset complications of the ketogenic diet for intractable epilepsy. *Epilepsia* 2004; 45:1116–1123.

39. Furth SL, et al. Risk factors for urolithiasis in children on the ketogenic diet. *Pediatr Nephrol* 2000;15:125–128.

40. Kwiterovich PO, et al. Effect of a high-fat ketogenic diet on plasma levels of lipids, lipoproteins, and apolipoproteins in children. *JAMA* 2003;290:912–920.

41. Vining EPG, et al. Growth of children on the ketogenic diet. *Dev Med Child Neurol* 2002;44:796–802.

42. Kossoff EH, Pyzik PL, Furth SL, Hladky HD, Freeman JM, Vining EPG. Kidney stones, carbonic anhydrase inhibitors, and the ketogenic diet. *Epilepsia* 2002;43:1168–1171.

43. McNally MA, Pyzik PL, Rubenstein JE, Hamdy RF, Kossoff EH. Empiric use of oral potassium citrate reduces symptomatic kidney stone incidence with the ketogenic diet. *Pediatrics* 2009;124:e300–e304.

44. Groesbeck DK, Bluml RM, Kossoff EH. Long-term use of the ketogenic diet. *Dev Med Child Neurol* 2006;48:978–981.

45. Kossoff EH, Turner Z, Bergey GK. Home-guided use of the ketogenic diet in a patient for over twenty years. *Pediatr Neurol* 2007;36:424–425.

46. Peterson SJ, Tangney CC, Pimentel-Zablah EM, Hjelmgren B, Booth G, Berry-Kravis E. Changes in growth and seizure reduction in children on the ketogenic diet as a treatment for intractable epilepsy. *J Am Diet Assoc* 2005; 105:718–725.

47. Ballaban-Gil K, Callahan C, O'Dell C, Pappo M, Moshe S, Shinnar S. Complications of the ketogenic diet. *Epilepsia* 1998;39:744–748.

48. Bergqvist AG, Schall JI, Stallings VA. Vitamin D status in children with intractable epilepsy, and impact of the ketogenic diet. *Epilepsia* 2007;48:66–71.

49. Martinez CC, Pyzik PL, Kossoff EH. Discontinuing the ketogenic diet in seizure-free children: risk factors and recurrence. *Epilepsia* 2007;48:187–190.

50. Worden LT, Turner Z, Pyzik PL, Rubenstein JE, Kossoff EH. Is there an ideal way to discontinue the ketogenic diet? *Epilepsy Res* 2011;95:232–236.

CHAPTER 54

Nursing Considerations in Epilepsy Treatment

Siobhan Hannan and Patricia Dean

▶ OVERVIEW

Epilepsy is often perceived as a frightening and stigmatizing disorder and its impact can be enormous. Some children outgrow their seizures, others achieve good seizure control, and some become refractory to medical treatment. Epilepsy often coexists with cognitive and behavioral problems.[1–6] Santilli (1993) describes the psychosocial factors as the spectrum of epilepsy[7,8] highlighting that while some children may have an uncomplicated course others are compromised or devastated by seizures (Table 54–1).

By adopting the role of patient advocate, educator, and counselor, epilepsy nurse specialists (ENSs) are able to develop a therapeutic relationship with patients to empower them to manage their epilepsy. Children and families often seek information to help them understand the condition. Providing information is not a one-way didactic process. Parents of children with epilepsy need the opportunity and time to ask questions and raise issues of concern, which due to time constraints, doctors may sometimes find difficult to provide. By providing good quality relevant information nurses can help families gain a greater sense of control, which is necessary for self-management and optimal quality of life (QOL). In the hospital, clinic, or community setting, nurses facilitate a close liaison with other professionals and coordinate the multidisciplinary service needed for children with epilepsy. The proactive and complementary role of the nurse specialist will minimize fragmented care and bring an integrated approach to the complex management of epilepsy patients.[9]

▶ THE ROLE OF THE NURSE IN THE MANAGEMENT OF EPILEPSY

How nurses become specialized and what role they have in the management of patients with epilepsy varies from country to country. There are no formal boards that certify nurses as epilepsy specialists. Their specialization comes from clinical experience and continuing education. They may work in the community or in hospital outpatient and inpatient settings. Clinical responsibilities may extend to drug studies, ketogenic diet programs, and vagus nerve stimulator clinics. ENSs with advanced degrees can diagnose and prescribe either as independent nonmedical prescribers or under a physician's supervision.

In the United Kingdom, National Institute of Clinical Excellence guidelines (NICE 2012) exist for the delivery of epilepsy services. This document provides a government framework for how nationally funded health services in epilepsy should be organized and delivered. Nursing care in the United Kingdom is organized into primary, secondary, and tertiary/quaternary care.[10] There are a plethora of epilepsy nursing titles and roles but broadly speaking, nurses who provide support to families with children with epilepsy in primary, secondary and tertiary/quaternary health care are referred to as ENSs.

In 2005, the Royal College of Nursing, United Kingdom produced a competency framework and guidance for pediatric ENS services.[11] This document defines the ENS role and outlines competencies required to progress from novice (in the specialty), to competent and onto expert (advanced) practitioner. ENSs are senior registered nurses with a first degree, who have or are working toward a Masters in Science in Epileptology, with clinical experience in epilepsy, acute neurology, and community nursing.[11] A summary of the ENS role in the United Kingdom is outlined in Table 54–2.

Nurses have a key role in the care of patients with chronic health problems. Managing medical illness involves more than managing medical problems. It entails managing psychological and social issues including helping patients develop strategies to adapt to their illness and alter their lifestyles. In pediatric epilepsy, the nurse is in a unique situation to be able to help the child and family cope with all aspects of the disorder. They can educate the family regarding the pathophysiology of seizures, treatment options, and medication side effects. Nurses can alleviate fears surrounding seizures by teaching parents and caretakers what to do during a seizure. They can also support families to cope with the complicated and devastating challenges of epilepsy.

Buelow (2006) looked at stressors of parents of children with epilepsy and intellectual disability. She

► **TABLE 54-1. THE SPECTRUM OF EPILEPSY**

Operational Category	Descriptors
Uncomplicated	Seizures controlled Minimal side effects of medication No concomitant neurologic problems Rare psychosocial or functional problems, usually Short lived Good supports Treatment: usually primary care providers
Compromised	Seizures controlled; occasional "breakthrough" seizures Variable side effects of medicine No serious neurologic problems or deficits Psychosocial or functional problems affect quality of life Variable supports Treatment: medical re-evaluation warranted, increased Support and periodic psychosocial and educational interventions
Devastated	Seizures uncontrolled Polytherapy; side effects of medicines present but tolerated Concomitant neurologic problems or deficits Psychosocial or functional problems affect quality of life Limited or strained supports Treatment: comprehensive epilepsy team for seizures, psychosocial problems, and education: frequent revaluation needed; surgical and other alternative therapy options considered

Source: Data from Shafer PO, Salmanson E. Psychosocial aspects of epilepsy. In Schachner SC, Schomer DL, (eds), *The Comprehensive Evaluation and Treatment of Epilepsy*. San Diego: Academic Press, 1997; p. 93 and Santilli N. The spectrum of epilepsy. *Clin Nurs Pract Epilepsy* 1993;1:4–7.

identified five categories/sources of stress, namely: concern about the child; communication with health care providers; interactions with the school; and support in the community. She found that families rarely discuss all their problems with their physicians. She concluded that an important step in helping parents is to assess stressor and psychosocial care needs. As many stressors arise from a child's medical condition, nurses are in a unique position to help parents address these sources. Buelow suggests a list of potential parental stressors (Table 54–3). She argues that strategies for assisting parents should include assessing the problem, educating when appropriate, and referring to other professionals when necessary.

Since the nurse cannot realistically solve all the family's problems, another important strategy is to simply be a good listener to enable parents to share their frustrations.[12] Nurses can fulfill their role as educator, counselor, and patient advocate by helping patients and families gain insight into the effects of epilepsy. Through the provision of relevant information they can help families gain a greater sense of power and control, which is necessary for self-management and optimal QOL.[13]

Appleton and Sweeney (1995) examined the impact of the ENS role on the management of pediatric epilepsy over a 12-month period. The authors defined the role as providing information and advice on epilepsy type, seizure management, medications, and the influence of lifestyle on seizure control. The nurse also offered counseling and support through a combination of clinic and visits to home and school. To evaluate the impact of these services a questionnaire was administered to 30 parents of children with epilepsy prior to the appointment of the nurse specialist, and to a separate group of parents after a single home visit by the ENS. The authors concluded that the establishment of this role led to an improvement in the management of children and quality of service provided for families through an increased understanding of epilepsy and its treatment. In addition, the service facilitated a close liaison with schools, community health personnel, and support groups dispelling misunderstanding and stigma in the local community surrounding epilepsy.[14]

A randomized, controlled trial by Helde and colleagues (2005) tested the hypothesis that structured epilepsy nursing improves QOL in adult patients with epilepsy. One hundred and fourteen patients with refractory epilepsy were randomly assigned to either an intervention or control group. The intervention group was offered one day of group education with nurse follow up in clinic, plus telephone consultations and nurse counseling. All patients in the study completed the QOLIE-89 questionnaire before randomization and after 2 years. QOL measures in the intervention group were significantly improved from inclusion to completion of the study. The authors concluded that a structured nurse-led intervention program provided by an ENS resulted in a significant improvement in QOL of patients with epilepsy.[15]

National guidelines for epilepsy services exist within the United Kingdom, but not in other countries such as the United States and Australia. Although the role of epilepsy nursing in other health care systems is not as formally defined as in the United Kingdom, clinical experience suggests that the contribution of epilepsy nurses is universal. Nurses are responsible for improving health outcomes not only of the patient's acute illness but also simultaneously providing coordinated care that will improve the health status related

▶ **TABLE 54–2.** ROLE OF THE UK EPILEPSY NURSE SPECIALIST

Epilepsy Nurse Specialist	Primary/Secondary Care	Tertiary/Quaternary Care
Base	• In the community with links to a district general hospital (within a geographical catchments area).	• In a hospital or outpatient department offering specialist epilepsy services for difficult to treat epilepsy within a geographical area (tertiary) or nationally (quaternary).
Aims	• To promote good practice in the assessment, diagnosis, treatment, and care of families with children with epilepsy. • To ensure the coordination and continuity of local care.	• To improve access to medical management advice regarding difficult to treat epilepsy. • To provide expert knowledge, information and management advice to professionals/families. • To reduce the number of follow-up outpatient appointments and acute admissions to hospital.
Nursing interventions	• Family advocate, acting as first point of contact for families and local health and education professionals. Liaison between agencies to ensure continuity of care. • Home and school visits • Health education teaching in schools • Run nurse led community clinics • Support consultant led outpatient clinics • Link families into respite care, social services, counseling, and psychology as required • Referral to tertiary health services as required	• Provide expert information; regarding complex medical care and investigations • Run nurse led outpatient clinics • Support consultant led outpatient clinics • In patient management and coordination of investigations and care during hospital admissions • Telephone consultations with parents • Management of clinical queries from professionals, including; community pediatricians, GP's, and community-based ENS • Liaison with primary and secondary services
Intended outcomes	• Decreased stigma and misinformation surrounding diagnosis of epilepsy • Reduction in social impact on child/family • Increased school attendance • Safety; appropriate rescue treatment plan for prolonged seizures	• Improved quality of complex epilepsy management/care • Streamlined and coordinated patient journey • Reduced number of acute admissions into hospital • Cost improvement: extended role of the ENS results in reduction in number of doctor hours required to maintain a specialist epilepsy service

Source: From Hannan S, Cross JH, Scott RC, Harkness W, Heyman I. The effects of epilepsy surgery on emotions, behaviour, and psychosocial impairment in children and adolescents with drug-resistant epilepsy: a prospective study. *Epilepsy & Behavior* 2009;15(3):318–324.

to their chronic condition.[16] Regardless of the country or medical system they practice in, specialist nurses are valuable members of the multidisciplinary team needed for the management of pediatric epilepsy patients.

▶ THE EPILEPSY MONITORING UNIT

Concurrent visualization of seizures on video and electroencephalography (EEG) has enabled clinicians to accurately define and diagnose seizures and conditions mimicking seizures, and localize seizure origin in potential candidates for epilepsy surgery. This has created important management issues for the nurse specialist responsible for coordinating patient care in the epilepsy-monitoring unit (EMU). The aim of video EEG monitoring is to capture events and nurses must have a clear understanding of their patients' seizure type and frequency. They must intervene and support patients and their families. Nursing and EEG technologist input are required to facilitate optimal EEG recording whilst ensuring the admission is tolerable for the child and family.

EMU or telemetry unit admission criteria are similar in most pediatric epilepsy programs. They include evaluation for epilepsy surgery, diagnostic evaluation of seizure type, or events that are potentially epileptic in origin, treatment of refractory epilepsy with specialized treatment regimes such as adrenocorticotropic hormone (ACTH) or the ketogenic diet and evaluation for language regression or Landau–Kleffner syndrome.[17] Inpatients often have complicated epilepsy with comorbid behavioral, cognitive, and developmental problems requiring multidisciplinary management. Although the entire team educates and supports families, the EMU nursing staff spends the most time with families.

▶ **TABLE 54–3. SOURCES OF STRESS FOR PARENTS AND CHILDREN WITH EPILEPSY**

Category Subcategory	
Concerns about the child	Future and transition issues
Behavior problems	
Consequences of seizures	
Communication with healthcare Providers	Medication problems
Need for information	
Time to diagnosis	
Changes in family relationships	Marital relationship
Sibling relationships	
Leisure time activities	
Support from extended family	
Interactions with school	Communication
Transition issues	
Child safety	
Socialization	
Support within the community	Work issues and financial considerations
Family counseling and respite care	

Source: From Buelow J, McNelis A, Shore C, Austin J. Stressors of parents of children with epilepsy and intellectual disability. *J Neurosci Nurs* 2006;38(3):147–154.

THE EMU EXPERIENCE

The ENSs' role in the multidisciplinary team consists of education and support. A primary responsibility of the ENS is to prepare families and children for the EMU experience. This may occur in the ambulatory clinic, by telephone prior to admission, or by mailing a detailed information package.

Upon arrival in the EMU, the ENS insures a smooth and nontraumatic evaluation process. It is important to discuss the EMU protocol with the family. For example, if medication is to be reduced or discontinued, parents must accept that this increases the likelihood of heightened seizure frequency or severity. Support and encouragement throughout the admission are, therefore, critical. EMU nurses are responsible for ictal single-photon emission computed tomography (SPECT) injections. Nurses are optimally suited to ensure an accurate and timely isotope injection but must follow established protocols outlining procedural details, training, and safety requirements.[18,19]

EMU SAFETY

Safety in the EMU is a primary nursing responsibility. There are few specific guidelines for nurses in the pediatric setting despite its critical importance to the patient. In contrast, much has been written about physical safety and the effects of drug withdrawal in adult

▶ **TABLE 54–4. PHYSICAL SAFETY MEASURES IN AN EMU**

Side rails in up position at all times
Thick padded side rails to help prevent injury
Thick carpeting or some type of soft flooring
Furniture with rounded corners and padding of sharp areas can be employed
Bathroom doors open both ways in case patient falls and blocks the door

Source: From Sanders PT, Cysyk BJ, Bare MA. Safety in long-term EEG/video monitoring. *J Neurosci Nurs* 1996;28(5):305–313.

and pediatric settings,[17,20–23] the nursing care of children with intracranial electrodes and safe administration of radioactive isotopes for SPECT studies.[19,24]

A recent article by Perkins and Buchhalter (2006) outlines a plan of optimal patient care in a pediatric EMU, highlighting the importance of educating both nursing staff and families about safety measures.[25] These studies are not evidence-based but offer examples of best practices from the authors' own institution.

Seizures are often associated with an increased risk of injury particularly from falls. Sanders and colleagues (1994) examined the number of falls per inpatient days in the EMU at Johns Hopkins Hospital, Baltimore, United States. They recorded 8 falls per 1000 patient days as compared to an overall Department of Neuroscience fall rate of 5.2 falls per 1000 patient days. Based on their experience, the authors' suggest five safety precautions to implement in EMU rooms to reduce the risk of patient injury (Table 54–4).[26]

This study was based on an adult population and the authors' suggest there may be additional issues to consider when caring for pediatrics patients, as children are potentially more spontaneous and less aware of consequences than adults. This is particularly relevant for the cognitively impaired or hyperactive child. Ideally the ENS and nursing staff should assess potential safety problems with each child and work with parents to minimize risks. However, there is no substitute for an adult presence in the room and children regardless of age should not be left alone. Parents should be informed prior to admission of the need for a family member to remain with the patient at all times.

MEDICATION WITHDRAWAL

An important nursing consideration within the EMU is the tapering or withdrawal of medications to induce seizures. Nursing staff must be aware that a reduction in antiepileptic medication (AED's) may increase the frequency and/or severity of seizures and increases the risk for status epilepticus.[23,26]

Each child's care plan should be individualized based on the number of seizures required for the purpose of the investigation. The care plan should also include an emergency or rescue plan outlining how and when to intervene if seizures increase in frequency or severity. Some institutions have set protocols while others require notification of the physician after each seizure. If seizures are interfering with function or stressing the child and family, the doctor should be informed and a new plan established.[24]

▶ INVASIVE INTRACRANIAL EEG MONITORING

Children undergoing presurgical evaluation for epilepsy surgery may require invasive (intracranial) EEG monitoring with subdural grids and strips or depth electrodes prior to resective surgery. Preparation of the child and family may be shared with other disciplines but is a primary responsibility of the ENS. The child and parents must understand the sequence of events and expectations. Parents should be made aware of postoperative discomfort associated with periorbital edema, headache, and vomiting. They should have an opportunity to ask questions and receive support with their decision making. The more parents know the less anxious they will be and more able to assist in the management of their child.[24]

When preparing children and their families, it is important to use language appropriate to developmental age and culture.[27] Properly prepared children show less fear and are better equipped to deal emotionally with hospital procedures.[28]

▶ CLINICAL ASSESSMENT

The development of clinical procedure guidelines[29] provide nurses with a useful tool to inform and assist in the management of potential complications postimplant such as infection, increased intracranial pressure, hemorrhage, or an increase in seizure severity and/or frequency (Fig. 54–1). Decreased sensory awareness needs to be carefully assessed to distinguish between normal postictal drowsiness and an altered level of consciousness. This assessment is more challenging when the patient is an infant, preverbal, or nonverbal child. Therefore, it is important for nurses to complete a good baseline assessment and formulate an individualized patient care plan. Clinical procedure guidelines are a useful tool for nurses as they outline logical decision-making procedures for problem solving thereby facilitating the safe and appropriate delivery of care.

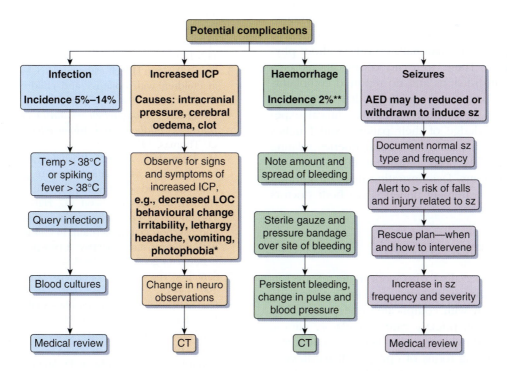

Figure 54–1. Invasive intracranial EEG monitoring algorithm for managing potential complications. From: Hannan S, Cross JH, Scott RC, Harkness W, Heyman I. The effects of epilepsy surgery on emotions, behaviour, and psychosocial impairment in children and adolescents with drug-resistant epilepsy: a prospective study. *Epilepsy & Behavior* 2009;15(3):318–324.

▶ ADVANCED NURSING PRACTICE

Advanced nursing practice helps meet the complex care demands of patients with complicated epilepsy. "Substitution of care" implies a shift of care, responsibilities and tasks so that good quality of care is provided by the most appropriate health care provider at the lowest cost level. Substitution takes place when clinical responsibilities shift from medical specialists to nurses.[30] Two epilepsy studies suggest that "substitution of care" may be beneficial to both doctors and patients. In a randomized clinical trial, Ridsdale et al (1997) tested the feasibility and consequences of nurse-run epilepsy clinics in primary care. In this trial, the intervention group was offered an appointment at a clinic with a nurse with specialist training in epilepsy. The control group received standard care by a general practitioner or specialist. The authors concluded that nurse-run clinics for patients with epilepsy were feasible and well attended. Furthermore, such clinics could significantly improve the level of advice and drug-management recorded.[31]

Letourneu (2003) examined the impact on patient care of utilizing neurology nurses to answer clinical calls from patients traditionally fielded by physicians. They documented the number of calls, diagnosis of patients, reasons for calling, and call duration. The most common patient diagnosis for the calls was epilepsy (63.5%). Most were about medical administration issues (28.4%). Long telephone calls (>10 minutes) were strongly associated with a diagnosis of epilepsy. Nurses managed more than half the calls without physician assistance. There were no complications as a result of their instructions and no reported complaints from parents. The authors concluded that nurses with advanced neurology training, extensive clinical experience, and knowledge of their patients and families were competent at managing clinical queries relating to prescription refills, dose adjustment, test results, and worsening symptoms. Demonstrating that "substitution of care" can be extremely beneficial to both doctors and patients.[32]

▶ CONCLUSIONS

Epilepsy nurses specialists who work in acute care settings, neuroscience, or epilepsy specialties often only encounter children with complicated epilepsies, while nurses who work in primary care, ambulatory clinics, or community settings are more likely to encounter children with varying forms of epilepsy. Regardless of the practice setting or the severity of the epilepsy, ENSs are essential to the appropriate management and care of these patients. Pediatric nurses in all practice settings must be capable of supporting patients and families who live with this chronic disorder.

ENSs have a central role in both the acute care and long-term management of epilepsy patients and their families. They are well placed to promote good practice in the assessment, diagnosis, treatment, and care of young people with epilepsy. Specialist nurses need to be knowledgeable about epilepsy investigations and therapies in order to help guide families with making choices about their child's care. They must recognize where their patients fit within the spectrum of epilepsy and individualize their care accordingly. Nurses in all clinical settings must be able to recognize different seizure types and help insure the child is diagnosed accurately. Nurses must also know how and when to intervene when a seizure occurs. Most importantly they must take the lead in education and provide ongoing support to the family and child.

"Knowing" the patient and their family is central to epilepsy specialist nursing. By adopting the role of patient advocate, educator, and counselor, ENSs are able to develop a therapeutic relationship with patients in order to empower them to manage their epilepsy and achieve an optimal QOL.

REFERENCES

1. Davies S, Heyman I, Goodman R. A population survey of mental health problems in children with epilepsy. *Dev Med Child Neurol* 2003;4:292–295.
2. Dean P. The pediatric patient with newly diagnosed epilepsy: planning for a lifetime. *Adv Stud Nurs* 2005;3(4) 113–119.
3. Hoare P, Mann H. Self esteem and behavioural adjustment in children with epilepsy and children with diabetes. *J Psychosom Res* 1994;38:859–869.
4. Livingston S. *Comprehensive Management of Epilepsy in Infancy, Childhood and Adolescence.* Springfield Illinois: CC Thomas, 1972.
5. Mc Dermott S, Mani S, Krishnaswami S. A population based analysis of specific behaviour problems associated with childhood seizures. *J Epilepsy* 1995;8:110–118.
6. Hannan S, Cross JH, Scott RC, Harkness W, Heyman I. The effects of epilepsy surgery on emotions, behaviour, and psychosocial impairment in children and adolescents with drug-resistant epilepsy: a prospective study. *Epilepsy & Behavior* 2009;15(3):318–324.
7. Santilli N. The spectrum of epilepsy. *Clin Nurs Pract Epilepsy* 1993;1:4–7.
8. Shafer PO, Salmanson E. Psychosocial aspects of epilepsy. In: Schachner SC, Schomer DL (eds), *The Comprehensive Evaluation and Treatment of Epilepsy.* San Diego: Academic Press, 1997; p 93.
9. Kwan I, Ridsdale L, Robbins D. An epilepsy care package: the nurse specialist's role. *J Adv Nurs* 2006;32(3):145–152.
10. NICE Clinical Guideline 137: The Epilepsies. *The Diagnosis and Management of the Epilepsies in Adults and Children in Primary and Secondary Care.* National Institute for Clinical Excellence ISBN, 2012; pp.1–117.

11. United Kingdom Royal College of Nursing. *Competency Framework and Guidance for Paediatric Epilepsy Nurse Specialists.* 20 Cavendish Square, London: RCN, 2005.

12. Buelow J, McNelis A, Shore C, Austin J. Stressors of parents of children with epilepsy and intellectual disability. *J Neurosci Nurs* 2006;38(3):147–154.

13. Saburi GL, Mapanga KG, Mapanga MB. Perceived family reactions and quality of life of adults with epilepsy. *J Adv Nurs* 2006; 38(3)156–166.

14. Appleton E, Sweeney A. The management of epilepsy in children: the role of the clinical nurse specialist. *Seizure* 1995;4:287–291.

15. Helde G, Bovim G, Brathen G, Brodtkorb E. A structured, nurse-led intervention program improves quality of life in patients with epilepsy: a randomized, controlled trial. *Epilepsy Behav* 2005;7(3):451–457.

16. Williams A, Botti M. Issues concerning the on-going care of patients with comorbidities in acute care and post-discharge in Australia: a literature review. *J Adv Nurs* 2002; 40(2):131–140.

17. O'Dell C, Lightstone L, Maloney-Lutz K, Clements P, Mancini A, Moshe S, Shinnar S. Issues related to caring for infants to adults on an integrated epilepsy unit. *J Neurosci Nurs* 1998;30(2):124–128.

18. Davis RT, Treves ST, Packard AB, Farley JB, Amoling RK, Ulanski JS. Ictal perfusion brain SPECT in pediatric patients with intractable epilepsy: a multidisciplinary approach. *J Nucl Med Technol* 1996;24(3):219–222.

19. Huntington NA. The nurse's role in the delivery of radioisotope for ictal SPECT scan. *J Adv Nurs* 1999; 31(4):208–215.

20. Burneo JG, Vezina W, Romsa J, Smith BJ, McLachlan RS. *Can J Neurosci Nurs* 2007;34(2):225–229.

21. Allen L, Morris G, Lathrop L. Seizure safety in long term monitoring. *Epilepsia* 1994;35(Suppl 8):105.

22. Calaguire S, Gates J, Goodermont K. Prevantion of injury on the adult epilepsy unit. *Epilepsia* 1995;36(Suppl 4):92.

23. Dewar S, Passaro E, Fried I, Engle J Jr. Intracranial electrode monitoring for seizure localization: indication, methods and prevention of complications. *J Neurosci Nurs* 1996;28(5):280–284,289–292.

24. Sanders PT, Cysyk BJ, Bare MA. Safety in long-term EEG/video monitoring. *J Neurosci Nurs* 1996;28(5):305–313.

25. Dean P. Grids for kids: the pediatric patient undergoing invasive extraoperative EEG monitoring. *J Neurosci Nurs* 1994;26(6):352–356.

26. Gilbert KI. Evaluation of an algorithm for treatment of status epilepticus in adult patients undergoing video/EEG monitoring. *J Neurosci Nurs* 2000;32:101–107.

27. Perkins AM, Buchhalter JR. Optimizing patient care in the pediatric monitoring unit. *J Neurosci Nurs* 2006;30(6):416–421.

28. Sclare I, Waring M. Routine venipucture: improving services. *Pediatr Nurs* 1995;7(4):23–27.

29. Lutz W. Helping hospitalized children and their parents cope with painful procedures. *J Pediatr Nurs* 1986;1(1):24–32.

30. Temmink D, Francke AL, Hutten JB, Huda Huijer A. Innovations in the nursing care of the chronically ill: a literature review from an international perspective. *J Adv Nurs* 2000;31(6):1449–1458.

31. Ridsdale L, Robins D, Cryer C, Williams H. Feasibility and effects of nurse run clinics for patients with epilepsy in general practice: randomized control trial. *Br Med J* 1997; 314:120–122.

32. Letourneau M, Mac Gregor D, Dick P, McCabe E, Allen A, Chan V, MacMillian L, Golomb M. Use of a telephone nursing line in a pediatric neurology clinic: one approach to the shortage of subspecialists. *Pediatrics* 2003;112(5):1083–1087.

SECTION X
Surgical Treatment

CHAPTER 55

Surgery for Focal Epilepsy—Why and When?

J. Helen Cross, Philippe Kahane, and Elaine Wyllie

▶ OVERVIEW

Epilepsy surgery, by definition is the removal of an area of brain with the aim of alleviating seizures. In order to proceed, evaluation needs to be undertaken to determine whether seizure onset can be localized to one area, and whether that area is functionally silent. In the majority, the aim is to alleviate seizures with no deterioration in function.

There are no current randomized studies in children demonstrating the superiority of surgery over medical treatment for this group of patients. However, many nonrandomized studies strongly suggest that epilepsy surgery may produce seizure freedom in a substantial number of nonidiopathic focal epilepsy (NIFE) cases, regardless of age or cause. The evidence base now suggests that 40%–80% will become seizure free. This figure is dependent on underlying pathology (less likely in developmental malformations and cryptogenic cases) and extent of resection. Therefore, surgery is now established in the routine management of children with presumed lesional focal epilepsy, and criteria for referral and evaluation for pediatric epilepsy surgery have been recently proposed.[1]

▶ SURGERY IN CHILDREN NOT ONLY AIMS AT SEIZURE ALLEVIATION

Children should not be referred for surgery as a "last resort." The rate of cognitive and behavioral comorbidity associated with early onset of epilepsy is high, and early cessation of seizures likely leads to improved neurobehavioral outcome. The concept of "epileptic encephalopathy" implies ongoing cognitive impairment as a result of underlying epileptic activity and may be potentially reversible. Longitudinal data on cognitive outcome are lacking due to the absence of standardized assessments over the lifespan and lack of a control group.

There is some evidence of stable postoperative intelligence quotient (IQ) suggesting at least an unchanged developmental trajectory that may be related to duration of epilepsy rather than ultimate seizure outcome. Brain plasticity and relocalization of function are additional factors that are influenced by age and type of surgery.

▶ SURGERY IN CHILDREN IS NOT THE VERY LAST OPTION

There is no minimal age for surgical referral. All children under the age of 5 years with a definitive magnetic resonance imaging (MRI) lesion are potential surgical candidates. Should seizure control be achieved with medication a conservative wait period is indicated. Children older than the age of 5 years with a definitive lesion may be left to determine response to anticonvulsants but failure of two medications in children with apparent focal seizures should be prompt referral for assessment. Delayed surgical referral depends on adequacy of neurodevelopmental progress. As a rule, all children suffering from pharmacoresistant focal epilepsy should be evaluated at a specialized epilepsy center if they exhibit behavioral and cognitive dysfunction.

The number of antiepileptic drugs (AEDs) utilized and duration of the epilepsy are of strict importance in the decision to perform epilepsy surgery in adults for epilepsy. In contrast, the pediatric evaluation is influenced by a variety of additional factors such as type of epilepsy and prognosis for seizure freedom. For instance, the likelihood of favorable surgical outcome is lower in nonlesional cases but the absence of a brain lesion does not exclude definitive surgical possibilities.

▶ SURGERY IN CHILDREN DIFFERS FROM SURGERY IN ADULTS

PRESURGICAL WORKUP

Once the history of disabling medically refractory focal seizures is clearly established—which requires at least a good description of seizure semiology, repeated interictal electroencephalographic (EEG) data, and an optimal MRI scan—the principal goal for resective epilepsy surgery is the identification and accurate localization of the epileptogenic zone. To answer this question, many investigations are available, but their use must be decided in a stepwise fashion based on the individual anatomo-electro-clinical features of each patient (Fig. 55–1). Not surprisingly, topographic diagnosis in children may prove challenging for several age-related issues.

1. Interictal EEG abnormalities may be diffuse and the EEG may need to be repeated over time to better define focal abnormalities that only appear or become more evident during evolution. Also, the coexistence of age-related "benign spikes" with other focal abnormalities may erroneously conduct to the diagnosis of multifocal epilepsy.

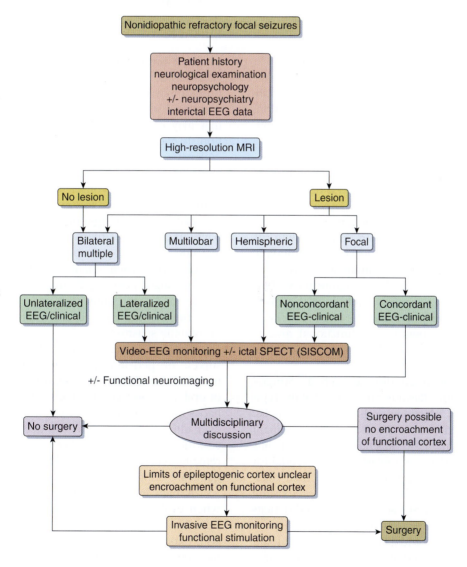

Figure 55–1. Algorithm for assessment of children with focal epilepsy for surgery.

2. The collection of precise information on seizure semiology is often difficult, especially in young children. Notably, description of the initial symptom, when found, is much less detailed than in adult patients, and the level of awareness is rarely possible to evaluate.

3. Focal seizures in children can manifest in very unusual clinical presentations, when compared to classical adult patterns. Ictal symptomatology may pass almost unnoticed or be particularly "explosive." Very young children often exhibit global motor signs that may mask the focal character of the seizures, or which precedes the more clearly focal semiology, as it is typically the case with epileptic spasms.

4. The clinical expression of focal seizures at a given age may evolve with time under the influence of many factors such as progression of brain maturation, increasing ability of children to describe subjective feelings, and treatment.

SURGERY TYPE

Although a significant number of children undergo surgery to remove a localized brain area, more commonly children often undergo lobar or multilobar resection; approximately one third will have a hemidisconnection, whether hemispherectomy or hemispherotomy.[2]

Children considered for hemidisconnection usually have a preexistent congenital hemiplegia due to structural abnormality of the contralateral hemisphere. Presurgical assessment is aimed at lateralisation of seizure onset, and any risk for functionality. Early seizure onset is often associated with complex patterns of language representation, especially if language is represented in the normal dominant hemisphere. Affected children may not evidence significant verbal/nonverbal discrepancy on neuropsychological evaluation. Remarkably, hemispherectomy is often associated with little change in cognitive or functional assessment although a visual field defect is inevitable if not already present.

Children with acquired disease such as Sturge–Weber syndrome and Rasmussen's encephalitis typically suffer greater functional postoperative deficits. Hemispheric procedures in children with dominant hemisphere involvement in Rasmussen's Encephalitis require careful consideration regarding the potential for of relocalization of language function. The final decision rests on the risk-benefit assessment of preexisting cognitive compromise versus surgically induced deficits and the prevention of future deterioration.

Children who are candidates for focal/multilobar resection (or disconnection) should have seizures arising from one area of the brain, which can be safely resected without functional consequence. Functionality is in turn determined by the region of brain involvement, the structural abnormality on neuroimaging and the pattern of representation of cognitive function.

In the presence of a discrete structural lesion in a silent cortical region, surgical planning is relatively straightforward. Removing the lesion is possible without further investigation, if there is concordance between the lesion, the clinical semiology, and interictal scalp EEG data. Video-EEG recording of seizures recording provides further confirmation of the epileptogenic zone.

In the presence of poorly defined lesions, lesions that encroach on motor or language cortex, or discordant findings, invasive EEG monitoring helps determine the extent of surgery. Intracranial EEG recording is almost always necessary in MRI-negative cases.

In all pediatric surgical candidates, the aims of the family must be carefully explored to ascertain that they have realistic expectations.

INFANCY

Children presenting with focal epilepsy often have a catastrophic course. Demonstration of focal seizure onset a may be challenging. Young infants may present with focal seizures and evolve through infantile spasms that may or may not be lateralized in their presentation. In view of the devastating effect that early onset epilepsy may have on ongoing neurodevelopment (Jonas et al, 2005), potential surgical candidates should be considered early; onset under the age of 2 years is particularly correlated to low long-term IQ.[3,4]

Data on the long-term outcome of children who have undergone surgery reveal maintenance of the learning trajectory postoperatively. The greatest gains are observed when seizure freedom is achieved, and after a longer postsurgery interval.[5] In children under the age of 3 years, gains were more likely if surgery was performed under the age of 1 year, and with a history of infantile spasms.[6]

The International League Against Epilepsy (ILAE) survey of pediatric procedures for epilepsy (2004) revealed that although two-thirds of children had onset of epilepsy less than the age of 2 years, only one-third had surgery within two years of seizure onset.[2] However, although major gains can occur with early seizure cessation, the primary goal of pediatric epilepsy surgery remains seizure freedom, as likely neurodevelopmental gains are unpredictable.

A high index of suspicion should be entertained when evaluating a child with medically resistant focal seizures. Assessment should be performed by a team with expertise in epilepsy Ictal semiology and the EEG may be difficult to interpret in young children;[8,9] focal seizures may occur in specific epilepsy syndromes may be apparent. Certainly all children with a focal or lateralized structural brain abnormality should be referred for surgical consideration at diagnosis, even though response to medication may be unclear at that point. It is also has to be considered that incomplete myelination may make MRI difficult to interpret; just as abnormalities may not become apparent until myelination is complete, lesions may also "disappear" despite being apparent on early scans as myelination progresses.[10]

Case 1

An 8-month-old boy presents with a history of asymmetric spasms. His first seizure occurred on day 1; his mother reported both his legs would draw up flexed, and he would look uncomfortable. This was originally diagnosed as infantile colic, but by 4 weeks of age the movements became more prominent and increased in frequency. They evolved into recognizable spasms; asymmetric posturing with head turning to the left then right, with fisting of the right hand. Clusters would occur on waking, for up to 20 minutes five to six times per day. Some reduction was noted with vigabatrin with subsequent resolution with steroids. At 8 months, he demonstrates a left-hand preference with evidence of a right hemiparesis, and visual inattention. MRI revealed left hemimegalancephaly (see Fig. 55–2).

Despite apparent seizure control, developmental assessment at 7 months suggested right visual field loss, right hemiplegia with nonverbal skills at 2–3 months age equivalent across all scales. His EEG showed evolution from asymmetric burst to continuing spike–wave discharges over the left hemisphere.

Although clinical seizures remain controlled, his EEG was markedly abnormal and he remained developmentally delayed. Neurological examination revealed a right hemiplegia and right visual field defect, with inattention of vision to the right. He is at high risk for return of seizures, and for continued developmental compromise. Hemidisconnection was offered to reduce the risk of recurrent seizures and optimize neurodevelopmental outcome. Twelve months following surgery he remains seizure free on medication and is at a 6-month developmental level.

Case 2

A 22-month-old boy presented at age 15 months with a first seizure. He was found motionless and staring in his buggy; he was hypotonic when lifted. This lasted a few minutes. An episode of abnormal jerking movements was noted the following day. Further episodes consisted of "head nods," singly or in clusters. Although he retained awareness, in some episodes he had a puzzled expression on his face, and in protracted clusters would tremble. At time of assessment he was experiencing 2–3 clusters per day, each involving 5–10 "spasms."

His neurodevelopment was normal until the time of seizure onset. Three months after seizure onset he underwent a marked regression of cognitive skills to a 6-month developmental level with loss of social interaction. There was a clinical suggestion of left visual inattention. He was treated with vigabatrin, levetiracetam, and oxcarbazepine without success.

MRI revealed an area of focal cortical dysplasia in the right mid temporal region. Interictal EEG showed multifocal sharp waves on a slow background, with variable asymmetry. A burst suppression pattern was evident in sleep (Fig. 55–3) with no consistent lateralization of seizure onset on ictal EEG recording. Semiology was also variable, but consistently included behavior arrest consistent with a temporal lobe onset prior to clusters of "spasms." Subsequent MRI evaluation demonstrated abnormality of the entire right temporal lobe extending posteriorly into the occipital region.

This case illustrates early onset catastrophic epileptic encephalopathy with focal onset. There was little likelihood of response to medication. Seizure onset was compatible with the MRI lesion, felt to be multilobar. Therefore, he proceeded to right tempo-occipital resection, maximizing chance of seizure freedom with

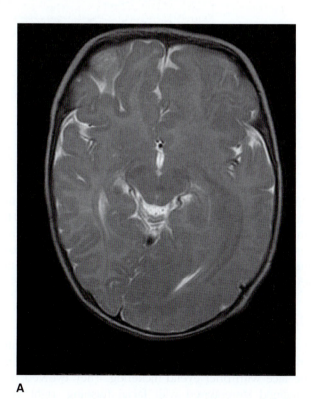

A

Figure 55–2. Magnetic resonance imaging (MRI) (**A**) and electroencephalography (EEG) (**B**) of case 1; MRI shows enlarged left hemisphere, with poor gyral pattern and gray–white contrast, demonstrating left hemimegalancephaly. EEG shows almost continuous spike activity over the left posterior quadrant. *(continued)*

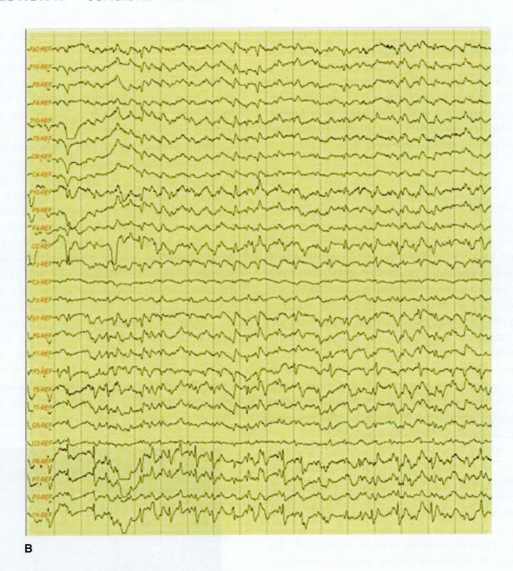

B

Figure 55–2. *(Continued)*

counseling for a definite visual field defect, and unpredictable prognosis for cognitive outcome. He underwent a right temporo-occipital disconnection and remains seizure free postoperatively at 12 months, off medication, with increased interest and developmental level.

Case 3

A 4-month-old girl presents with a history of seizure onset soon after birth. Episodes involved flushing of the face with brief eyelid flickering. They evolved but remained stereotyped with facial flushing, right versive head deviation, right arm and leg flexion, and left limb extension. This sequence was followed by four limb clonic movements for 20–30 seconds. Seizures were occurring 8–10 times daily at time of assessment. She had been treated with phenobarbitone with no response, followed by phenytoin, vigabatrin, carbamazepine, and topiramate. She was bright, alert, and sociable, having smiled at 8 weeks.

An interictal EEG showed persistent discharges over the right central electrodes (C4, C6). An MRI showed the suggestion of an abnormality in the form of "advanced" myelination in a similar central position (Fig. 55–4).

Video-EEG revealed stereotyped attacks with subtle asymmetry to the motor component of the seizures with the left limbs always moving slightly prior to the right. Ictal EEG revealed focal seizure onset at C4–C6 (see Fig. 55–5). Ictal single-photon emission computed tomography (SPECT) showed right central hyperperfusion.

In view of the persistent nature of her seizures, and the presence of a structural lesion she was referred for resective surgery. As the margins of the lesion were poorly defined on MRI, and close to motor cortex, she underwent subduralelectrode implantation. A 48-contact grid was placed on the neocortex; seizures were

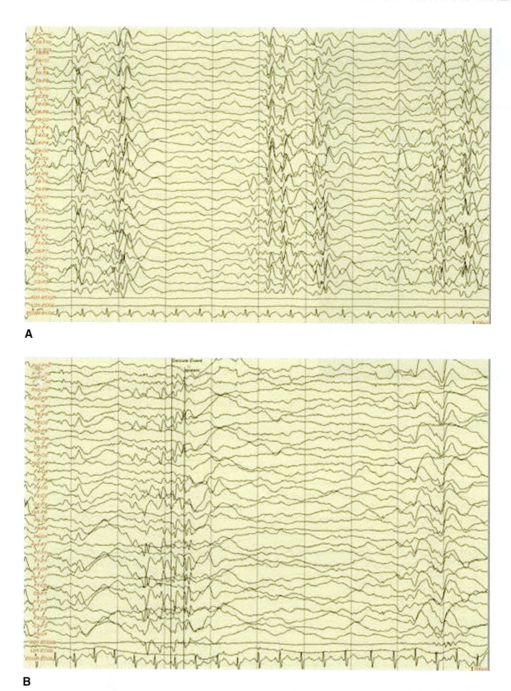

Figure 55–3. Interictal electroencephalography (EEG) of case 2 (**A**) demonstrating burst suppression pattern seen in sleep, and spasm with lateralizaiton to the left on ictal recording (**B**). A dysplastic lesion of whole temporal lobe on the right with extension into the occipital lobe is demonstrated on magnetic resonance imaging (**C**). *(continued)*

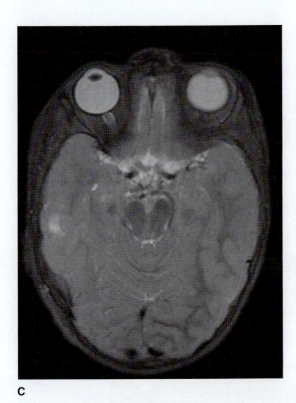

C

Figure 55–3. *(Continued)*

recorded from a localized area and sensorimotor cortex was defined. A localized resection was possible preserving motor cortex. She remains seizure free for five years following resection, with no neurological deficit.

Mid-Childhood

Children within this age group may not have the same catastrophic onset as younger children, but drug resistance may still be readily apparent early in the natural history. Further, ongoing seizures may still impact learning and psychosocial development. Consequently, early recognition of potential surgical candidates is of the utmost importance.

Certain syndromes are more likely to be problematic in this age range; Rasmussen's syndrome typically presents in mid childhood. Further age-related changes are associated with more problematic epilepsy at this stage, for example, continuous spike-and-waves in slow wave sleep, and hemipolymicrogyria.[11] The possible benefits of surgery require careful evaluation and the risks and likely benefits must be discussed with the family prior to surgical decision. It is more likely that functionality is already established by this stage, and a

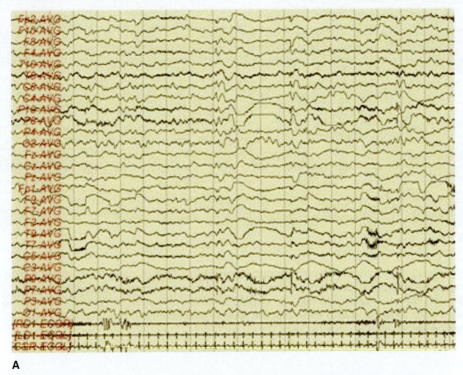

A

Figure 55–4. Electroencephalographic (EEG) recordings (**A, B**), magnetic resonance imaging (MRI) (**C**) and ictal single-photon emission computed tomography (**D**) of case 3. Interictal EEG (**A**) demonstrates focal spikes over the right central electrodes. An ictal recording shows definite lead from the same electrodes. MRI (**C**, transverse section) shows apparent enhanced myelination in the right central region but is ill defined (arrow). An injection of ECD during a seizure with subsequent scan showed hyperperfusion in this area (**D**, coronal sections, arrow). *(continued)*

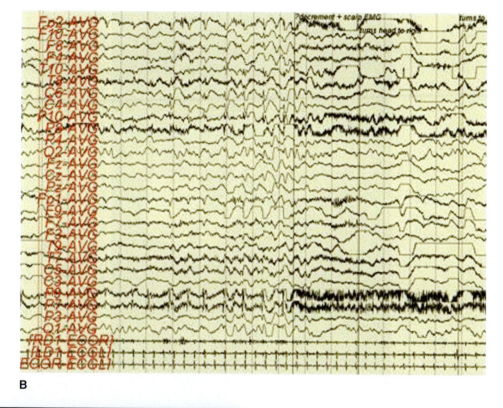

B

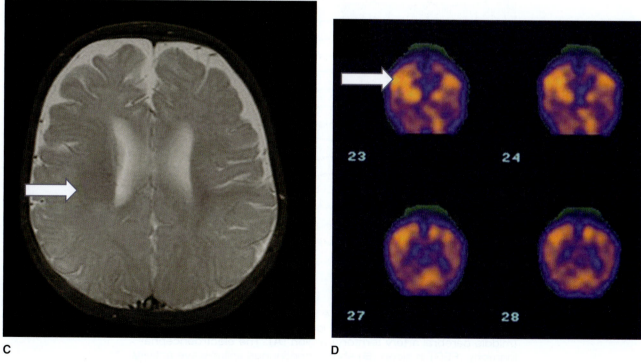

C

D

Figure 55–4. *(Continued)*

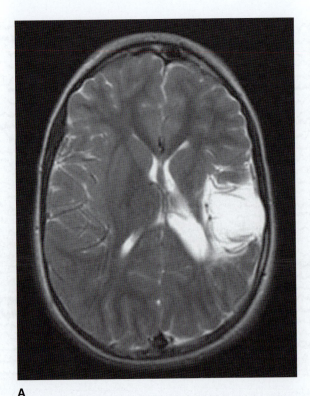

A

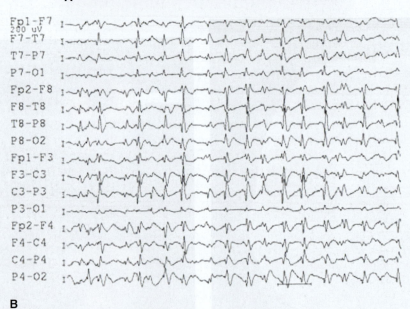

B

Figure 55–5. Magnetic resonance imaging of the brain at 8 years of age of case 4 showing an old ischaemic infarct in the left central (middle cerebral artery territory) region (**A**). The electroencephalography (EEG) in sleep (**B**) shows continuous spike-wave activity. The EEG at the start of an epileptic seizure (**C**) with staring and unresponsiveness is nonlateralizing. *(continued)*

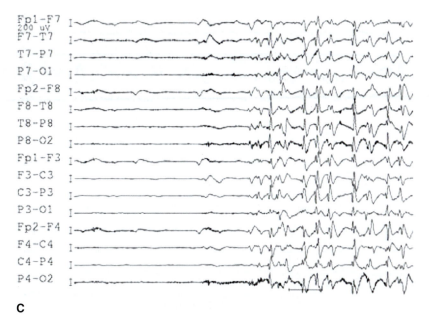

C

Figure 55–5. *(Continued)*

later onset of epilepsy has little impact on relocalization. However, earlier seizure onset and location of pathology should be taken into consideration. There is a high prevalence of behavior disorder both in children with temporal[12] and extratemporal epilepsy (Colonelli et al submitted.

Case 4

This 8-year-old girl presented with a right hemiparesis and loss of fine finger movement at the age of 8 months of, without visual field deficit. Medically refractory epilepsy developed at 6 years of age, with nocturnal (secondarily) generalized tonic–clonic seizures lasting 2–3 minutes occurring twice a month, and epileptic staring with arrest of activity, unresponsiveness, and lip smacking for 10–20 seconds occurring 10 or more times per day. MRI showed encephalomalacia consistent with perinatal left middle cerebral artery infarction (Fig. 55–6A), and EEG revealed generalized ictal and interictal epileptiform discharges on EEG (Fig. 55–6B, C), with slow spike–wave complexes and electrographic status epilepticus in sleep (ESES). Failed antiepileptic medications included carbamazepine, lamotrigine, levetiracetam, and valproate. The ketogenic diet and a course of prednisone produced no benefit.

She subsequently manifested severe cognitive and behavioral problems. She became distractible, with poor focusing. Neuropsychological assessment at the age of 8 years indicated overall cognitive functioning at about the age of 2-year level.

A functional hemispherectomy was performed without perioperative complications. She had no worsening of hemiparesis after surgery troublesome. She has

been seizure free for 22 months, and the postoperative EEG showed complete resolution of her generalized epileptiform discharges and ESES. Parents and teachers have noted dramatic improvement in behavior, cognition, language, judgment, and learning.

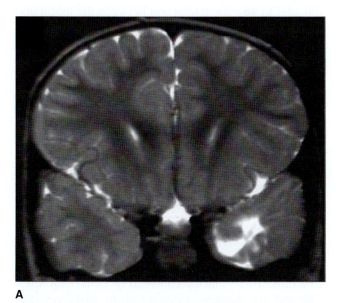

A

Figure 55–6. Magnetic resonance imaging coronal section (**A**) of case 5 showing the lesion in the left mesial temporal region. Sleep electroencephalography (**B**) shows continuous spiking over the left temporal electrodes. *(continued)*

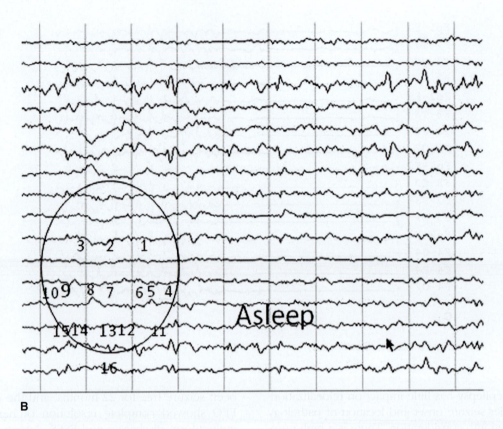

B

Figure 55–6. *(Continued)*

This case illustrates that a surgically remediable unilateral congenital or early acquired epileptogenic lesion may present with diffuse EEG manifestations, presumably due to an early interaction between the lesion and the developing brain. This may be seen not only during infancy (infantile spasms and hypsarrhythmia), but also later in childhood (generalized slow-spike-wave and other patterns). The critical factor appears to be *the age at which the lesion occurred*, rather than the age at which the child presents for surgery. In carefully selected children with a congenital or early-acquired unilateral epileptogenic lesion, surgery should not be delayed due to ongoing generalized epileptiform discharges including ESES. In some cases surgery may be able to shorten the ESES and epileptic encephalopathy, and lead to improved developmental outcome.

Case 5

A 5-year-old girl experienced her first seizure at age 4 months. These initially consisted of behavioral arrest with oral automatisms occurring up to 10–12 per day. Seizure control was established at the age of 2 years with carbamazepine. Early development was normal with plateauing between ages 15–22 months. She subsequently did progress but at the age of 26 months was at a 12–16 month level with language and behavioral concerns. MRI revealed a left mesial temporal lesion suggestive of a dysembryoplastic neuroepithelial tumor (see Fig. 55–6). Interictal awake EEG was normal; interictal sleep EEG showed continuous spikes in the left temporal eregion. A formalized developmental assessment was not possible due to her marked attentional impairment.

Despite being seizure free, her continuing developmental concern, sleep EEG abnormality and requirement for ongoing medication prompted a parental decision to proceed to left temporal resection, despite uncertainty regarding postoperative cognitive and behavioral status. She was subsequently weaned from medication and showed marked developmental gains over the next 5 years with no recurrence of seizures. At this time, her full scale IQ was f 82, compared to 60 1 year postoperatively.

Although seizure control should always remain the predominant aim of epilepsy surgery, the likely is the relationship of continuing epileptiform activity to cognitive dysfunction. In this scenario, the low risk of surgery and its potential benefits were felt to outweigh the risks.

Case 6

A 10-year-old girl presented at the age of 2 years in status epilepticus presumed due to enterovirus encephalitis.

At the age of 4 years, her mother noticed episodes of vacant staring occurring several times per week, associated with behavioral arrest. At the age of 7 years, she began to experience more obvious events where she would suddenly become unresponsive, with hand automatisms.

At evaluation, she described episodes beginning with a "scary" feeling, an inability to talk, and trembling of her hands. Some episodes would evolve to unresponsiveness associated with swallowing, mouthing, and lip smacking. Automatisms involving the hands were also noted. Episodes lasted 45 seconds to 2 minutes followed by confusion and incoherent speech.

MRI revealed a focal cortical dysplastic lesion in the pars opercularis of the left inferior frontal gyrus and hippocampal sclerosis (Fig. 55–7). The ictal EEG demonstrated a wide field of seizure onset over the left hemisphere. Eight AEDs produced little benefit. Neuropsychological testing demonstrated intact cognition with average memory and academic attainment.

While the ictal semiology was consistent with a mesial temporal onset, and hippoocampal sclerosis, but the EEG was not localizing. Invasive EEG recording helped determine the epileptic source and absence of functional activity. A subdural grid was placed over the dysplastic region and a depth electrode was inserted into the left hippocampus. Seizure onset was confirmed from the left hippocampus and absent functionality was demonstrated from the dysplastic lesion. A left temporal lobe resection and lesionectomy were performed. Two years following surgery, she is seizure free off medication, with no neurological deficit.

OLDER CHILDHOOD

Although many of the children who are surgical candidates in this age group experienced seizure onset in early childhood, seizure frequency is often variable, with either periods of remission, or a later seizure onset of epilepsy.[13] Children coming for surgery in this age group are more likely to have underlying developmental pathology (either focal cortical dysplasia or tumors) and undergo focal rather than multilobar resections.[2] Recent data reviewing adults who had undergone temporal lobe resection in childhood showed longer term cognitive improvement more than 6 years following surgery. Further there was definitive psychosocial improvement compared with controls who had not undergone surgery.[14]

Children with acquired pathology require careful consideration to optimally time surgery. For example, timing of surgery in Rasmussens syndrome (discussed in detail in Chapter 37); is based on the rate of progression, the hemisphere involved and relocation of function.

Case 7

A 12-year-old girl had her first febrile seizure at the age of 12 months characterized by eye rolling and unresponsiveness lasting several minutes followed by generalized jerking. The entire episode lasted 15 minutes. Subsequent seizures started at the age of 6 years and were characterized by a warning (feeling scared, unable to think properly), staring, swallowing, and fiddling with her hands. She could hear but not speak during episodes, and had no recollection of events. After each seizure she becomes nauseated, may vomit and has word finding difficulties. By the time of referral she had unsuccessfully tried four medications, although at the age of 7 years had a 2.5-year period seizure free on carbamazepine.

She attended a mainstream school, progressing although demonstrating particular problems with languages. Her interictal EEG recording (Fig. 55–8A) revealed focal slowing with discharges in the left temporal lobe that enhanced in sleep. MRI (Fig. 55–8B) demonstrated changes compatible with left hippocampal sclerosis. Two brief stereotyped episodes were recorded on video-EEG that were similar to the description of her semiology- and consisted of a warning followed by behavioral change with oral and hand automatisms. Postictal expressive aphasia was also noted. Neuropsychology assessment showed intellectual ability and visual memory within the average range for her age, but she had difficulty with word knowledge, verbal comprehension, and verbal memory. She underwent a left temporal resection, counseled for small chance of further word difficulties. After 4 years she remains seizure free with no discernable increased cognitive deficit.

The seizure semiology and EEG were compatible with left temporal lobe seizure onset, with mesial temporal onset consistent with the left hippocampal sclerosis seen on MRI. Her neuropsychological profile was also consistent with the pathology suggesting a low risk of further impairment from temporal resection. One could argue that additional video telemetry was unnecessary given the structural abnormality. Adult epilepsy surgical series suggest this may not be required if the semiology is typical, interictal abnormalities point to anterior and basal temporal electrodes, and the neuropsychological profile is coherent with the side of the lesion. Further this case illustrates that mesial temporal lobe epilepsy is not necessarily an adult disease and can be recognized easily in children.

Case 8

A 14-year-old boy was referred with a 12-year history of seizures. His first seizure had been an afebrile tonic–clonic seizure, but he subsequently experienced periods of behavioral arrest lasting from seconds to up to

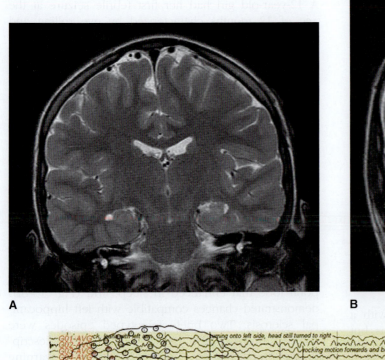

A

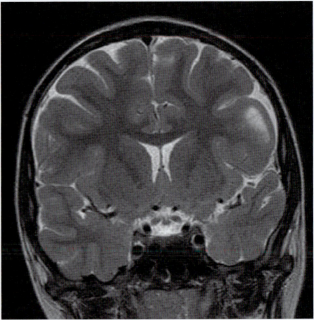

B

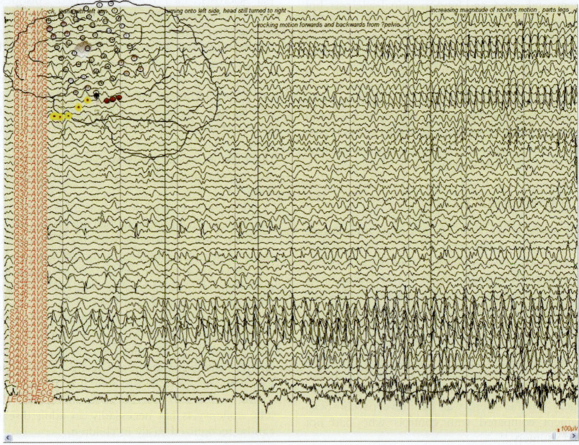

C

Figure 55–7. A Coronal T2 magnetic resonance imaging of case 6, showing left hippocampal sclerosis (**A**) and the area of high signal in the left frontal cortex (**B**) suggestive of cortical dysplasia.
(**C**) Invasive electroencephalographic recording of seizure from case 6. Seizure onset appears
from anterior temporal strip (yellow) with engagement of depth into hippocampus, with later
involvement of grid in region of dysplastic lesion.

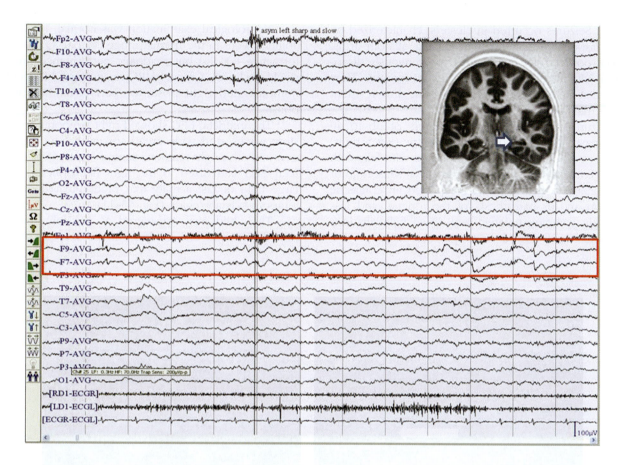

Figure 55–8. Coronal T1 magnetic resonance imaging of case 7 (inset), showing a small left hippocampus compatible with hippocampal sclerosis (arrow). Interictal electroencephalography shows spikes over the left anterior quadrant.

20 minutes. At evaluation he was having 2–3 episodes per day where he would experience a warning (described as a feeling in his right arm), fumble, lose color, remain aware, but become noncommunicative for 30 seconds to 5 minutes. These episodes have persisted despite treatment with phenytoin, sodium valproate, oxcarbazepine, and levetiracetam. MRI revealed an area of focal cortical dysplasia left the posterior superior temporal gyrus (see Fig. 55–9). The possibility of epilepsy surgery had been discussed with the local team but dismissed in view of likely language localization and the extent of the lesion. He never had a protracted period of seizure freedom however, further, although of average intellect in mainstream school he had word finding difficulty and hesitance of language, having lost ground at school over the preceding 4 years.

Interictal EEG showed mild slowing of the background, with occasional discharges in the left temporal region in sleep. Ictal recording revealed three semiologically similar seizures, two demonstrating attenuation at onset and one demonstrating right fronto-temporal discharges late in the event. Motor functional MRI revealed motor activation distant to the lesion. Language functional

MRI revealed left hemisphere dominance without activation in the lesion.

Following full discussion, it was felt seizure semiology was compatible with seizure onset from the lesion. However, language representation in close proximity to the lesion could not be excluded. He proceeded to invasive EEG monitoring with a 48-contact grid placed over the lesion, and an anterior temporal strip. Seizure onset was demonstrated around the lesion, with language function on stimulation superior to the lesion (Fig. 55–9). The area was removed successfully with no increased deficit. Two years following surgery, he is seizure free off medication, planning trips abroad with the school.

This case illustrates that decision making about the likelihood of a lesion being resectable should be made by the surgical team; little can be lost by an evaluation without proceeding to surgery. Much can be lost by waiting.

Case 9

This 13-year-old right-handed girl started her epilepsy at the age of 3 years. Psychomotor development was normal. Seizures occurred in clusters, characterized by brief episodes of bilateral tonic raising of both arms, without postictal deficit. Seizures spontaneously disappeared without treatment within a few months. They recurred at the age of 9 years and became drug-resistant despite trials of seven different AEDs.

Seizures consisted of daily clusters of up to 40 brief "spasm-like" episodes of asymmetric (left > right) tonic contraction of the arms, associated with falls with "convulsions." There was neither postictal sensorimotor nor language deficit. The child reported an epigastric sensation and/or paresthesia of the tongue, and less frequently complex unlateralized visual hallucinations that sometimes followed the tongue sensation.

Neurological examination was normal. Intellectual abilities were in the normal range (verbal IQ: 100, performance IQ: 94) but academic performance progressively declined. A repeat MRI was normal; 18-FDG-PET demonstrated right posterior perisylvian hypometabolism.

The interictal EEG showed right temporal posterior slow waves, and widespread spikes that were prominent over the right temporo-central region (Fig. 55–10). Ictal EEG lateralized to the right hemisphere, with a large field of fast activity that predominated over the temporo-sylvian region (Fig. 55–11).

The child was considered as possibly surgically remediable and she underwent stereotactic intracer-

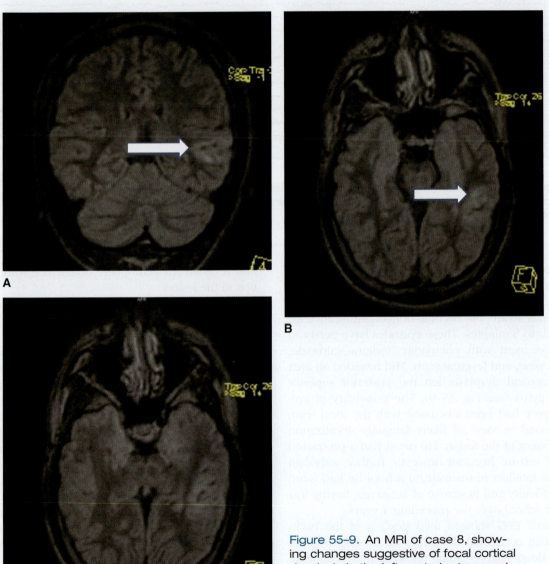

Figure 55–9. An MRI of case 8, showing changes suggestive of focal cortical dysplasia in the left posterior temporal cortex. Figure 55–9B shows the placement of the grid over the area, and focal onset of seizures from immediately inferior to this lesion. *(continued)*

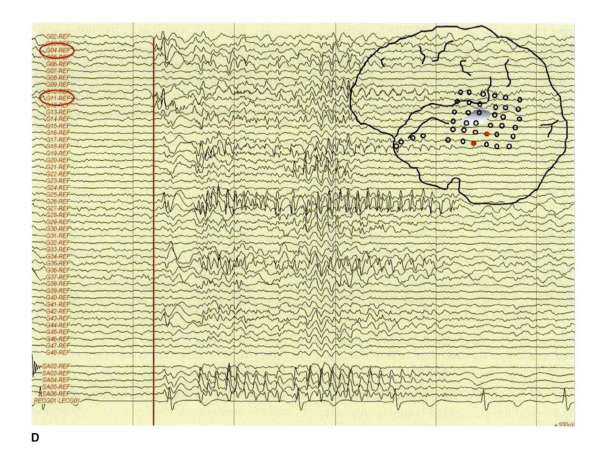

D

Figure 55–9. *(Continued)*

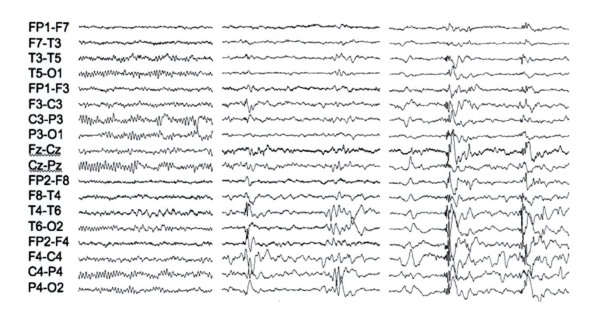

Figure 55–10. Interictal electroencephalography from case 9, showing right temporal posterior slow waves, as well as more widespread spikes that seem more prominent over the right temporo-central region.

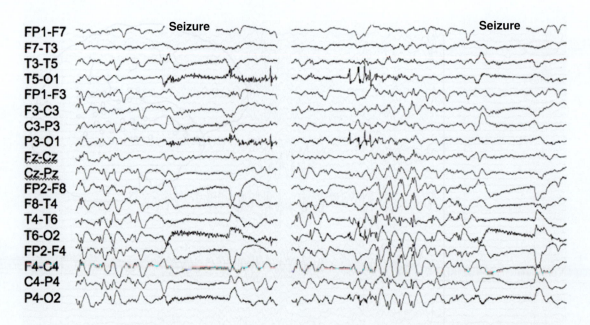

Figure 55–11. Ictal electroencephalography from case 9, lateralizing to the right hemisphere, with a widely extended fast activity that predominates over the temporo-sylvian region.

ebral EEG (SEEG) recordings. The implantation strategy (Fig. 55–12) favored the perisylvian cortex (paresthesia of the tongue, epigastric sensation, 18-FDG PET findings), with additional electrodes exploring also the posterior temporal region (complex visual hallucinations, posterior temporal slow waves and spikes), as well as the sensori-motor and premotor cortices (bilateral asymetric tonic contraction). It was not considered necessary to monitor the left hemisphere, as there was a clear right-side predominance of interictal and ictal EEG abnormalities.

Interictal EEG spike-and-waves complex were recorded from the temporo-occipital region (Fig. 55–13). During periods that preceded seizure occurrence, bursts of fast oscillations were recorded over the suprasylvian opercular cortex (Fig. 55–14). They progressively spread to additional electrodes before triggering a cluster of seizures from the fronto-parietal operculum, insula, temporo-occipital junction, and premotor cortex (Fig. 55–15). The seizure cluster terminated with prolonged bilateral tonic contractions of the arms followed by secondary tonic–clonic generalization (Fig. 55–16). Further analysis of SEEG data suggested seizure origin from the fronto-parietal operculum before spreading to insular cortex, the temporo-parietal junction, and premotor cortex (Fig. 55–17).

Based on SEEG findings, a tailored resection of the right frontal and parietal operculum was performed (Fig. 55–18). Pathological examination of the resected tissue did not find any clear abnormalities, except a few ectopic neurons. Seizures recurred 1 month after surgery (brief tonic contractions of both legs) that were nocturnal, and much less frequent (1–2 clusters per

months). They disappeared several months later. The child is now seizure free for 2 years. Academic performance increased into the normal range, and antiepileptic drugs have been reduced.

This case illustrates that MRI-negative cases can be successfully treated by limited cortical resection. Yet, it illustrates that "spasm-like" episodes do not represent a contraindication to surgery, even in the absence of brain lesion. Despite major advances in neuroimaging, the rate of MRI-negative cases among surgically treated patients is around 15%.[15] These cases are undoubtedly the most challenging in terms of presurgical assessment, and invasive recordings are often required, especially in extratemporal locations. Successful localization of MRI-negative cases although challenging, can be achieved similar to lesional MRI cases, as recently showed in series of patients who underwent a SEEG investigation[15] or other invasive EEG.[17] However, not all MRI-negative cases are surgically remediable, and a working hypothesis concerning the site(s) of seizure onset should be in place before undertaking an invasive evaluation.

▶ SUMMARY

The range of epilepsy surgery in childhood is wide. The primary outcome remains one of seizure control; however, secondary gains may be achievable including improvement in cognitive outcome. However, each child requires careful evaluation in a comprehensive epilepsy center, to determine the optimal way forward including the timing of such intervention. Determination of possible surgical candidates is often challenging; therefore,

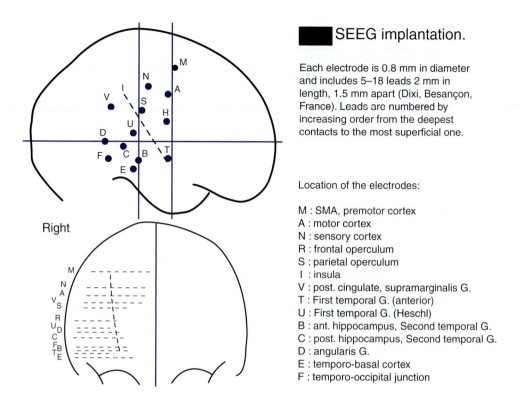

SEEG implantation.

Each electrode is 0.8 mm in diameter and includes 5–18 leads 2 mm in length, 1.5 mm apart (Dixi, Besançon, France). Leads are numbered by increasing order from the deepest contacts to the most superficial one.

Location of the electrodes:

M : SMA, premotor cortex
A : motor cortex
N : sensory cortex
R : frontal operculum
S : parietal operculum
I : insula
V : post. cingulate, supramarginalis G.
T : First temporal G. (anterior)
U : First temporal G. (Heschl)
B : ant. hippocampus, Second temporal G.
C : post. hippocampus, Second temporal G.
D : angularis G.
E : temporo-basal cortex
F : temporo-occipital junction

Figure 55–12. Implantation strategy for electrodes for case 9.

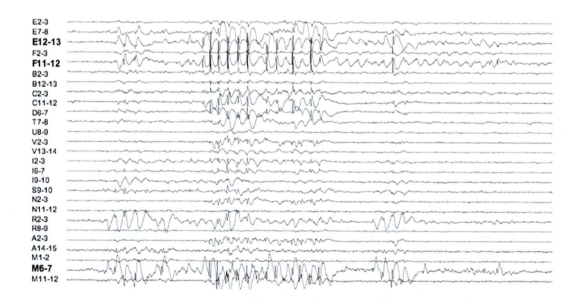

Figure 55–13. From the implanted electrodes, interictal electroencephalographic spike-and-waves complex were mainly seen over the temporo-occipital region.

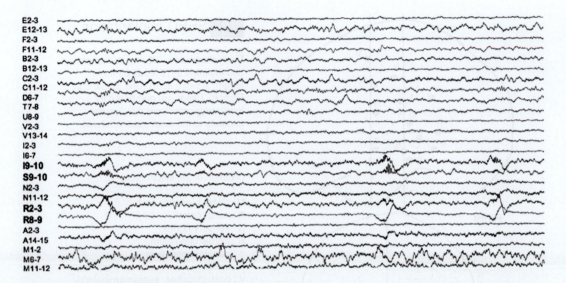

Figure 55–14. Burst of fast oscillations were recorded over the supra-sylvian opercular cortex prior to seizure onset.

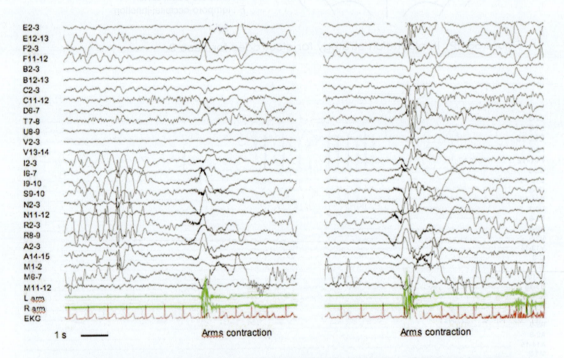

Figure 55–15. Fast oscillations progressively extended over additional electrodes before to give rise to a cluster of seizures involving the fronto-parietal operculum, the insula, the temporo-occipital junction, and the premotor cortex.

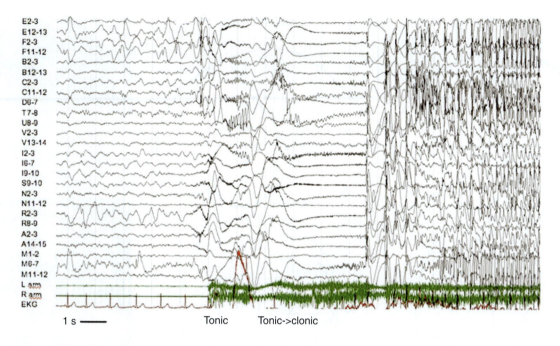

Figure 55–16. The cluster ended by a more prolonged episode with bilateral tonic contraction of the arms followed by a secondary tonic–clonic generalization.

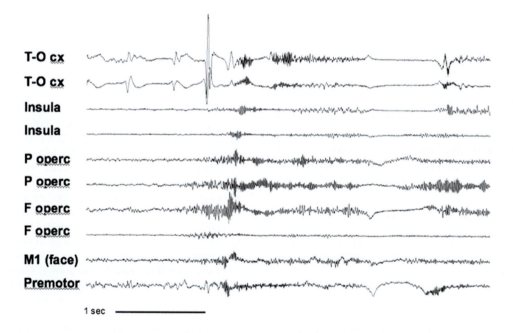

Figure 55–17. A fine analysis of stereoelectroencephalography data in case 9 suggested that the episodes originated from the fronto-parietal operculum before to spread very quickly to the insula, the temporo-parietal junction, and the premotor cortex.

Interictal findings   Ictal findings

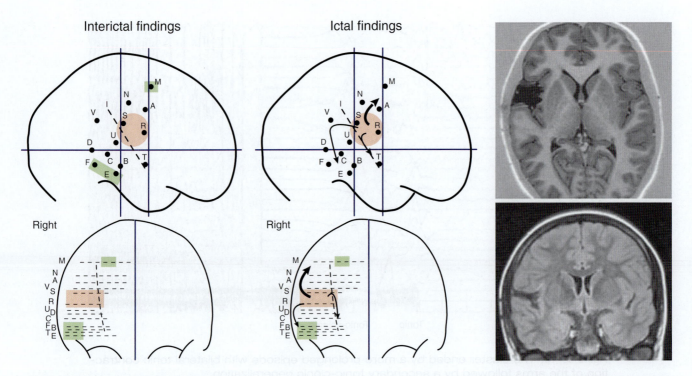

Figure 55–18. The tailored resection of the right frontal and parietal operculum that resulted from analysis of the stereoelectroencephalography data.

guidance should be followed as to when to refer children for specialist epilepsy opinion, including all children presenting under 2 years with epilepsy, all with an apparent unilateral lesion, as well as children failing to respond to two optimal medications. Also, attention must be paid to cognitive decline in children suffering from focal seizures, even if the response to medication is positive. Further, the outcome aims should be carefully evaluated with the family to determine expectations. Much can be gained from an early referral for epilepsy surgery; much can be lost by waiting.

REFERENCES

1. Cross JH, et al. Proposed criteria for referral and evaluation of children with epilepsy for surgery. *Epilepsia* 2006;47: 952–959.
2. Harvey AS, Cross JH, Shinnar S, Mathern GW. Seizure syndromes, eitiologies and procedures in paediatric epilepsy: a 2004 International Survey. *Epilepsia* 2008;49:146–155.
3. Cormack F, Cross JH, Vargha-Khadem F, Baldeweg T. The development of intellectual abilities in temporal lobe epilepsy. *Epilepsia* 2007;48:201–204.
4. Vasconcellos E, et al. Mental retardation in pediatric candidates for epilepsy surgery: the role of early seizure onset. *Epilepsia* 2001;42(2):268–274.
5. Freitag H, Tuxhorn I. Cognitive function in preschool children after epilepsy surgery: rationale for early intervention. *Epilepsia* 2005;46:561–567.
6. Loddenkemper T, Holland KD, Stanford L, Kotagal P, Bingaman W, Wyllie E. Developmental outcome after epilepsy surgery in infancy. *Pediatrics* 2007;119:930–935.
7. Cross JH, et al. Proposed criteria for referral and evaluation of children for epilepsy surgery: recommendations of the Subcommission for Paediatric Epilepsy Surgery. *Epilepsia* 2006;47:952–959.
8. Wyllie E, et al. Temporal lobe epilepsy in early childhood. *Epilepsia* 1993;34:859–868.
9. Korff CM, Nordli DR. The clinical-electrographic expression of infantile seizures. *Epilepsy Res* 2006;70S:S116–S131.
10. Eltze C, Chong WK, Harding B, Cross JH. Focal cortical dysplasia in infants; some MRI lesions almost disappear with maturation of myelination. *Epilepsia* 2005; 46: 1988–1922.
11. Guerrini R, et al. Multilobar polymicrogyria, intractable drop attack seizures and sleep related electrical status epilepticus. *Neurology* 1998;51:504–512.
12. Mclellan A, et al. Psychopathology in children undergoing temproal lobe resection—a pre and postoperative assessment. *Dev Med Child Neurol* 2005;47:666–672.
13. Berg AT, et al. How long does it take for epilepsy to become intractable? A prospective investigation. *Ann Neurol* 2006; 60:73–39.
14. Skirrow C, Cross JH, Cormack F, Harkness W, Vargha-Khadem F, Baldeweg T. Long-term outcome after temporal lobe surgery in childhood: intellectual gains are correlated with brain volume change. *Neurology* 2011;76:1330–1337.
15. Tonini C, et al. Predictors of epilepsy surgery outcome: a meta-analysis. *Epilepsy Res* 2007;62:72–87.
16. McGonigal A, et al. Stereoelectroencephalo-graphy in presurgical assessment of MRI-negative epilepsy. *Brain* 2007;130:3169–3183.
17. Jayakar P, et al. Epilepsy surgery in patients with normal or nonfocal MRI scans: integrative strategies offer long term seizure relief. *Epilepsia* 2008;49:758–764.

CHAPTER 56

Surgery for Catastrophic Epilepsies: When and Why?

Brian Neville

The term catastrophic epilepsy is applied to children with epilepsy who present with some of the following characteristics:

- Urgent need for treatments.
- Onset in early life.
- There is commonly a major loss of cognitive and behavioral functions, which may be profound.
- There is relatively high mortality.

The combination of sudden onset of seizures and massive regression may resemble an acute brain illness and be mistakenly diagnosed as having "encephalitis." Careful review of the history and investigations should show no positive evidence of parenchymal brain disease and the time course may show fluctuations of function relating to seizure severity even if only over a few weeks.

▶ INDICATIONS FOR SURGERY

The term "catastrophic" has been particularly useful in the context of potentially surgically treatable epilepsies.[1,2] The term implies that seizures per se are causing the deterioration, that is, it is an epileptic encephalopathy as defined in the 2001 ILAE epilepsy classification[3] and that early intervention for seizures, be it medical or surgical, may arrest or even reverse some of the loss of skills.[4] It may, however, be difficult to accurately define the contribution of seizures and causative pathological process, which serves as the basis for case selection and management (Fig. 56–1). The imperatives for surgical intervention are:

- The seizure disorder is caused by a focal abnormality, which may be a discrete or hemispheric lesion.
- Resistance to antiepileptic drug (AED) treatment.
- The lesion is resectable with minimal hazard.
- The chances of natural remission are small.

Catastrophic epilepsy surgery should be performed as early as possible with the aim of allowing the child as many seizure-free years of childhood as possible; the ultimate goal is to minimize cognitive and behavioral impairments. Too often, several years pass between the early presentation with epilepsy and surgery.[5] It is common to successfully surgically treat children of 8 years or more who have presented in the first year of life with infantile spasms, but it may take several years to recognize that the child has a surgically treatable epilepsy.

The reasons for delaying surgical intervention are numerous and include lack of awareness that the child has a surgically treatable epilepsy or temporary seizure remission. There is also a tendency to unsuccessfully try multiple AEDs.[6] In some cases, accurate localization of the epileptogenic zone may be challenging in the first year of life.

Many children with lesional epilepsy who present with infantile spasms rapidly regress at seizure onset and remain delayed, even with successful treatment. The correlates of epileptic encephalopathy are poorly understood but clearly involve cognitive and behavioral network dysfunction distant from the lesion. Early regression is easily overlooked and a careful history and review of family photographs/movies is often helpful. Assessment instruments appropriate for young regressed children are therefore essential.

▶ NONSURGICAL CATASTROPHIC EPILEPSY SYNDROMES

The first priority is to identify syndromes that present with early severe seizure onset and regression that are not surgically treatable.

- *Severe (malignant) migratory partial seizures of infancy.* This recently described disorder presents with the abrupt onset of focal motor seizures with major autonomic features in the first 6 months of life.[7] Although seizures initially begin at one focus, other brain regions rapidly become involved leading to widespread shifting focality of seizure semiology and EEG features. Progressive cognitive and motor impairment

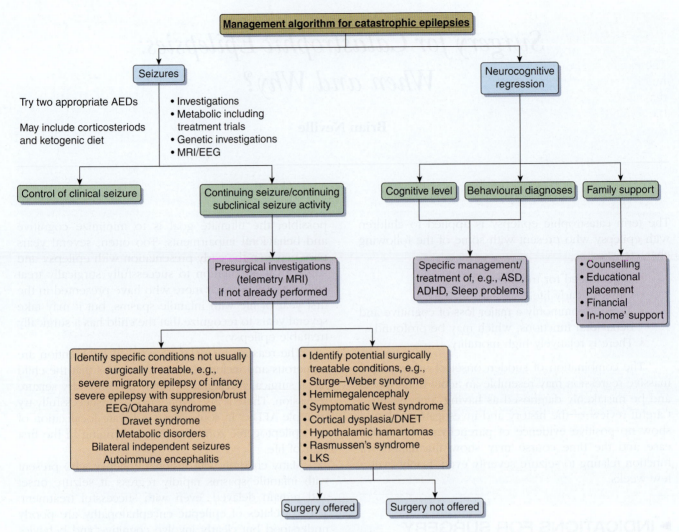

Figure 56–1. Management algorithm for catastrophic epilepsies.

(hypotonia and pyramidal signs) and acquired microcephaly typically follow. This disorder is usually easy to distinguish from a potentially surgically treatable epilepsy except perhaps at initial presentation.

• *Severe neonatal epilepsies with suppression—burst EEG/Ohtahara syndrome.* Ohtahara syndrome presents with seizures, mostly tonic spasms from the first 2–3 months of life and a suppression-burst EEG.[8] Partial seizures including hemiconvulsions are common. The course is severe with high seizure frequency, slow development, severe motor delay, and high mortality. It is clear that despite its rarity, this syndrome is the end point for several pathologies, which include malformations and nonketotic hyperglycinemia.[9] Rarely malformations such as hemimegalencephaly are amenable to surgical treatment. While this occurs rarely, it should be considered in all presenting cases.

• *Dravet's syndrome* typically presents with complex febrile seizures in the first 6 months of life, followed by multiple seizure types and regression beginning around 1 year of age.[10] About 80% have abnormalities in the SCN1A gene.[11] Hippocampal sclerosis is occasionally noted but the seizure semiology, regression, and EEG abnormalities suggest widespread brain involvement.

• Metabolic causes of epilepsy, for example, pyridoxine/pyridoxal phosphate dependent,[12] phenylketonuria,[13] GLUT1 deficiency,[14] biotinidase deficiency.[15] Infants with early onset seizures should be given a trial of pyridoxine/pyridoxal phosphate and biotin (or the enzyme measured) and have their blood glucose, calcium, magnesium, CSF glucose and urinary amino acids and organic acids measured. This group of disorders typically first presents with abnormal development followed by regression at an early age.

▶ OPERABLE CATSTROPHIC EPILEPSY SYNDROMES

The explosive onset of seizures with regression is commonly lesionally based. There are several syndromes that are best dealt with individually as surgery may only be possible in some.

- *Sturge–Weber syndrome.* Not uncommonly a baby with a typical port-wine stain naevus presents with repeated or prolonged focal seizures, acquired hemiplegia, and reduced consciousness indicating developmental regression. MRI reveals evidence of cerebral cortical rim ischemia apparently caused by inadequate vascular reserve to cope with the increased metabolic rate of severe seizures.[16] Prolonged seizures typically occur without warning and the stage at which surgery should be offered is not yet agreed.

In a baby with a skin naevus, it seems appropriate to perform gadolinium-enhanced MRI early to see if a pial naevus is present. Unilateral or hemispheric or lobar/multilobar involvement suggests a potential resective surgical option. An antiepilepsy drugs administered prior to clinical seizures, although there is no evidence that it prevents a severe episode and low-dose aspirin is commonly given. The most difficult problem is how to offer surgery early enough to usefully prevent further damage as well as stopping seizures. Many procedures are performed when the child has a dense hemiplegia and severe cognitive impairment. While this outcome is not inevitable, inflicting a hemiplegia and possibly some cognitive impairment by surgery following the onset of seizures is not an easy decision.

- *Hemimegalencephaly.* Children with hemimegalencephaly may present with sudden onset of severe hemiepilepsy and regression in which case urgent surgical referral is appropriate, even while AEDs are being tried. Development may not proceed if clinical seizures stop but subclinical seizure activity continues. However, many patients with hemimegalencephaly have intrauterine seizure onset and are already regressed and hemiplegic at birth. Cognitive outcome even after very early surgery is usually poor.[2]
- *Infantile spasms/West Syndrome.* The characteristic epileptic spasms usually begin between ages 4 and 6 months. In addition to runs of many spasms, there is regression of visual and social behavior. Spasms are sometimes preceded by focal seizures, which may give a clue to the source. Where there is no evidence of underlying pathology with normal MRI and previous development, seizure response to corticosteroids and/or vigabatrin is usually favorable, but cognitive

outcome is still often poor.[17] It is important to perform EEG monitoring to ascertain that the EEG has normalized and the spasms have stopped. The results of medical treatment for patients with an abnormal MRI, previous slow development or focal seizures are generally unfavorable and patients typically exhibit a high rate of intractability and psychosocial morbidity.[18] A particularly high rate of autism spectrum disorders is always combined with cognitive impairment.[19] It should not take more than 2–3 weeks of medical treatment with the earlier two drugs to diagnose medical unresponsiveness and begin presurgical investigations.

An underlying lesion, for example, dysembryoplastic neuroepithelial tumor, tuberous sclerosis, cortical dysplasia, hypoxic/ischemia, or infectious disorder may be recognized in the MRI. Solitary lesions in this setting should be considered urgently for resection once two AEDs have failed. In cases of tuberous sclerosis, studies of seizure semiology, video/EEG, and ictal SPECT may assist in localizing the epileptogenic tuber. The role of serotonin PET is unclear.[20]

The spectrum of hypoxic/ischemic lesions and rapid onset of severe epilepsy include children with severe pre- or perinatal cerebral damage. In these cases, pathologic changes are often bilateral and are not usually surgically amenable. When the MRI scan is normal, imaging data should be reviewed in the light of the clinical evidence as clinical findings could change their interpretation. Occasionally, a lesion may be present on an early scan and "fade" as myelination proceeds.[21]

Earlier studies of "MR negative" West syndrome showed significant yield of abnormal PET scans, which led to successful surgery.[22] It seems likely that higher field strength MRI now reveal lesions; FDG PET is an important option in cases with focal features and a negative MRI. The causes of infantile spasms include conditions that can damage the cerebral cortex in early life, many of which involve bilateral pathology.

- *Focal cortical dysplasia and dysembryoplastic neuroepithelial tumors (DNET).* When a child under age 1 year presents with recent onset focal seizures and MRI shows a well-defined lesion in resectable cortex in, for example, temporal lobe neocortex with the characteristics of a DNET, surgical treatment should be urgently planned. This initial presentation typically progresses to a severe seizure disorder accompanied by cognitive and autistic regression.[23] This clinical scenario is highly predictable unless clinical seizures and subclinical seizure activity are stopped by initial medication.

Dysplastic malformations are the commonest in cases of early surgery and often present with the sudden onset of severe seizures and regression. The dysplastic cortex may not be apparent on the initial sMRI but ultimately recognized by careful review. There is often uncertainty about the full extent/margins of the lesion and invasive monitoring may be required for accurate characterization. MRI negative focal catastrophic epilepsy will almost always require invasive monitoring if the clinical history and video/EEG data suggest a reasonably confined area of the cortex. Ictal fMRI, magnetoencephalography, and positron emission tomography may provide additional confirmation of focality. Cognitive assessments of children with lesional early onset seizures show high rates of severe cognitive impairment.[24]

- *Acute mesial temporal epilepsy.* Simple mesial temporal sclerosis (MTS) can rarely present with explosive seizure onset in early life. Several conditions may present with a mesial temporal lesion and/or epilepsy syndrome. These include:
  - Dravet's syndrome and GLUT1 deficiency (see earlier). The seizure semiology and developmental progress should distinguish both of these nonsurgically treatable conditions.
  - Rasmussen's syndrome may begin as an acute mesial temporal syndrome but imaging may not be typical of MTS. However, it occasionally happens that a mesial temporal resection in this setting shows pathology typical of Rasmussen's.[25] Seizure remission is often temporary, and further surgery can be planned as needed.
  - Viral encephalitis, particularly herpes simplex typically presents with fever, reduced consciousness, seizures, and CSF pleocytosis. The MRI commonly shows asymmetric but bilateral involvement and mandates prompt antiviral treatment.
  - Patients occasionally present with the explosive onset of focal usually mesial temporal epilepsy which progresses to chronic intractable epilepsy with MTS.[26] Such patients may come to surgery but the results are not as good as with MTS preceded by febrile status epilepticus, suggesting bilateral or more widespread involvement. It is generally assumed to result from viral encephalitis.
  - Fever-induced refractory epileptic encephalopathy in school-aged children (FIRES) may resemble the previous group, but the sequence of fever, very frequent seizures with mesial temporal and opercular features, and status epilepticus progressing rapidly to chronic intractable epilepsy are characteristic.[27] The clinical and EEG features indicate bilateral involvement and therefore are not considered candidate for epilepsy surgery.

- *Hemiconvulsion-hemiplegia syndrome.* This early onset syndrome of fever, prolonged hemiseizures and permanent hemiplegic and cognitive impairment is not treated with surgery in the acute phase for early surgery, although it may be offered at a later age for intractable hemiepilepsy.[28]
- Encephalitis related to anti-NMDA antibodies has been mainly described in adults with a catastrophic onset of epilepsy and motor, cognitive, and behavioral impairments. Voltage-gated potassium channel antibody encephalitis is mainly a bilateral limbic encephalitis.
- Increasingly, pediatric cases and patients without ovarian tumors are being described and if correctly identified, are managed by immunotherapy.[29]
- *Hypothalamic hamartomas.* These masses of ectopic gray matter cause a rare form of epilepsy usually presenting in the first 2 years of life. Seizures may present in the newborn and are characterized by mirthless laughter or occasionally crying. The symptoms may not be recognized as epileptic and initially may lack EEG correlates. A wide range of seizure types develop subsequently. Gelastic seizures commonly disrupt cognitive and social development.[30]

The temporal lobe is often a target for seizure activity. However, SPECT scans and needle electrodes will confirm that the hamartoma is the source of the seizure but these investigations are not required in a typical patient. Several surgical approaches are used for accessible lesions that are penduculated into the interpeduncular cistern or third ventricle or have a clear line of separation. These include transcallosal, lateral (pterional), and endoscopic approaches but excision is rarely complete and should be performed in a center with experience in this disorder. Gamma knife has been used for lesions that are not approachable by conventional techniques. There are significant side effects of surgery that include somnolence, weight gain, panhypopituitarism, diabetes insipidus, and loss of drive.[31] AEDs should be given a fair trial and the balance between the effects of the seizure disorder and surgery should be carefully assessed.

- Landau–Kleffner Syndrome (LKS) and continuous spike wave in slow-wave sleep (CSWS). LKS is an epilepsy syndrome that presents after age 2 years with loss of language comprehension, speech and frequent wider cognitive, autistic and behavioral regression, which may amount to "disintegrative psychosis."[32] Clinical seizures occur at presentation in approximately 80% of patients but are often mild. Regression is associated with high rates of epileptic activity in sleep particularly in the superior temporal gyrus and perisylvian region. No lesion is apparent on MRI. The main treatment is medical, particularly with corticosteroids. Children with predominantly (90%) unilateral discharges as judged by telemetry and magnetoencephalography have been treated with multiple subpial transections under corticographic control.[33] The results are partial and improvements may be in the psychiatric domain rather than aphasia.[34] Multiple subpial transections are less effective than excisional surgery for lesional epilepsy but the main outcome measure for LKS is not seizure relief but recovery from the language deficit.

LKS is now regarded as fitting into a wider range of epilepsies, both lesional and nonlesional, in which high rates of epileptic activity in slow-wave sleep are associated with cognitive and psychosocial regression.[35] Regression can be difficult to treat medically although corticosteroids and/or benzodiazepines may be effective. If there is a surgically treatable lesion, surgery should be urgently considered. The procedure of wide subpial transections for very extensive epileptic activity has not been generally accepted.

► COGNITIVE AND BEHAVIORAL ASSESSMENT

A crucial aspect of working with young children with severe epilepsy is multidisciplinary cognitive and behavioral assessment. Most children are low functioning but their selective impairments, for example, language function, autism spectrum disorder, attention deficit hyperactivity, coordination and obsessive compulsive disorders, and violent behavior are important factors in the presurgical assessment. It is important to identify medically treatable aspects of behavior (e.g., ADHD) and measure the effects of surgery. Thus, developmental psychology, psychiatry, and relevant therapists are an essential part of an epilepsy surgery program for children.

Since reversing major regression is unlikely, parental counseling regarding parental expectations for surgery is indicated.[36] It is important to recognize the desperate and vulnerable state of many parents who had the normal baby they were expecting and who responded to them. Then, within a short-time seizures began and the baby with whom they were bonding is "lost" and replaced by an unresponsive, unhappy child with intractable seizures. In these circumstances, it is important that while recognizing the urgency, parents have the opportunity to fully understand the evidence. This may be given in small amounts, at short intervals with a member of the team to listen to their concerns. A written account of the proposed surgery is important.

There are parent support groups for several of these conditions, which may be accessed. If a young child is severely regressed with a high rate of seizures/seizure activity, they may reveal their behavioral problems if successfully relieved of seizures by medical or surgical treatment.

There is increasing evidence of improved development following surgery[37,38] but this must be balanced by the recognition that severe regression is rarely reversible with the exception of some patients with LKS. Thus, the major aim is early seizure relief, so that the majority of the child's childhood and later life will not be dominated by seizures. However, the rate of seizure relief ranges from below 50% in hemispherectomy for hemimegalencephaly to over 80% in the same procedure for other pathologies.

It is therefore clear that we are either operating too late to prevent or reverse regression or surgery is not sufficient to achieve this end. As suggested earlier, we must be looking for young children, particularly under 1 year with operable focal epilepsy and begin to treat them urgently to attempt to prevent regression.

REFERENCES

1. Arsanow RF, et al. Developmental outcomes in children receiving resection surgery for medically intractable infantile spasms. *Dev Med Child Neurol* 1997;39:430–440.
2. Jonas R, et al. Cerebral hemispherectomy; hospital course seizure, developmental, language and motor outcomes. *Neurology* 2004;62:1712–1721.
3. Engel J Jr. A proposed diagnostic scheme for people with epileptic seizures and with epilepsy: Report of the ILAE Task Force on Classification and Terminology. International League Against Epilepsy (ILAE). *Epilepsia* 2001;42:796–803.
4. Duchowny M, et al. Epilepsy surgery in the first three years of life. *Epilepsia* 1998;39:737–743.
5. Harvey AS, Cross JH, Shinnar S, Mather GM, The Paediatric Epilepsy Surgery Survey Taskforce. Defining the spectrum of international practice in paediatric epilepsy surgery patients. *Epilepsia* 2008;49:146–155.
6. Kwan P, Brodie MJ. Early identification of refractory epilepsy. *New Eng J Med* 2000;342:314–319.
7. Coppola G, Plouin P, Chiron C, Robain O, Dulac O. Migrating partial seizures in infancy: a malignant disorder with developmental arrest. *Epilepsia* 1995;36:1017–1024.
8. Ohtahara S, et al. The early infantile epileptic encephalopathy with suppression-burst: developmental aspects. *Brain Dev* 1997;9:371–376.
9. Schlumberger E, Dulac O, Plouin P. Early infantile syndrome(s) with suppression-burst: nosological considerations. In: Roger J, Bureau M, Dravet C, Dreifuss FE, Perret A, Wolf P (eds), *Epileptic Syndromes of Infancy, Childhood and Adolescence*. London: John Libbey, 1992; 2nd edn: pp. 35–42.
10. Dravet C, Roger J, Bureau M, Dalla Bernardina B. Myoclonic epilepsies in childhood. In: Akimoto H, et al (eds),

Advances in Epileptology:. XIIIth Epilepsy International Symposium. New York: Raven Press, 1982; pp. 135–140.

11. Claes L, Del-Favero J, Ceulemans B, Lagae L, Van Broeckhoven C, De Jonghe P. De novo mutations in the sodium-channel gene SCN1A causes severe myoclonic epilepsy of infancy. *Am J Hum Genet* 2001;68:1327–1332.

12. Baxter P. Vitamin responsive conditions in paediatric neurology: a clinical approach. In: Baxter P (ed), *International Review of Child Neurology Series.* London: Mac Keith Press, 2001; pp. 166–174.

13. Poley JR, Dumermuth G. EEG findings in patients with phenylketonuria before and during treatment with a low phenylalanine diet and in patients with some other inborn errors of metabolism. In: Holt KS, Coffey VP (eds), *Some Recent Advances in Inborn Errors of Metabolism.* Edinburgh: Churchill Livingstone, 1968; pp. 61–69.

14. Pascual JM, Wang D, Leucmberri B, Wang H, Mew X, Yang R, DeVivo DC. GLUT1 deficiency and other glucose transporter diseases. *Eur J Endocrinol* 2004;150:627–633.

15. Wolf B, et al. Biotinidase deficiency: the enzymatic defect in late-onset multiple carboxylase deficiency. *Clin Chim Acta* 1983a;135:273–281.

16. Aylett SE, Neville BGR, Cross JH, Boyd S, Chong WK, Kirkham FJ. Sturge–Weber syndrome: cerebral haemodynamics during seizure activity. *Dev Med Child Neurol* 1999;41(7):480–485.

17. Koo B, Hwang PA, Logan WJ. Infantile spasms: outcome and prognostic factors of cryptogenic and symptomatic groups. *Neurology* 1993;43:2322–2327.

18. Chevrie JJ, Aicardi J. Le prognostic psychique des spasms infanties traités par l'ACTH ou les corticoïdes. Analyse statistique de 78 cas suivis plus d'un an. *J Neurol Sci* 1971;12:351–357.

19. Rikonen R, Amnell G. Psychiatric disorders in children with earlier infantile spasms. *Dev Med Child Neurol* 1989;23:747–760.

20. Chugani HT, et al. Surgery for intractable infantile spasms: neuroimaging perspectives. *Epilepsia* 1993;34:764–771.

21. Eltze CM, Chong WK, Bhate S, Harding B, Neville B, Cross H. Taylor-type focal cortical dysplasia in infants: some MRI lesions almost disappear with maturation of myelination. *Epilepsia* 2005;46:1988–1992.

22. Chugani HT, et al. Infantile spasms I: PET identifies focal cortical dysgenesis in cryptogenic cases for surgical treatment. *Ann Neurol* 1990;27:406–413.

23. Raymond AA, Halpin SFS, Alsanjari N, Cook MJ, Kitchen ND, Fish DR, Stevens JM, Harding BN, Saravilli F, Kendall B, Shorvon SD, Neville BGR. Dysembryoplastic neuroepithelial tumour: features in l6 patients. *Brain* 1994;117:461–475.

24. McLellan A, Davies S, Heyman I, Harding B, Harkness W, Taylor D, Neville BGR, Cross JH. Psychopathology in children with epilepsy before and after temporal lobe resection. *Dev Med Child Neurol* 2005;47:666–672.

25. Honavar M, Janota I, Polkey CE. Histological heterogeneity of dysembryoplastic neuroepithelial tumour: identification and differential diagnosis in a series of 74 cases. *Histopathology* 1999;34:342–356.

26. Neville BGR, Scott RC. Severe memory impairment in child with bihippocampal injury after status epilepticus. (*Letter*) *Dev Med Child Neurol* 2007;49:396–399.

27. Mikaeloff Y, Jambaque I, Hertz-Pannier L. Devastating epileptic encephalopathy in school-age children (DESC): a pseudo-encephalitis. *Epilepsy Res* 2006;69:67–69.

28. Gastaut H, Vigouroux M, Trevisan C, Régis H. Le syndrome Hémiconvulsions-Hémiplégie-Epilepsie (syndrome HHE). *Rev Neurol* 1957;97:37–52.

29. Dalmau J, Lancaster E, Martinez-Hernandez E, Rosenfeld MR, Balice-Gordon R. Clinical experience and laboratory investigations in patients with anti-NMDAR encephalitis. *Lancet Neurol* 2011;10:63–74.

30. Berkovic SF, et al. Hypothalamic hamartoma and seizures: a treatable epileptic encephalopathy. *Epilepsia* 2003;44: 969–973.

31. Procaccini E, Dorfmüller G, Fohlen M, Bulteau C, Delalande O. Surgical management of hypothalamic hamartomas with epilepsy: the steroendoscopic approach. *Neurosurgery* 2006;59:336–344.

32. Landau WM, Kleffner FR. Syndrome of acquired aphasia with convulsive disorder in children. *Neurology* 1957;7: 523–530.

33. Morrell F, Whistler WW, Bieck TP. Multiple subpial transection: a new approach to the surgical treatment of focal epilepsy. *J Neurosurg* 1989;70:231–239.

34. Robinson RO, Baird G, Robinson G, Smirnoff E. Landau–Kleffner syndrome: course and correlates with outcome. *Dev Med Child Neurol* 2001;43:243–247.

35. Cross JH, Neville BG. The surgical treatment of Landau–Kleffner syndrome. (Fifty years of Landau–Kleffner syndrome). *Epilepsia* 2009;50:63–67.

36. Taylor DC, Neville BGR, Cross JH. New measures of outcome needed for the surgical treatment of epilepsy [editorial]. *Epilepsia* 1997;38:625–630.

37. Freitag H, Tuxhorn I. Cognitive function in pre-school children after epilepsy surgery: rationale for early intervention. *Epilepsia* 2005;46:561–567.

38. Loddenkemper T, Holland KD, Stanford LD, Kotagal P, Bingaman W, Wyllie E. Developmental outcome after epilepsy surgery in infancy. *Pediatrics* 2007;119: 930–935.

CHAPTER 57

Vagus Nerve Stimulation

Prakash Kotagal

► INTRODUCTION

There is widespread consensus that recurrent epileptic seizures need treatment and the first line of treatment invariably involves use of antiepileptic drugs (AEDs). However, experience from several large studies has shown that only about two-thirds of patients can be controlled satisfactorily with AEDs either as monotherapy or combination therapy.[1,2] The remaining patients have medically refractory epilepsy and should be evaluated at an epilepsy center to determine if they may be candidates for excisional epilepsy surgery. Of this group approximately 25% will be offered a resection (personal observation), still leaving a sizeable proportion of patients without effective medical control. Seizures in medically refractory patients have a major impact on quality of life (QOL), and may result in injuries or even death.[3] Treatment options consist of additional trials of AEDs, ketogenic diet, or vagus nerve stimulation (VNS therapy). Deep brain stimulation remains investigational. Figure 57–1 outlines a treatment algorithm showing the diagnostic and therapeutic approach to a patient with epilepsy.

In 1987, the Food and Drug Administration (FDA) approved VNS therapy for the adjunctive treatment of partial onset seizures in patients 12 years and older. It has not undergone testing in clinical trials for patients younger than 12 or patients with other seizure types; however, postmarketing experience indicates that VNS is useful in such situations.

► MECHANISMS OF ACTION

VNS therapy stimulates the left vagus nerve that carries both myelinated and unmyelinated efferent (80%) and afferent (20%) fibers. The parasympathetic efferents are mostly unmyelinated and not much influenced by vagal nerve stimulation. The rationale for choosing the left vagus nerve is that it has fewer cardiac fibers supplying the SA node (although right side VNS implantation has been performed). However, McGregor et al have shown that right-sided VNS implantation is also safe and efficacious.[4] Ascending fibers from the vagus nerve reach the nucleus of the Tractus Solitarius; from there widespread projections reach the limbic, reticular, and autonomic regions of the brain as well as other brain stem nuclei like the locus coeruleus and raphe magnocellularis that CSF influence serotonin and norepinephrine levels.[5] Lesioning the LC appears to abolish the antiepileptic effect of VNS.

VNS in monkeys was shown to abort generalized convulsive seizures induced with pentylenetetrazole; this effect persisted beyond the time of actual stimulation.[6,7] Studies in humans have shown reduction of interictal spike discharges and prolongation of the interspike interval.[8] In addition, VNS is accompanied by a bilateral increase in blood flow to the thalamus, the hypothalamus, and the insular cortex and a bilateral decrease in blood flow to the amygdala, hippocampus, and posterior cingulate gyri. The reduction in thalamic blood flow was shown to correlate with seizure reduction.[9,10] GABA receptor plasticity may also contribute to reduced epileptogenesis.[11] In patients with depression, VNS increased glucose metabolism in the orbitofrontal cortex, cingulate gyrus, and insula.[12]

► INDICATIONS

Currently, the only FDA-approved indication is for treatment of patients 12 years and older with partial onset seizures (with or without secondary generalization) that are refractory to antiepileptic medications. Off-label use, (i.e., not approved by the FDA) in younger age groups and for other seizure types and epilepsy syndromes has been reported extensively in the literature. VNS therapy has also been investigated in adult patients with treatment-resistant depression.

► TECHNICAL PROCEDURE

The VNS therapy system consists of an implanted device or generator with electrodes or leads that attach to it. The generator contains a lithium battery and microprocessor sealed inside a titanium case (Fig. 57–2). The device delivers intermittent stimulation to the vagus nerve using preprogrammed settings that are adjusted using a programming wand attached to a handheld computer (Fig. 57–3). When placed over the device, the programming wand transmits the device settings magnetically.

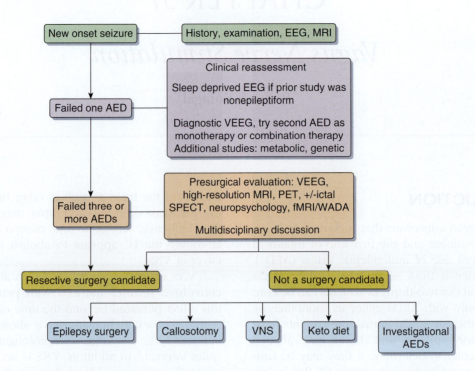

Figure 57–1. Treatment algorithm showing the diagnostic steps and therapeutic approach to a patient with epilepsy.

The generator can also be programmed to deliver a preset stimulus by bringing a small handheld magnet close to the device for 2–3 seconds and then removing it. This allows the patient (or nearby caregiver) to manually activate the device when he/she experiences an aura or the onset of a seizure. In about half, the patients magnet stimulation may abort a seizure, shorten its duration, and permit quicker recover after the seizure.

Typically the surgeon makes two incisions: one just below the left clavicle subcutaneously for device placement and a second horizontal incision in the neck bringing the lead (tunneled subcutaneously) from

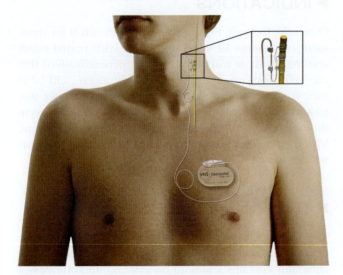

Figure 57–2. Schematic diagram of the device placement in the chest and lead around the left vagus nerve. The inset shows three spirals attached to the nerve: the cathode is proximal, anode distal and allowed to coil around the nerve; the lowermost or third loop is the anchoring tether. © Cyberonics

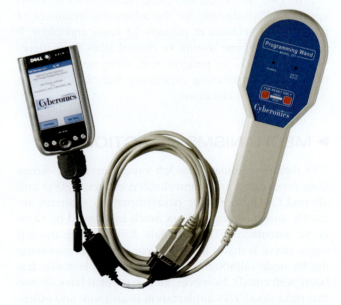

Figure 57–3. Programming wand and handheld computer used for interrogating and programming the vagus nerve stimulator. © Cyberonics

the device. In infants with little subcutaneous fat, the device may be placed in the soft tissue of the belly. The vagus nerve is exposed as it lies in the carotid sheath. The two stimulating leads are placed around the vagus nerve with the cathode proximal and anode distal and allowed to coil around the nerve; a third loop acts as the anchoring tether. A loop of wire is generally left in the chest to provide strain relief.

The original models 100 and 101 had two-pin leads whereas the Model 102 is a single-pin lead. Newer models have an expected battery life of 7–10 years, up from 3–5 years for the Model 100. Battery life is influenced by stimulus parameters and the lead impedance. The newest Model 103, the Demipulse® generator has a smaller footprint and advanced circuitry.

The device and lead are tested in the operating room before and after implantation and a lead test is carried out. There have been occasional reports of bradycardia or cardiac asystole during lead testing that is done with a higher current of 1 mA (compared to a lower starting current of 0.25 mA used for initial programming); however, patients can safely continue using the VNS.[13,14] The surgical procedure takes 2 hours or less and patients usually go home the same day or next morning. Absorbable sutures are used. Incisional pain is usually mild and patients may report a ticking sensation or cough when the device cycles on intermittently. The device may be turned on at the time of implantation or at an outpatient visit in 2 weeks.

▶ STIMULATION PARAMETERS AND PARADIGMS

Although there are differences in practice from one physician to another, the usual approach is generally to increase stimulus current stepwise every 3–4 weeks to a current intensity between 1and 2.5 mA (maximum allowable by the software is 3.5 mA). Next, the off-time is shortened from 5 to 3 minutes. Subsequently, one may try a signal frequency of 25 Hz or 20 Hz. If the patient has difficulty tolerating the stimulation due to coughing,

choking sensation, or dysphagia, the pulse width can be shortened from the usual 500 to 250 or 130 microseconds although the latter setting may be less than fully effective. With each stimulus current increase, the magnet current is also increased, keeping it 0.25 mA above the stimulus current—this allows the patient to receive a stronger current at the time of a seizure and may have the added benefit of allowing the patient to become habituated to this higher current. After each adjustment in the office, it is prudent to ask the patient to wait 30–60 minutes to make sure they are tolerating the new settings. Response to the changes in VNS settings take 2–4 weeks to take full effect, so more frequent adjustments at shorter intervals are not likely to help.

The ratio of the ON time plus 2 seconds ramp-up and 2 seconds ramp-down time divided by the OFF time is called the Duty Cycle (Fig. 57–4). The duty cycle should be kept below 40% (maximum allowable is 50%) to avoid the excessive stimulation and possible nerve damage. The ramp-up and ramp-down times help reduce patient perception of the intermittent nature of the vagus nerve stimulation. Table 57–1 shows commonly used settings found to be efficacious.

Device malfunction leading to excessive or continuous stimulation leading to vocal cord injury is exceedingly rare. In case of extreme discomfort, the patient can turn off the device by affixing the hand-held magnet to the chest overlying (with tape) until they can be evaluated in the doctor's office. At each visit, a diagnostic check should be performed that gives additional information regarding model number, serial number, date of implantation, how long the device has been in use, number and time of magnet activations, lead impedance, and whether the battery is approaching the end of its useful life.

The VNS programming software displays a number called DC–DC code as a measure of lead impedance, expressed as a numerical value between 0 and 7 with each number equivalent to 2000 ohms. A DC–DC code of 0, 1, or 2 (impedance <4000 ohms) is desirable whereas a number higher than 4 indicates problems with the lead interface, a fractured lead, or surrounding

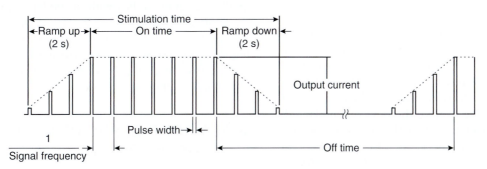

Figure 57–4. Diagram illustrating the various parameters, which may be adjusted for VNS therapy.

► **TABLE 57-1.** TYPICAL DEVICE SETTINGS USED FOR VNS THERAPY IN CHILDREN AND ADOLESCENTS. IN ADDITION, MAGNET-ACTIVATED SETTINGS ARE ALSO PREPROGRAMMED WITH THE CURRENT TO BE DELIVERED AND ITS DURATION. STIMULUS INTENSITY IS NORMALLY INCREASED IN STEPS OF 0.25 mA AT EACH VISIT TO AVOID PATIENT DISCOMFORT

Parameter	Typical Settings	Range
Stimulus intensity	1–2.5 mA	0.25–3.5 mA
Signal frequency	25 or 30 Hz	1–30 Hz
Pulse width	250 or 500 µs	130, 250, 500, 750, or 1000 µs
Signal on time	30 s	7–60 s
Signal off time	5 min	0.2 –180 min

fibrosis. Higher lead impedance results in inadequate stimulation to the nerve with loss of efficacy and faster depletion of the battery. Documentation of the settings and changes made at each visit should be carefully recorded. At each visit, the device is interrogated to verify the settings (if they have changed from what was programmed at the last visit, the cause needs to be investigated)—this has been known to occur when the device battery is nearing its End of Service (EOS). Similarly, the device should be interrogated just prior to the end of the office visit.

AEDs are not generally reduced during the initial months after VNS implantation. As seizures become better controlled, gradual withdrawal of ineffective AEDs may be possible. The majority of patients will need to remain on one AED, although rare patients may elect to be on VNS as their sole epilepsy therapy.

An indication that the battery is nearing the end of its useful life may take the form of:

1. an increase in seizures for which no other explanation such as noncompliance or a fall in AED levels;
2. device settings noted to be different from settings programmed at the previous visit (this occurs because the device attempts to deliver the same current intensity at the expense of other parameters);
3. during interrogation, the programming software flashes an "End of Service" message, which occurs when the device has about 3 months of useful life left.

If the VNS device battery is nearing the "End of Service" and the patient and doctor choose to continue VNS therapy, it is preferable to replace the device without waiting for the battery to be completely discharged as there could be a delay or loss of efficacy.[15] About 70% of patients choose to have the device reimplanted, which is much higher than that the retention rate for most AEDs.[16] Diagnostic checks are also recommended to be performed every 6 months: *normal mode testing* is done with the current intensity already being used while the *lead test* is done at 1 mA. It should be remembered that if the patient is presently at a lower current intensity, the lead test may cause undue patient discomfort.

► SAFETY CONCERNS

Since magnetic signals are used to program the VNS device settings, exposure to magnetic fields would cause the device to turn on and deliver a "magnet stimulation." Therefore prior to the patient undergoing a MRI scan, the VNS device has to be turned off by adjusting both the stimulus current and magnet current to zero (and turned back to the previous settings after the MRI scan). This still does not prevent electrical currents being induced in the lead if subjected to a changing magnetic field. According to the manufacturer "magnetic resonance imaging (MRI) should not be performed with a magnetic resonance body coil in the transmit mode. The heat induced in the Lead by an MRI body scan can cause injury. If an MRI should be done, use only a transmit-and-receive type of head coil. MRI compatibility was demonstrated using a 1.5T General Electric Signa Imager with a Model 100 only."[17] Implanting a VNS device will generally preclude patients from functional MRI studies as they are typically done in 3T machines. However, Sucholeiki et al showed that it is possible to perform functional MRI studies on a patient who has a VNS using a 1.5 Tesla scanner.[18]

These limitations should be discussed with the patient and family before proceeding with VNS implantation. It is recommended that patients first have good quality imaging studies with an epilepsy protocol and a presurgical evaluation to identify whether they would be suitable candidates for resective surgery that has a higher chance of seizure-free. Diathermy should not be used during surgical procedures in a patient implanted with the VNS therapy system.

► ADVERSE EFFECTS AND COMPLICATIONS

Complications of the implantation procedure are relatively uncommon and usually minor. Superficial or deep infections occur in about 3%–5% of patients.[19–21] Mild cases resolve with antibiotic treatment but the majority of patients require device and lead removal. Lead fractures, sometimes the result of external trauma to the neck may require lead replacement. Rare reports of vocal cord paralysis are mentioned. Incorrect placement of the lead has resulted in shoulder twitching or torticollis.[22–24]

In the initial few weeks following implantation, patients may complain of throat discomfort, hoarseness, or coughing when the device cycles on but these invariably resolve down. A change in voice quality during stimulation is often present long term in most patients. Instances of device failure are extremely rare. Increased drooling and dysphagia are common in patients with preexisting difficulties. Shortening the pulse width from 500 to 250 or 125 microseconds may help. Sleep apnea or worsening of sleep apnea symptoms has also been noted. Although generally mild, care should be taken to screen for sleep apnea prior to implantation and if found to treat that prior to implantation. Lowering stimulus frequency, shortening pulse width, and decreasing stimulus intensity are beneficial.[19,25] Sleep apnea symptoms may respond to CPAP therapy.[26] A few patients report dyspnea without any change in pulmonary function.

▶ EFFICACY OF VNS

Efficacy was demonstrated in two randomized, placebo-controlled double-blind trials (EO3 and EO5), which showed a median seizure reduction of 24.5% with high stimulation versus 6.1% for the low stimulation group. Fifty percent seizure reduction was noted in 31% of the high-stimulation group compared with 13% for the low-stimulation group when evaluated at 3 months.[27,28] Longer term follow-up of this cohort showed improving efficacy up to 24 months, with 35% of patients experiencing at least a 50% seizure reduction and 20% had at least 75% seizure reduction.[29] These studies included adolescents as well as adults.

DiGiorgio et al compared three stimulation paradigms: a conventional 30 seconds on per 3 minutes off, 30 seconds on per 30 seconds off, and 7 seconds on per 14 seconds off (rapid cycling). The number of patients showing more than 50% seizure reduction was the same in all three arms, but there were more patients showing a 75% reduction in the group receiving 30 seconds on per 3 minutes off; they also showed a response as early as 1 month compared to the other two groups. The authors concluded that a more conventional paradigm is superior initially but a rapid cycling should be instituted if there is not a good response by 3 months.[30] Labiner and Ahern have extensively reviewed the various therapeutic parameter settings for VNS.[31] Morris

retrospectively analyzed the effect of magnet stimulation in patients who had been enrolled in the clinical trials. Magnet stimulation resulted in seizure termination for 22% of patients and seizure diminution for 31% of patients.[32]

A retrospective, multicenter study of 125 children and adolescents (41 younger than 12 years) showed median seizure reduction of 51% at 3 months and 6 months. Similar seizure reduction was noted in children younger than 12 years.[33] This group included patients with partial and generalized epilepsies. Response was better in those with symptomatic generalized epilepsy and patients who had failed corpus callosotomy or other epilepsy surgeries. The median value for stimulus current was only 1.25 mA. Improvements in QOL were also seen and unrelated to seizure response. Murphy et al reported 100 children who received VNS therapy. Forty-five percent had more than 50% seizure reduction and 18% had no seizures for the last 6 months of the study.[34] Several other series have also reported more than 50% of patients having greater than 50% seizure reduction.[20,35]

A retrospective study of 42 children and adolescents from our center examined results with VNS therapy.[36] Twenty patients (43.5%) had more than 75% seizure-frequency reduction while five patients (10.1%) were seizure-free for more than 6 months by their last follow-up. No response (<50% seizure reduction or worsening) was noted in 19/46 (41.3%). We noted that younger children responded better than adolescents, who in turn did better adults reported in the literature—perhaps a reflection of brain plasticity. Similarly, Saneto[37] reported 43 children younger than 12 years, of whom more than half had 50% seizure reduction and 37% had 90% seizure reduction. Janszky et al noted that the absence of bilateral interictal epileptiform discharges correlated with a favorable outcome.[38]

Wilfong found good results in 6/7 girls with Rett's syndrome.[39] Patients with Tuberous Sclerosis also appear to do quite well with more than half achieving a 90% seizure reduction.[40,41] However, not all reports of VNS therapy in childhood epilepsy are favorable; Parker and colleagues noted that only 4/16 children had a worthwhile seizure reduction, although a much larger percentage reported improvement in QOL domains.[42] Kossoff has observed that children on the ketogenic diet receiving vagus nerve stimulation do better than with either therapy alone suggesting a synergistic effect.[43] Vagus nerve stimulation and corpus callosotomy both produced good seizure reduction in patients with Lennox–Gastaut syndrome.[44] Since corpus callosotomy is a major and irreversible procedure, it is preferable to try VNS first. A similar argument may be made for children with refractory epilepsy due to hypothalamic hamartoma in whom surgery carries major operative risks.[45] VNS was also been found efficacious for patients with medically resistant primary generalized epilepsy.[46,47]

A unique and remarkable aspect of VNS therapy is the finding that a large number of patients show improvement in mood, alertness, and interaction following implantation, even if they have not had a significant seizure reduction. This could be due to improved mood, fewer seizures, improvement in sleep architecture, and reduction of interictal spiking.[48–50]

► WHAT IF VNS THERAPY FAILS

Typically, it takes about 1 year for the epileptologist to make stepwise increments in current intensity, then change the on/off settings and finally to adjust signal frequency before it can be concluded that VNS therapy is ineffective. This concept is analogous to AED therapy where gradual introduction of a drug and titration to maximally tolerated doses is recommended. It has been shown that over a period of 24 months more patients show a decrease in seizures. Not uncommonly when the device is turned off at the request of the patient or physician, seizure exacerbation occurs 2–4 weeks later, suggesting that VNS therapy was probably having a therapeutic effect. Some patients undergo explanation of the device prior to undergoing high-resolution MRI studies as part of an evaluation for resective epilepsy surgery. Removal of the lead is tedious and difficult due to the presence of surrounding fibrosis but can be done safely in most instances.[51]

► ECONOMIC CONSIDERATIONS

Vagus nerve stimulation is not first-line therapy and most neurologists considering VNS therapy should have tried at least two or more AEDs and documented that the patient indeed has intractable epilepsy. A presurgical evaluation and good quality MRI should be done to determine whether resective epilepsy surgery is possible. Many such patients have disabling seizures impacting their QOL and resulting in frequent emergency room visits or hospitalizations, leading to high direct and indirect costs for care. VNS device and lead implantation costs about $25,000 to $30,000, the cost of hardware accounting for most of the expense. Frequent visit are needed, especially in the first 2 years. The longevity of the device battery and leads has to be taken into account as well, given that the average battery life is approximately 7 years, depending upon the settings. Several studies have shown that medical costs decrease following VNS implantation making this a cost-effective therapeutic intervention.[52]

► SUMMARY

Vagus nerve stimulation is a well-established epilepsy treatment for children and adults with intractable epilepsy. Patients whose seizures are not coming under control should undergo careful evaluation to verify that they indeed have epilepsy and have been treated appropriately with AEDs. A presurgical evaluation is advisable to find whether resective epilepsy surgery would not be a better option. Patients should have good quality imaging with epilepsy protocols and screened for sleep apnea before being implanted with a VNS device. VNS therapy is unique in that it is effective for a wide variety of epilepsies in both young children and adult patients and unlike AEDs is free of cognitive, behavioral side effects, or metabolic consequences.

REFERENCES

1. Kwan P, Brodie MJ. Early identification of refractory epilepsy. *N Engl J Med* 2000;342:314–319.
2. Kwan P, Sperling MR. Refractory seizures: try additional antiepileptic drugs (after two have failed) or go directly to early surgery evaluation? *Epilepsia* 2009;50(Suppl 8): 57–62.
3. Beghi E. Accidents and injuries in patients with epilepsy. *Expert Rev Neurother* 2009;9:291–298.
4. McGregor A, Wheless J, Baumgartner J, Bettis D. Right-sided vagus nerve stimulation as a treatment for refractory epilepsy in humans. *Epilepsia* 2005;46:91–96.
5. Ben-Menachem E, et al. Effects of vagus nerve stimulation on amino acids and other metabolites in the CSF of patients with partial seizures. *Epilepsy Res* 1995;20:221–227.
6. McLachlan RS. Suppression of interictal spikes and seizures by stimulation of the vagus nerve. *Epilepsia* 1993;34: 918–923.
7. Takaya M, Terry WJ, Naritoku DK. Vagus nerve stimulation induces a sustained anticonvulsant effect. *Epilepsia* 1996;37: 1111–1116.
8. Koo B. EEG changes with vagus nerve stimulation. *J Clin Neurophysiol* 2001;18:434–441.
9. Henry TR, et al. Brain blood flow alterations induced by therapeutic vagus nerve stimulation in partial epilepsy I. Acute effects at high and low levels of stimulation. *Epilepsia* 1998;39:983–990.
10. Henry TR, et al. Acute blood flow changes and efficacy of vagus nerve stimulation in partial epilepsy. *Neurology* 1999;52:1166–1173.
11. Marrousu F, et al. Correlation between GABA (A) receptor density and vagus nerve stimulation in individuals with drug-resistant partial epilepsy. *Epilepsy Res* 2003;55: 59–70.
12. Conway CR, Sheline YI, Chibnall JT, George MS, Fletcher JW, Mintun MA. Cerebral blood flow changes during vagus nerve stimulation for depression. *Psychiatry Res* 2006;146:179–184.
13. Asconape JJ, et al. Bradycardia and asystole with the use of vagus nerve stimulation for the treatment of epilepsy: a rare complication of intraoperative device testing. *Epilepsia* 1999;40:1452–1454.

14. Ali II, Pirzada NA, Kanjwal Y, Wannamaker B, Medhkour A, Koltz MT, Vaughn BV. Complete heart block with ventricular asystole during left vagus nerve stimulation for epilepsy. *Epilepsy Behav* 2004;5:768–771.

15. Vonck K, Dedeurwaerdere S, De Groote L, Thadani V, Claeys P, Gossiaux F, Van Roost D, Boon P. Generator replacement in epilepsy patients treated with vagus nerve stimulation. *Seizure* 2005;14:89–99.

16. Ben-Menachem E. Vagus-nerve stimulation for the treatment of epilepsy. *Lancet Neurol* 2002;1:477–482.

17. Safety information. http://www.vnstherapy.com/Epilepsy/hcp/resourcecenter/safetyinformation.aspx, 2007.

18. Sucholeiki R, Alsaadi TM, Morris GL 3rd, Ulmer JL, Biswal B, Mueller WM. fMRI in patients implanted with a vagal nerve stimulator. *Seizure* 2002;11:157–162.

19. Khurana DS, Reumann M, Hobdell EF, Neff S, Valencia I, Legido A, Kothare SV. Vagus nerve stimulation in children with refractory epilepsy: unusual complications and relationship to sleep-disordered breathing. *Childs Nerv Syst* 2007;23:1309–1312.

20. Kabir SM, Rajaram C, Rittey C, Zaki HS, Kemeny AA, McMullan J. Vagus nerve stimulation in children with intractable epilepsy: indications, complications and outcome. *Childs Nerv Syst* 2009;25:1097–1100.

21. Air EL, Ghomri YM, Tyagi R, Grande AW, Crone K, Mangano FT. Management of vagal nerve stimulator infections: do they need to be removed? *J Neurosurg Pediatr* 2009;3:73–78.

22. Smyth MD, et al. Complications of chronic vagus nerve stimulation for epilepsy in children. *J Neurosurg* 2003;99:200–203.

23. Wheless JW. Vagus nerve stimulation therapy in pediatric patients: use and effectiveness. In: Pellock JM, Bourgeois BFD, Dodson WE, Nordli DR, Sankar R (eds), *Pediatric Epilepsy: Diagnosis and Therapy.* Demos Medical, 2008; 3rd edn: pp. 811–827.

24. Patwardhan RV, Stong B, Bebin EM, Mathisen J. Grabb PA. Efficacy of vagal nerve stimulation in children with medically refractory epilepsy. *Neurosurgery* 2000;47:1357–1358.

25. Holmes MD, Chang M, Kapur V. Sleep apnea and excessive daytime somnolence induced by vagal nerve stimulation. *Neurology* 2003;61:1126–1129.

26. Hsieh T, Chen M, McAfee A, Kifle Y. Sleep-related breathing disorder in children with vagal nerve stimulators. *Pediatr Neurol* 2008;38:99–103.

27. The Vagus Nerve Stimulation Study Group. A randomized clinical trial of chronic vagus nerve stimulation for treatment of medically intractable epilepsy. *Neurology* 1995;45:224–230.

28. Handforth A, et al. Vagus nerve stimulation of partial-onset seizures: a randomized active-control trial. *Neurology* 1998; 51:48–55.

29. DeGiorgio CM, et al. Prospective long-term study of vagus nerve stimulation for the treatment of seizures. *Epilepsia* 2000;41:1195–1200.

30. DeGiorgio C, Heck C, Bunch S, Britton J, Green P, Lancman M, Murphy J, Olejniczak P, Shih J, Arrambide S, Soss J. Vagus nerve stimulation for epilepsy: randomized comparison of three stimulation paradigms. *Neurology* 2005;65:317–319.

31. Labiner DM, Ahern GL. Vagus nerve stimulation therapy in depression and epilepsy: therapeutic parameter settings. *Ann Neurol Scand* 2007;115:23–33.

32. Morris GL. A retrospective analysis of the effects of magnet-activated stimulation in conjunction with vagus nerve stimulation therapy. *Epilepsy Behav* 2003;4:740–745.

33. Helmers SL, et al. Vagus nerve stimulation therapy in pediatric patients with refractory epilepsy: retrospective study. *J Child Neurol* 2001;16:843–848.

34. Murphy JV, et al. Vagal nerve stimulation in refractory epilepsy: the first 100 children receiving vagal nerve stimulation at a pediatric epilepsy center. *Arch Pediatr Adolesc Med* 2003;157:560–564.

35. Shahwan A, Bailey C, Maxiner W, Harvey AS. Vagus nerve stimulation for refractory epilepsy in children: More to VNS than seizure frequency reduction. *Epilepsia* 2009;50: 1220–1228.

36. Alexopoulos AV, Kotagal P, Loddenkemper T, Hammel J, Bingaman WE. Long-term results with vagus nerve stimulation in children with pharmacoresistant epilepsy. *Seizure* 2006;15:491–503.

37. Saneto RP, Sotero de Menezes MA, Ojemann JG, Bournival BD, Murphy PJ, Cook WB, Avellino AM, Ellenbogen RG. Vagus nerve stimulation for intractable seizures in children. *Pediatr Neurol* 2006;35:323–326.

38. Janszky J, Hoppe M, Behne F, Tuxhorn I, Pannek HW, Ebner A. Vagus nerve stimulation: predictors of seizure freedom. *J Neurol Neurosurg Psychiatry* 2005;76: 384–389.

39. Wilfong AA, Schultz RJ. Vagal nerve stimulation for the treatment of epilepsy in Rett syndrome. *Dev Med Child Neurol* 2006;48:683–686.

40. Parain D, et al. Vagal nerve stimulation in tuberous sclerosis complex patients. *Pediatr Neurol* 2001;25:213–216.

41. Major P, Thiele EA. Vagus nerve stimulation for intractable epilepsy in tuberous sclerosis complex. *Epilepsy Behav* 2008;13:357–360.

42. Parker APJ, et al. Vagal nerve stimulation in epileptic encephalopathies. *Pediatrics* 1999;103:778–782.

43. Kossoff EH, et al. Combined ketogenic diet and vagus nerve stimulation: rational polytherapy? *Epilepsia* 2007; 48:77–81.

44. You SJ, Kang HC, Ko TS, Kim HD, Yum MS, Hwang YS, Lee JK, Kim DS, Park SK. Comparison of corpus callosotomy and vagus nerve stimulation in children with Lennox–Gastaut syndrome. *Brain Dev* 2008;30:195–199.

45. Murphy JV, Wheless JW, Schmoll CM. Left vagal nerve stimulation in six patients with hypothalamic hamartomas. *Pediatr Neurol* 2000;23:167–168.

46. Farrag A, Pestana E, Kotagal P. Vagal nerve stimulation for refractory absence seizures. *Epilepsia* 2002;43(Suppl 7): 79–80.

47. Ng M, Devinsky O. Vagus nerve stimulation for refractory idiopathic generalised epilepsy. *Seizure* 2004;13:176–178.

48. Hallbook T, Lundgren J, Kohler S, Blennow G, Stromblad LG, Rosen I. Beneficial effects of vagus nerve stimulation in children with therapy resistant epilepsy. *Eur J Ped Neurol* 2005a;9:399–407.

49. Hallbook T, Lundgren J, Stjernqvist K, Blennow G, Stromblad LG, Rosen I. Vagus nerve stimulation in 15 children with therapy resistant epilepsy; its impact on

cognition, quality of life, behaviour and mood. *Seizure* 2005b;14:504–513.

50. Hallbook T, Blennow G, Lundgren J, Stromblad LG, Rosen I. Long term effects on epileptiform activity with vagus nerve stimulation in children. *Seizure* 2005c;14:527–533.

51. Espinosa J, Aiello MT, Naritoku DK. Revision and removal of stimulating electrodes following long-term therapy with the vagus nerve stimulator. *Surg Neurol* 1999;51: 659–664.

52. Boon P, D'Havé M, Van Walleghem P, Michielsen G, Vonck K, Caemaert J, de Reuck J. Direct medical costs of refractory epilepsy incurred by three different treatment modalities: a prospective assessment. *Epilepsia* 2002; 43:96–102.

CHAPTER 58

Comorbidities of Surgical Treatment

Ailsa McLellan

▶ INTRODUCTION

Epilepsy surgery is an extremely effective therapeutic option for many children with drug-resistant epilepsy. In medically resistant children, the likelihood that further antiepileptic drugs (AEDs) will significantly reduce seizure frequency is less than 10%, whereas surgery leads to seizure freedom in 40–90% of appropriately selected cases, depending on the degree of resection, underlying pathology, and operative procedure. In addition, other positive postoperative outcomes are arguably considered more important and include enhanced development and behavior and improved quality of life.

Epilepsy surgery is not without risk and there is a rare risk of mortality, which must be weighed against the risk of mortality of continual seizures and potential benefits of successful surgery. There are also several surgical complications, some of which may be anticipated, such as a visual field defect following hemispherectomy, whereas others are unexpected. Rarely, there may be postoperative deterioration in other comorbid domains, namely behavior, cognition, and quality of life, all of which have significant implications for the child and family. This chapter will address the mortality and comorbidities associated with epilepsy surgery in children.

▶ MORTALITY

Historically, there has been a significant risk of mortality associated with neurosurgery in children, including epilepsy surgery. However, with improved surgical technique, anesthesia and postoperative care, the development of dedicated epilepsy surgery centers, and availability of new techniques of evaluation, this risk is now very low and generally estimated at 0–2%.[1] Children are at higher risk of mortality in epilepsy surgery than adults. Most reports of mortality in pediatric epilepsy surgery describe isolated cases in large surgical series.[2–5]

Causes of early postoperative death include infections, hydrocephalus, dehydration, hemorrhage, and allergic reactions. Most mortalities related to epilepsy surgery occur in children younger than 3 years.[4] Infants have a greater risk due to their relatively small blood volume and the development of coagulopathy following hemorrhage in surgery.[6,7] Young hemispherectomy candidates have the highest mortality. Anatomical hemispherectomy is associated with even greater mortality due to intraoperative blood loss and of the potential for late hemosiderosis (resulting from numerous acute and chronic hemorrhages from the fragile capillaries in the subdural membrane), obstructed hydrocephalus, bleeding into the hemispherectomy cavity, and progressive brain stem shift.[8] Newer functional hemispherectomy techniques involving initial tissue removal followed by disconnection of remaining structures require a shorter operating time and are associated with reduced blood loss and are therefore associated with lower mortality and morbidity than anatomical hemispherectomy procedure. However, risk of mortality in hemispherectomy remains higher than for other epilepsy surgery procedures. Hemispherectomy for hemimegalencephaly is associated with the highest risk of mortality compared with other pathologies (Rasmussen's, infarct/ischemia) due to the more complex surgery (related to the enlarged megalencephalic hemisphere and distorted anatomical landmarks), longer operative time, and greater blood loss.[3]

The overall low risk of mortality from epilepsy surgery must be balanced against its benefits (seizure freedom, improved development/cognitive potential, and enhanced quality of life) and risk for death due to chronic epilepsy. Children with epilepsy have a high standardized mortality rate reported at 7–13.2.[9] Children with epilepsy die for a variety of reasons but most commonly as a result of comorbid neurological deficits rather than as a direct result of their epilepsy.[10,11] There are no studies comparing long-term mortality rates in surgically versus medically treated pediatric patients; thus, it is unclear whether successful surgery actually reduces mortality for children with epilepsy. Several adult studies have addressed this issue, but the data is conflicting. However, overall it is widely believed that mortality rates are lower and approach normal mortality rates in patients who are seizure free postoperatively[12] than in patients with continuing seizures.

All families should therefore be counseled about the risk of mortality prior to surgery, albeit small overall and appropriate emphasis given to families of children who are at higher risk, that is, children younger than 3 years who are undergoing hemispherectomy, particularly for hemimegalencephaly.

▶ SURGICAL MORBIDITY

All epilepsy surgery procedures are associated with blood loss, which varies by procedure. Blood loss during focal or lobar resection is approximately 200 to 500 mL, whereas losses in anatomic hemispherectomy often exceed 1500 mL.[7] Infants are at particular risk of significant blood loss for several reasons. First, the volume of cardiac output to the brain is proportionally larger in infants than in older children due to the larger ratio of brain weight compared with body weight. Second, the circulating blood volume in infants is much smaller than in older children and adults. Third, infants more commonly undergo extensive hemispheric surgery, which is associated with larger relative blood loss. When an infant has had significant blood loss, there is a higher probability of postoperative coagulopathy and further hemorrhage. Blood loss is managed with volume replacement, blood transfusion, and, in the case of large hemorrhage, with concomitant use of other blood products.

Epilepsy surgery has an overall infection rate of 2–3%. Infections include wound infections, meningitis, and osteomyelitis of the bone flap. Most wound infections are managed with antibiotics, but it may occasionally be necessary to debride or re-explore the wound. Should osteomyelitis develop, it may be necessary to remove the bone flap and perform a cranioplasty. Chronic invasive monitoring is associated with higher rates of infection ranging from 2% to 16%.[13]

Invasive monitoring is associated with cerebrospinal fluid (CSF) leaks in 19–33% of patients, 2–14% experience cerebral edema, 0–16% develop subdural hematoma, and 9% have an intracerebral hemorrhage. Figure 58–1 shows an intracranial hematoma overlying a subdural grid. Isolated cases of permanent neurological morbidity and death have been reported.[14] However, the complications of invasive monitoring need to be balanced against the benefits of epilepsy surgery for this selective group, and though rates of complications are higher than for children having resective surgery without invasive monitoring, significant improvements in seizure outcome are reported in up to 80% of cases.[15]

Neurological complications of epilepsy surgery can be broadly classified into anticipated neurological sequelae or unexpected neurological morbidity. Neurological deficits resulting from resections involving sensorimotor and visual cortex are generally anticipated and discussed with the family prior to surgery. Many unanticipated neurological deficits such as those related to edema are transient and may fully recover with time.

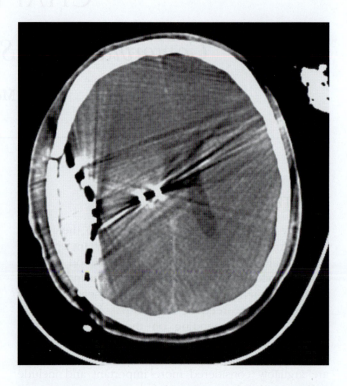

Figure 58–1. Intracranial hematoma overlying a grid.

Typical anticipated neurological sequelae following hemispherectomy include homonymous hemianopia (if not present preoperatively), quadrantanopic field defects following temporal lobectomy, hemiparesis (if not already present) in hemispherectomy, and deterioration in hand function (if well preserved prior to hemispherectomy).

After focal resection, 0–10% of patients have permanent sequelae including hemiplegia, homonymous hemianopia, quadrantanopia, and dysphasia.[1] Some children experience a worsening of their hemiparesis after hemispherectomy while others may be unchanged or improved.[16,17] Children undergoing corpus callosotomy before puberty do not develop the typical disconnection deficits experienced by one-third of adults.[18] However, teenagers may experience this syndrome, particularly after total callosotomy, but this often improves over time.

Greater plasticity of the central nervous system allows young children to better compensate for surgically induced deficits. However, although surgery to language dominant cortex should be avoided, it may be necessary in patients with tumors and/or hemispherectomy of the dominant hemisphere in Rasmussen's encephalitis. Reorganization of language, due to brain plasticity, to the nondominant hemisphere occurs robustly after surgery in early childhood, diminishes with advancing age, but may still be possible in adolescents.[19]

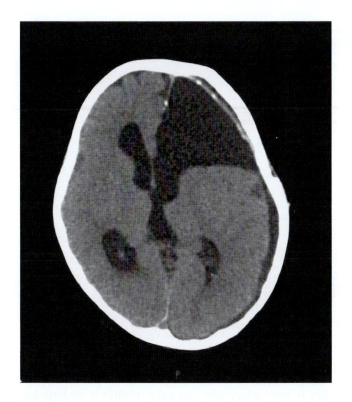

Figure 58–2. Hydrocephalus occurring after a left frontal resection.

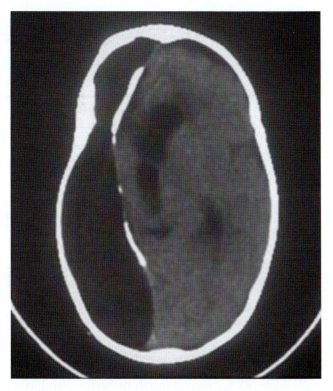

Figure 58–3. Hydrocephalus following anatomical hemispherectomy.

Single cases of hydrocephalus have been observed rarely after focal resections.[20,21] Figure 58–2 shows hydrocephalus occurring after a left frontal resection. Hemispherectomy is associated with higher rates of hydrocephalus and 8–33% of children will require shunt placement.[1] Hydrocephalus was much more common after anatomical hemispherectomy (Fig. 58–3) and the advent of hemispherectomy or functional hemispherectomy has greatly reduced this problem.

▶ POSTOPERATIVE SEIZURES

Acute postoperative seizures (APOSs) occurring in the first 7–14 days after surgery are thought to be due to local phenomena as a result of surgery, that is, hemorrhage and edema. The occurrence of postoperative seizures is often disappointing for the families and children but is not necessarily associated with a poor postoperative outcome. While children with APOS experience lower rates of postoperative seizure freedom, there is still a reasonable chance of a favorable surgical outcome. A report of 148 children undergoing epilepsy surgery found APOS in 25% of cases; 51% of these children had good long-term seizure control compared with 81% of children who had not experienced APOS.[22]

Further management options must be considered if seizures continue after the period of postoperative recovery (Fig. 58–4). Reevaluation for epilepsy surgery is appropriate for some children. Figure 58–5 demonstrates an incomplete frontal dissection in a child who underwent a functional hemispherectomy but continued to experience seizures. Completion of the dissection led to the child becoming seizure free. Other management options include change in AED regimen, institution of the ketogenic diet, or vagal nerve stimulator. Families and children require significant support in this situation.

▶ PSYCHOPATHOLOGY

Children with epilepsy have increased rates of mental health problems (28–58%) compared with the general population (7–9%) and children (11–12%) with chronic illnesses outside the central nervous system.[23,24] Psychiatric disorders can be more problematic than the seizures themselves and hugely impact quality of life. The range of psychiatric diagnoses seen in children with epilepsy includes conduct disorders, emotional disorders, attention deficit hyperactivity disorder, and pervasive developmental disorders. Children with structural brain abnormalities are at even higher risk with reported rates of 58% with a psychiatric diagnosis.[23] Children undergoing epilepsy surgery often have gross

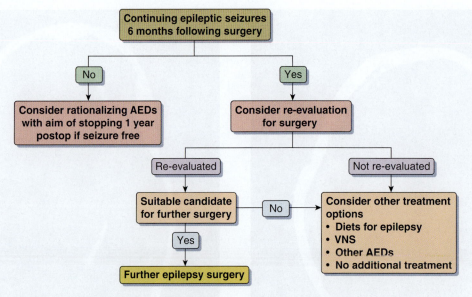

Figure 58–4. Algorithm for management of continuing epileptic seizures following surgery.

structural brain abnormalities and are therefore at especially high risk for mental health problems. Psychiatric disorders are reported in up to 83% of adults coming to epilepsy surgery[25] and up to 72% of children awaiting temporal lobectomy.[26]

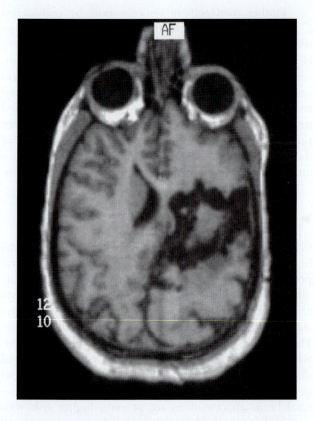

Figure 58–5. Incomplete frontal dissection following functional hemispherectomy.

While behavior may improve postoperatively,[26–28] this is not universally the case. Children undergoing hemispherectomy have better postoperative behavioral outcomes than children undergoing temporal lobectomy. Devlin reported improvement in behavior in 92% of children posthemispherectomy who had preoperative behavioral problems. Five children experienced new-onset behavioral problems postoperatively who had not previously experienced difficulties. The emergence of behavioral problems was not related to good seizure outcome as two children were seizure free and two had greater than 75% reduction in seizures.

Children undergoing temporal lobe resections have higher rates of preoperative psychiatric diagnoses than children with extratemporal lesions.

In a study of 60 children undergoing temporal lobectomy,[26] 83% of children had a psychiatric diagnosis at some stage—72% preoperatively and 72% postoperatively. The range of psychiatric disorders is summarized in Table 58–1. New psychiatric diagnoses emerged postoperatively in 22 (37%) and psychiatric symptoms deteriorated postoperatively in 15 (25%). There was no relationship between the emergence of new psychiatric diagnoses and seizure control as had been reported in an adult study of temporal lobectomy and mental health[29] or indeed a small series of 16 children undergoing temporal lobectomy.[28] Twenty percent of children developed emotional disorders postoperatively, the majority of who had normal cognition and were seizure free.

There is little information about postoperative psychiatric outcome after extratemporal lesions in children, but rates of mental health problems are lower than for

▶ **TABLE 58–1.** DSM-IV DIAGNOSIS PREOPERATIVELY, POSTOPERATIVELY, AND TOTAL AT ANY POINT IN CHILDREN UNDERGOING TEMPORAL LOBE SURGERY FOR EPILEPSY

Diagnoses	Preoperative (Total 60)	Postoperative (Total 57)	Affected at Any Time
PDD	23 (38%)	21 (37%)	23 (38%)
ADHD	14 (23%)	13 (23%)	16 (27%)
ODD/CD	13 (22%)	12 (21%)	16 (27%)
DBD	24 (40%)	25 (42%)	30 (50%)
Emotional disorder	5 (8%)	12 (21%)	15 (25%)
Eating disorder	1 (2%)	2 (4%)	2 (4%)
Conversion disorder	1 (2%)	1 (2%)	2 (4%)
Psychosis	0	1 (2%)	1 (2%)

PDD, pervasive developmental disorder; ADHD, attention deficit hyperactivity disorder; ODD/CD, oppositional defiant disorder/conduct disorder; DBD, disruptive behavior disorder.
From McLellan A, Davies S, Heyman I, et al. Psychopathology in children with epilepsy before and after temporal lobe resection. *Dev Med Child Neurol* 2005;47(10):666–672.

children undergoing temporal lobectomy. One study (JH Cross, PhD, written communication) has shown that in children undergoing extratemporal resections, one or more psychiatric diagnoses were present in 31/71 (44%) children preoperatively and 32/71 (45%) postoperatively. Mental health problems improved postoperatively in 8 (11%) children; in, 5 (7%) completely resolved; in 6/71 (9%) children with no preoperative diagnosis, a DSM-IV diagnoses evolved postoperatively. The nature of the psychiatric diagnoses is summarized in Table 58–2.

Children and families must be carefully counseled about mental health outcomes after epilepsy surgery and psychiatric assessment should be an integral part of a comprehensive epilepsy surgery program. Close liaison between the psychiatrist in the comprehensive epilepsy surgery program and local psychiatric services is crucial, as the local team will take the lead role in providing ongoing assessment and management of any mental health problems and link in more effectively to local pediatric services and education.

▶ NEUROPSYCHOLOGY

Cognitive impairment is common in children with epilepsy, and rates of learning disability in children undergoing epilepsy surgery are very high.[30–32] A major goal of epilepsy surgery is to improve overall cognitive development; however, there is little supporting prospective evidence. Some case series report improvement in developmental outcome, particularly after epilepsy surgery at a young age and in seizure-free patients, but there is a need for long-term prospective confirmation. The majority of children having epilepsy surgery do not have any significant change in their cognitive skills postoperatively.[1,33,34] There are, however, some reports of declines in cognitive skills and these will be reviewed by procedure.

The cognitive outcome following temporal lobe surgery for epilepsy has been examined more thoroughly than neuropsychological outcomes following other epilepsy surgery procedures. Several studies report no significant cognitive deterioration after temporal lobe

▶ **TABLE 58–2.** DSM-IV DIAGNOSES PRE- AND POSTOPERATIVELY IN CHILDREN UNDERGOING EXTRATEMPORAL RESECTIONS

Diagnoses	Preoperative, n (%)	Postoperative, n (%)	Lost Diagnosis Postop	Developed Diagnosis Postop	No Change
ADHD	4 (6)	7 (10)	0	3	4
ODD/CD	9 (13)	10 (14)	0	1	9
DBD (NOS)	4 (6)	4 (6)	1	1	3
Change of behavior due to a general medical condition	9 (13)	6 (9)	4	1	5
Emotional disorder	10 (14)	12 (17)	0	2	10
ASD	9 (13)	10 (14)	0	1	9
Other major disorder	2 (3)	3 (4)	0	1	2

ADHD, attention deficit hyperactivity disorder; ASD, autistic spectrum disorder; ODD/CD, oppositional defiant disorder/conduct disorder; DBD, disruptive behavior disorder; NOS, not otherwise specified.
From JH Cross, PhD, written communication.

resection.[1,35] However, despite the absence of demonstrable change in postoperative IQ, some children do not perform as well at school following surgery. Some children undergoing left-sided temporal lobe procedures for epilepsy experience deterioration in verbal learning performance and recall compared with preoperative levels[36,37]; children undergoing amygdalohippocampectomy appear to be at particular risk. However, significant recovery in verbal memory performance may occur 1 year postoperatively.[36] In contrast, postoperative deterioration in verbal memory in adults following left temporal lobe tends to persist.

One study comparing children and adults undergoing left temporal lobe surgery for epilepsy demonstrated that while adults and children both experienced deterioration in verbal learning capacity postoperatively, only the children recovered to their preoperative level 1 year following surgery. This was attributed to their greater plasticity and compensational capacity.[38]

Studies of cognitive outcome following hemispherectomy reveal little change from preoperative level with some reports of improvements or lack of continued developmental deterioration.[3,16,32] Rarely, patients experience minor deterioration in cognition.

There is limited data regarding neuropsychological outcome after extratemporal resection. Reports of neuropsychological outcome following frontal lobe resection suggest no significant deterioration in cognitive skills or language as long as Brodmann area 44 is avoided.[39] Further studies reveal small decreases in working memory and visuoconstructive skills following frontal lobectomy particularly in children who presented at an older age with epilepsy and underwent surgery in late childhood.[33] Parietal lobe and occipital lobe resection is less common, and information about the cognitive sequelae of surgery is extremely limited. Cognitive comorbidities following surgery in these regions are not clearly reported and larger studies are required to draw firm conclusions about risk of possible complications.

Neuropsychological function following corpus callosotomy is often enhanced, but there are isolated reports of deterioration in speech and verbal memory particularly in individuals with crossed dominance (e.g., right handedness and right hemisphere dominance for language)[40,41] and this might be a relative contraindication to a total callosotomy.

Significant persistent deterioration in neuropsychological profile is therefore unusual after epilepsy surgery in children. It is, however, important to have comprehensive neuropsychological evaluations pre- and postoperatively to detect specific cognitive defects that may not be identified on routine neuropsychology assessments, and which may have significant impact on school performance.

► QUALITY OF LIFE

There is an increasing understanding of health-related quality of life (HRQOL) for children with epilepsy. Children with epilepsy have poorer HRQOL than controls or children with nonneurological chronic health problems such as asthma;[42] these issues persist into adult life. Severity and duration of epilepsy, comorbidities (cognitive, behavioral, neurological), and number of AEDs are factors that particularly impair HRQOL[1] and are associated with medical intractability in surgical candidates.

There is an expectation that successful epilepsy surgery would improve HRQOL, but the evidence is controversial. Several studies demonstrate improvement in HRQOL if the child is seizure free following surgery,[43,44] but others reveal no change in HRQOL in children undergoing epilepsy surgery, even in children who become seizure free, compared with children with medically intractable epilepsy who were not surgical candidates.[34] The strongest predictor of HRQOL was baseline level of function.

Patients undergoing temporal lobe surgery later in life have a higher incidence of psychosocial, behavioral, and educational difficulties than patients undergoing earlier surgery.[45] While this observation supports the concept that earlier surgery might be associated with better psychosocial outcome, even epilepsy that has remitted in adult life may negatively impact HRQOL. Individuals with childhood epilepsy that remitted and were off AEDs had similar rates of employment and socioeconomic status as controls but lower rates of marriage and childbirth.[46] However, their HRQOL was better than those who continued to have epilepsy and were on AEDs.

There are difficulties in interpreting and comparing studies of HRQOL in children due to methodological problems and the numbers of different assessment tools used. This is an important area that requires further evaluation. Parents and children should be counseled that while an improvement in HRQOL may emerge postoperatively, this might not be the case, particularly in children with significant neurological and cognitive comorbidities.

► SUMMARY

Epilepsy surgery in children is an effective and generally safe treatment. There are many benefits of epilepsy surgery for children in addition to seizure control, including improved development, psychosocial function, and quality of life. There are, however, a number of morbidities associated with epilepsy surgery related to surgical complications, neurological sequelae, and negative impact of surgery on behavior and cognition, which may have detrimental effects on quality of life.

It is important that children are assessed for epilepsy surgery in a comprehensive epilepsy surgery program by a multidisciplinary team and families appropriately counseled about these risks.

REFERENCES

1. Spencer S, Huh L. Outcomes of epilepsy surgery in adults and children. *Lancet Neurol* 2008;7:525–537.
2. Wyllie E, Comair YG, Kotagal P, Bulacio J, Bingaman W, Ruggieri P. Seizure outcome after epilepsy surgery in children and adolescents. *Ann Neurol* 1998;44:740–748.
3. Jonas R, Nguyen S, Hu B, Asarnow RF, LoPresti C, Curtiss S, de Bode S, Yudovin S, Shields WD, Vinters HV, Mathern GW. Cerebral hemispherectomy. Hospital course, seizure, developmental, language and motor outcomes. *Neurology* 2004;62:1712–1721.
4. Steinbok P, Gan PYC, Connolly MB, Carment L, Sinclair DB, Rutka R, Aronyk K, Hader W, Ventureyra E, Atkinson J. Epilepsy surgery in the first 3 years of life: a Canadian survey. *Epilepsia* 2009;50(6):1442–1449.
5. Paolicchi JM, Jayakar P, Dean P, Morrison G, Prats A, Resnick T, Alvarez L, Duchowny M. Predictors of outcome in pediatric epilepsy surgery. *Neurology* 2000;54(3):642–647.
6. Carson BS, Javedan SP, Freeman JM, Vining EP, Zuckerberg AL, Lauer JA, Guarnieri M. Hemispherectomy: a hemidecortication approach and review of 52 cases. *J Neurosurg* 1996;84(6):903–911.
7. Piastra M, Pietrini D, Caresta E, Chiaretti A, Viola L, Cota F, Pusateri A, Polidori G, Di Rocco C. Hemispherectomy procedures in children: haematological issues. *Childs Nerv Syst* 2004;20(7):453–458.
8. Falconer MA, Wilson PJ. Complications related to delayed haemorrhage after hemispherectomy. *J Neurosurg* 1969;30:413–426.
9. Appleton RE. Mortality in paediatric epilepsy. *Arch Dis Child* 2003;88:1091–1094.
10. Callenbach PMC, et al. Mortality risk in children with epilepsy: the Dutch study of epilepsy in childhood. *Pediatrics* 2000;107:1259–1263.
11. Camfield CS, Camfield PR, Veugelers PJ. Death in children with epilepsy: a population-based study. *Lancet* 2002;359:1891–1895.
12. Tellez-Zenteno JF, Dhar R, Hernandez-Ronquillo L, Wiebe S. Long-term outcomes in epilepsy surgery: antiepileptic drugs, mortality, cognitive and psychosocial aspects. *Brain* 2007;130:334–345.
13. Johnston JM Jr, Mangano FT, Ojemann JG, Park TS, Trevathan E, Smyth MD. Complications of invasive subdural electrode monitoring at St. Louis Children's Hospital, 1994–2005. *J Neurosurg* 2006;105:(5):343–347.
14. Hamer HM, Morris HH, Mascha EJ, Karafa MT, Bingaman WE, Bej MD, Burgess RC, Dinner DS, Foldvary NR, Hahn JF, Kotagal P, Najm I, Wyllie E, Lüders HO. Complications of invasive video-EEG monitoring with subdural grid electrodes. *Neurology* 2002;58(1):97–103.
15. Onal C, Otsubo H, Araki T, Chitoku S, Ochi A, Weiss S, Logan W, Elliott I, Snead III OC, Rutka JT. Complications of invasive subdural grid monitoring in children with epilepsy. *J Neurosurg* 2003;98(5):1017–1026.
16. Devlin AM, Cross JH, Harkness W, Chong WK, Harding B, Vargha-Khadem F, Neville BG. Clinical outcomes of hemispherectomy for epilepsy in childhood and adolescence. *Brain* 2003;126(Pt 3):556–566.
17. Basheer SN, Connolly MB, Lautzenhiser A, Sherman EM, Hendson G, Steinbok P. Hemispheric surgery in children with refractory epilepsy: seizure outcome, complications, and adaptive function. *Epilepsia* 2007;48(1):133–140.
18. Bogen JE. The callosal syndrome. In: Heilman KM, Valenstein E (eds), *Clinical Neuropsychology.* New York: New York University Press, 1985; pp. 308–359.
19. Loddenkemper T, Wyllie E, Lardizabal D, Stanford LD, Bingaman W. Late language transfer in patients with Rasmussen encephalitis. *Epilepsia* 2003;44(6):870–871.
20. Smyth MD, Limbrick DD Jr, Ojemann JG, Zempel J, Robinson S, O'Brien DF, Saneto RP, Goyal M, Appleton RE, Mangano FT, Park TS. Outcome following surgery for temporal lobe epilepsy with hippocampal involvement in preadolescent children: emphasis on mesial temporal sclerosis. *J Neurosurg* 2007;106(3, Suppl):205–210.
21. Maton B, Jayakar P, Resnick T, Morrison G, Ragheb J, Duchowny M. Surgery for medically intractable temporal lobe epilepsy during early life. *Epilepsia* 2008;49(1):80–87.
22. Park K, Buchhalter J, McClelland R, Raffel C. Frequency and significance of acute postoperative seizures following epilepsy surgery in children and adolescents. *Epilepsia* 2002;43(8):874–881.
23. Rutter M, Graham P, Yule W (eds). A neuropsychiatric study in childhood. *Clinics in Developmental Medicine.* London: Heinemann, 1970; Vol. 35/36.
24. Davies S, Heyman I, Goodman R. A population survey of mental health problems in children with epilepsy. *Dev Med Child Neurol* 2003;45:292–295.
25. Taylor DC. Mental state and temporal lobe epilepsy. A correlative account of 100 patients treated surgically. *Epilepsia* 1972;13:727–765.
26. McLellan A, Davies S, Heyman I, Harding B, Harkness W, Taylor D, Neville BG, Cross JH. Psychopathology in children with epilepsy before and after temporal lobe resection. *Dev Med Child Neurol* 2005;47(10):666–672.
27. Lendt M, Helmstaedter C, Kuczaty S, Schramm J, Elger C. Behavioural disorders in children with epilepsy: early improvement after surgery. *J Neurol Neurosurg Psychiatry* 2000;69(6):739–744.
28. Danielsson D, Rydenhag B, Uvebrant P, Nordborg C, Olsson I. Temporal lobe resections in children with epilepsy: neuropsychiatric status in relation to neuropathology and seizure outcome. *Epilepsy Behav* 2002;3:76–81.
29. Blumer D, Wakhlu S, Davies K, Hermann B. Psychiatric outcome of temporal lobectomy for epilepsy: incidence and treatment of psychiatric complications. *Epilepsia* 1998;39(5):478–486.
30. Vasconcellos E, Wyllie E, Sullivan S, Stanford L, Bulacio J, Kotagal P, Bingaman W. Mental retardation in pediatric candidates for epilepsy surgery: the role of early seizure onset. *Epilepsia* 2001;42(2):268–274.

31. Freitag H, Tuxhorn I. Cognitive function in preschool children after epilepsy surgery: rationale for early intervention. *Epilepsia* 2005;46(4):561–567.

32. Pulsifer MB, Brandt J, Salorio CF, Vining EP, Carson BS, Freeman JM. The cognitive outcome of hemispherectomy in 71 children. *Epilepsia* 2004;45(3):243–254.

33. Lassonde M, Sauerwein HC, Jambaqué I, Smith ML, Helmstaedter C. Neuropsychology of childhood epilepsy: pre- and postsurgical assessment. *Epileptic Disord* 2000; 2(1):3–13.

34. Smith ML, Elliott IM, Lach L. Cognitive, psychosocial, and family function one year after pediatric epilepsy surgery. *Epilepsia* 2004;45(6):650–660.

35. Westerveld M, Sass KJ, Chelune GJ, Hermann BP, Barr WB, Loring DW, Strauss E, Trenerry MR, Perrine K, Spencer DD. Temporal lobectomy in children: cognitive outcome. *J Neurosurg* 2000;92(1):24–30.

36. Gleissner U, Sassen R, Lendt M, Clusmann H, Elger CE, Helmstaedter C. Pre- and postoperative verbal memory in pediatric patients with temporal lobe epilepsy. *Epilepsy Res* 2002;51(3):287–296.

37. Szabó CA, Wyllie E, Stanford LD, Geckler C, Kotagal P, Comair YG, Thornton AE. Neuropsychological effect of temporal lobe resection in preadolescent children with epilepsy. *Epilepsia* 1998;39(8):814–819.

38. Gleissner U, Sassen R, Schramm J, Elger CE, Helmstaedter C. Greater functional recovery after temporal lobe epilepsy surgery in children. *Brain* 2005;128(Pt 12):2822–2829.

39. Lendt M, Gleissner U, Helmstaedter C, Sassen R, Clusmann H, Elger CE. Neuropsychological outcome in children after frontal lobe epilepsy surgery. *Epilepsy Behav* 2002;3(1): 51–59.

40. Spencer SS. Corpus callosum section and other disconnection procedures for medically intractable epilepsy. *Epilepsia* 1988; 29(Suppl 2):S85–S99.

41. Cendes F, Ragazzo PC, da Costa V, Martins LF. Corpus callosotomy in treatment of medically resistant epilepsy: preliminary results in a pediatric population. *Epilepsia* 1993;34(5):910–917.

42. Austin JK, Smith MS, Risinger MW, McNelis AM. Childhood epilepsy and asthma: comparison of quality of life. *Epilepsia* 1994;35(3):608–615.

43. Zupanc ML, dos Santos Rubio EJ, Werner RR, Schwabe MJ, Mueller WM, Lew SM, Marcuccilli CJ, O'Connor SE, Chico MS, Eggener KA, Hecox KE. Epilepsy surgery outcomes: quality of life and seizure control. *Pediatr Neurol* 2010;42(1):12–20.

44. Van Empelen R, Jennekens-Schinkel A, van Rijen PC, Helders PJM, van Nieuwenhuizen O. Health-related quality of life and self-perceived competence of children assessed before and up to two years after epilepsy surgery. *Epilepsia* 2005;46(2):258–271.

45. Mizrahi EM, et al. Anterior temporal lobectomy and medically refractory temporal lobe epilepsy of childhood. *Epilepsia* 1990;37:753–757.

46. Sillanpaa M, Haataja L, Shinnar S. Perceived impact of childhood-onset epilepsy on quality of life as an adult. *Epilepsia* 2004;45(8):971–977.

INDEX

Page numbers followed by *b*, *f* and *t* indicate boxed material, figures and tables respectively.

N